The Injured Athlete

Third Edition

The Injured Athlete

Third Edition

Editor

David H. Perrin, Ph.D., A.T.C.
Professor
Curry School of Education
University of Virginia
Charlottesville, Virginia

Illustrations by Birck Cox
Photography by Daniel Grogan

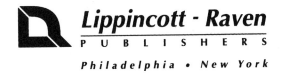

Lippincott - Raven
PUBLISHERS

Philadelphia • New York

Acquisitions Editor: Danette Knopp
Developmental Editor: Anne M. Sydor
Manufacturing Manager: Tim Reynolds
Production Manager: Kathleen Bubbeo
Production Editor: Carolyn Foley
Cover Designer: Joseph DePinho
Indexer: Dorothy Hoffman
Compositor: CJS-Tapsco
Printer: Maple Press

Printed and bound in the United States of America

9 8 7 6 5 4 3 2 1

Library of Congress Cataloging-in-Publication Data

The injured athlete.—3rd ed. /editor, David H. Perrin;
    illustrations by Birck Cox.
        p.   cm.
    Includes bibliographical references and index.
    ISBN 0-397-51534-0
    1. Sports injuries. 2. Sports medicine. I. Perrin, David H.,
1954–
    [DNLM: 1. Athletic Injuries—therapy. 2. Physical Education and
Training—methods. 3. SportsMedicine—methods. QT 261I56 1999]
RD97.I55 1999
617.1'027—dc21
DNLM/DLC
for Library of Congress   98-26849
                                                                     CIP

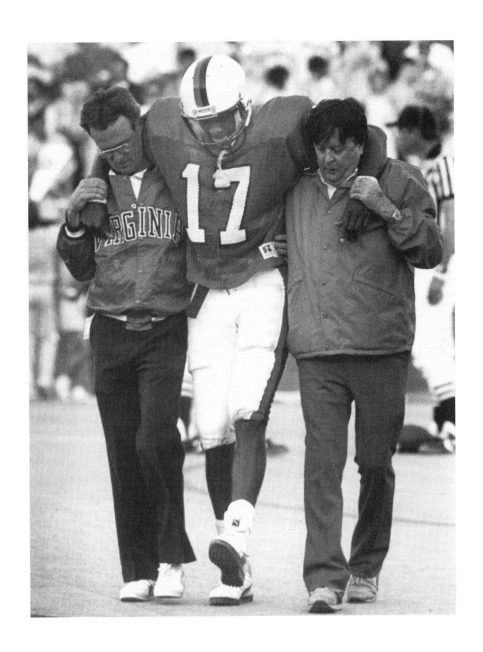

*To University of Virginia athletic trainer Joe H. Gieck, Ed.D.,
A.T.C., P.T., and team physician Frank C. McCue III, M.D., sports
medicine pioneers for nearly four decades.*

Contents

Section I: Prevention and Rehabilitation

Section II: Evaluation and Management

Contributors

Lorraine J. Armstrong, M.D.   *Senior Staff, Department of Pediatrics, Henry Ford Medical Center—Pierson, 131 Kercheval Avenue, Grosse Pointe, Michigan 48236*

Michael E. Brunet, M.D.   *Department of Orthopaedics, Tulane University, 1432 Tulane Avenue, New Orleans, Louisiana 70112*

Robert C. Cantu, M.D.   *Instructor, Department of Surgery, Boston University School of Medicine; Chief, Neurosurgery Service, Emerson Hospital, 131 Old Road to Nine Acre Corner, Concord, Massachusetts 01742*

Anthony Decker, M.Ed., A.T.C., C.S.C.S.   *Athletic Department, University of Delaware, Newark, Delaware 19716*

Martin A. Fees, M.S., P. T., A.T.C, C.S.C.S.   *Department of Health and Exercise Science, Gettysburg College, Bream Hauser Wright Field House, Gettysburg, Pennsylvania 17325; Clinical Director, Joyner Sportsmedicine Institute, 39 North Fifth Street, Gettysburg, Pennsylvania 17325*

Brian L. Fong, M.D.   *Clinical Assistant Professor, Department of Orthopaedics, Tulane University Medical Center, 1430 Tulane Avenue, New Orleans, Louisiana 70112-2699*

Susan Foreman, M.Ed., A.T.C., M.P.T.   *Instructor, Curry School of Education and Department of Orthopaedic Surgery; Associate Athletic Trainer, Department of Athletics, University of Virginia, McCue Center on Massie Road, P.O. Box 3785, Charlottesville, Virginia 22903*

Bruce M. Gansneder, Ph.D.   *Curry School of Education, University of Virginia, Charlottesville, Virginia 22903*

Michael Gaudette, M.S., P.T., O.C.S.   *Regional Director of Operations, Joyner Sportsmedicine Institute, 601 Perimeter Drive, Suite 110, Lexington, Kentucky 40517*

Joe H. Gieck, Ed.D., A.T.C., P.T.   *Director of Sports Medicine, Department of Athletics, and Professor, Curry School of Education; Professor of Clinical Orthopaedics, Department of Orthopaedics, University of Virginia, Charlottesville, Virginia 22903*

Henry T. Goitz, M.D.   *Assistant Professor, Department of Orthopaedic Surgery, Case Western Reserve University, Cleveland Ohio 44106; and Senior Staff, Athletic Medicine, Department of Orthopaedic Surgery, Henry Ford Medical Center—Lakeside, 14500 Hall Road, Sterling Heights, Michigan 48313-2195*

Keith E. Griffin, M.D.   *Copperfield Internal Medicine, 390 Copperfield Boulevard, Concord, North Carolina 28025*

Susan Grossman, Ed.D., M.S.W., L.C.S.W.   *Director of Prevention Services, Institute for Substance Abuse Studies, University of Virginia, #1 Boar's Head Lane, Charlottesville, Virginia 22903*

Elizabeth G. Hedgpeth, Ed.D., R.N.   *Sport Psychology Consultant, Mindset–Attitude, 2429 Perkins Road, Durham, North Carolina 27706*

Mark R. Hutchinson, M.D.   *Assistant Professor of Orthopaedics and Sports Medicine, Director of Sports Medicine Services, Department of Orthopaedics, University of Illinois at Chicago, 901 South Wolcott Avenue, M/C 844, Medical Sciences South, Chicago, Illinois 60612-7342*

Mary Lloyd Ireland, M.D.   *Team Physician, Eastern Kentucky University, Richmond, Kentucky 40475; President and Orthopaedic Surgeon, Kentucky Sports Medicine Clinic, 601 Perimeter Drive, Lexington, Kentucky 40517*

Kirk L. Jensen, M.D.   *Assistant Clinical Professor, Division of Orthopaedic Surgery, San Francisco General Hospital and the University of California, San Francisco, 100 Potrero Avenue, Room 3A36, San Francisco, California 94110; Staff Physician, Department of Orthopaedic Surgery, Summit Medical Center, 350 Hawthorne Avenue, Oakland, California 94609*

S. D. Steen Johnsen, M.D.   *Fellow of Sports Medicine, Institute for Bone and Joint Disorders, 3320 North Second Street, Phoenix, Arizona 85012*

David M. Kahler, M.D.   *Associate Professor, Department of Orthopaedic Surgery, University of Virginia Health Sciences Center, Charlottesville, Virginia 22908*

Frank C. McCue III, M.D.   *Alfred R. Shands Professor of Orthopaedic Surgery and Plastic Surgery of the Hand, Director, Division of Sports Medicine and Hand Surgery, Department of Orthopaedic Surgery, Team Physician, Department of Athletics, University of Virginia School of Medicine, Box 243, Charlottesville, Virginia 22908*

Russell R. Pate, Ph.D.   *Professor and Chairman, Department of Exercise Science, University of South Carolina, Columbia, South Carolina 29208*

David H. Perrin, Ph.D., A.T.C.   *Professor, Curry School of Education, University of Virginia, 405 Emmet Street, Charlottesville, Virginia 22903*

Morris M. Pickens, Ph.D.   *President, Carolina Performance Enhancement, 152 Alexander Circle, Columbia, South Carolina 29206*

Robert J. Rotella, Ph.D.   *Memorial Gymnasium, University of Virginia, Charlottesville, Virginia 22903*

Ethan N. Saliba, Ph.D., A.T.C., P.T.   *Head Athletic Trainer, Department of Athletics, University of Virginia, P.O. Box 3785, Charlottesville, Virginia 22903*

Thomas Sweeney, M.D., Ph.D.   *Department of Orthopaedic Surgery, Sarasota Memorial Hospital, 1921 Waldemere Street, Suite 609, Sarasota, Florida 34239*

Scott Urch, M.D.   *Orthopedic Sports Medicine Fellow, Methodist Sports Medicine Center, Thomas A. Brady Clinic, 1815 N. Capitol Avenue, Suite 600, Indianapolis, Indiana 46202*

Arthur Weltman, Ph.D.   *Professor, Department of Human Services—Medicine, University of Virginia, 203 Memorial Gymnasium, Charlottesville, Virginia 22903; Director of Exercise Physiology Laboratory, General Clinical Research Center, University of Virginia Health Sciences Center, Box 410, Charlottesville, Virginia 22908*

Amelia L. Williams, Ph.D.   *Medical Writer and Editor, Th'Inkwell Writing and Editing, 128 Wildwood Trail, Afton, Virginia 22920*

Gaylord S. Williams, M.D., F.A.C.S.   *Associate Professor, Department of Plastic Surgery, University of Virginia Health Sciences Center and University of Virginia Hospitals, Box 376, Charlottesville, Virginia 22908*

Richard I. Williams, M.D., M.S.   *Team Orthopaedic Physician, Tennessee Technological University, Upper Cumberland Orthopaedics and Sports Medicine, 404 North Hickory Avenue, Cookeville, Tennessee 38501*

Preface

I am honored to serve as Editor for the Third Edition of *The Injured Athlete,* edited in its first two editions by Daniel N. Kulund, M.D. Dr. Kulund deserves a great deal of credit for having the vision to create this much needed reference for primary care and orthopaedic team physicians, certified athletic trainers, and sport physical therapists.

This edition of *The Injured Athlete* has been substantially reorganized, and most of the chapters are either new or have undergone major updating and revision. The book is now organized into two sections: Section I, Prevention and Rehabilitation, and Section II, Evaluation and Management.

The first section, Prevention and Rehabilitation, focuses on the key elements necessary for safe participation in sports. Chapter 1, "Preparation for Athletic Participation," and Chapter 2, "Medical Concerns of the Athlete", present guidelines for musculoskeletal and medical preseason screening of athletes. A regrettable yet very real issue facing athletes at all levels of participation is the use and abuse of recreational and performance-enhancing drugs. The University of Virginia's Institute for Substance Abuse Studies, with support from the National Collegiate Athletic Association, has developed a model substance abuse education and testing program for athletes. The key elements of this program, which incorporates the development and use of student-athlete mentors, are presented in Chapter 1. The University of Virginia's substance abuse policy is included as Appendix C.

Chapter 3, "Designing Strength and Conditioning Programs," and Chapter 4, "Principles of Strength Training," address the cardiovascular and musculoskeletal needs of athletes participating in sports requiring high levels of aerobic and anaerobic fitness. Chapter 4 is written by two authors with combined expertise in athletic training, physical therapy, and strength and conditioning. They address the transition from the rehabilitation facility to the strength room, and provide guidelines for the design of safe strength-training programs for athletes.

In spite of our efforts toward prevention, physical activity carries an inherent risk of injury. Chapter 5, "Principles of Therapeutic Exercise," provides general guidelines for the rehabilitation of musculoskeletal injuries. A progression from pain relief to the return of strength, flexibility, proprioception, and endurance, to functional activities, and ultimately to return to competition, is provided. Chapter 6, "Therapeutic Modalities in Rehabilitation of Athletic Injuries," discusses how heat, cold, electrotherapy, and other modalities can influence the healing process during injury rehabilitation. The authors of this chapter teach the most comprehensive modalities course I know to our graduate students in athletic training and sports medicine at the University of Virginia. They have presented the theory, indications, and contraindications of this essential component of injury rehabilitation.

The physical aspects of injury prevention and rehabilitation are usually far more straightforward than those involving the athlete's psyche. However, the injured athlete requires both physical and psychological well-being before a safe return to participation can be achieved. With this in mind, Chapter 7, written by expert sport psychologists, discusses the psychology of athletic injury and rehabilitation. The authors present guidelines for clinicians to facilitate effectively an athlete's transition through each phase of injury rehabilitation.

The accurate documentation of athletic injuries and a knowledge of the appropriate research designs to study injury epidemiology and the effectiveness of management protocols is essential to a comprehensive sports medicine program. The final chapter of Section I, "Research Methods and Injury Surveillance in Sports Medicine," is written by an expert in research design and statistics who has learned the language of sports medicine.

Section II, Evaluation and Management, is written by an eminent group of physicians who are experts in the medical specialties of neurosurgery, plastic surgery, and orthopaedics. These chapters address the etiology and management of the most common athletic injuries to the head, face, neck, trunk, and extremities. Where appropriate, related anatomic considerations for injury evaluation and surgical treatment are presented and expertly illustrated.

Chapters 9 and 10, written by a plastic surgeon and a neurosurgeon respectively, cover injuries to the face, head, and neck. Athletic injuries to these regions can have a devastating impact; the authors have succinctly identified the injuries that carry the potential for a catastrophic outcome. They also address the role of protective equipment, classification of injury, and criteria for returning to competition.

The remaining chapters are written by orthopaedic surgeons who offer a wealth of experience as team physicians and medical care providers for physically active people of all ages. The authors discuss athletic injury mechanisms and treatment, and also provide modifications and guidelines necessary for a safe return to competition.

I have retained a substantial University of Virginia influence in this updated version of *The Injured Athlete*. Several of the contributors are either current or past faculty or fellows with the University of Virginia School of Medicine and/or the Curry School of Education at the University of Virginia. I also invited experts from beyond the grounds of the University of Virginia to contribute in a significant way to the Third Edition. The University of Virginia offers a master's degree program in athletic training, a doctoral program in sports medicine, and sports medicine fellowship training in orthopaedic surgery and primary care medicine. These academic programs have served as the basis for the content of this book.

I trust you will find this information useful for your work as a team physician, athletic trainer, or sport physical therapist.

David H. Perrin

Acknowledgments

I am indebted to several people at Lippincott–Raven Publishers. Jim Ryan invited me to take the reins from Daniel N. Kulund for the third edition of *The Injured Athlete*. Danette Knopp, editor, assumed the project from Jim Ryan, and I am grateful for her persistence and enthusiasm for the book. Anne Sydor, developmental editor, expertly tied together the loose ends and moved the book to production. Carolyn Foley, production editor, is responsible for overseeing the transformation from manuscript to bound book.

Dan Grogan, photographer, and Birck Cox, artist, are largely responsible for the many illustrations found throughout the book. Both stepped up to the plate when I needed them most in the final phases of developing the book.

The contributors are nationally recognized for their respective areas of expertise in sports medicine. I thank each of the authors for their substantial contribution to *The Injured Athlete, Third Edition,* and for their patience with the development of the final product.

Finally, I thank my students and colleagues at the University of Virginia for providing the stimulation and support to pursue my scholarly work in athletic training and sports medicine. These people, in combination with the grounds of the University of Virginia, provide an exceptional environment in which to pursue one's professional goals and dreams.

The Injured Athlete, Third Edition,
edited by D. H. Perrin.
Lippincott–Raven Publishers, Philadelphia © 1999.

CHAPTER 1

Preparation for Athletic Participation

Joe H. Gieck, David H. Perrin, Susan Grossman, and Amelia L. Williams

Physical activity, by its very nature, invites injury. Each year, millions of participants in recreational and organized sports sustain an injury to the musculoskeletal system. Professional and intercollegiate athletes receive comprehensive sports medicine services from a team of professionals that include a team physician, an athletic trainer, and a host of other medical specialists and allied health care providers. Unfortunately, the majority of participants in interscholastic sports do not receive comprehensive sports medicine care, yet the number of injuries sustained by athletes at this level is astounding. The National Athletic Trainers' Association (NATA) began a three-year injury surveillance study in 1995 to determine the trends of high school injuries in ten sports (17). The study includes boys' football, basketball, wrestling, baseball, soccer, and girls' basketball, field hockey, volleyball, softball, and soccer. Results from the first phase of this research have revealed that 39% of varsity high school football players were injured during the 1995 season. More than 23% of high school soccer players, regardless of gender, sustained an injury during the 1997 season. Two players on every high school basketball team in the country, regardless of gender, were likely to be injured during the 1996 to 1997 season. Unfortunately, high school athletes do not have the same comprehensive medical coverage enjoyed by professional and collegiate athletes. This same NATA study documents that fewer than 42% of U.S. high school athletic programs have certified athletic trainers.

Sports medical care for physically active people not involved in organized sports is available through the many sports medicine clinics that have proliferated throughout the United States over the past decade. These facilities are typically staffed with sport physical therapists and occasionally certified athletic trainers.

SPORTS MEDICINE TEAM

The primary members of the sports medicine team are a team physician and an athletic trainer. The team physician is usually a family practitioner, a pediatrician, or an orthopaedic surgeon, and is ultimately responsible for the athletes' health care. The team physician should be committed to setting up comprehensive programs for preseason evaluation, conditioning, health education, and injury prevention, treatment, and rehabilitation. The American Orthopaedic Society for Sports Medicine (AOSSM) and the American Medical Society for Sports Medicine (AMSSM) are organizations for orthopaedic surgeons, family practitioners, and pediatricians having an interest in serving as team physicians (see Appendix A: Sports Medicine Organizations).

When a physician becomes a team doctor, it is often a labor of love. He or she should, however, insist on an agreement with school officials that delineates the role of the team physician. The institution must, in turn, vest the physician with the authority to make medical judgments relating to student-athletes' participation in interscholastic or intercollegiate sports. Since the health of the athletes will be the primary concern, the team physician must be the final word on all medical decisions regarding participation in athletics.

Good communication is essential, and for this reason the team physician should meet with athletes (and their parents in interscholastic sports) before the start of the season. A suit-conscious public may have the notion that protective equipment always prevents injury and may therefore charge negligence if an athlete is injured. This notion can be dispelled at the preseason meeting if the limitations of protective equipment are explained. All participants should be advised in writing of the inherent risks of participating in competitive athletics. Athletes and parents should also be told how the physician, athletic trainer, and coach propose to reduce as much as possible the occurrence of athletic injury.

J. H. Gieck, D. H. Perrin, S. Grossman, and A. L. Williams: Curry School of Education and Institute of Substance Abuse Studies, University of Virginia, Charlottesville, Virginia 22903

TABLE 1.1. *Performance domains of the certified athletic trainer*

Prevention of athletic injuries
Recognition, evaluation, and immediate care of athletic injuries
Rehabilitation and reconditioning of athletic injuries
Health care administration
Professional development and responsibility

From the National Athletic Trainers' Association Board of Certification.

The certified athletic trainer comprises the other essential component of the primary sports medicine team, and functions under the direction of the team physician. The roles and responsibilities of a certified athletic trainer are explained in Table 1.1. The National Athletic Trainers' Association (NATA) is the professional organization for athletic trainers (see Appendix A: Sports Medicine Organizations). The Joint Review Committee on Athletic Training Education (JRC-AT) of the Commission on Accreditation of Allied Health Education Programs (CAAHEP) accredits approximately 100 entry level athletic training curricula in colleges and universities throughout the country (see Appendix B: List of Accredited Entry Level and Graduate Athletic Training Education Programs). Thirteen graduate programs are accredited by the NATA and provide opportunities for certified athletic trainers to obtain an advanced master's degree in athletic training. The NATA Board of Certification sets the standards and conducts the certification process for athletic trainers. In addition, many states have either certification, registration, or licensure for athletic trainers.

Several other medical and allied health care specialists comprise the remainder of the sports medicine team and play an essential role in the prevention, treatment, and rehabilitation of athletic injuries. Certified strength coaches design and supervise year-round strength and conditioning programs for athletes that prevent injury and optimize performance. The National Strength and Conditioning Association (NSCA) is the professional organization for these individuals, and oversees the process that leads to a Certified Strength and Conditioning Specialist (CSCS). Sport physical therapists specialize in evaluation and rehabilitation of the musculoskeletal system. The Sports Physical Therapy section of the American Physical Therapy Association offers a process that leads to the Sports Certified Specialists (SCS). Sport psychologists optimize coping and compliance during the rehabilitation process. Nutritionists, massage therapists, exercise physiologists, podiatrists, chiropractors, dentists, and a host of other medical specialists all play a role in the delivery of sports medicine services to athletes.

PRESEASON MUSCULOSKELETAL EXAMINATION

All athletes should receive a comprehensive medical and musculoskeletal examination before authorization to participate in competitive athletics is granted. The details of the medical examination are discussed in Chapter 2. The musculoskeletal examination is designed to identify prior injuries and any deficiencies in joint stability, strength, and flexibility.

Cervical Spine

Cervical length should be measured with a tape measure from the occiput to the vertebra prominens, which is the spinous process of C-7. The neck circumference is then measured just below the larynx and the neck motion checked. The athlete first must lower the chin to the chest with the mouth closed, because an open mouth will add about 15 degrees to the flexion. If there is a gap of one finger width between the athlete's chin and chest, there will be 10 degrees of restricted motion.

To check cervical extension, the athlete should lean the head backwards until the forehead is parallel to the ceiling, a position that yields 35 degrees to 50 degrees of cervical extension. For lateral flexion testing, the athlete should bend the head toward the shoulder without shrugging. This measurement depends on the athlete's musculature, which can block movement, but 40 degrees to 45 degrees of lateral flexion is desirable. For measurement of cervical rotation, the athlete should turn the head as far as possible to each side, and should be able to nearly align the chin with each shoulder.

Shoulder

In the preparticipation setting, the shoulder examination is a general one, although any suspicion of impingement, rotator cuff tear, or instability should be confirmed through the more definitive examination techniques described in Chapter 11. Prior subluxation or dislocation may account for apprehension during overhead activities or a feeling that the arm has suddenly gone "dead." In such cases, radiographs may show a compression fracture in the humeral head (a Hill-Sach lesion) or calcification at the anteroinferior part of the labrum that may indicate a labral tear (Bankart lesion). The athlete may say that the shoulder "pops or grinds." These sounds may indicate a deranged acromioclavicular joint or a torn rotator cuff. "Pops, snaps, or clunks" may signify that a torn glenoid labrum is being caught between the humeral head and the glenoid or that the biceps tendon is subluxing. The character and location of pain may aid the examiner in arriving at a diagnosis. A deep ache at night may indicate a rotator cuff tear, whereas a stabbing or burning pain is more characteristic of bursitis or tendinitis.

If the history reveals a past injury to the shoulder, the uninvolved shoulder should be examined and compared to the injured side. The examination of an athlete's shoulder may be more difficult than a nonathlete's shoulder because of muscular hypertrophy in the trained individual. Atrophy, however, will be more evident to the examiner. The shoulders should be examined with the athlete standing, supine, and then prone. With the athlete standing, any shoulder drop or muscle atrophy should be noted, although a lower dominant side shoulder is a normal finding. The athlete is then asked to abduct the shoulders while the examiner feels the inferior angle of each scapula. Normally the scapula will begin to move upward and outward at about 45 degrees of glenohumeral abduction. In contrast to the normal shoulder girdle movement, the athlete will hike a painful, weak, or injured shoulder. The examiner can next assess the athlete's general shoulder strength and well-being with resisted abduction and adduction (Fig. 1.1 A and B). Shoulder rotation can be assessed with Apley's tests of adduction-internal rotation and abduction-external rotation. To examine for winging of the scapula, the athlete is asked to push against a wall (Fig. 1.2 A). Winging indicates a weak serratus anterior muscle, injury to the long thoracic nerve, or both. The acromioclavicular joint is close to the surface and easily observed and palpated. Pain indicative of acromioclavicular joint sprain, or "separation" may be elicited by horizontally adducting the shoulder across the front of the torso.

With the athlete supine, the shoulder is abducted to 90 degrees with the elbow bent. The examiner then presses gently at the wrist to rotate both shoulders externally while comparing range of motion. A throwing athlete will normally have more external rotation at the expense of some internal rotation when compared to the nondominant side (see Fig. 1.2 B). Finally, with the athlete prone and the arm hanging over the side of the table, the examiner holds the scapula fixed and abducts the shoulder to 90 degrees. By externally rotating and internally rotating the shoulder, contractures of the glenohumeral joint may be

noted. Further, in this position the shoulder is relaxed and the rotator cuff easily palpated.

Elbow

The carrying angle of the elbow is usually about 20 degrees of valgus. Some flexion deformity will usually be found in the elbows of pitchers, tennis players, and boxers. Occasionally the forearm of a little league baseball pitcher may lack full supination. The medial and lateral epicondyles should be palpated for presence of inflammation resulting from "tennis elbow" (lateral epicondylitis) or "little league elbow" (medial epicondylitis).

Lumbar Spine

The distance between C-7 and S-1 should be measured while the athlete is standing erect. The athlete then forward flexes, and the change in distance between the two points is measured. A difference of about 10 cm is normal, and a measurement of less than 10 cm is a sign of decreased flexibility of the lower back. If the bending measurement remains about the same as when erect, ankylosing spondylitis should be suspected. A natural curve should also occur during forward flexion (Fig. 1.3 A). If the athlete has tight hamstring muscles, the lower back will flatten during forward bending.

A sit and reach test may be used to determine general spinal flexibility. Lordosis (swayback) increases an athlete's susceptibility to lower back strain, and when this condition is present, postural exercises should be prescribed to help alleviate the lordotic posture. Leg-length inequality may be uncovered by placement of the examin-

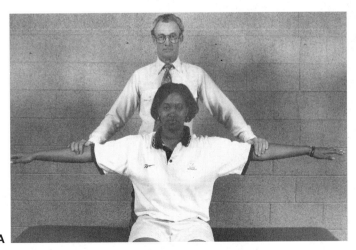 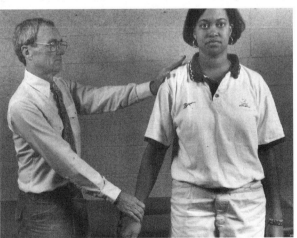

A   **B**

FIG. 1.1. To determine general shoulder strength, the examiner resists abduction (**A**) and then resists adduction (**B**).

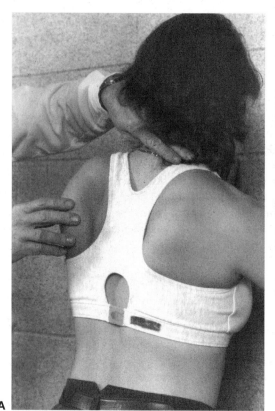

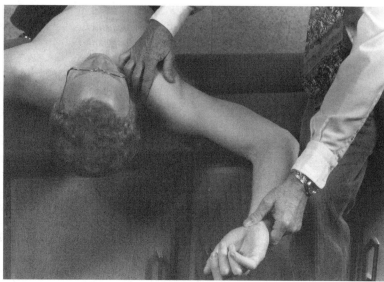

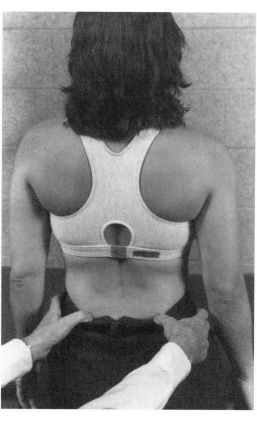

FIG. 1.2. A: The examiner feels for winging of the scapula as the athlete does a wall push-up. **B:** With the athlete supine, the examiner checks for limited external rotation.

A

B

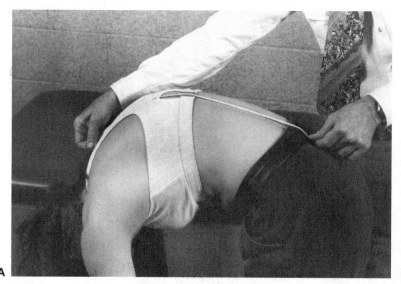

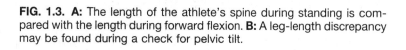

A

B

FIG. 1.3. A: The length of the athlete's spine during standing is compared with the length during forward flexion. **B:** A leg-length discrepancy may be found during a check for pelvic tilt.

er's hands on the athlete's iliac crests and noting whether the hands are at the same level (see Fig. 1.3 B).

Scoliosis

The preparticipation examination is a good occasion to screen for scoliosis or lateral spinal curvature. This condition is seen primarily in 9- to 14-year-old girls, who may even have a substantial curve that their parents have not noticed. Because secondary curves may balance the head in line with the pelvis, the spine may not at first glance appear curved. The early detection of scoliosis is essential so that proper bracing, and when necessary, surgery can be performed to prevent large curves that may affect cardiopulmonary function and decrease in life expectancy. When checking for scoliosis, the level of the shoulders should be ascertained before checking elbow height. Waist and flank symmetry are observed, and the athlete then bends forward to have alignment of the spinous processes and the symmetry of the thorax examined.

Youngsters with vertebral epiphysitis (Scheuermann's disease) have standing lateral spine radiographs that show vertebral wedging and undulation of their vertebral endplates. The wedging produces a round back deformity that may be progressive. These athletes should avoid activities that develop the pectoral muscles, which can exacerbate the humpback deformity. Progression of the deformity is combated by postural and back extensor strengthening exercises, and when necessary, by bracing.

Hips

Hip flexor strength may be tested with the athlete in a sitting position with arms crossed to avoid accessory muscle involvement. The knee is then lifted by flexing the hip against the examiner's resistance. Hip adductor tightness

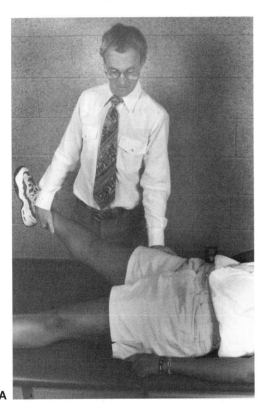

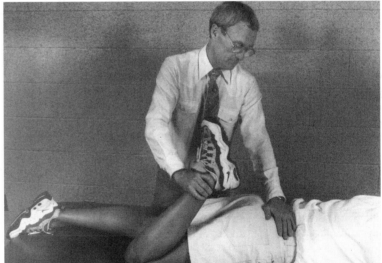

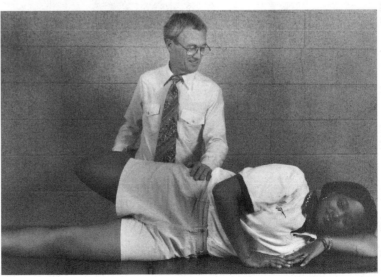

FIG. 1.4. The examiner checks for adductor tightness (**A**), a tight rectus femoris (**B**), and a tight iliotibial band (**C**).

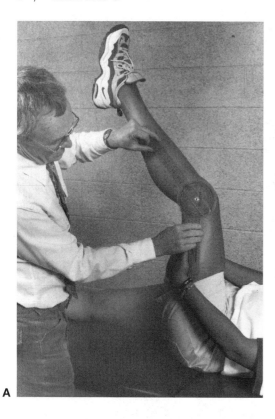

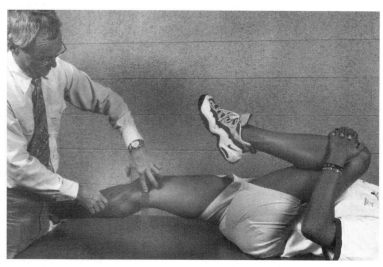

FIG. 1.5. Measurement of hamstring flexibility with a goniometer. **A:** Note how the athlete maintains 90 degrees of hip flexion by grasping the thigh. **B:** To measure flexibility of the iliopsoas, the athlete pulls the opposite knee toward the chest and the heel toward the hip. The distance from the back of the tested knee to the table is then measured.

(Fig. 1.4 A) is than assessed by abducting the athlete's hips while permitting no hip external rotation. When the knee and toes are pointing toward the ceiling, each lower extremity should abduct about 45 degrees.

Flexion of the relaxed hip with some knee extension is indicative of rectus femoris tightness, a muscle that crosses both the hip and knee joints. The athlete first maximally flexes the knee, then the examiner passively flexes the knee further to see if the anterior superior iliac spine on the same side rises from the table. This movement normally occurs at about 130 degrees of knee flexion, but if the pelvis rises earlier it is indicative of rectus femoris tightness (see Fig. 1.4 B).

Iliotibial Tract

The iliotibial tract traverses from the pelvis to the tibia. In a runner, tightness of this band may lead to lateral hip and knee pain. To test for tightness, the athlete must lie on the side with the tested limb raised (see Fig. 1.4 C). The back is flattened by flexing the lower hip and the

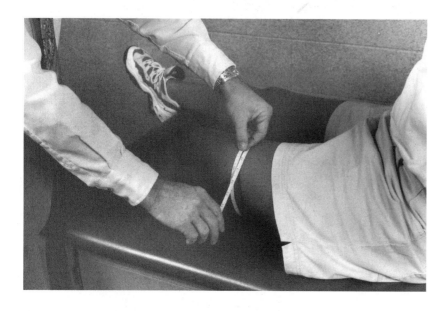

FIG. 1.6. The circumference of the thigh is measured approximately 18 cm (7 inches) above the knee joint.

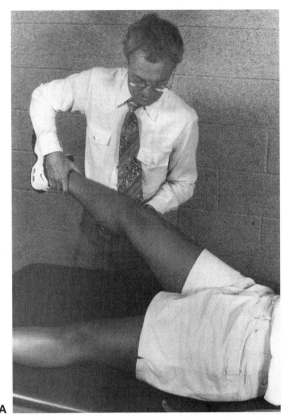

A

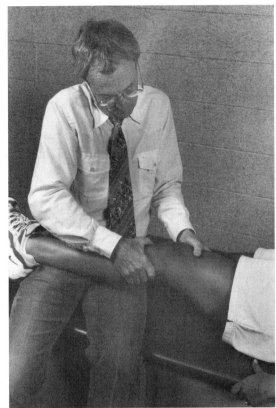

C

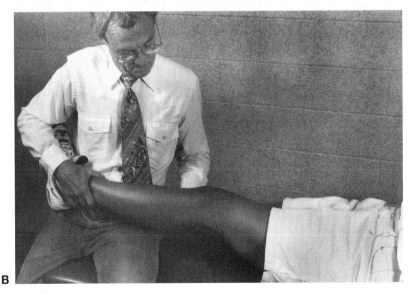

B

FIG. 1.7. Stress tests for integrity of the medial collateral ligament (**A**), the lateral collateral ligament (**B**), and the Lachman's test for integrity of the anterior cruciate ligament (**C**).

tested knee then flexed to 90 degrees, the hip extended, and the knee pressed down toward the table. If the band is not tight, the knee should reach the table without extending. Alternatively, the lower knee may be flexed, with the tested limb allowed to drop. The foot will normally fall below the level of the table if the band is not tight.

Knee

The athlete's hamstring muscles demand evaluation because tightness or weakness can lead to muscle strain. Tight hamstring muscles can also alter normal patellofemoral biomechanics, leading to anterior knee pain. A neutral pelvis is needed for hamstring muscle testing, but tight hip flexors will arch the lower back and tilt the pelvis anteriorly. To establish a neutral position, a pillow should be placed under the athlete's thigh to flatten the lower back. The opposite thigh is placed flat on the table to fix the pelvis and to keep it from rotating. The tested hip is flexed to 90 degrees, and the athlete then actively extends the knee (Fig. 1.5 A), aiming for terminal knee extension. The degrees from complete extension are noted as the amount of hamstring tightness.

To test for tightness of the iliopsoas, the athlete flexes the opposite knee to the chest and the heel to the hip. The distance from the knee to the table is measured and noted as the amount of iliopsoas tightness (see Fig. 1.5 B).

The skeletal configuration of the knees should be assessed, with any excessive genu valgus (knock-knees), varus (bowlegs), or recurvatum (hyperextension) noted. Patella position and tracking should also be examined for any abnormalities. Thigh circumference should be assessed about 18 cm above the knee joint and around the joint itself (Fig. 1.6). Bilateral discrepancies of greater than 2.5 cm may be indicative of muscular alienation

resulting from pathology of the joint or neuromuscular system.

The major ligaments providing stability to the knee should also be assessed. The collateral ligaments can be quickly assessed with valgus (medial collateral) and varus (lateral collateral) stress tests, and the Lachman's test can be used to confirm integrity of the anterior cruciate ligament (Fig. 1.7 A–C). KT1000 knee arthrometry is also useful in documenting the range of anterior translation of the tibia (21) (Fig. 1.8). This baseline information can be helpful in diagnosing a potential injury to the anterior cruciate ligament at a later date.

Ankle

Normal ankle range of motion is essential to injury-free athletic performance. For example, a restriction of ankle dorsiflexion can predispose the athlete to inversion sprain. Ankle motion should range from 10 to 20 degrees dorsiflexion to about 50 degrees of plantar flexion. Dorsiflexion is first tested with the knee flexed to 90 degrees to measure the soleus component of the triceps surae complex. The knee is then fully extended and ankle dorsiflexion retested to measure the gastrocnemius portion. To test ankle dorsiflexion more dynamically, the athlete can be asked to crouch and lean forward while attempting to maintain the heels on the floor. The distance from the heel to the floor becomes the measure of ankle dorsiflexion restriction (Fig. 1.9). All athletes, especially those with tight heel cords, should stretch on a stair step or incline board.

Feet

The feet should be evaluated for excessive pronation, pes planus (flat foot), and pes cavus (high arched foot).

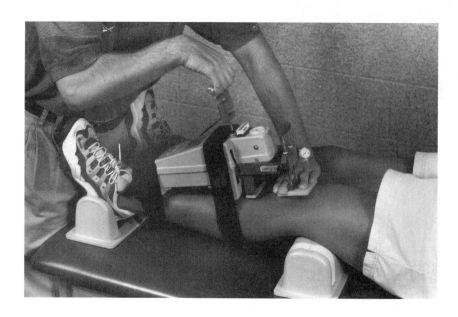

FIG 1.8. Use of a KT1000 knee arthrometer to quantify the amount of anterior translation of the tibia on the femur.

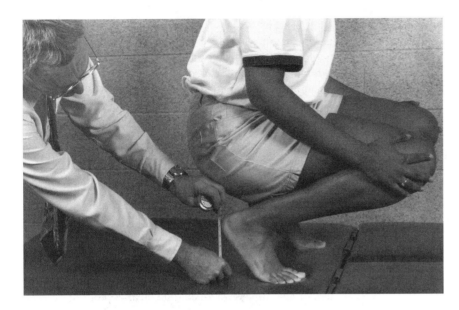

FIG 1.9. Measurement of calf flexibility with the athlete in the squatting position. The distance from the heel to the table is the amount of restricted motion.

Any corns, warts, blisters, fungi, and ingrowing toenails should be identified and treated. All athletes should be encouraged to invest in footwear that is appropriate for their particular athletic endeavor.

ATHLETIC ACTIVITY IN THE HEAT

As early fall and late spring practices necessitate participating in weather of high heat stress, and with artificial turfs compounding the problem, it is wise for all personnel to review the literature pertaining to the problems associated with heat. Between 1955 and 1990 there were 84 reported deaths due to heat stroke in athletes participating in football alone (1).

It is important to remember that humidity must be considered in heat stress as cases of fatal heat stroke have been recorded in an environment of 64°F with a humidity reading of 100% (9). In hot humid weather, when skin temperature is high and/or evaporation is decreased, adequate transfer of heat from the body to the environment may not occur (2). Most literature does not take humidity into account when discussing heat illness.

Physiologic Response to Heat

The nervous control and coordination of thermoregulation is located in the hypothalamus (4). Heat conservation and heat dissipation are subcenters in the hypothalamus that regulate the body's reaction to cold and heat, heat dissipation being regulated by cutaneous vasodilation and sweating (2). Increased blood temperature from the periphery causes the hypothalamus to respond to the environmental temperature. Sensitive hypothalamic receptors and indirect afferent impulses of the thermoreceptors are responsible for this response. Other centers for homeosta-

sis located in the hypothalamus are: water balance, vasomotor, and humoral activities. Body temperature of up to 110°F in heat stroke can damage the central nervous system resulting in dizziness and mental confusion (14). The athlete with a defective hypothalamus is most susceptible to heat disorders.

The results of heat disorders are most pronounced on the cardiovascular system. The heart must pump a greater supply of blood in order to cool the body. For each degree of rectal temperature increase, there is a 7% additional demand for oxygen to maintain body processes. As a result, the heart must increase its blood supply also to the lungs. As is sometimes the result, particularly in the unacclimated, heat stroke results as the cardiovascular system is overloaded (14). There is circulatory failure attributable to the exhaustion and cessation of the myocardium. Pulse rate is said to be an indicator of cardiovascular response with a resting rate of 110 per minute associated with tolerable body temperature.

Body fluid lost through perspiration and not replaced is derived mainly from interstitial fluid that is osmotically drawn by the plasma to keep plasma water content normal. During heat stress, secretion from the pituitary gland of an antidiuretic hormone can conserve fluid by the reabsorption of water in the renal tubules, thus diminishing urine flow. One hundred fifty liters of fluid or more may pass through the kidneys with only 1.5 liters excreted, and not reabsorbed back into the body. Salt in the perspiration is conserved, after a period of acclimation, by adrenocortical activity providing for its reabsorption in the kidneys. Na^- and Cl^- are the ions primarily responsible for maintaining the water content of the extracellular compartment. A potassium deficit may arise as this sodium conserving process increases the loss of potassium from the body (14). Large quantities of water are lost in heavy daily activities and up to 20 gm of salt may accompany this fluid loss (1 gm being 15 grains). During these activities, athletes are able to regain their fluid balance only by rehydrating after the activity. *Fluid may be lost more rapidly than it can be taken in during exercise.* Thirst accounts for only 50% of body needs. The sensation of thirst doesn't occur until the athlete has lost 2% of his body weight. Table 1.2 lists the effects of dehydration.

Heat is gained or lost through the following means: conduction, radiation, convection, and evaporation (2,14). Conduction may cause a rise in body heat of a football player through his contact with hot pads and helmets. The drinking of cool water causes the body to lose heat by conduction as this water must be warmed to body temperature. Cold water empties more rapidly from the stomach as the cooler temperature increases the smooth muscle activity. Sweat loss is often more than a quart per hour whereas maximum replacement may be less than a quart per hour.

Surrounding temperatures may cause a rise in body heat from radiation. Athletes can gain as much as 250 cal per hour in the sun (radiation), but the wearing of white clothing reduces this gain by one-half (14). Hot air flow increases body temperature through convection means.

When the environmental temperature is below 87°F (skin temperature), 70% of body heat is lost through radiation, conduction, and convection, and 30% by evaporation (2). Once the temperature rises above 87°F, heat is added to the body temperature, as heat is supplied more rapidly to the body than can be eliminated by evaporation (perspiration). In areas of high heat stress, sweating provides the primary protective mechanism of the body against overheating. As the humidity rises, the amount of body heat lost by evaporation decreases to almost zero at 100% humidity (19). With an exchange of cool air by ventilation, the heat elimination of convection and evaporation is greatly increased. Hot air exchange may often offset the benefits of evaporative cooling.

Heat Disorders

The classification of heat disorders are: circulatory instability, water and electrolyte balance disorders, and

TABLE 1.2. *Effects of dehydration*

- Decreased anaerobic capacity
- Decreased aerobic capacity
- Decreased gastric emptying
- Decreased sweat rate
- Decreased skin blood flow
- Decreased splanchnic and renal blood flow
- Decreased blood volume
- Increased heart rate
- Increased body temperature at which sweating begins
- Increased core temperature
- Increased incidence of gastric distress

From refs. 1 and 16.

heatstroke or heat hyperpyrexia (2,8,14). Of these, one group may predispose to another. Circulatory instability is often characterized by heat syncope or fainting. Other symptoms are light-headedness, dizziness associated with postural change, long standing, or exercise, nausea and weakness (24). As football linemen are constantly changing postural movements, they are particularly susceptible to heat syncope, a form of exercise-induced heat exhaustion. In circulatory instability, peripheral vasodilation takes place with tendency toward venous pooling and hypertension. There is an immediate drop in pulse blood pressure with a rise in pulse rate. Recovery is rapid if the athlete spends a few minutes in a reclining position (14).

In disorders of water and electrolytes that lead to heat edema, water depletion heat exhaustion, salt depletion heat exhaustion, and heat cramps, unlimited access to the ingestion of water and electrolytes is the major preventative of heat illness. Frequent and clear copious urine flow is a sign of adequate hydration. Heat edema results in swelling of the feet and ankles during early exposure to heat. This is probably because of the pooling of blood in the area (14).

Heat affects performance of individuals and there is a direct correlation between heat and minor injuries, illnesses, and irritability. Studies have shown 15% decrease in weight lifting when the temperature was elevated from 68°F to 75°F. Manual dexterity also shows a deterioration. Heat, however, seems to decrease man's willingness to work rather than his capacity to work (14).

Hyperthermia needs greater attention in the young. They have fewer sweat glands than do adults, as many as 40% fewer, therefore, they can eliminate metabolic heat less efficiently. They also will require more exposures to heat stress for acclimatization to take place (14).

Other individuals susceptible to heat disorders are: the aged, obese, unacclimated, the salt depleted, the dehydrated whether from vomiting, diarrhea, or alcohol, and those with diabetes and cardiovascular disorders. The physically unfit, those just recovering from a febrile illness, and those with a prior history of heat illness are also prone to heat illness. Some individuals seem to be genetically predisposed to heat illness whereas others seem impervious to heat illness even though they may be obese and in poor physical condition (14,16).

Football is the organized sport where heat illness is most pronounced as heavy equipment preventing heat loss is worn. Wrestling is a sport that dehydrates through weight loss and attention to heat illness is important in this sport even though it is performed in the winter (2). The implications for athletes is clearly seen.

The individual who is highly competitive and overenthusiastic should be watched carefully during periods of heat stress as the athlete is often the one doing more than the rest of the team. Consequently the athlete is overtaxing his system in the heat and is usually the player with the uniform that is dry at the end of practice as he has exhausted his perspiration. As the individual matures, the athlete learns to pace himself and thus doesn't suffer the effects of heat as does the inexperienced.

Heat Exhaustion

Water depletion heat exhaustion often occurs early and is caused by a loss of body fluid from diarrhea as well as sweat loss. Rectal temperature increases, as does pulse rate and respiration leading to hyperventilation. The skin becomes hot and inelastic, cheeks hollow, eyes sunken, and the victim exhibits symptoms of tingling, paraesthesia, restlessness, hysteria, giddiness, and uncoordination. Water depletion heat exhaustion sometimes leads to cyanosis, hypertension, circulatory and urinary failure, heat stroke, coma, and death (2). Hyperventilation is a signal in water depletion heat exhaustion that the body is not being cooled rapidly enough and that heat stroke may be rapidly approaching.

There is an early weight loss of 2% that may be followed by a severe 7% weight loss (14). Rehydration in a cool area is necessary. Salted drinks are of no use in this instance and may compound the problem.

Cutaneous blood flow decreases drastically as exhaustion appears during exercise in heat, thus jeopardizing the ability of the body to dissipate heat from the skin. As a result the athlete may become hypothermic and begin shivering. Slow runners in cool weather thus become hypothermic with a resultant excess heat loss.

Although water depletion heat exhaustion and salt depletion heat exhaustion may coexist (Table 1.3), the chemical picture of the latter is somewhat different (W. R. Butham, personal correspondence, September 9 and 23, 1966). A large intake of unsalted fluid predisposes to salt depletion heat exhaustion. Less water is reabsorbed from the renal tubules and water depletion is secondary.

Salt depletion heat exhaustion generally progresses over 3 to 5 days with a normal or slightly elevated temperature. Symptoms are: cool clammy skin, weariness, headache, nausea, vomiting, diarrhea, or constipation, and muscular cramps. Cramps from heat stress are caused by water intoxication into the intracellular fluid resulting in dilution of the sodium chloride content. In areas of high humidity, the skin classically is warm and moist as evaporation is ineffective.

The use of intravenous fluids is most helpful in the individual who suffers heat injury, either salt or water depletion. Body weight is instantly regained and the individual returned to practice much earlier.

Heat Stroke

Heat stroke and heat hyperpyrexia are the result of thermoregulatory failure that too often results in death. Physical exercise is the most common cause in this type of reaction to heat stress and may occur in 30 minutes of heavy exercise progressing from water depletion heat exhaustion. There is a primary failure in the production of sweat by water depletion, the fatigue of the sweating apparatus being unknown. A 4% to 5% body-weight loss results in a 20% to 30% decline in hard muscular work and a 7% body-weight loss often results in heat stroke (14).

It is postulated that circulatory collapse from high output leads to cardiac failure, and cessation of sweating from increased venous pressure. Sweating shuts down to prevent further dehydration (16). Heat stroke often progresses from water depletion heat exhaustion (8).

The individual may have sudden coma onset, delirium, central nervous system disturbance, convulsions, disorientation, incontinence, involuntary limb movements, plus the usual milder symptoms of heat stress. The skin, usually hot and dry, may be pale and cool. Temperature will be high. Cyanosis and lack of pupil coordination and reaction to light may be noticed. The pulse rate is often above 130 per minute with a rapid, labored, gasping respiration of 35 per minute. Renal failure and shock may develop in the individual.

Rapid effective cooling is the treatment for heatstroke and heat hyperpyrexia. The heatstroke patient is unconscious, irrational, with a temperature of 105°F plus, whereas the heat hyperpyrexia individual is conscious, rational, and has 105°F temperature. If the temperature is reduced within an hour to 102°F the cooling is usually effective. If cooling is not effective, heatstroke is fatal to between 20% and 75% of the cases, depending on complications. Heat hyperpyrexia fatality rate is about 5%. Untreated cases of both are fatal (14).

TABLE 1.3. *Difference in water versus salt depletion heat exhaustion*

Water	Salt
Urgency of thirst	Slight or no thirst
Predisposes to heat stroke	Does not predispose to heat stroke
High intake of salt without water danger	High intake of water without salt dangerous
May occur immediately	Generally progresses 3–5 days
Fatigue less prominent	Fatigue prominent
Muscle cramps absent	Muscle cramps present
Vomiting usually absent	Vomiting and diarrhea present
Skin inelastic, usually dry	Skin, clammy, moist
Temperature high	Temperature near normal
Death occurs generally as a consequence of heatstroke	Death rare
Treat by cooling and saline	Treatment by cooling and rehydration drinks
Chills	Anorexia
Hyperventilation	Frontal headache

Various modalities for cooling may be used. If practical, submersion in cold water is the most effective means of temperature reduction (2). A special slatted table designed to spray cool water (44°F) on all sides of the patient is effective (14). So also is the use of wet sheets, and use of the "cold blanket" in heart surgery (2). Probably the most practical of all is the use of a fan blowing across the athlete lying on a slotted deck lounger while at the same time vigorously massaging the extremities with cool wet towels. Care should be taken not to over-chill as shock and/or shivering (vasoconstriction) may occur. The extremities should be massaged to promote circulation. Medication may be administered by medical personnel to depress the hypothalmic center for heat to promote vasodilation, and to prevent shivering. Aspirin is of no effect as you are dealing with a defective heat loss mechanism.

Prevention

Water is the major preventive of heat illness. As long as the athlete is adequately hydrated heat illness will usually be of a minor consequence (24).

The magnitude of increase in core temperature, heart rate, and the decline in stroke volume are directly related to dehydration. Ingesting fluid in proportion to sweat loss best maintains cardiovascular function and prevents body temperature from rising too high (24). The ingestion of fluid reduces the rise in body temperature by promoting higher skin blood flow (2,14).

Thirst accounts for only 50% of body needs. The sensation of thirst doesn't occur until the athlete has lost 2% of body weight. At 4% weight loss there is a 30% decrease in work capacity (2).

The act of drinking stimulates heat loss by maintaining the sweat rate. Sweating is known to increase immediately following drinking in dehydrated subjects (14).

The acclimated individual tolerates dehydration better than the unacclimated. Voluntary fluid consumption increases with acclimation (14). After about two weeks the sweat rate then returns to near normal. With this massive dehydration, cool water or a saline solution (1 to 2 tsp salt/gal) should be available on a continuous basis during exercise (19). The athlete should also drink 16 oz of fluid prior to competition. With increased pressure of copious amounts of cold fluid in the gut, absorption is drastically increased due to the resultant increase of smooth muscle activity (16). In addition, cold water reduces body temperature through conduction (5).

During activity, athletes are able to regain their fluid balance only by rehydrating after the activity. Fluid may be lost more rapidly than it can be consumed during exercise. Sweat loss is often more than a quart per hour, whereas maximum replacement may be less than a quart per hour (16).

A 6% to 10% carbohydrate mixture in water optimizes fluid absorption and effectively supplies carbohydrate to working muscles. Sport drinks average between 6% and 10%, and are recommended over soft drinks, which tend to have carbohydrate levels about 12% to 14%. The higher level found in sodas and fruit drinks can slow fluid absorption, and thus it is not recommended to consume these drinks while exercising. A weak carbohydrate solution also aids in delaying exhaustion as exercise in heat increases glucose needs (5). If water is drunk in addition to electrolyte drinks, the carbohydrate content is usually not a concern as the water is diluting the carbohydrate drink.

The use of weight charts is beneficial to document the individual's weight status. Athletes should be encouraged to drink fluids to get their weight back from dehydration levels before the next practice. One pint of water is one pound. Another indicator of adequate hydration is urine color. Dark urine indicates dehydration whereas clear urine indicates the athlete is getting adequate fluids (5).

Exercise in heat is a must for full development of physical adaptation to heat. Acclimation to heat allows an individual to effectively work in heat of 80°F, whereas the physically unfit cannot perform in environments much above 65°F to 75°F. For full benefits of acclimation, two sessions of 2 hours daily are best employed. One session should be during the heat of the day and one when the weather conditions are cool. Longer sessions only put excessive strain on the athlete. Most acclimation occurs in 4 to 7 days and is usually complete in 12 to 14 days (2,14,24). Effects of acclimation however become lost within a few days unless exposure to heat is repeated at least every 4 days. Deaths usually occur in the first 3 to 5 days among the dehydrated who may lose 20 or more pounds during a practice. Heat illness may be accumulative so be aware of those showing increasing effects of the heat.

When the athlete becomes acclimated, the rectal temperature and pulse rate recede to near normal from an initial increase during heat stress. Cardiac output, blood volume, and venous tone are increased. Less blood is needed by skeletal muscle; therefore, the skin can get more blood to the surface for body cooling. The basal metabolic rate is reduced. The initial sweat rate may increase up to several liters per hour for improved cooling capacity. Increased sweating reduces the need of skin blood flow for heat transfer and results in a lowering of core temperature (14,24).

The acclimated individual will tolerate dehydration better than the unacclimated, but will drink more as voluntary fluid consumption increases with acclimation. After about 2 weeks the sweat rate returns to near normal. With this massive dehydration, cool water or a saline solution (1 to 2 tsp salt/gal) should be available every 30 to 90 minutes of exercise. However, it is recommended that the athlete have access to unlimited water at all times. The athlete should drink several glasses of fluid just prior to competition. Increased pressure of cold fluid in the gut increases absorption.

Contrary to some beliefs, the athlete needs added salt in the diet, by tablets if necessary, during periods of high heat stress. Sodium concentration in sweat rises sharply as the rate of sweat production increases. This is explained by the fact that the sodium concentration of sweat at its site of formation in the secretory coil of the gland is closely similar to that in plasma water. At low sweat rates there is time for sodium reabsorption to occur as the precursor fluid passes along the duct. However, at high flow rates, there is insufficient contact time for sodium reabsorption to occur, and as a consequence, the concentration of sodium in the final sweat is much higher. Even when the body is rehydrated water stimulates urine production and the body simply will not retain all of its needed fluid. The addition of sodium to the diet preserves thirst drive, decreases hyponatremia, increases absorption of fluids, and helps maintain body fluid during exercise (20).

Five to 15 gm of salt per day may be needed at the start of the acclimation process for the individuals who lose 3% or more of their body weight through perspiration. Vitamin C, potassium, and calcium are useful to the diet at this time also. It has been suggested that potassium deficiency leads to depressed muscular activity (2). Tablets are available containing salt, potassium dextrose, ascorbic acid, and calcium to prevent an excess loss of any of the above.

There is no benefit in using electrolyte solutions for the individual with a normal diet and participating in activities except possibly marathon runners. Some commercial electrolyte solutions have such a high concentration of sugar that they actually interfere with the emptying of the gastrointestinal tract. A 10% glucose concentration decreases gastric emptying by one-half. The primary aim of any replacement fluid is to maintain blood volume, and water does this best. No more than 2.5 mg/100 mL of sugar is indicated. Soft drinks need 3:1 dilution with water; Gatorade, 2:1. Endurance events over 60 minutes,

however, benefit from the intake of a dilute carbohydrate drink (5% to 8% carbohydrate) as the carbohydrates delay exhaustion.

Players should weigh out and in for each practice and these charts examined for athletes losing 3% body weight in 24 hours. These are the candidates for heat illness, and ideally should be excluded from practice (8,9). Those with episodes of heat illness should be excluded from practice as well for 24 hours. Also, exclude those with minor heat problems for 24 hours. Vomiting and diarrhea further dehydrate the body and should be contraindications for heavy workouts in the heat (14). Clothing should be light, loose, and white whenever possible. Mesh or net jerseys further help in body cooling. A cold shower taken prior to competition will also increase the body's resistance to heat.

The use of the wet bulb globe thermometer (WBGT) or sling psychrometer is a useful index as to the number of salt and fluid breaks and the length of practice times (14) (Fig. 1.10, Table 1.4). The WBGT is preferred over the sling psychrometer as it takes a measure of radiant heat into account. In many instances the physically fit and acclimated athlete has participated above these standards without any seemingly ill effects. Table 1.5 provides guidelines for practice intensity based on findings of the universal WBGT index. Table 1.6 provides practice guidelines for the fit and acclimated athlete. The recommendations for the fit and acclimated athlete are for a 2-hour practice session once daily. No more than one 2-hour practice session a day should be undertaken in the heat, even for athletes preacclimated to heat. The use of managers to give each group continuous and unlimited cold fluids is to be considered the ideal. The differences in the recommendations of the universal and acclimated index should be noted. Physical fitness tests measuring endurance (e.g., timed 300 shuttle runs) at the beginning of hot weather training will indicate to the athletic trainer who is in poor physical condition and thus is a candidate for heat illness. It is unfortunate that these individuals are not motivated enough to report in good condition. They

TABLE 1.4. *WBGT index for outdoor activities (wet bulb global temperature)*

Range	Signal flag	Activity	Wet bulb temperature guide	
82–84.9	Green	Alert for possible increase in index	Under 60°F	No precaution necessary
			61–65°F	Alert all participants, especially heavy weight losers
85–87.9	Yellow	Active practice curtailed (unacclimated athletes)	66–70°F	Insist that appropriate fluids be given in the field
88–89.9	Red	Active practice curtailed (all athletes—except most acclimated)	71–75°F	Alter practice schedules to provide rest periods every 30 min, plus above precautions
90+		All training stopped, skull session—demonstrations	76°F and up	Practice postponed or conducted in shorts
			Whenever relative humidity is 97% or higher, great precaution should be taken.	

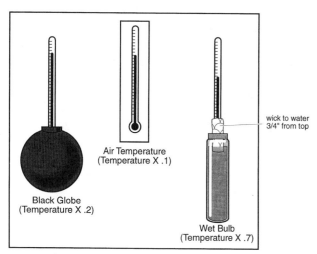

Components of the WBGT Instrument

FIG. 1.10. Use of a wet bulb globe thermometer (WBGT) to determine safe exercise intensity.

Explanation of above diagram and how to assemble the components of the WBGT instrument:

A 1/2″ metal rod is driven into the ground to support the unit. Placed across the top is a 10″ section of 2 × 4 lumber sanded and sprayed with aluminum paint. A standard outdoor thermometer is fixed to a flat side of the 2 × 4 trunk piece. Two support brackets of 1/2″ diameter are bent at right angles 1 1/2″ from one end to fit into holes drilled in top of trunk piece. The distal end of each is bent into a slight upward concavity to hold suspension cord of the black globe and the wet bulb units. The black globe is a spherical 5″ or 6″ copper float bulb, the threaded nipple of which is sawed off and a 3/8″ hole drilled. 1 copper cuff (1″ section sawed from scrap piece of 3/4″ copper tubing) is soldered so that the drilled hole is centered in the cuff. A standard chemical thermometer with a 3″ emersion line is fitted through a #1-hole rubber stopper up to the 10-degree mark on the thermometer. This unit is then sprayed flat black with Rust-O-Leum after masking the thermometer. This black globe unit is then suspended from the bracket by a loop of nylon line taped to the cuff. The wet bulb consists of a plastic bottle sprayed with aluminum and also suspended by a nylon line loop taped to the neck of the bottle. Also suspended from the bracket is another chemical thermometer with a 6″ wick up to the 3″ emersion line. (A wick can be cut from a "boot lace" and fixed in place with white thread wound and tied near the top.) The supporting lines for the bottle and thermometer should have such a length that the mercury bulb at the bottom of the thermometer clears the top of the bottle by 3/4″.

often may only train 30 minutes per day in hot weather but when they are in two-a-day sessions 4 to 5 hours of training are required. Athletes in poor condition should probably be worked by themselves or in selective drills until they are ready to participate. The use of rubber sweat suits is to be condemned for obvious reasons. Weight loss should be no more than 2 pounds per week.

A common early practice conditioning mistake is to overwork the athlete. The poorer the physical condition, the less work the athlete is able to tolerate. Here is another

TABLE 1.5. *Recommendations for exercise intensity based on findings of the universal WBGT index*

During acclimation
  82–85-light exercise
  83–85-no exercise, instruction in shade
  >85-all activity discontinued
After acclimation (10 days)
  >85 strenuous exercise stopped
  >88 all exercise stopped
Other precautions
  Stop activity if wet bulb within 3° of dry
  Remove football pads if WB within 3° of dry
  Read every 30 min

instance where the cardiovascular physical fitness test plays an important part in determining the amount of physical conditioning necessary. Conditioning done past the point of fatigue only results in an overall decline in fitness as food stores are depleted. Once liver and muscle glycogen stores are exhausted, usually about the third or fourth day two-a-day session, work capacity rapidly diminishes (5). Thus by the first game the question often is not who is in the best shape, but who is the least tired and worn out. Hard practices should not be held but every 48 hours. The same holds true for after practice conditioning as it takes at least 48 hours to replenish carbohydrate stores (5).

As a result, the unfit, unacclimated, obese athletes worked harder with their restricted diets are prime candidates for heat illness. Any athlete exhibiting signs and symptoms of heat illness should be immediately withdrawn from activity, for 12 to 24 hours.

The ideal diets for exercise in the heat are high in carbohydrates, as carbohydrates are high in water content. Plus glycogen stores release 3 gm of water for every gram of glycogen burned. Proteins require a great amount of water for digestion, thus adding to fluid imbalance. Heavy meals prior to exercise are contraindicated so that maximum circulation may be used for cooling (5).

It is important for the athlete to maintain his/her normal calorie intake. The intake of large amounts of fluids leads to loss of appetite and thus diarrhea and vomiting. The

TABLE 1.6. *Exercise recommendations based on the physically fit and acclimated WBGT index*

Attire break	Duration of exercise	WBGT	Length of water
Full pads	45 min	84 or below	5 min
Full pads	45 min	84–85	10 min
Full pads	30 min	85–88	10 min
or			
Helmet, shoulder pads, shorts, shoes	30 min	85–89	5–10 min
Practice canceled		90	

athlete should drink just enough fluid to satiate his thirst prior to eating. After he has eaten a good meal, he then may take on extra fluids. Coffee and tea are diuretics and should be avoided for obvious reasons.

Alcohol is to be avoided during periods of heat stress as it causes dehydration and increases the metabolic load (2,14). All medications should be evaluated for possible deleterious effects. Medications that reduce sweating are phenothiazines, which include the major tranquilizers; antihistamines; diuretics such as chlorothiazide, and anticholinergics such as atropine and belladonna, usually taken for the treatment of gastrointestinal disorders. Athletes taking diuretics for control of high blood pressure should be closely observed (2). Sedatives and haloperidol, which decreases thirst recognition, are also contraindicated in periods of high heat stress.

Air conditioning with dehumidifiers for off-practice hours benefits acclimation as the body processes don't have to constantly be active cooling the body (2,14). Sweating is reduced so dehydration is not as much of a problem. Skin disorders from chronic wetness are also avoided, and the athletes are better able to rest in a cool environment, thus diminishing the fatigue element and additional cardiovascular strain.

All personnel dealing with heat should be familiar with the prevention and treatment of heat disorders, and yearly review of existing literature is to be encouraged. With the use of sound practices, athletes will be able to compete safely in times of heat stress.

A SUBSTANCE ABUSE PREVENTION AND TESTING MODEL FOR COLLEGE STUDENT ATHLETES

College athletes not only face the usual stresses of college life and young adulthood, but they also face the pressures and risks associated with competitive performance (22). National studies show that although college athletes abuse alcohol and drugs at lower rates than other students (3), they are not immune to the high-risk atmosphere of the college campus. On the contrary, as Pinkerton notes, their experience as athletes creates some special vulnerabilities to substance abuse:

> Athletic participation at the college level creates major personal and emotional demands on the sports participant. Although many accommodate and successfully navigate this period, others are at risk and succumb to a variety of stress-producing circumstances . . . (18).

The unique pressures, expectations, and day-to-day living arrangements that student-athletes encounter have led researchers to suggest that this population may require specialized or "targeted" alcohol and other drug (AOD) abuse prevention programming (3,15). Athletes not only face the usual stresses of college life and young adulthood, but they also face risks and pressures associated

with competitive performance (11,23). Svendsen and Griffin list a number of reasons athletes may be particularly vulnerable to AOD use (Table 1.7).

Replacing the "Dreaded Drug Talk"

Although many colleges and universities in the 1990s established fairly sophisticated drug-testing programs for their student athletes, their approach to substance abuse prevention education lacked comparable sophistication. Too often the approach consisted of a single, annual "Dreaded drug talk" in which a speaker, such as a recovering athlete-addict or a law enforcement officer detailed the negative social, financial, and legal consequences of substance abuse and exhorted the students to "just say no." No one attempted to evaluate student reactions to these programs. The athletic trainer strives to effect quality programs, but because of severe lack of time and lack of education of substance abuse, is often at a loss to bring about the changes necessary to initiate a comprehensive program.

In 1989, the head athletic trainer at the University of Virginia suggested to the athletic director a revision of substance education programs. It was proposed that student athletes, with some guidance and structure, be given a voice in their substance abuse prevention programs. The athletic director approved and the head athletic trainer contacted the associate director of Prevention Programs at the Institute of Substance Abuse Studies (ISAS), and together they designed a more comprehensive substance abuse prevention program for varsity athletes. The resulting peer-based education program, later known as the SAM (student athlete mentor) program, was implemented during the 1989 to 1990 school year with the assistance of a grant from the Department of Education/Funds for the Improvement of Post-Secondary Education program. The SAM peer education program is now a crucial component of the Athletic Department's prevention/education program (12).

Research has identified several applications in which peer helping is most successful, including substance abuse prevention (13). An interactive style and the use of peers in design and implementation have also been shown to be particularly effective in preventing alcohol abuse by

TABLE 1.7. *Reasons for athlete vulnerability to alcohol and other drug use*

Athletes are very visible and vulnerable to criticism from fans, coaches, and teammates
Athletes face a time limited career due to age and/or injury
Participation in sports often involves inconsistent scheduling
There is a clear connection in our society between sports and alcohol use

From ref. 23.

college women (7). The same study suggests that the relational approach to substance abuse prevention, which includes peer participation and a focus on affective and connected learning, may best be tried in single-sex groups (such as college athletic teams).

Although there are a number of different models for successful peer helping programs (10), V. Alex Kehayan points out that most training programs for peer helpers should "emphasize group building, communication/barriers, empathy rapport building, behavioral warning signals requiring professional referral, personal support skills and limit setting, ethics and group management skills" (13).

Typical peer programs focus on a one-on-one, student-to-student approach to AOD prevention. In such programs, college students may be enlisted as volunteers, hired to facilitate campus-wide functions, or given the responsibility of planning campus-wide prevention activities for students. Although more effective than top-to-bottom, administrator-to-student AOD prevention programs, there are some problems with this model. Many existing peer prevention programs operate under the assumption that self-selected, volunteer peer educators will be accepted by students as peers simply because they too are students. This approach does not take into account that college environments are comprised of a number of subcultures (e.g., athletic teams, fraternities, sororities, and ethnic or minority group organizations) that have specific needs, issues and concerns relating to alcohol and other drug abuse. Therefore, student peer educators outside a student subculture may be less successful in influencing the belief systems or behaviors of students inside a student subculture than a member of that subculture. Since college student athletes are more likely to turn to peers than professional counselors for help with problems, and given the lifestyle issues and stresses that differentiate them from their nonathlete compatriots, it made sense for ISAS to design a program that uses athletes' teammates as the primary network for their own proactive prevention and education program.

The SAM Program

The overall goal of the SAM program is to create a safer social environment in which substance abuse and the negative consequences of substance abuse are reduced or eliminated. The SAM program involves athletes in prevention, education, and early referral for counseling and/or evaluation for AOD abuse and other health-related problems. The focus of the program is to help student athletes make healthy choices and to promote a community of caring within the team and department. Implementation of the program includes three main areas: selection, training, and ongoing activities.

Selection

Prior to selecting the student athlete SAMs, the SAM program directors invite all varsity coaches to attend their own training session. The coaches' session explains the goals of the SAM program, gives the coaches the latest data on alcohol and other drug use at the institution, and gives them some pointers on how they can actively support their teams' SAMs.

Ideally, athletes are recruited for the program at team meetings beginning in the spring semester, through a balloting process. Students are asked to select representatives from their team who have already demonstrated the ability to be a "natural helper"—one who is easy to talk to, conveys nonjudgmental attitudes, and has a caring personality. Teams are reminded that SAMs are not watchdogs, waiting to turn in their friends, but are instead people who will listen to friends' concerns, recognize problem behaviors, and identify team-wide health concerns.

Although the primary focus of the SAM program is AOD abuse prevention, it is clear that as natural helpers, the elected SAMs might be contacted by their teammates about other issues, for example, sexual assault, sexually transmitted diseases, or eating disorders. In order to be effective helpers, the elected SAMs have to be comfortable with the idea of helping in this broader capacity. During the selection process, therefore, we encourage the team to select individuals who possess the characteristics essential to their role as a SAM, not just their friends or even those who show leadership on the court or athletic field. SAMs become an internal resource for their team, examining the areas they feel are important to their teams and assisting in the design of programs or services that address these areas.

Training

Once chosen, SAMs are required to complete two training sessions totaling at least 5 hours. The goals of the training sessions, which are conducted and evaluated by ISAS staff, are to make the SAMs more aware of the status-quo, that is, of the expressed or implicit attitudes toward drinking and drug-taking within the athletic department and the university and to teach them skills necessary to initiate proactive and reactive responses to health-related concerns within that environment.

The training, which is conducted in small groups, is designed to be both interactive and thought-provoking. As the content has varied from year to year it has become clear that the training must provide the students with certain core information and skill-building exercises in order for them to be effective SAMs. ISAS surveys show that alcohol use far outstrips the use of other drugs on the University of Virginia campus. Therefore the focus in the brief training time available is on alcohol. SAMs are referred to the extensive SAM manual for information about other drugs, current statistics on their use, physiologic and psychologic effects, and referral suggestions/phone numbers. The core components of the two training sessions are presented in Table 1.8.

The elements in Table 1.8 have been presented in different forms as coordinators seek to develop training modules that can be mixed and matched to keep continuing training interesting for the students and trainers. Trainers have found that students usually have little concrete information about the physiologic and psychologic effects of alcohol. Data on absorption-rate factors, the significance of family histories of substance abuse, definitions of heavy drinking and how tolerance is developed can help SAMs respond knowledgeably when discussing AOD abuse with their peers in both formal and informal settings. Since most reported incidents of rape at most institutions involve alcohol, information about acquaintance rape is also included in training and follow-up activities.

Despite developing creative solutions to risky behavior associated with AOD abuse, many SAMs find it hard to accept that they might intervene once they observe such behavior. An important part of training, then, involves providing them with some active listening skills and communications skills and asking them to role-play situations in which they might intervene with a peer, or ways to respond to comments and queries by teammates.

After training, SAMs are expected to take proactive prevention measures at parties and other social occasions, to be available for teammates who might want to discuss any number of issues, and to give or arrange one prevention presentation for the whole team. Topics that SAMs have chosen to address in team presentations include alcohol and other drug abuse, sexual assault and alcohol, eating disorders, and nutrition.

TABLE 1.8. *Core components of the student-athlete mentor training sessions*

- An exercise to address personal attitudes about substance use and abuse.
- An explanation of the program and the athletes' roles as SAMs.
- An exercise to convey AOD information and institution-specific data.
- More comprehensive information on alcohol and other drugs, communications techniques and referral sources in a comprehensive manual given to each SAM.
- Discussions of enabling, the need for firm and publicized policies, current laws and regulations, and issues of concern to student athletes (e.g., underage drinking, liability, drinking and driving, alcohol-induced sexual activity, and problem drinking).
- Exercises that address values clarification, communication, active listening and decision-making skills, intervention techniques and leadership styles.
- Evaluation of the training session to assess additional training needs.

Ongoing Support

ISAS provides additional support services that include follow-up training sessions, assistance in program development, and monthly meetings. As an example of such support, when information about the characteristics of adult children of alcoholics (ACOAs) led several student athletes to realize that they fell into this category, they requested help in starting their own ACOA group, since their training schedules conflict with the meeting times for self-help groups conducted by the student health center.

A SAM council was established in the second year of the program to make suggestions for improving the program and offer additional leadership opportunities for SAMs who had been involved in the previous year. In November 1994 a university-wide computer news list to which all SAMs are subscribed was initiated. This list gives SAMs instant access via personal computer to updated statistics, notices about meetings, and questions or suggestions on handling certain situations from other SAMs. Many of the SAMs are also involved in a cooperative mentorship program working with high-risk 9th graders at a local high school. Since college athletes serve as role models for other students and local youth and often become involved in professional or intramural coaching later on, their involvement in substance prevention has a positive ripple effect.

Outcomes

Six years spent developing and modifying the SAM program have resulted in a number of positive outcomes. The program is directly responsible for positive changes in athletic department policies. A department-wide alcohol policy was developed after SAMs pointed out the lack of uniform alcohol regulations. Representatives from all areas of the athletic department (administrators, coaches, athletic trainers, and students) met to develop the department's now uniform and well-publicized alcohol and other drug policy.

In 1994 to 1995 the program's 59 SAMs served 21 athletic teams, 30 student athletic trainers, and the 100 members of the Pep Band—a total of 680 students. After the first 2 years of the SAM program, data from pre- and post-tests administered to SAMs show that students were almost twice as likely to have taken positive actions to change enabling myths/stereotypes about AOD use after becoming SAMs than before entering the program. SAMs, after being in the program for 9 months, reported a general decrease in the frequency of having one drink, two drinks, or five drinks in a row during the past 2-week period. In addition, students were over three times less likely to report behaving in ways they later regretted because of alcohol use after entering the SAM program than before (6). In 1992 to 1993 exit evaluations filled out by

11 of 30 SAMs, the responses to the question "what has been your impression of your impact on your team?" included nine positive responses ranging from "Positive. I really feel I have been a role model for our team," to "I do not think I made a major impact but I do think that I made a difference."

One of the key outcomes of the SAM program so far is the lesson that the attitude of athletic department administrators and coaches is crucial to the success of the program. At University of Virginia the support of administrators has been strong, and generally the program enjoys strong support among coaches. For some coaches the idea of the team acting autonomously to elect it own SAM is clearly threatening. Program coordinators have found that a few coaches are not yet persuaded by the natural helpers model. Some more resistant coaches have suggested that the program should be run by "professionals, not student athletes" or feel that the program "is a lot of show with not much accomplished." As an example of this resistance, the program coordinator describes how the coach of a major revenue sport decided to "give" the SAM position to a student who did not play regularly, thinking that this athlete might have more energy for the role, or might need to be given a role in order not to feel left out of contributing to the team. In another example cited, a coach selected as a SAM a team member known to have an alcohol problem, thinking that SAM training might help that individual. However, knowing their teammate's drinking habits, the team members were unable to take seriously the idea of this individual serving as the team's "prevention specialist." Occasionally coaches send unintentional double messages to players, supporting the team SAM, but out of habit allowing of-age members to drink to celebrate a win on the road. Rather than alienate these coaches (who are the exception rather than the rule) by insisting on elections, the program coordinator decided to acquiesce in having the coach select the team SAMs, hoping that if the program succeeded and both the coach and the team members became more comfortable with

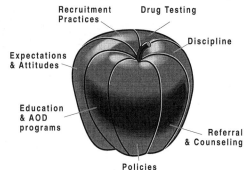

APPLE
Athletic Prevention Programming and Leadership Education

FIG. 1.11. Slices of the APPLE model representing components of an athletic department and how they interrelate.

the program and confident that it served a positive purpose, the SAMs would eventually be chosen by election.

Coaches of the women's teams and the women athletes themselves have been more enthusiastic about the program and about the natural helping/supportive role of the SAM in caring for and nurturing her team. Coordinators speculate that the relational model of peer helping comes more easily to the women athletes who have been socialized such that "self-esteem is tied to the capacity to engage and maintain" empathic relationships (7).

The program as a whole appears to be meeting the needs of those who become SAMs. Many SAMs have remained active in the program for two or three years. Overall, the SAM program provides a unique opportunity for student-athletes (1) to get more involved in the development of need-specific prevention programs for their team, (2) to elicit small group discussions that confront the traditions that perpetuate enabling, (3) to educate their peers on how to create a safe environment to prevent the negative consequences of AOD abuse in social situations, and (4) to serve as a resource to their team, offering a willing ear, recognizing the "red flags" of a potential

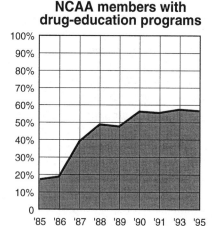

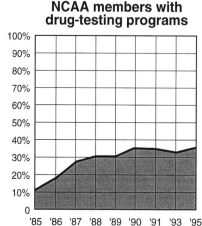

FIG. 1.12. Percent of NCAA members with drug-education and drug-testing programs.

Drug tested for:

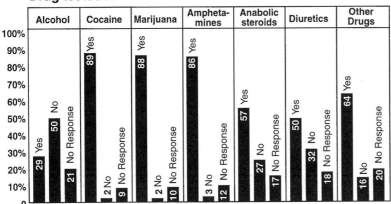

FIG. 1.13. Classification of drug tested for by NCAA member institutions

substance abuse problem and knowing when to refer a peer for professional consultation.

The APPLE Conference

After the formation and initial pilot year of the SAM program, the head athletic trainer in conference with student athletes recognized the need for a more comprehensive education/prevention approach in the athletic department. Further collaboration took place with the ISAS and others to devise a proactive approach that could address and include members from the entire athletic department. The athletic prevention programming and leadership (APPLE) model was developed to show this comprehensive approach. The APPLE model reflects the need for athletic departments to be actively involved in developing policies for education and prevention programs. As illustrated in Fig. 1.11, there are seven "slices" to the model that represent the components of an athletic department and the ways they interrelate. The APPLE model presents specific guiding principles for each of the seven slices of the apple. These guiding principles are designed to provide clear, precise, and achievable goals for athletic departments.

Substance Abuse Testing: Philosophy and Technique

The number of National Collegiate Athletic Association (NCAA) schools with AOD education and testing programs has steadily increased since 1985 (Figs. 1.12 and 1.13). The NCAA tests for substance abuse in football and track and field on a random sample, yearly basis for all Division I schools. Some of the drugs for which substance testing occurs include alcohol, cocaine, marijuana, amphetamines, anabolic steroids, diuretics, among other drugs. The primary purpose of a substance abuse testing program should be to identify abusers for follow-up counseling and rehabilitation. A positive test should result in disciplinary measures, but the athlete should have

the opportunity to receive assistance without loss of a grant-in-aid or team dismissal for the first offense. The athletic department thus demonstrates to the athlete a goal of help rather than punishment.

Development of a substance abuse testing program should consider the steps listed in Table 1.9.

Program integrity is essential to the success of a substance abuse testing program. In this regard, written policies should be developed, in consult with legal counsel, that address issues related to privacy rights, and local, state, and federal statutes. The written policies should be developed with input from athletic department administrators, student athletes, and members of the student health and dean of student's offices. Participation of the student-athlete is perhaps the most important element in development of written policies. Student participation leads to empowerment and reinforces the notion that the athletic department's sanctioned program has not been developed in an adversarial manner. Table 1.10 lists seven essential points in the development of written policies.

The written policies should be provided to the student-athlete and his/her parents prior to enrollment and matriculation at the institution. The athlete should sign an acknowledgment of receipt and understanding of the established policies, and these documents should be kept for the duration of the athlete's matriculation at the institution. The athlete should also read and sign a waiver agreeing to submit to substance abuse testing under the terms delineated in the written policies document.

Additional details specific to the substance abuse test-

TABLE 1.9. *Steps in development of a substance abuse testing program*

- Consult the institution's legal counsel
- Develop written policies
- Have waiver forms signed by athletes
- Develop the logistics of the testing program
- Identify key personnel to deal with positive tests
- Develop a committee to review all aspects of the program on a regular basis

TABLE 1.10. *Points to consider for the development of substance abuse program written policies*

- Outline the purpose of the program.
- Identify the program's participants including who will be tested and who will administer the program.
- Explain methods to be followed for the program.
- Identify the substances to be tested.
- Outline the frequency of testing and/or conditions under which testing will occur, e.g., random sample, unannounced, and announced testing.
- Clearly delineate the sanctions against those who test positive.
- Identify the counseling and rehabilitative services for those who test positive.

ing program are addressed in Table 1.11. To further assist the reader in the development of a substance abuse policy, the program used by the University of Virginia can be found in Appendix C.

The athletic trainer often oversees the administration of the substance abuse testing program. Coaches should also be involved in test administration, especially with respect to the recording and securing of specimens. Table 1.12 is a suggested delineation of the responsibilities of the team coach.

Successful defense of a legal challenge to a positive drug test necessitates documentation that the chain of custody of the specimen has been properly handled at all times. Observation of the specimen collection must occur by someone above reproach as this is one of the greatest areas of contention with substance abuse program litigation. To this end, an institution's police department can be an invaluable supplement to the role provided by the athletic trainer and coach.

Specimens should be stored in a locked refrigerator prior to delivery to the laboratory. Moreover, a reputable

TABLE 1.11. *Details specific to a substance abuse testing program*

- Who will be responsible for overseeing the testing procedures?
- Who will observe collection of the specimen?
- Who will record and secure the specimens?
- Where will the specimens be stored and secured?
- What is the courier system to the laboratory for analysis?
- What are the qualifications of the laboratory and what analytical procedures will be used?
- What is the cost of the regular screening procedures, and what is the cost of including anabolic steroids?
- What is the accuracy of testing and the rate of false-positive and false-negative screening?
- How will false-positive findings be identified and handled?
- What is the length of time from collection to notification?
- Who will be advised of the procedures and results after results are obtained?

TABLE 1.12. *Responsibilities of the coach in specimen collection*

1. Provide a team roster to ensure testing of all team members and managers
2. Obtain the following testing materials from the athletic training room:
   - specimen containers
   - specimen numbers
   - specimen security tape
   - chain of custody bags
   - drug test roster
3. Ensure the following test procedures for each team member:
   - record member's name on the drug roster, and place one small specimen number beside the name
   - place the other small specimen number on the chain of custody sheet
   - place the large specimen number on the specimen container
   - give the specimen container to the athlete who will have the specimen collection witnessed by the institution's police
   - receive specimen container back from athlete
   - record the date, time, and initial receipt of the container
   - ensure the name, face, and number of the container
   - place the cup into the chain of custody bag
   - return all materials to the athletic training room
4. Important considerations:
   - No more than two specimen containers should be checked out beyond those collected
   - The athlete must be either within viewing of the coach or institutional police officer or the specimen is rendered invalid
   - If the athlete is unable to provide a specimen, the coach must regain possession of the specimen container until a specimen can be provided
   - If the athlete is unable to provide a specimen at the scheduled collection time, one must be provided prior to any further athletic participation
   - Specimens will be discarded if there is any question of validity as a result of any variation in the aforementioned procedures

individual should be responsible for delivery of specimens to the lab.

Several factors should be considered in the selection of a laboratory. The state of the art in analysis is gas chromatography/mass spectrometry, with the latter providing the definitive results. As such, selection of a laboratory with these capabilities is highly recommended. Table 1.13 lists other factors that should be considered in the selection of a laboratory.

A successful substance abuse program should include a sound prevention and testing program that involves the student-athlete. The substance abuse testing policies should be well founded in a legal system, should be sound in steps of policy organization and administration, and should be inclusive of all professionals involved in the decision-making process. With adherence to the steps provided in this chapter, the development and administration

TABLE 1.13. *Factors to consider in the selection of a laboratory for a substance abuse testing program*

- Is the instrumentation used for analysis state of the art?
- What is the reputation of the lab and what other organizations offer their recommendation?
- What is the turnaround time for results of the analyses?
- Is the cost of the analyses reasonable without comprising accuracy and integrity?
- What is the laboratories' accuracy record and rate of false-positive and false-negative tests?

of an effective and ethically sound program can be accomplished.

REFERENCES

1. Allman FL. The effects of heat on the athlete. *J Med Assoc (GA)* 1992;81:307–310.
2. Hunter-Griffin LY, ed. *Athletic training & sports medicine*. Rosemont, IL: American Academy of Othopaedic Surgeons, 1991:850–857.
3. Anderson WA, Albrecht RR, McKeag DB, Hough DO, McGrew CA. A national survey of alcohol and drug use by college athletes. *Phys Sportsmed* 1991;19(2):91–104.
4. *Man, sweat & performance*. Becton, Dickinson & Company, 1969.
5. Costill DL, Miller JM. Nutrition for endurance sport: carbohydrate and fluid balance. *Int J Sports Med* 1980;1:2–14.
6. Evaluation Report: Student Assistant/Athlete Mentor Program, IPSE Grant #P183A00058 (unpublished report). Research and Evaluation Division, Institute for Substance Abuse Studies, University of Virginia, June 1992.
7. Gleason N. Preventing alcohol abuse by college women: a relational perspective. *J Am College Health* 1994;43:15–24.
8. Gieck JH. Heat & activity. Athl Train. *JNATA* 1974;9:78–81.
9. Gieck JH. Athletic activity in the heat. In: Kulund D. *The injured athlete*, 2nd ed. Philadelphia: JB Lippincott Co, 1988.
10. Gould J, Lomax AR. The evolution of peer education: where do we go from here? *J Am College Health* 1993;41:235–240.
11. Grossman SJ, Gieck JH. A model alcohol and other drug peer education program for student athletes. *J Sport Rehab* 1992;1:337–349.
12. Grossman SJ, Gieck JH, Freedman A, Fang WL. The athletic prevention and leadership education (APPLE) model: developing substance abuse prevention programs. *J Ath Train* 1993;28:137–144.
13. Kehayan VA. Peer helping: a powerful force. *Student Assistance J* 1992;32(Nov/Dec):20–24.
14. Leithead CS, Lind AR. *Heat stress and heat disorders*. Philadelphia: FA Davis Co, 1964.
15. Martin H, Thrasher D. Chemical dependency and treatment of the professional athlete. In: Lawson GW ed. *Alcoholism and substance abuse in special populations*. Rockville: Aspen Publishers, 315–349, 1989.
16. Murray R. The effects of consuming carbohydrate-electrolyte beverages on gastric emptying and fluid absorption during and following exercise. *Sports Med* 1987;4:322–351.
17. National Athletic Trainers' Association, 2952 Stemmons Freeway, Suite 200, Dallas, TX 75247.
18. Pinkerton RS, Hinz L, Barrow JC. The college student athlete: psychological considerations and interventions. *J Am College Health* 1989;37:218–226.
19. Prentice TA, Garmel GM, Auerbach PS. Environment dependent sport emergencies. *Med Clin North Am* 1994;78(2):305–325.
20. Pitts GC, Johnson RE, Consolazio FC. Work in the heat as affected by intake of water, salt, & glucose. *Am J Physiol* 1944;142:253–259.
21. Rijke AM, Perrin DH, Goitz HT, McCue FC. Instrumented arthrometry for diagnosing partial versus complete anterior cruciate ligament tears. *Am J Sports Med* 1994;22:294–298.
22. Rotella RJ. Achievement and stress in sport: research findings and practical suggestions. In: Straub WF, ed. *Sport psychology: an analysis of athlete behavior*. Ithaca, NY: Movement Publications, 1980.
23. Svendsen R, Griffin T. *Alcohol: choices and guidelines for college students*. Overland Park, KS: National Collegiate Athletic Association, 1990.
24. Zachazowski JE, Magee DJ, Quillen, WS. Athletic injuries & rehabilitation. Philadelphia: WB Saunders, 1996:264–271.

The Injured Athlete, Third Edition,
edited by D. H. Perrin.
Lippincott–Raven Publishers, Philadelphia © 1999.

CHAPTER 2

Medical Concerns of the Athlete

Keith E. Griffin

OVERVIEW

Athletics, both organized or recreational, team or individual, are one of the most ubiquitous and unchanging aspects of our society, and consequently help to define and enrich our culture. A majority of individuals receive enjoyment and self-fulfillment from participation in athletics of one form or another. Identification with individual sports teams, whether high school, college, or professional, can be extremely intense and durable and often take precedence over almost every other facet of life. Televised sporting events routinely reach millions of viewers and generate enormous revenues. Given their special place in our society, it is not surprising that athletics have carved out a niche in the practice of medicine.

Sports medicine, as the name implies, deals primarily with the medical concerns of the athlete. When one considers that the term athlete can refer to the 5-year-old playing soccer, the 19-year-old college varsity football player, the pregnant aerobics enthusiast, the middle-aged recreational tennis player, or the elderly person who enjoys a daily "constitutional" walk, it becomes apparent that the scope of sports medicine spans the entire spectrum of medical illness. Obviously, it would be impossible to cover this entire topic in a chapter of this size; therefore, the scope must be narrowed. The discussions that follow will deal primarily with athletes as they are thought of in the traditional sense; that is, young, healthy, and active people free of underlying chronic illness. Those athletes who do not meet this description need to be evaluated and treated based upon their exercise capacity and the nature and severity of any underlying medical conditions.

PREPARTICIPATION ISSUES

Prior to engaging in any strenuous activity, it is important for the potential athlete to be evaluated for any underlying medical problems, which may be important for a variety of reasons (41,48). The condition might interfere with the ability to fully participate in the chosen sport, increase the risk of serious injury, or potentially lead to serious medical complications including death. In addition to these medical concerns, the reduction of legal liability has become an increasingly important rationale, particularly as it relates to organized competition. In addition, the preparticipation evaluation allows the opportunity for general medical evaluation and disease prevention in a healthy young population that may be unlikely to seek medical care otherwise. For these reasons, the preparticipation physical examination has become increasingly important and most physicians are likely to be requested to complete a clearance form at one time or another. Recently, through the combined efforts of the American Medical Society for Sports Medicine, American Academy of Family Physicians, American Academy of Pediatrics, American Orthopedic Society for Sports Medicine, and the American Osteopathic Academy of Sports Medicine, there has been published a monograph that attempts to standardize the preparticipation clearance process and provide guidance in making decisions regarding ability to play (7). This publication is an excellent reference and should be obtained by those physicians who deal frequently with preparticipation clearance.

The preparticipation clearance generally involves both a medical history and physical examination. Of these, the history is usually the most important as careful screening can often give important clues to the presence of underlying problems in otherwise apparently healthy athletes. The physical exam can then be used to confirm these suspicions and occasionally will pick up unsuspected problems such as heart murmurs and hypertension.

There are several questions of logistics related to preparticipation physical examinations that are important to address. The evaluation should ideally be performed at least 6 weeks prior to the beginning of the season in order

K. E. Griffin: Copperfield Internal Medicine, Concord, North Carolina, 28025

to allow time for any concerns elicited to be properly addressed and evaluated. The frequency of exams is somewhat dependent upon the age and condition of the athlete and is an issue of some debate. High school age or younger athletes should probably be evaluated completely every year as their bodies are rapidly changing during the process of maturation. College aged athletes are less likely to develop intercurrent medical problems. The National Collegiate Athletic Association (NCAA) therefore recommends that all varsity college athletes be thoroughly screened upon initial admission into the program with a history and physical examination and then subsequently have a yearly screening medical history with a directed physical examination only if the history raises any concerns (52). Those athletes with previously identified medical problems should be reevaluated on a yearly basis. Older athletes (over 35 years) should be individually assessed as to the need for repeat evaluations.

The other major logistical question regards the form of the screening. The two most frequent types of evaluations are mass group screening or individual office-based assessments. Both forms have advantages and disadvantages as listed in Table 2.1. The office-based examination allows for better physician-patient interaction; however, for reasons of time and expense group screenings are very popular and common, particularly among high school programs. If the group screening method is used, it is imperative that the cardiovascular examination be done in a quiet area and that the athletes have an opportunity to ask questions and raise concerns in a private situation during the process. It is also important that one physician be identified as having the final word in the clearance of any athlete for participation.

History

As mentioned above, the medical history is extremely important in the evaluation of all potential athletes. Since most significant problems are found by performing a careful history, it is imperative to obtain all the important information. The use of prepared questionnaires can help ensure thoroughness and consistency of data collection. In younger athletes, it is necessary that the parents be involved in preparing the answers to the questionnaire. Figure 2.1 is the health history form used at the University of Virginia, which has been modified from a similar published form. The questions address almost all of the important problems that might preclude or interfere with athletic participation. Particular emphasis should be placed upon the cardiovascular portion of the history since the vast majority of sudden death events in athletes are related to cardiac conditions. Any positive answers require further investigation by the physician, including laboratory and diagnostic evaluation as necessary, prior to clearance. Immunizations should be up to date, particularly tetanus and measles. Tetanus should be updated every ten years, and a second measles booster vaccination should be documented (2). Eating disorders are very common among young women and should be approached with a high index of suspicion, although this information is rarely volunteered directly.

Physical Examination

The physical examination should emphasize those areas most likely to be of significant concern (particularly the cardiac examination) as well as those areas that the medical history identifies as a potential problem. Figure 2.2 is the standard physical examination form used at the University of Virginia. The height, weight, blood pressure, and visual acuity can be obtained by nursing personnel and the musculoskeletal evaluation can be performed by athletic trainers if available. The remainder of the examination should be performed by a physician.

Usually the most important component of the physical examination revolves around the cardiac evaluation, given its role in the identification of athletes at risk for sudden cardiac death. The general appearance of the athlete can be important, most commonly as relates to Marfan's syndrome. Marfan's is a genetic connective tissue disorder

TABLE 2.1. *Potential advantages and disadvantages of office-based and station-screening preparticipation physical examinations (PPEs)*

Office-based PPE	Station-screening PPE
ADVANTAGES	ADVANTAGES
Physician-patient familiarity	Use of specialized personnel
Continuity of care	Efficient and cost effective
Opportunity for counseling	Good communication with school athletic staff
Ease of scheduling any necessary testing	Opportunity for performance testing
DISADVANTAGES	DISADVANTAGES
Many athletes don't have a primary care physician	Noisy, hurried environment
Limited time for appointments	Lack of privacy
Varying knowledge of and interest in sports medicine problems	Difficulty following up on any medical problems and
Greater cost	concerns
Lack of communication with school athletic staff	Lack of communication with parents

UNIVERSITY OF VIRGINIA
ATHLETIC DEPARTMENT
PRE-PARTICIPATION PHYSICAL EXAMINATION
1994

HISTORY   Date _____

Name _____ Sex _____ Age _____ Date of Birth _____

Sport(s) _____ _____ _____

Home Physician _____ _____ _____
                                        Address   Phone

                                                                          YES   NO
1. Have you ever been hospitalized ?... ☐   ☐
    Have you ever had surgery?... ☐   ☐
2. Are you presently taking any medications or pills?................................. ☐   ☐
3. Do you have any allergies (medicine, bees, other insects)?.................... ☐   ☐
4. Have you ever passed out during exercise ?... ☐   ☐
    Have you ever been dizzy during or after exercise?............................. ☐   ☐
    Have you ever had chest pain during or after exercise?....................... ☐   ☐
    Have you ever had high blood pressure ?.. ☐   ☐
    Have you ever been told you have a heart murmur?............................ ☐   ☐
    Have you ever had racing of your heart or skipped heartbeats?........... ☐   ☐
    Has anyone in your family died of heart problems or a sudden death before 50?................. ☐   ☐
5. Do you have any skin problems (itching, rashes, acne)?....................... ☐   ☐
6. Have you ever had a head injury?... ☐   ☐
    Have you ever been knocked out or unconscious?.............................. ☐   ☐
    Have you ever had a seizure?... ☐   ☐
    Have you ever had a stinger, burner, or pinched nerve?.................... ☐   ☐
7. Have you ever had heat or muscle cramps?... ☐   ☐
    Have you ever been dizzy or passed out in the heat?........................ ☐   ☐
8. Do you have trouble breathing or do you cough during or after activity?............ ☐   ☐
9. Do you use any special equipment (pads, braces, neck rolls, eye guards, etc.)?.............. ☐   ☐
10. Have you had any problems with your eyes or vision?......................... ☐   ☐
11. Have you ever had a significant injury to the following bones or joints?............ ☐   ☐
    ☐ Head   ☐ Shoulder   ☐ Thigh   ☐ Neck   ☐ Elbow   ☐ Knee   ☐ Chest
    ☐ Shin/Calf ☐ Back   ☐ Wrist   ☐ Ankle   ☐ Hip   ☐ Hand   ☐ Foot
12. Have you ever had mono?.. ☐   ☐
13. Do you have any chronic medical illnesses (diabetes, asthma, kidney problems, etc.)?........ ☐   ☐
14. Have you ever had an eating disorder, or do you have any concerns about your eating habits? ☐   ☐
15. Do you or any of your family members have sickle cell trait or sickle cell disease? .... ☐   ☐
16. When was your last tetanus shot?_____ When was your last measles immunization ?_____
17. (for women only)
    When was your first menstrual period?_____ When was your last menstrual period?_____
    What was the longest time between your periods last year?_____
    Are you now or have you ever been pregnant? _____

EXPLAIN ALL YES ANSWERS BELOW (attach additional sheets if necessary)

_____
_____
_____
_____
_____
_____

I hereby state that, to the best of my knowledge, my answers to the above questions are correct.

Signature of Athlete _____ Date_____

Signature of Parent/Guardian_____ Date_____

FIG. 2.1. Preparticipation physical examination health history form.

that has skeletal, ocular, and cardiovascular effects on the patient. From the athletic perspective, the major concerns are cardiac because of the risk of aortic regurgitation and aortic dissection that can lead to sudden death. Suspicion of Marfan's is based upon the presence of tall stature, long fingers (arachnodactyly), pectus excavatum, kypho-

scoliosis, and dislocation of the eye lens. These patients require echocardiography as part of their overall evaluation.

The examining physician should have a good understanding of cardiac physiology and examination techniques. Peripheral pulses should be palpated to rule out

PHYSICAL EXAMINATION   DATE_____

Height_____   Weight_____   B/P _____/_____   Pulse _____

Vision R 20/ _____   L 20/ _____   Corrected :   Y   N

	Normal	Abnormal Findings
HEENT exam		
Neck		
Lungs		
Cardiac		
Pulses		
Abdominal		
Genitalia (Males)		
Hernia (Males)		
Musculoskeletal		
Dermatologic		
Neurologic		

PREVENTION

__TSE (males)   _ annual GYN exam (females)   _ Seat Belts   _ alcohol & drugs

_ safe sex   _ eating disorders   _ Sickle cell trait & heat illness

Assessment:_____

_____

_____

_____

_____

Clearance: A: Cleared
                       B: Cleared after completing evaluation/rehabilitation for: _____
                       C: Not Cleared   Due to: _____

Student Health Physician: _____   Date: _____

Signature of physician: _____

Reviewed: _____

FIG. 2.2. Physical examination form noting height, weight, blood pressure, pulse, visual acuity, findings of the medical exam and recommendation for participation.

coarctation of the aorta. Many young athletes will have benign, functional murmurs on auscultation, and it is dependent upon the examiner to accurately differentiate these patients from those with significant cardiac problems. The physician should listen to the heart while the patient is sitting up as this position minimizes benign flow murmurs and can accentuate the murmur of hypertrophic cardiomyopathy. The valsalva maneuver should be performed in all patients while listening to the heart as this will usually increase the murmur of hypertrophic cardiomyopathy. Those patients found to have a suspicious murmur should be referred for echocardiography to confirm the finding and determine severity.

Laboratory Testing

There has been much debate regarding the use of routine screening tests in the preparticipation physical evaluation. For instance, in the past it was very common for urinalysis to be performed on all prospective athletes. This practice has subsequently been challenged as not being cost-effective since it often leads to extensive workups in healthy young people and only very rarely discovers true renal pathology (55,78). Currently routine screening urinalysis is not recommended. In addition, the utility of other screening tests such as hematocrit, CBC, ferritin, sickledex, blood chemistries, and lipid profiles in young, healthy, and asymptomatic athletes is low and they are therefore not recommended. It may be advisable to screen for anemia in women engaging in endurance running events due to the high prevalence in this population.

Following the highly publicized deaths of Hank Gathers and Reggie Lewis from cardiac conditions, some authorities have recommended the use of routine cardiac evaluation including echocardiography, EKG, and stress testing. These tests have not been shown to be effective at reducing risk in this setting and obviously increase the cost and complexity of screening greatly (78). They are therefore not recommended unless the history or physical examination raise concerns the patient may be at increased risk of cardiovascular problems.

Prevention

For many if not most young athletes, the preparticipation examination is the only formal contact with a physician other than for acute care of illness. For this reason, the preparticipation examination represents an excellent opportunity to provide preventative health advice to patients who may otherwise not receive it. The physical exam form used at the University of Virginia also utilizes a checklist for discussion of preventative issues. Seat belt use is encouraged since the leading cause of death and disability in the young adult population is automobile accidents. Testicular self examination is discussed and taught during the genital examination of male athletes. This is emphasized due to the fact testicular cancer is the most common type of malignancy in young men and is usually curable if found early. Likewise, all young women are encouraged to have yearly gynecologic examinations with Pap smears, particularly if they have become sexually active. Eating disorders are a major problem in young athletic women with prevalence rates as high as 15% to 20%. These issues are discussed with an eye toward primary prevention. In addition, athletes should be encouraged to contact the physician or other appropriate personnel if they have any concerns about the eating habits of either themselves or their teammates.

Alcohol and drug abuse clearly represent a major health concern among young adults and should be addressed in order to educate athletes about potential consequences and problems that can result from irresponsible drinking or drug use. It is also important for the physician to attempt to identify those individuals who have existing problems with alcohol or drug abuse in order to provide counseling and possible referral to an appropriate treatment program. HIV and other sexually transmitted diseases are a major health concern in all sexually active young people. These issues are discussed with abstinence and condom use being emphasized as vitally important in preventing infection.

Clearance Issues

Once all the information has been acquired from the history, physical, and any indicated testing; the decision must be made regarding clearance of the athlete for participation in the desired sport. In most cases, the athlete will be found to be healthy and can be cleared without much contemplation or debate. Those athletes who are found to have conditions that could interfere with participation need to be individually assessed regarding the risk of an adverse outcome, the consequences of the potential problem, and the level of commitment to the sport by the athlete. An informed recommendation can then usually be given regarding the ability of the patient to participate in the chosen sport. Occasionally, specialty opinions may be required for evaluation of complicated problems.

Cardiovascular abnormalities are the most common serious problem identified in prospective athletes. In particular, the potential for sudden cardiac death is obviously of major concern and is one of the primary reasons for careful screening. Fortunately this event is a rare occurrence. In one survey, it was estimated that on average four cases of sudden cardiac death occur per 1 million athletes per year (1). Unfortunately, the ability to predict or prevent this tragic outcome is very limited, and the elimination of risk for sudden death during athletics is impossible at the present time. The use of screening echo and stress tests in young people considered to be at low risk is extremely controversial and prohibitively expensive. It has been estimated that in order to identify one athlete at risk for sudden cardiac death, 200,000 competitive athletes would require screening by these methods (24). Preparticipation examinations can often identify those athletes most at risk for sudden death and allow for proper management of these individuals. In particular careful screening by history and physical examination for Marfan's syndrome, hypertrophic cardiomyopathy, myocarditis, congenital anomalies of coronary arteries, and valvular lesions is imperative (46). A family history of sudden cardiac death at a young age also indicates a need for further evaluation since many causes of sudden death are hereditary. In older athletes (over 30), coronary disease becomes the most common cause of cardiac death and should be carefully searched for, often with treadmill testing (60). Despite the most careful and complete screening, there will continue to be the previously healthy individual who will be stricken by sudden death during athletic competition. This reality is difficult for athletes, the public, and physicians to accept, particularly when confronted directly by a tragic example. In this age of frequent litigation, the desire to ascribe blame for these occurrences is very strong, but in most instances the event could neither be predicted nor prevented.

For those athletes that are found to have a cardiac condition (be it congenital malformation, valvular disease, rhythm disturbance, coronary disease, or cardiomyopathy), the decision on whether or not to allow participation can be very complicated. Recently, the 26th Bethesda Conference, jointly sponsored by the American College of Cardiology and the American College of Sports Medicine, dealt specifically with athletic participation in the person with identified cardiac problems. The guidelines that were established by this conference have recently been published and represent an invaluable resource for all physicians who deal with these issues (3). The report offers comprehensive and clear recommendations regarding the types of activity that are not indicated for patients with specific cardiac problems. This conference summary rep-

TABLE 2.2. *Recommendations for participation in competitive sports*

	Contact		Noncontact		
	Contact/ collision	Limited contact/ collision	Strenuous	Moderately strenuous	Nonstrenuous
Atlantoaxial instability	NO	NO	YES*	YES	YES
*Swimming (no butterfly, breast-stroke or diving starts)					
Acute illnesses	*	*	*	*	*
*Needs individual assessment (e.g., contagiousness to others, risk of worsening illness)					
Cardiovascular					
Questions regarding participation should be referred to the recommendations of the 26th Bethesda Conference as discussed and referenced in the text					
Eyes					
Absence or loss of function of one eye	*	*	*	*	*
Detached retina	†	†	†	†	†
*Availability of American Society for Testing Materials approved eye guards may allow competitor to participate in most sports, but this must be judged on an individual basis					
†Consult ophthalmologist					
Inguinal hernia	Yes	Yes	Yes	Yes	Yes
Kidney (absence of one)	No	Yes	Yes	Yes	Yes
Liver (enlarged)	No	No	Yes	Yes	Yes
Musculoskeletal disorders	*	*	*	*	*
*Needs individual assessment					
Neurologic					
History of serious head or spinal trauma, repeated concussions or craniotomy	*	*	Yes	Yes	Yes
Convulsive disorder					
Well controlled	Yes	Yes	Yes	Yes	Yes
Poorly controlled	No	No	Yes†	Yes	Yes††
*Needs individual assessment					
†No swimming or weight lifting					
††No archery or riflery					
Ovary (absence of one)	Yes	Yes	Yes	Yes	Yes
Respiratory					
Pulmonary insufficiency	*	*	*	*	Yes
Asthma	Yes	Yes	Yes	Yes	Yes
*May be allowed to compete if oxygenation remains satisfactory during a graded stress test					
Sickle cell trait	Yes	Yes	Yes	Yes	Yes
Skin (boils, herpes, impetigo, scabies)	*	*	Yes	Yes	Yes
*No gymnastics with mats, martial arts, wrestling, or contact sports until clear					
Spleen (enlarged)	No	No	No	Yes	Yes
Testicle (absence or undescended)	Yes*	Yes*	Yes	Yes	Yes
*Certain sports may require protective cup					

Adapted from American Academy of Pediatrics. Committee on Sports Medicine. Recommendations for participation in competitive sports. *Pediatr* 1988;81:737–739.

TABLE 2.3. *Classification of sports*

Contact		Noncontact		
Contact/collision	Limited contact/ impact	Strenuous	Moderately strenuous	Nonstrenuous
Boxing	Baseball	Aerobic dance	Badminton	Archery
Field hockey	Basketball	Crew	Curling	Golf
Football	Bicycling	Fencing	Table tennis	Riflery
Ice hockey	Diving	Field (discus, javelin,		
Lacrosse	Field (high jump, pole	shot put)		
Martial arts	vault)	Running/track		
Rodeo	Gymnastics	Swimming		
Soccer	Horseback riding	Tennis		
Wrestling	Skating (ice, roller)	Weight lifting		
	Skiing (cross country,			
	downhill, water)			
	Softball			
	Squash/handball			
	Volleyball			

From American Academy of Pediatrics. Committee on Sports Medicine. Recommendations for participation in competitive sports. *Pediatr* 1988;81:737–739.

resents current standards of care and should be referred to when a physician is faced with these decisions.

For those athletes found to have medical problems that are not cardiovascular in nature, Table 2.2 can provide guidance for medical clearance. Table 2.3 breaks down the different sports into categories based on degree of exertion, contact potential, and relative aerobic versus anaerobic demands. This differentiation can then be utilized when referring to Table 2.2. Often an athlete who cannot be cleared for a particular sport can be redirected into a safer activity. Those athletes with problems not listed in the table need to be considered on an individual basis, often with specialty consultation. Most patients with unpaired organs can participate in athletic competition provided they use protective equipment as indicated. For legal purposes, it has become customary for the athlete to sign a liability waiver stating they understand and accept the risks involved and the consequences should the single organ be lost. In the case of legal minors, the parents should release liability. It is good practice to involve the parents in the discussion regardless of the patient's age, assuming the patient gives consent. Although the actual legal protection afforded by liability wavers is unproven, it does provide documentation of informed consent and demonstrates that potential complications were discussed prior to athletic participation.

The recent passage of the Americans with Disabilities Act has required some changes in the way athletic clearance issues are handled. Historically, physicians have been able to be very paternalistic and authoritarian in denying clearance to an athlete. Now it is often difficult to distinguish between protecting an athlete from a dangerous situation and discriminating against a patient with a handicap. The various questions regarding medical judgment, patient's rights, individual and institutional liability, and societal pressures are extremely complex and difficult to resolve. The specific circumstances surrounding this decision are important since there is a difference between the younger child involved with recreational team sport, the college athlete recruited and given a scholarship for his/her abilities, and the professional making a living through athletics. In those circumstances in which the physician feels participation is potentially dangerous but the patient strongly desires to play despite knowledge of the risks involved, the resulting conflict can be difficult to resolve, particularly when the possible consequences are severe. In the case of legal minors, the emphasis must lie on the well-being and safety of the child. Most parents are willing to accept the recommendation not to participate when confronted with the possibility of serious danger for the child. In older athletes who do not accept the recommendation of forgoing athletic competition, secondary medical and legal opinions may be required.

CARDIOLOGY

Hypertension

Hypertension is the most common cardiovascular abnormality among adults in this country and is consequently the most common cardiac problem seen in athletes. Blood pressure measurement should therefore be a required part of any preparticipation evaluation for athletics. The diagnosis and management of hypertension is a frequent problem confronting the sports medicine physician. The diagnosis of hypertension is confirmed when the patient's blood pressure is measured to be above certain threshold levels on at least three separate occasions. Proper sphygmomanometry technique is essential for proper diagnosis. A very common error relates to use of improperly sized blood pressure cuffs, particularly when the athlete has large biceps. Table 2.4 shows blood pressure levels considered to be elevated in various age groups and categorized into degrees of hypertension. Once an athlete has been diagnosed as having systemic hypertension, a decision regarding athletic eligibility needs to be made in addition to appropriate medical work-up and therapy. One study of over 10,000 athletes aged 11 to 19 years demonstrated that the leading cause of medical disqualification from athletics was the presence of hypertension (44). What criteria should be used for disqualification of the athlete with high blood pressure?

There is no convincing evidence that physical exertion is harmful in young, competitive athletes with mild to moderate hypertension and without other underlying cardiovascular abnormalities. In contrast, there is a large amount of literature that demonstrates a beneficial antihypertensive effect with regular physical activity (4,5). Regular aerobic exertion may normalize blood pressure in some patients with mild hypertension. Therefore, the benefits from regular exertion would appear to outweigh any risk in young patients with mild to moderate high blood pressure (47). Accordingly, those patients with stage 1 or 2 hypertension (as defined in Table 2.4) should not be restricted from athletic competition, assuming there is no known heart disease or end target organ damage (37). These athletes should have their blood pressure rechecked at 2- to 4-month intervals to follow the effects of exercise.

Those athletes with stage 3 or 4 hypertension are considered to be at higher risk of adverse outcomes and should be restricted from competition, particularly those sports that involve high static pressures such as wrestling or weight lifting, until their blood pressure is brought under control either by lifestyle changes or medication. These patients also require frequent follow-up and more extensive evaluation for possible secondary causes of hypertension. Older patients (over 35 years) with hypertension of any significant degree along with other coronary risk factors (male sex, smoking, diabetes, family history) should be considered for exercise stress testing prior to athletic clearance.

The medical evaluation and treatment of hypertension are topics well beyond the scope of this chapter. Some general points are important to make, particularly as relates to athletic populations. The initial evaluation of the hypertensive patient should be directed toward possible end target organ damage or a secondary cause of the elevated blood pressure. All hypertensive patients should have a thorough medical history and physical examination with particular emphasis placed upon fundoscopic exam to assess for retinal changes, cardiac exam to evaluate for possible murmurs, abdominal exam to assess for masses or bruits, and peripheral pulses to rule out coarctation of the aorta. Initial laboratory evaluation of the hypertensive patient should be directed toward screening for common

TABLE 2.4. *Classification of hypertension by age in children and adolescents*

	Magnitude of hypertension			
	Mild Stage 1	Moderate Stage 2	Severe Stage 3	Very severe Stage 4
Child (6–9 yr)[a]				
Systolic	120–124	125–129	130–139	≥140
Diastolic	75–79	80–84	85–89	≥90
Child (10–12)[a]				
Systolic	125–129	130–134	135–144	≥145
Diastolic	80–84	85–89	90–94	≥95
Adolescent (13–15)[a]				
Systolic	135–139	140–149	150–159	≥160
Diastolic	85–89	90–94	95–99	≥100
Adolescent (16–18)[a]				
Systolic	140–149	150–159	160–179	≥180
Diastolic	90–94	95–99	100–109	≥110
Adult (>18)[b]				
Systolic	140–159	160–179	180–209	≥210
Diastolic	90–99	100–109	110–119	≥120

These definitions apply to individuals who are not taking antihypertensive drugs and are not acutely ill. When the systolic and diastolic blood pressures fall into different categories, the higher category should be selected to classify that individual's blood pressure status. In adults, isolated systolic hypertension is defined as a systolic blood pressure of 140 mm Hg or more and a diastolic blood pressure of less than 90 mm Hg and staged appropriately. Blood pressure values are based on the average of three or more readings taken at each of two or more visits after the initial screening.

[a] These levels are adapted from the recommendations of the Second Task Force on Blood Pressure Control in Children (*Pediatrics* 79:1–25, 1987) to be consistent with the classification in adults.

[b] From the Fifth Report of the Joint National Committee on Detection, Evaluation and Treatment of High Blood Pressure (JNC V). *Arch Intern Med* 1993;153:154–183.

secondary forms and usually includes urinalysis, serum creatinine, serum potassium, complete blood count, and EKG. Cholesterol testing should also be considered in these patients. Since over 95% of hypertension is primary in nature and not due to other causes, extensive evaluation for secondary causes such as renal vascular disease, primary aldosteronism, pheochromocytoma, Cushing's syndrome, or adrenal hyperplasia is usually not necessary unless the history or physical exam raises suspicion. Other indications for more extensive diagnostic evaluation include treatment failure with appropriate medication, extremes of age (either under 25 years or new hypertension after age 55) or malignant hypertension (diastolic blood pressure over 120 mm Hg).

All patients with hypertension should be educated regarding life-style changes, which may help in blood pressure control. Frequent aerobic exercise is important but is usually not a major issue in the athletic population since most are very active already. Those hypertensive athletes participating in sports such as weight lifting or field events should be advised to add regular aerobic activity to their regimen. Dietary intake of sodium may play a role in some cases of hypertension, but sodium restriction should not be recommended to athletes frequently exposed to high temperature and humidity during competition, as it may increase the risk of dehydration and heat illness. Weight loss is usually encouraged, but this may be an impractical recommendation for an athlete whose sport relies on size and strength (e.g., football, weight lifting). Smoking should be discontinued in those few athletes who smoke. Smokeless tobacco is often a greater problem among the athletic population and should be strongly discouraged. Excessive use of alcohol can frequently be found in the adolescent or young adult with hypertension and should be investigated. Although it has recently been shown that moderate use of alcohol (two or fewer drinks a day) may be beneficial in the reduction of heart disease, it is at best problematic to make this recommendation to adolescents or young adults as the advice may be misinterpreted to condone irresponsible drinking in a group with an already high incidence of excessive alcohol use. The risks of serious or fatal injuries, health problems, and school or legal troubles are more consequential than any potential benefit in this age group.

Medical treatment of hypertension is a complicated subject with many issues regarding efficacy, expense, side effects, and relative benefits of various antihypertensive medications. These issues are frequently in flux and the treating physician must be informed and up to date as to the current treatment recommendations (19). Only a few major points will be made regarding antihypertensive medication and the athlete. The initial choice of treatment is based upon severity of hypertension, associated symptoms or comorbid illness, anticipated side effects, and cost. It is important to monitor response to whatever therapy is chosen and make adjustments as indicated.

One of the most frequently prescribed class of medications for initial treatment of hypertension are the diuretics. Since these drugs act primarily by reducing the patient's blood volume, they are usually not a good choice in athletes because of the increased possibility of dehydration, electrolyte imbalance, and heat illness during heavy exertion in hot, humid conditions.

β-blocking agents such as propranolol are also very frequently used for the initial medical treatment of hypertension. These drugs are often particularly effective in younger patients who have a higher adrenergic tone. Unfortunately, a significant percentage of athletes will complain of decreased exercise tolerance while on β-blocker therapy, primarily because of a decrease in maximal exertional heart rate and cardiac output. β-blockers should always be used with great caution, if at all, in patients with asthma. Like all antihypertensive medications, β-blockers can cause impotence in males, which can be very distressing to an affected patient. Despite these potential problems, most athletes will tolerate β-blockers well and they are a good first choice in many young patients with hypertension because of low cost and good efficacy. The athlete should be warned of potential side effects and then switched to a different agent should they occur.

Angiotensin converting enzyme inhibitors (ACE inhibitors) are a very effective class of antihypertensive. They have minimal side effects, which might interfere with athletic performance. They act as peripheral vasodilators primarily through suppression of the renin-angiotensin-aldosterone system but will reduce blood pressure even in patients without elevated renin. They tend to be somewhat less effective in black patients. The major side effect is the development in 4% of patients of a chronic nonproductive cough, which resolves once the medication is discontinued. The major drawback to their use is cost since they are much more expensive than older medications such as β-blocking agents. If the patient is able to afford one of these agents, they can be an excellent choice for hypertension control in the athlete.

Calcium channel blockers are another relatively newer class of antihypertensive agents that are increasingly being used, often as a first line therapy. They act by inhibiting the movement of calcium ions across the cell membrane, resulting in depression of mechanical contraction of myocardial muscle and vasodilation of peripheral vasculature, resulting in decreased blood pressure. They are very effective antihypertensives and tend to work very well in black patients. Like ACE inhibitors, they have very few side effects. There is some theoretical concern that these drugs, particularly verapamil, might decrease exercise tolerance because of reduction in cardiac output resulting from decreased myocardial contractility. In actual practice however, this effect is usually compensated for by peripheral vasodilitation and seldom presents a significant problem. As in ACE inhibitors, one of the major drawback of these agents is the expense of the medications.

Other antihypertensives such as reserpine, clonidine, guanabenz, alpha-blocking agents, hydralazine, and methyldopa are less frequently used in the younger athlete except in unusual circumstances and will not be discussed.

INFECTIOUS DISEASES

Upper Respiratory Infections

Upper respiratory infections (URI) are the most common acute illnesses in the United States. These illnesses are the most common cause of absences from school or work and Americans spend over $3 billion annually for over-the-counter medications to relieve their symptoms. They are also the most common illness athletes suffer from and can have a significant impact both on the performance of the individual and the success of the team.

The common cold is caused by any of over 200 different viruses, most commonly members of the rhinovirus, coronavirus, and adenovirus families. Each of these over 200 viruses is capable of causing infection in an individual patient, explaining why people are susceptible to innumerable colds during their lifetime and why the average adult suffers three to five colds per year. However, the average young athlete (and particularly the college student) probably gets even more than this because of the fact they have developed immunity to fewer individual viral causes, are exposed to multiple viruses from other parts of the country, spend large amounts of time in crowded, closed spaces (e.g., classrooms, buses, planes, locker rooms), and often share towels and drinking bottles. In addition, there is some research that possibly implicates high levels of exertion with decreased immune function and increased susceptibility to infection (23). Regardless of the causative virus, the symptoms of the common cold are similar and well known to all people.

Following an incubation period of 48 to 72 hours, a cold usually begins with mild malaise, rhinorrhea, sneezing, and a scratchy sore throat. Fever is unusual and, if present, rarely exceeds 100°F. Symptoms are worst on the third to fourth day and usually resolve by 1 week but can often persist for 2 weeks. Initially the nose is runny but as the illness progresses it will frequently become congested with thick tenacious mucus, which may be discolored because of dehydration. There is also, generally, a sensation of global sinus pressure. Not uncommonly, the patient will also develop a dry cough several days into the illness. These symptoms, in the absence of other findings or complaints, are expected and are not evidence of secondary bacterial infection. Having a URI does predispose a patient to developing a secondary sinusitis or otitis media. A careful initial assessment along with in-

structions given to the patient concerning worrisome symptoms will facilitate proper diagnosis of these conditions.

Despite great efforts, there is still no specific antiviral therapy for the common cold. Therapy is therefore supportive and based upon symptom relief. Bed rest is not necessary and patients should be encouraged to remain active unless they have a temperature over 100.5°F or have significant systemic complaints (in which case abstinence from exercise should be advised because of the possibility of underlying myocarditis secondary to coxsackie virus infection). Patients with URI should be advised not to exercise maximally or to the point of physical exhaustion as this may delay recovery. Aspirin, Tylenol, or ibuprofen are frequently used for relief of fever and muscle aches. Steam and nocturnal vaporizer usage can help to keep nasal secretions moist and liquid, particularly in the winter when heating systems tend to decrease ambient humidity. Hoarseness, should it occur, is treated by voice rest. Sore throat is a difficult symptom to completely relieve but can be helped by saltwater gargles, drinking lots of fluids, lozenges, topical anesthetics, and occasionally pain medication such as codeine. A vaporizer also can help with early morning sore throat because of mouth breathing of dry air at night.

Nasal congestion is best relieved by topical decongestants such as Afrin nasal spray. However, these preparations have been shown to have an addictive potential if used frequently for prolonged periods. The rebound effect of decongestive nasal sprays is probably overstated, but they should be utilized with caution. They can be very effective if utilized immediately prior to an athletic event to provide short-term relief of congestion that would interfere with performance. Oral decongestants (pseudoephedrine, phenylpropanalamine) are found in a wide variety of over-the-counter and prescription medications. The mechanism of action is to constrict blood vessels in the mucous membranes, thereby reducing swelling and mucous secretion. Guaifenesin is an expectorant that acts to thin the nasal secretions and help prevent the thick tenacious mucus that can block up sinuses and ears. A combination product of guaifenesin and a decongestant is often the most effective option for symptom relief. Antihistamines (Benadryl, Claritin, Allegra, Tavist) have only a marginal effect on symptom relief and often cause excessively dry and tenacious nasal secretions, which often makes the patient feel worse and possibly predisposes to secondary sinus or ear infections. Vitamin C has been extensively studied and no clear evidence of effectiveness in treatment or prevention of viral URIs has been demonstrated (13).

Antibiotics are clearly useless in the uncomplicated common cold. Frequently, the physician is placed under great pressure from the patient and other sources to overuse bacterial antibiotic therapy in viral illnesses. The truth is that undirected treatment of an illness in the hope it may help seldom benefits the patient and always carries risk. All antibiotics have side effects, which sometimes can be serious or even fatal. In addition, the growing problem of antibiotic resistance can be attributed to the misuse of antibiotic therapy. In the absence of clear indications of bacterial infection, they should be avoided.

Patients should be educated that transmission of infection can be minimized by frequent hand washing, by reducing hand to face contact, by covering mouth and nose when sneezing and by not sharing towels, drinks, and so on. Community water bottles should be avoided if possible to reduce transmission.

Influenza

Influenza (the flu) is a very common and debilitating viral illness, which occurs in epidemics every winter. It is caused by the influenza virus, most common is the group A strain, although B and C strains can also cause infection. The influenza virus is unusual in the fact that it undergoes spontaneous mutation very frequently. These mutations result in the altering of the virus so that the immune system is unable to recognize it, even if the patient has had the flu before. These mutations (called antigenic shifts) occur almost annually in the influenza A virus, which results in a flu epidemic every year usually between December and February. In the elderly or compromised patient, the flu can represent a serious and possibly fatal disease. In the healthy athlete, the flu is usually a self-limited but often incapacitating illness that can significantly impact athletic participation.

Influenza has a very characteristic course of infection, which usually allows for rapid clinical diagnosis, particularly during an epidemic. Following an incubation period of 2 to 3 days, the illness is usually characterized by abrupt onset of malaise, prostration, muscle aches, headache, and fever. The temperature is usually above 102°F and often as high as 105°F. Nasal congestion, sore throat, and dry cough typically begin a couple of days into the illness and worsen as the fever and prostration improve. In healthy adults, the acute illness usually resolves spontaneously over 4 to 5 days; however, the cough frequently persists for an additional 2 to 3 weeks, presumedly because of necrosis and subsequent healing of respiratory epithelium. During an epidemic, the accuracy of clinical diagnosis based upon these symptoms is excellent. Treatment consists primarily of rest, fluids, Tylenol or other antipyretic for fever control, and occasionally codeine or other analgesic for muscle aches or headaches.

It is often underappreciated that an effective therapy for influenza A is available. Although it is true that influenza is a self-limited disease that usually resolves without treatment or long-term sequela, the acute illness can be incapacitating. Amantidine and rimantadine are specific antiinfluenza viral medications that have been shown to significantly reduce the duration and severity of the pa-

tient's symptoms. If initiated within the first 48 hours of the illness, the length of the fever and systemic symptoms is reduced by 1 to 2 days (17). Often this benefit can be of major significance to the athlete who becomes ill during the sport season and treatment should therefore be considered for these patients. Amantidine is dosed at 100 mg bid for five days and is usually well tolerated but occasionally causes dizziness, nausea, and difficulty with concentration. Rimantadine is much more expensive but has fewer side effects and can therefore be used in patients who cannot tolerate amantidine. Amantidine and rimantadine can also be used as chemoprophylaxis to prevent illness during an influenza epidemic (15). Chemoprophylaxis should be considered under certain circumstances such as when a team has an important upcoming game or tournament during an influenza outbreak.

Influenza can also be prevented by use of influenza vaccine. This vaccine is formulated every year by the Center for Disease Control (CDC) and is based upon the predicted prevalent strains for the upcoming flu season. It is released in the fall of the year and is most effective if given before flu season begins. When there is good antigenic match between the vaccine and the actual prevalent influenza strains, the vaccine is very effective and most years it reduces the risk of infection by at least 70% (39). In addition, if a sufficient percentage of the population is vaccinated, there is a reduction in the number of susceptible individuals and the risk of an epidemic is attenuated. Offering the vaccine to those athletes who participate in their sport during the winter months is an effective means of reducing the illness' impact on an individual or athletic team. It should also be recommended to coaching staff, athletic trainers, and managers. Contrary to popular misconception, the influenza vaccine does not cause the flu. Sore arm and a low-grade fever are the most frequent side effects and are due to immune system activation (51). The vaccine should not be given to patients with hypersensitivity to eggs.

Pharyngitis

Sore throat (pharyngitis) is another very common complaint among athletes. Pharyngitis is caused by a wide variety of bacterial and viral pathogens including streptococci (strep), *Mycoplasma pneumonia*, chlamydia, gonorrhea, influenza, parainfluenza, herpes simplex, adenovirus, and infectious mononucleosis. Although the vast majority of sore throats are viral in origin and require only symptomatic treatment, it is extremely important to evaluate all complaints of sore throat completely to rule out a potentially dangerous illness such as peritonsillar abscess or mononucleosis with impending airway obstruction. Fortunately, these complications are rare and for practical purposes the two most important causes of sore throat that need to be identified are group A streptococci and infectious mononucleosis: strep, because it needs to be treated in order to prevent complications such as rheumatic fever, and mono because of the length of illness and impact on athletic participation.

Strep Throat

Group A streptococcal infection (strep throat) has an incubation period of 2 to 4 days, which is usually followed by the abrupt onset of sore throat, fever, malaise, and headache. Several clinical clues should alert one to the possibility of strep throat. First, strep is less likely to present with cough or nasal congestion and the presence of these usually suggests a viral etiology. The presence of a combination of temperature greater than 101°, tender anterior cervical adenopathy, and a tonsillar exudate is the classic description for strep throat; although surprisingly only 40% of patients with this symptom complex actually turns out to have strep on culture (the other 60% have one of the other causes of sore throat) (11). The absence of any of these three symptoms make strep very unlikely to be the cause and diagnostic testing with culture is not indicated. The presence of one or two of these symptoms make strep unlikely but possible. Since the only way to know for sure if a patient who presents with this scenario has strep throat is to have a positive diagnostic test, a throat culture or rapid strep test should be obtained and therapy directed based upon test results.

Treatment for strep is penicillin (or erythromycin if allergic to penicillin) for 10 days. The rationale for treating strep is to prevent complications such as tonsillar abscess, scarlet fever, glomerular nephritis, and rheumatic fever. Rheumatic fever used to be a common complication of strep throat that results in damage to the valves of the heart and subsequent long-term problems. It is much less common today than 40 years ago, at least partially because of appropriate antibiotic therapy. Antibiotics probably do not significantly impact on length of the illness itself. The sore throat itself is self-limited and lasts for 5 to 6 days. The management of the patient is based on presenting symptoms. Those patients that have all four symptoms of fever, absence of cough, adenopathy, and tonsillar exudate are likely to have strep pharyngitis and are started empirically on antibiotics without further testing (12). Those patients with two to three of the diagnostic symptoms have a rapid strep test performed. If the rapid strep test is negative or unavailable, a regular throat culture is performed. If the rapid strep test or culture is positive, the patient is treated. For those patients with only one diagnostic symptom, only those with tonsillar exudate are cultured with the rest being managed conservatively. Those patients without any of the above symptoms are not cultured, but are instructed to come back if their symptoms worsen. All patients with pharyngitis are urged to drink plenty of fluids, use saltwater gargles, take Tylenol or aspirin, and use lozenges or chloroseptic spray for sore throat relief.

Infectious Mononucleosis

Infectious mononucleosis (mono) is a systemic viral infection caused by the Epstein-Barr virus (EBV), a member of the herpes virus family. The illness is very common among teenage and young adults and is thus seen frequently among young athletes. The severity of symptoms in this illness vary from individual to individual with some patients having no symptoms at all at time of infection, whereas others have a severe, debilitating course that can drag on for months. The illness usually begins after a 1- to 2-month incubation period. Classically, patients present with sore throat (which can be impossible to distinguish from strep without a culture), lymphadenopathy, fever, splenomegaly, and a distinctive appearance to certain lymphocytes in the blood known as atypical lymphocytes. Some patients with mono may develop hepatitis and jaundice, whereas others may develop a peculiar skin rash, although still others may develop a hemolytic anemia or thrombocytopenia. Most patients with mono complain of fatigue ranging from mild to incapacitating. It is important to recognize that the disease can present in many different ways and is therefore not always easy to diagnose.

Diagnosis is usually made on clinical grounds and is often then confirmed by use of a specific blood test known as the monospot, which usually turns positive the second week of infection. Unfortunately, 10% to 20% of actual mono cases never develop a positive mono test (6). In addition, there are other viruses besides Epstein-Barr that can cause an illness that is clinically identical to mono but does not cause a positive monospot test. Therefore, the monospot test is not always accurate and diagnosis sometimes requires more specific testing such as Epstein-Barr or cytomegalovirus antibody titers.

Treatment of mono is entirely supportive and consists of adequate rest, fluids, Tylenol, sore throat therapy, and time. Antibiotics are not indicated for treatment and ampicillin/amoxicillin is actually associated with a high incidence of drug rash in these patients. Antivirals such as acyclovir have also not been shown to be effective. In patients with severe problems, such as impending airway obstruction from tonsillar hypertrophy or hemolytic anemia, prednisone is frequently used to improve symptoms but has little effect on the overall course of the illness. Patients should be periodically reexamined during the illness in order to follow symptoms and watch for potential complications. Patients should also be advised to avoid drinking alcohol while recovering from mono.

Patients are encouraged to remain as active as their symptoms allow but are instructed to avoid strenuous exercise while having fever, bad sore throat, or other acute problems. Once their symptoms improve, patients are allowed to gradually increase their activity as tolerated; however, patients are prohibited from contact sports and diving because of the possibility of splenic rupture. Mononucleosis patients are at increased risk for this complication because of enlargement of the spleen (45). Although the overall number of mono associated splenic ruptures is very low, the potential consequences of this problem can be catastrophic or fatal. Therefore, these patients should not be allowed to return to contact sports for 1 month and their abdominal examination is normal without evidence of splenomegaly (70). Abdominal ultrasound can help identify subclinical splenomegaly in those cases in which it may not be clear on the basis of physical exam (16). Even after they recover from the acute illness, many patients will continue to complain of excessive fatigue and decreased exercise performance for several months after the infection and may miss an entire season of competition.

Sinusitis

Sinusitis refers to a bacterial infection of one or more of the paranasal sinuses, which complicates about 0.5% (1 in 200) of viral URIs. These infections usually occur because of the fact that URIs cause inflammation of the mucous membranes lining the nose and sinuses and thus cause blockage of the small ostia, which allow the sinuses to drain normally. This leads to a backup of sinus secretions that can then become secondarily infected with bacteria. In most acute sinus infections, the major distinguishing symptom is pain over one or more of the sinuses, usually on one side of the face. This pain may be dull in the early stages but usually becomes throbbing as the infection progresses. The pain is usually made worse by leaning the head forward, coughing, or straining. Often maxillary sinus pain is felt in the upper teeth. The ''pressure'' that people often complain about during a URI is much less localized, frequently changes location, and either fails to worsen or improves with time. Other causes of facial pain such as tooth infection, migraine, or cluster headache need to be ruled out.

Diagnosis of sinusitis is usually made based on clinical presentation since the only way to definitively diagnose sinusitis is to perform a sinus puncture, which involves placing a needle through the surrounding bone and culturing the sinus material. This procedure is impractical in most instances. Symptoms that are suspicious for a bacterial sinus infection include the pain pattern mentioned previously, purulent nasal discharge, maxillary toothache, persistence of a ''cold'' for more than 2 weeks, and failure of symptoms to improve with appropriate decongestants. The physical exam consists of examining the ears, pharynx, nose, and teeth for other causes of the symptoms. Purulent drainage seen in the back of the throat is sugges-

tive of a possible sinus infection, but as a single symptom, is not diagnostic. Palpation of the sinuses frequently worsens the pain in sinusitis. Transillumination of the sinuses (shining a bright light through the sinuses) is helpful if the suspected sinus fails to transilluminate and the opposite side does. If any other results are obtained, the test is not very reliable. In questionable cases, sinus x-rays can be diagnostic but are expensive. The most important factors for clinical diagnosis are the presence of maxillary toothache, purulent secretions noted on examination, poor response to decongestant therapy, abnormal transillumination, and a history of colored nasal discharge (79). The presence of four or more of these predictors strongly suggests sinusitis, two or fewer makes sinusitis less likely, and three represents a toss-up. As a practical consideration, the presence of three or more of these predictors could warrant treatment.

Treatment of bacterial sinusitis consists of steam, humidity, decongestants, pain relief, and antibiotics. Although most sinus infections resolve spontaneously without antibiotic treatment, it is common practice to treat in order to reduce risk of complications such as meningitis or chronic sinusitis. The antibiotic usually chosen initially is amoxicillin but because of the worsening problem of bacterial resistance to antibiotics, the infection often requires stronger and more expensive drugs such as Ceftin or Augmentin. For the penicillin allergic patient, erythromycin or Bactrim are used. The antibiotics should be taken for at least 10 days and usually 2 weeks to prevent recurrence with resistant organisms.

Bronchitis

Acute bronchitis is an inflammatory condition of the trachea-bronchial tree that results from respiratory infections primarily because of common cold viruses, influenza, adenovirus, pertussis, *Mycoplasma pneumonia*, or chlamydia. The illness is characterized by cough, with or without sputum production, persisting longer than expected (usually 1 to 2 weeks) after the onset of a URI. It is almost impossible to distinguish between the various causes of bronchitis. It is clear, however, that the majority of coughs in healthy nonsmoking young people with clear lung sounds are due to postviral inflammation of the airways, and not coexistent bacterial infection. This means that almost all otherwise healthy athletes with coughs require time to allow the body to heal itself as the major therapy for recovery. It is important to rule out other causes of cough such as asthma or pneumonia. In the absence of fever, shortness of breath, abnormal lung sounds, or chest pain, the recommended approach is to avoid antibiotics and use mild cough suppressants such as Robitussin DM. If the athlete is having trouble sleeping at night because of coughing, a preparation containing codeine can aid in obtaining adequate rest. Additional symptomatic measures include fluids, steam, or other cough suppressants such as Tessilon Perles.

Unfortunately, there is no easy test to determine who might have mycoplasma or other bacterial pathogens as the cause of their bronchitis. Since the majority of coughs are self-limited and of viral origin, antibiotics should not routinely be used in cases of acute bronchitis (31,54). Unfortunately, many patients have developed the expectation that antibiotics should be given to them when they have bronchitis because of over-prescribing in the past. This author usually insists on 1 or 2 weeks of conservative management prior to considering prescribing antibiotics. If antibiotics are used to treat a persistent cough, erythromycin or doxycycline should be chosen to cover the possibility of mycoplasma. Inhaled bronchodilators (as used in asthma) have been shown to provide symptomatic relief in some cases of bronchitis (36). If the patient has chest pain, shortness of breath, fever, or abnormal lung sounds on examination, an x-ray should be obtained to rule out pneumonia. Coincidentally, erythromycin is probably the best choice of antibiotic for the young patient who develops a community-acquired pneumonia.

BLOOD-BORNE PATHOGENS

Human Immunodeficiency Virus

The human immunodeficiency virus (HIV) epidemic is a source of anxiety for most people, and the athletic community is not immune to these concerns. The saga of Magic Johnson's revelation of his illness and retirement, followed by his controversial and aborted return to competition illustrates the depth of fear this illness generates. More recently, the announcement by Greg Louganis that he has AIDS, and his competition in the 1992 summer Olympics with knowledge of his illness, has refocused the public's attention on athletes and HIV. The fact that he bled into the pool after hitting his head certainly increases concerns in many athletes regarding risk of transmission from competition with an HIV-positive athlete. Many sports, such as football, wrestling, boxing, and basketball, involve very close contact and have a high incidence of bleeding episodes. Concern about blood and infection makes it very difficult to separate the emotional nature of this epidemic from the medical understanding of the disease and how it is spread.

The HIV virus is a retrovirus that attacks the infected person's immune system, specifically the CD4 lymphocytes, resulting in an inability to fight off other infections. The end result is the acquired immunodeficiency syndrome (AIDS). Many people infected with HIV will remain asymptomatic for many years and are able, during this time, to live normal active lives. Most experts believe that eventually all patients infected with HIV will develop AIDS, which is uniformly fatal. In the United States esti-

mates are that 40,000 to 50,000 adults are newly infected with HIV each year. It is estimated that over one million people in the United States are infected with HIV presently (10).

It must be assumed, based on the overall prevalence of the disease, that athletes who are HIV positive but not identified as such are currently competing in organized sports at all levels (29). Given this assumption, the fact that there has never been a conclusive case of HIV transmission during athletic competition is good evidence that the risk of this occurrence, although probably not zero, is so "infinitesimally small" as to completely defy estimation (33). Despite this reassuring statistical analysis, many athletes have fear and anxiety about possible infection during competition and consequently would possibly not participate with an athlete who is known to be HIV positive. In Texas, high school basketball games have been canceled because teams did not want to play against a student who was known to be HIV positive. In addition, there has been some debate concerning the utility of testing all athletes for HIV prior to competition. The handling of these issues must balance the real but greatly exaggerated fear of infection, the extremely low actual risk, the practicalities of policy institution, the medical privacy of the HIV-positive patient, and the potential legal issues involved.

Currently, almost all athletic organizations do not require HIV testing for athletes. An exception is the state of Nevada that requires that all boxers be tested (63). The International Olympic Council recently upheld their policy of not requiring testing following the Greg Louganis revelation. Most authors feel that the extremely low risks involved do not justify the potential for invasion of privacy that would be implied by routine testing. It has been pointed out, however, that the routine drug screening that is commonly done on many levels of athletics involves a similar invasion of privacy. Voluntary testing and counseling are an acceptable means of assessing HIV risk that does not infringe on athletes' privacy rights.

The problems involved in dealing with the athlete known to be HIV positive are many, difficult, and largely unexplored. Should the athlete be allowed to compete? Should the teammates and opponents be made aware of the athlete's HIV status? Should different sports be considered differently in regards to how HIV-positive athletes are counseled? The legality of excluding HIV-positive patients from competition is at best untested. The Americans with Disabilities Act of 1990 prohibited discrimination against people with HIV, and thus does not allow for exclusion of athletes from competition unless there exists a medically sound basis to do so. Since there has never been a confirmed case of HIV transmission related to sports participation, it is difficult to make the argument that risk of infection to other athletes constitutes a legitimate reason for exclusion. The NCAA has stated that student-athletes should not have their athletic participation limited based solely on being HIV positive (52).

Another issue regarding HIV positive patients involves whether participation in athletics can hasten the progress of the disease and therefore be harmful to the patient. It has been shown that moderate exercise may in fact be beneficial for the asymptomatic HIV patient. Unfortunately, there has never been a study regarding the effect of intense training and competition for the elite athlete with HIV. In general terms, if the athlete is asymptomatic and without evidence of deficiencies in immune system function, then athletic participation in patients with HIV infection has not been shown to be harmful and should be permitted. However, the athlete should be counseled that it is unclear what possible risks to long-term health high level athletic participation might entail. Patients with symptoms or other evidence of severe disease such as low CD4 counts (less than 200) or AIDS defining illnesses need to be individually assessed regarding ability to participate.

Hepatitis B

The other major infectious blood-borne pathogen of concern in athletics is hepatitis B (HBV). In reality, because of the fact that the virus levels are higher in blood and that the virus is much better able to survive outside the body for longer periods of time, hepatitis B is of more concern for possible transmission during sports than HIV. As opposed to HIV, there have been documented instances of HBV transmission during athletic contact. This occurred among Sumo wrestlers in Japan.

The majority of adults with acute HBV infection do not develop a clinical illness but have an asymptomatic course with complete recovery. As the name implies, the main consequence of infection with this virus is hepatitis or inflammation of the liver. This usually presents as jaundice, right upper quadrant tenderness, nausea, vomiting, dark urine, and malaise. Twenty-five percent of patients infected with HBV will develop clinical hepatitis and a small number of these patients (less than 1%) will develop fulminant hepatitis, which carries a high mortality rate. In addition, approximately 5% to 10% of infected patients will develop chronic HBV infection, which can ultimately lead to cirrhosis and hepatic failure. These patients are also at greatly increased risk of developing hepatocellular carcinoma. It is estimated that there are over 1 million chronic carriers of HBV in the United States and nearly 5,000 deaths from resulting cirrhosis or hepatocellular carcinoma each year (56). HBV is therefore a potentially severe, life-threatening infection that warrants consideration along with HIV as a blood borne pathogen.

The incubation period for HBV ranges from 40 to 140 days. Initially during infection titers of surface antigen (HBsAg), as well as liver enzymes alanine transferase (ALT) and aspartate transferase (AST), are high. As the disease progresses, surface antigen levels fall and are replaced by specific antibodies. The earliest antibody to appear is IgM to the core antigen of the virus (IgM anti-HBc). Finding IgM anti-HBc and surface antigen (HBsAg) in the serum together is diagnostic of acute HBV infection. Eventually IgM anti-HBc is replaced by IgG anti-HBc. The clearance of HBsAg may take several weeks and is accompanied by the appearance of anti-HBs. This antibody is protective and gives the patient lifelong immunity to further HBV infection. In patients who develop chronic HBV infections HBsAg is not cleared within 6 months of diagnosis. Knowledge of this usual chain of events is important in determining those patients at risk of passing the infection to others. Patients found to have anti-HBs antibody have either been immunized or have cleared the infection and pose no risk of infection. Those patients with acute infection are most contagious because of high viral titers in their blood. Patients with chronic hepatitis B remain contagious for a prolonged period.

Patients with acute HBV should not be allowed to participate in athletics until the acute hepatitis has resolved. They should be reminded that HBV can be spread through sexual contact and should also be warned not to share toothbrushes and razor blades with others. Those patients who recover and develop anti-HBs are at no risk of infecting others and can resume all activities without further follow-up. The 5% to 10% of patients who develop chronic HBV infection represent a problem not unlike that of patients with HIV. They are potentially infectious to others, but the risk of transmission during sports is too low to accurately quantify. Currently, most experts do not feel this risk is high enough to warrant disqualification from athletics. The NCAA does not recommend limiting participation solely on the basis of chronic HBV infection, except in the case of wrestling in which the risk of transmission is the highest (52). Affected patients should be told of the potential for transmission to other athletes, particularly those whose sports involve close contact and frequent bleeding such as football and basketball. It may be reasonable to offer the hepatitis B vaccine to athletes participating in these sports in order to reduce their risk of infection. The vaccine is fairly expensive and requires three injections over a 6-month period for full efficacy. The vaccine should be strongly recommended to athletic trainers and physicians frequently exposed to blood.

Universal Precautions

Because of the fact that these infections can be completely asymptomatic, most athletes with HIV or HBV infection are probably unaware of their condition and potential infectiousness. Certainly their teammates, coaches, and competitors will be unable to know their condition. It therefore becomes imperative to treat every episode of bleeding during athletic competition as a potential source of infection. This concept is known as universal precautions and should be followed by physicians, athletic trainers, coaches, and players alike. The NCAA has published recommendations for universal precautions that have been modified to cover athletic events.

1. Pre-event preparation includes proper care for existing wounds, abrasions, cuts, or weeping wounds that may serve as a source of bleeding or as a port of entry for blood-borne pathogens. These wounds should be covered with an occlusive dressing that will withstand the demands of competition. Likewise, care providers with healing wounds or dermatitis should have these areas adequately covered to prevent infection to or from a participant. Student-athletes may be advised to wear more protective equipment on high risk areas, such as elbows and hands.

2. The necessary equipment and/or supplies important for compliance with universal precautions should be available to caregivers. These supplies include appropriate gloves, disinfectant bleach, antiseptics, designated receptacles for soiled equipment and uniforms, bandages and/or dressings, and a container for appropriate disposal of needles, syringes, or scalpels.

3. When a student-athlete is bleeding, the bleeding must be stopped and the open wound covered with dressing sturdy enough to withstand the demands of activity before the athlete may continue participation in practice or competition. Current NCAA policy mandates the immediate, aggressive treatment of open wounds or skin lesions that are deemed potential risks to transmission of disease. Participants with active bleeding should be removed from the event as soon as is practical. Return to play is determined by appropriate medical staff personnel. Any participant whose uniform is saturated with blood, regardless of the source, must have that uniform evaluated by appropriate medical personnel for potential infectivity and changed if necessary before return to participation.

4. During an event, early recognition of uncontrolled bleeding is the responsibility of officials, coaches, and medical personnel. In particular, student-athletes should be aware of their responsibility to report a bleeding wound to the proper medical personnel.

5. Personnel managing an acute blood exposure must follow the guidelines for universal precaution. Sterile latex gloves should be worn for direct contact with blood or body fluids containing blood. Gloves should be changed after treating each individual participant and after glove removal, hands should be washed.

6. Any surface contaminated with spilled blood should be cleaned in accordance with the following procedure: With gloves on, the spill should be contained in as small an area as possible. After the blood is re-

moved, the surface area of concern should be cleaned with an appropriate decontaminate.

7. Proper disposal procedures should be practiced to prevent injuries caused by needles, scalpels, and other sharp instruments or devices.

8. After each practice or game, any equipment or uniforms soiled with blood should be handled and laundered in accordance with hygienic methods normally used for treatment of any soiled equipment or clothing before subsequent use. This includes provisions for bagging the soiled items in a manner to prevent secondary contamination of other items or personnel.

9. Finally, all personnel involved with sports should be trained in basic first aid and infection control, including the preventive measures outlined previously (4).

Following these guidelines routinely should significantly reduce the risk of accidental transmission of blood-borne pathogens among the athletic population.

RESPIRATORY

Asthma

Asthma is a chronic respiratory condition characterized by inflammation, reversible airway obstruction, and hypersensitivity of the airways of the lung to various stimuli such as allergens, environmental irritants, viral respiratory infections, cold air, or exercise. The majority of symptoms are due to constriction of the medium-sized airways with resultant decrease in the ability of the patient to move air through the lungs. It most commonly presents as shortness of breath, chest tightness, wheezing, and/or unexplained cough and can therefore obviously interfere with athletic performance. For practical purposes, a subset of asthma is frequently described as exercise-induced asthma. Although these categories probably represent an artificial division of the same disease continuum, the diagnostic and treatment strategies differ enough between the two that it is logical to consider them separately. The patient with exercise-induced asthma will have symptoms almost exclusively with physical exertion, particularly during cold weather and in air with low humidity. The patient with chronic forms of asthma will tend to have difficulties throughout the day, although exercise will frequently exacerbate symptoms. Pathologically, the differences between the two types of asthma lies in the degree of underlying airway inflammation, with exercise-induced asthma patients typically having a lesser degree of chronic airway inflammation.

The diagnosis of asthma can range from straightforward to difficult depending upon the patient's presentation. When the patient complains of severe shortness of breath, has obvious wheezing on exam and the symptoms improve rapidly with therapy it is relatively easy to make the diagnosis. However, asthma can present as only a mild cough at night or during physical exertion; therefore, it is important to have a high index of suspicion when an athlete presents with pulmonary complaints. On physical examination, asthma patients will often demonstrate rhinitis, nasal polyps, or other signs of allergy symptoms. The lung exam frequently (but not always) demonstrates musical wheezing breath sounds. The intensity of the wheezing does not always correspond to the severity of the asthma. Patients will also frequently demonstrate a prolonged phase of expiration because of airflow obstruction. Patients with exercise induced asthma will often have completely normal examinations while at rest, but if examined following strenuous activity will frequently develop wheezing or other physical signs.

The diagnosis of asthma rests on the demonstration of reversible airway obstruction on objective pulmonary testing. Most patients with daily asthma symptoms should have complete pulmonary function testing with spirometry both in order to diagnose and to determine the severity of their disease. Patients with asthma will demonstrate a decreased FEV1 (forced expiratory volume in 1 second), which is a standard measure of the amount of air the patient is able to exhale during the first second of maximal exhalation. The combination of a decreased FEV1 with a normal vital capacity (the total amount of air moved during forced exhalation) indicates that airway obstruction is present. If the obstruction is shown to be reversible by bronchodilator treatment, the diagnosis of asthma is made. In patients with exercise-induced asthma, spirometry testing may be normal while at rest, which can lead to confusion and misdiagnosis. These athletes should be tested following a provocative exercise challenge. A simple method involves the use of a simple hand-held peak expiratory flow meter. This device measures the maximum rate of airflow during forced expiration, which usually provides a reasonable correlation with the FEV1 in most circumstances. The normal peak flow for an individual patient is determined from nomograms and is based upon the patient's sex, height, and age. In the athlete with suspected exercise-induced asthma, a baseline peak flow rate is initially obtained. It is vitally important that the patient use maximal effort during exhalation. The athlete is then instructed to run or exercise on a stationary bike until the asthma symptoms develop. A peak flow rate is then obtained while the patient is having symptoms. A reduction of 15% between the two measurements confirms the diagnosis (49), however, sometimes smaller changes can be significant if the patient's symptoms are consistent with asthma and treatment improves the problem.

Treatment of asthma is based upon alleviation of symptoms and prevention of acute exacerbations. Asthma is a chronic condition that tends to wax and wane in patients and can be managed but not cured. The goals of therapy are to maintain near normal pulmonary function rates, maintain normal activity and exercise levels, prevent chronic symptoms such as cough or shortness of breath, prevent asthma exacerbations, and avoid adverse effects from asthma medications (26). Athletes with asthma are in almost all cases able to compete in their sport with good management of their symptoms if they are able to comply with effective treatment regimens.

The mainstay of asthma therapy are the bronchodilators, primarily the inhaled β-adrenergic agonists such as albuterol. These medications act by inducing the relaxation of the constricted smooth muscles in the airways and consequently relieve symptoms of airway obstruction. They have a rapid onset of effect; and in many cases of mild asthma they can completely abort an asthmatic attack. Inhaled bronchodilator represents the primary treatment of acute asthma and the primary prevention for exercise-induced asthma. It is vitally important that patients receive detailed instruction in the proper usage technique for the inhaler. Basically this involves exhaling completely, opening the mouth wide, placing the inhaler approximately one inch from the mouth, and activating the inhaler at the same time a slow, deep breath is initiated. Many asthma patients make the mistake of inhaling very rapidly during usage, which has the effect of depositing the medication on the back of the throat instead of the airways. Patients who have difficulty with inhaler technique can benefit from the use of a spacer device that allows easier ability to administer the medication.

The dosage of inhaled bronchodilator therapy is usually two puffs every 4 to 6 hours as needed for symptoms. Patients should be informed that these medications do not need to be used routinely if they remain asymptomatic. The exception to this rule is patients with exercise induced asthma in which the bronchodilator is being used as a preventive therapy. These patients should be instructed to take two puffs of the inhaler 15 to 30 minutes prior to engaging in maximal exertion. The athlete should then engage in gentle calisthenics and warm up during the interval prior to competition. The athlete should keep the inhaler handy should symptoms occur during the activity. For many patients with mild or exercise-induced asthma, β-adrenergic inhalers and education will be all the therapeutic intervention required. Patients who experience daily asthma symptoms or whose exercise-induced asthma is not well controlled with preperformance treatment need to be placed on additional therapy to control symptoms. This is particularly important in light of recent concerns that daily or excessive bronchodilator therapy can contribute to worsening long-term asthma control (62).

Prophylactic asthma medications are for the most part aimed at alleviating the underlying inflammation of the airways and preventing bronchial constriction. For patients with chronic asthma symptoms, the primary class of medications used for this purpose are inhaled corticosteroids such as beclomethasone or triamcinolone. These medications act topically in the airways to reduce the underlying inflammation that contributes to the pathogenesis of asthma. Since these steroids act topically, they have a much lower incidence of side effects than systemic steroids and can be used for indefinite periods of time in patients. They are extremely effective in reducing or even eliminating episodes of wheezing or other asthmatic symptoms in patients with chronic asthma (18). These effects usually require 1 to 2 weeks of continual therapy to occur, and patients should be alerted that they will not notice any short-term or immediate improvement with these inhalers (as opposed to the β-adrenergic inhalers that provide almost immediate relief). If the patient will use a steroid inhaler regularly (two to four puffs, two to four times daily, titrated based upon response) they will often be rewarded with dramatic improvement in their asthma symptoms. Some patients who have significant problems only during short predictable periods of the year (e.g., spring for a patient with pollen allergies) can add a steroid inhaler to their regimen only during those time periods, whereas others will require their use year round. Since exercise-induced asthma has less underlying airway inflammation, steroid inhalers are less effective and the use of other forms of prophylactic treatment such as cromolyn is recommended. In patients with a severe asthma exacerbation, a short course of oral steroids (such as prednisone 50 mg a day for 7 to 10 days) may be required to improve symptoms. This dosing regimen has been shown to have similar efficacy and no greater side effects than more traditional steroid tapers (53). It has the advantage of simplicity and hopefully improved patient compliance.

The other major preventive treatment for asthma is cromolyn, which is also administered as an inhaler. The mechanism of action for cromolyn is not completely understood, but it appears to interact with the mast cells in the mucosa of the lung. The mast cells contain histamine and other allergic mediators that induce bronchospasm when released. Cromolyn acts by stabilizing the mast cell to prevent release of these chemicals, thus alleviating asthma symptoms. This medication is particularly useful in patients with exercise-induced asthma. In most cases of refractory exercise-induced asthma, cromolyn should be the first medication added to β-adrenergic therapy. The usual initial dose for cromolyn is two puffs four times a day, which can then be titrated downward based upon response. For patients with exercise-induced asthma, an alternative technique would be to administer two puffs 30 minutes prior to exercise as is done with β-adrenergics. It should be emphasized to the athlete that the medication is only of benefit if used on a consistent basis and often takes several weeks to have full effect. Other asthma medications such as theophylline tend to be less frequently used in athletes and will not be discussed further.

Allergies

Seasonal allergies, commonly known as hay fever, are a common complaint among athletes because of the amount of time spent outdoors during the height of pollen season. Allergy symptoms are due to an IgE mediated inflammatory response to one or more airborne allergens. The symptoms of hay fever are well known to most people and consist of nasal congestion, sneezing, itchy eyes, scratchy throat, fatigue, and cough. Often patients with asthma will have exacerbation of their symptoms during allergy season. Seasonal allergies are usually due to plant pollen although other patients may have year-round allergy symptoms because of dust, molds, pets, or cockroaches. In very general terms, spring allergies are due to flowering trees, summer allergies are due to grasses, and fall allergies are due to ragweed. Different regions of the country experience varying types and degrees of pollen production and patients may have only minimal symptoms while living in one area but develop problems following a move.

The diagnosis of hay fever is largely based on clinical presentation, particularly during the height of an allergy season. Physical examination will often reveal dark circles under the eyes because of venous congestion. The nasal mucosa is often edematous with a pale-blue coloration and the turbinates are often coated with clear, thin secretions. The family history should be taken for history of allergies. Gram stain of the nasal secretions will often reveal eosinophils, the presence of which suggests an allergic etiology. Specific allergen testing can help to pinpoint the exact allergy source, but is frequently not required if symptoms are easily controlled.

The initial step in the treatment of allergy symptoms is an attempt at the avoidance of the offending allergen. Limiting outdoor activity during pollen season is usually recommended but this is often impossible for an athlete. The use of air conditioners can help, particularly in areas of high humidity. Commercial smoke and pollen filters are also available. Patients with indoor allergies to mold, dust, or cockroaches should frequently clean house, use bare floors in lieu of carpeting (particularly in the bedroom), and frequently clean humidifier reservoirs. Smoke can exacerbate symptoms and should be avoided.

Drug treatment of allergies usually attempts to strike a balance between alleviation of symptoms and side effects of therapy. The mainstay of therapy are the antihistamines. There are many different classes of antihistamines, and a patient may experience better relief from one class than another. Antihistamines are effective at relieving itching, sneezing, and rhinorrhea but are often less effective at relieving symptoms of nasal congestion. Combining the antihistamine with a decongestant such as pseudoephedrine can often provide effective relief from this symptom. Most antihistamines have sedation as their major side effect and this can be a particularly troubling symptom for the athlete. Patients who experience excessive sedation with one class of antihistamine can be tried on a different class to assess response. However, frequently they will need to be placed on one of the newer nonsedating antihistamines such as Allegra or Claritin. These drugs do not cross the blood-brain barrier and consequently usually do not typically cause sedation. They are no more effective than traditional antihistamines and are very expensive.

Second-line medication for allergy symptoms that are not controlled by antihistamines and/or decongestants usually consists of the addition of nasally inhaled corticosteroids such as beclomethasone. These drugs work by inhibiting the inflammatory response and can often provide significant relief of symptoms. The potency of topical steroids exceeds that of antihistamines, decongestants, and cromolyn (51). They must be used routinely to provide maximal benefit and the dosage can be titrated up or down depending upon the response. Using corticosteroids in the form of a topical nasal spray helps to prevent the complications (such as Cushing's syndrome, avascular necrosis, or adrenal suppression) that can arise from long-term use of systemic steroids. Cromolyn is also frequently used in refractory allergy symptoms. Cromolyn theoretically works by stabilizing the mast cell to prevent histamine release. It is administered as a nasal spray. Rarely, a short course of systemic steroids may be required in order to control severe allergy symptoms. Desensitizing allergy shots are often used in patients with persistent allergies. They tend to be more desirable in patients with year round allergies because of molds, dander, or cockroaches. Allergy shots are very expensive and it is difficult to predict their efficacy. Allergy shots should therefore only be considered in patients that have failed a reasonable attempt at medical therapy.

HEMATOLOGY

Sickle Cell Trait

It used to be felt that patients with sickle cell trait were at no increased risk for problems during physical activity. There has been strong recent evidence that under the proper circumstances these patients can have red cell sickling with resultant cramping, rhabdomyolysis, acute renal tubular necrosis and occasionally sudden death. Since approximately 8% of African-Americans are carriers of Hemoglobin S, a significant population of athletes are at risk for these potential complications. The great majority of these patients remain asymptomatic and have no problems with athletic participation or performance. However, when exercising strenuously in conditions of high heat, high humidity, and/or high altitude, these patients are at risk for possible intravascular sickling and resultant complications (66). This is particularly a problem when the patient is in early exercise conditioning or when there is a recent change in altitude or climatic conditions.

Some authors have recommended routine screening for sickle cell trait among all athletes of black and Mediterra-

nean descent whose sport involves prolonged exertion in conditions of high humidity, heat, or altitude (8). Those athletes identified to have sickle cell trait can then be given detailed instructions regarding warning symptoms (cramping, back pain, excessive muscular fatigue), the necessity for adequate hydration during exercise, and increased risk while exercising during an acute viral illness or while suffering from a lack of sleep. In addition, the medical staff would be more alert to potential sickling problems in those athletes known to have the trait; and consequently, might be able to provide necessary treatment sooner.

Because of the fact that the actual risk for complications is very low and that an athlete who tests positive for the sickle cell trait would not be discouraged from athletic participation, routine laboratory testing of all athletes is certainly debatable based on expense and possible stigmatization of an otherwise normal individual. For these reasons the NCAA does not recommend routine laboratory screening for sickle cell trait (52). An alternate and acceptable approach would involve voluntary testing and routine counseling of all athletes at time of the preparticipation examination regarding this condition. Included in this discussion would be the warning symptoms, the need for adequate hydration, the importance of a gradual increase in conditioning exercises, and the need for caution in times of high heat, humidity, or increased altitude. The coaching and athletic training staff should also be educated about this problem in order to design appropriate preseason training regimens. In particular the tradition of early maximal practices without access to water or rest breaks should be condemned and eliminated. Athletes should be frequently reminded to take adequate fluids, and rest periods should be incorporated into the practice schedule. Practice time should be curtailed during times of high heat or humidity as based on wet bulb thermometer readings. Athletes who develop worrisome symptoms should be carefully evaluated with the possibility of sickle cell trait kept in mind. Education of athletes, coaching staff, athletic trainers, and medical staff along with close monitoring of practice conditions should minimize the risk of serious problems.

Anemia

Anemia is a frequent complaint among athletes, primarily because anemia has become synonymous with fatigue. Although most athletes complaining of fatigue will not have anemia, true anemia is relatively common among healthy young athletes, particularly females. It is estimated that the incidence of iron deficiency anemia is around 6% for adult women and adolescents in this country (73). Iron deficiency anemia is much less common among males. Athletes are usually discovered to be anemic during evaluation for an unrelated medical problem or during investigation for complaints of fatigue or decreased exercise performance. The evaluation of anemia requires careful assessment as to the likely cause and judicious laboratory testing to confirm suspicions.

Anemia is defined as low hemoglobin blood levels, normally defined as below 14 g/dL in males and 12 g/dL in females. These cutoffs may not be accurate in elite athletes, particularly those engaging in endurance sports. These athletes commonly will have slightly lower hemoglobin levels because of an increase in blood volume. This effect does not represent a true anemia, since the total red cell mass is not decreased and the mean red cell volume is normal. The effect is dilutional and is due to an increase in the blood plasma volume. This "pseudoanemia" may be of benefit to the athlete since it may provide extra fluid for heat loss because of sweating and it increases the stroke volume of the heart, which improves aerobic capacity. Since this pseudoanemia is a normal response and not indicative of any problem, it is important not to label these athletes as having anemia. The cutoff for true anemia in elite athletes is therefore lower than normal; 13 g/dL for males and 11 g/dL for females. Hemoglobin levels below these cutoffs have a 95% chance of representing true anemia (21).

The most common cause of true anemia among healthy athletic populations is due to iron deficiency. Iron is a trace mineral that is necessary for the production of hemoglobin. In the absence of adequate iron stores, hemoglobin synthesis is impaired and anemia results. The anemia of iron deficiency is described as being microcytic (small red blood cells) and hypochromic (pale red cells). Typically the mean corpuscular volume (MCV) is less than 80 in iron deficiency anemia, an important clue as to etiology. Iron deficiency occurs when iron intake in the diet is less than iron loss from the body. Women are much more prone to develop iron deficiency because of monthly menstrual blood losses. Because of these menstrual losses, the recommended daily dietary allowances (RDA) is almost twice as high for women as men (18 mg/day and 10 mg/day, respectively). Many women, particularly those who avoid red meat, have a difficult time obtaining this much iron in their diet. Men are more likely to develop iron deficiency because of gastrointestinal blood loss from benign or malignant lesions. In addition, iron deficiency can occasionally occur because of gastrointestinal blood losses as has been shown to occur in runners (71). This loss is felt to be secondary to bowel ischemia. In addition, poor dietary habits as well as frank eating disorders are commonly seen among many athletes with iron deficiency.

Over the course of time, iron deficiency progresses in stages. The first stage occurs when the body's bone marrow iron stores are depleted. This can be recognized by a low serum ferritin (less than 12 ng/dL). Otherwise the patient appears healthy with normal blood counts. This stage does not affect athletic performance. The second stage occurs after several months of iron depletion and is characterized by impaired iron transport. This is identified by a low serum iron, increased total iron binding capacity (TIBC) and decreased transferrin saturation. The hemoglobin remains normal and the athlete remains asymptomatic. The third stage occurs several weeks later and is characterized by the development of a true anemia and symptoms. The diagnosis of iron-deficiency anemia rests upon the demonstration of the combination of anemia and reduced iron stores (usually indicated by low ferritin). Treatment consists of iron supplementation. Ferrous sulfate 325 mg three times a day is the typical treatment. Although the anemia improves fairly quickly with iron replacement, it is important to continue therapy until iron stores are depleted (evidenced by ferritin less than 20 ng/mL), which takes several months (34).

Other causes of anemia in the athlete are much less common. Destruction of red cells because of pounding of the feet while running ("footstrike hemolysis") is frequently listed as a cause of athletic anemia, but is very seldom a significant problem. However, it can contribute to the severity of other anemias. Anemia is seen not infrequently during acute illnesses such as mono because of red cell hemolysis or bone marrow suppression. Although rare, other causes of anemia such as B_{12} deficiency, hemolysis, aplastic anemia, and leukemia must be in the differential for the athlete presenting with low hemoglobin.

RENAL

Hematuria

Hematuria, or blood in the urine, is a common problem among athletes and can be due to a variety of underlying causes. These can range from benign postexertional hematuria, which requires no treatment, to potentially serious problems such as kidney stones, glomerulonephritis, and bladder or renal malignancies. The proper management of the athlete with hematuria is dependent upon the performance of a careful history, physical examination, and urinalysis with further testing reserved for only those cases that remain questionable as to etiology. It is important to note that normal individuals will have blood in their urine up to 1,000 red blood cells per mL, which would account for over 2 million red cells in the urine per day. Hematuria is commonly defined as greater than 3 red blood cells per high power microscopic field, which corresponds to the upper limit of normal (74). For clinical purposes, hematuria is often described as either microscopic hematuria or gross hematuria.

Microscopic hematuria usually is not associated with any symptoms and is most often discovered on urinalysis performed during investigation of other problems or as a routine screening test. As discussed under the section on preparticipation issues, eliminating the urinalysis as part of the preparticipation physical examination will reduce the number of unnecessary evaluations for benign hematuria. Microscopic hematuria is very common. In one study 13% of otherwise normal adult men were shown to have asymptomatic microscopic hematuria (50). It is even more common among athletes, with 20% of marathon runners demonstrating hematuria following completion of a race (68). It is felt that in most cases of exercise-related hematuria, the source of bleeding is the bladder mucosa because of the trauma of running, although the site may occasionally be the kidney itself (30). In most cases in which strenuous exertion precedes the presence of hematuria, the urine will be clear of red cells following 1 to 2 days of rest. In most athletes with asymptomatic hematuria not related to blunt trauma, this course of management is an appropriate first step. If the urine clears rapidly and completely with rest, then further evaluation is not required (22). In cases in which hematuria is not related to exercise, the urine fails to clear with rest, or hematuria recurs, further evaluation becomes necessary to determine the etiology.

Gross hematuria refers to the presence of visible blood in the urine. Athletes will often present to the athletic trainer or team physician with great anxiety after experiencing an episode of gross hematuria. They require reassurance as well as appropriate evaluation. The causes of gross hematuria are similar to those for microscopic hematuria. If the episode occurs soon after strenuous exertion, a repeat urinalysis in 24 to 48 hours can be very helpful. As in microscopic hematuria, if the urine completely clears with rest, further evaluation is probably unnecessary and the patient should be advised to return if symptoms recur. If the episode of hematuria cannot be related to exertion or fails to clear rapidly on subsequent urinalysis, then more extensive testing is required.

In cases of persistent hematuria, the history can often give clues as to underlying etiology. Patients with gross hematuria are frequently able to describe the character of the blood in the urine. If bleeding occurs with the initial urine stream, a urethral source such as urethritis or intraurethral papilloma is likely. Blood noticed at the end of urination suggests the prostate as the source. Bleeding observed throughout the urination is suspicious for bladder, ureter, or kidney problems. If blood clots are seen, the bleeding is occurring below the glomerulus. Large clots suggest the bladder as a source whereas small or thin and stringy clots are more likely to be from the ureters or collecting system. Dysuria and urinary frequency suggest cystitis, especially in females. A history of colicky flank pain points to the possibility of a kidney stone. Additional historical clues would be the presence of easy bruising or bleeding gums (bleeding dyscrasia), recent strep infection (glomerulonephritis), family history of sickle cell disease, and use of nonsteroidal antiinflammatory agents or anticoagulants. In addition, the use of pyridium, rifampin, or other medications can change the color of urine and be mistaken for hematuria. Beet juice can have a similar effect.

Patients with persistent hematuria, which remains unexplained after history and physical examination, require further testing. The urine and urine sediment should be carefully examined for clues. The presence of red cell casts suggests possible glomerulonephritis. A positive dipstick analysis for hemoglobin without red cells seen on microscopic exam is usually due to myoglobinuria or hemoglobinuria. Fragmented or misshapen red cells suggest the glomerulus as the source. Patients should have renal function checked with serum blood urea nitrogen (BUN) and creatinine levels. The choice of imaging study often depends upon the patient's age and history. Younger patients (under 35 years) are usually evaluated initially with an intravenous pyelogram (IVP) or renal ultrasound. Older patients have a higher incidence of bladder cancer and are usually initially screened with cystoscopy followed by IVP or ultrasound. Definitive treatment recommendations depend on the underlying source of the hematuria.

Proteinuria

Proteinuria, like hematuria, was a frequently encountered problem in athletes when urinalysis was a routine part of the preparticipation evaluation. It is encountered less often when the urinalysis is not required but is often seen when urine is ordered for evaluation of an unrelated problem. Proteinuria is defined as greater than 150 mg of protein in the urine per day and usually consists of albumin. Protein loss occurs at the level of the glomerulus. In most cases, mild proteinuria in an otherwise healthy athlete occurs only following heavy exercise and is due to transient changes in renal blood flow. This scenario is benign and does not lead to renal failure. However, there are many potentially serious causes of proteinuria that need to be ruled out in these cases. Similar to the evaluation of hematuria, the initial step involves repeat urinalysis following 24 to 48 hours of rest. If the proteinuria has resolved, no further testing is necessary. Persistence of proteinuria requires further testing.

Renal function should be evaluated with serum BUN creatinine. A 24-hour urine collection should be initiated to quantify total protein loss and creatinine clearance. If the 24-hour protein exceeds 150 mg, then proteinuria is confirmed. In otherwise healthy, asymptomatic patients, the next step is to rule out orthostatic proteinuria. This is characterized by proteinuria that occurs while the patient is in an upright position with its disappearance while in the recumbent position. It is diagnosed by demonstrating that urine collected during the evening hours while the patient is recumbent has less than 75 mg of protein and the total 24-hour urine protein loss is less than 1.5 gm. Orthostatic proteinuria is benign and does not require further evaluation (28). Patients with nephrotic range proteinuria (3.5 grams or greater) or proteinuria, which persists during recumbency, require further testing by a nephrologist and often undergo kidney biopsy.

GASTROENTEROLOGY

Diarrhea

Diarrhea refers to an increase in the frequency and fluid volume of the bowel movement. In the vast majority of cases, diarrhea begins abruptly, lasts only 1 to 2 days, and resolves on its own without further problems. However, it is important to remember that there are some very serious causes of diarrhea that need to be ruled out in the patient presenting with this complaint. Basically, there are four major mechanisms of diarrhea. First is osmotic, which occurs when the patient eats a poorly absorbed material that causes fluid to be retained in the lumen of the colon. The most common of these disorders is lactose intolerance, which usually occurs in blacks and Asians, because of the absence of the enzyme lactase. This enzyme is responsible for breaking down the sugar found in milk and therefore these patients develop diarrhea and gas after eating milk or milk products. The second cause of diarrhea is secretory diarrhea, which refers to increased secretion of water and electrolytes by the intestine. This is usually caused by either viral infection or food poisoning because of a toxin made by bacteria. Laxatives and other drugs can also cause this form of diarrhea. The third cause is exudative, which refers to the sloughing off of protein, blood, or mucus from the bowel wall. Most serious causes of diarrhea fall into this category and include such conditions as invasive bacterial infection, amoebic dysentery, ulcerative colitis, Crohn's disease, and certain tumors. The fourth cause of diarrhea is motility disorders such as the irritable bowel syndrome. Runners will often have urgent bowel movements prior to or even during a race, which are related to a motility disorder as well (72).

The majority of diarrhea in the young patient is due either to viral infection or ingestion of a preformed bacterial toxin commonly known as "food poisoning." Both usually present with frequent, watery diarrhea, which initially begins rather abruptly. There may be some mild abdominal cramping, but usually no severe pain. Fever is also rare. Nausea and vomiting are frequently seen in these conditions. The patient may know friends suffering from similar problems, or may have eaten unusual or poorly prepared foods the day or two before. The presence of fever, blood, or mucus in the stool, severe abdominal pain, recent foreign travel or camping trip, or systemic symptoms suggest a more serious cause such as bacterial

or parasitic infection and need to be fully evaluated by a physician. The recent use of antibiotics suggests the possibility of a bacterial etiology because of *Clostridium difficile* overgrowth. It is important to remember that treating these more serious infectious causes of diarrhea with Immodium or other motility drug can result in the infection becoming worse.

If the patient has a watery diarrhea and none of the worrisome symptoms above, then it is reasonable to treat with Immodium AD (loperamide) to slow the gut down and decrease the amount of diarrhea. This is given as two capsules initially and then one capsule after each loose stool up to ten a day. This treatment can also be effective in runners with pre-event stool urgency. Other drugs such as lomotil do not offer any additional efficacy and have more side effects. The main goal of therapy is to avoid dehydration. The patient should be encouraged to drink plenty of fluids; water, flat soda, or a sports drink will do for most mild cases of diarrhea. In more severe cases a standard oral rehydration fluid such as Pedialyte should be used. The patient is instructed to watch his or her urine. If the urine becomes dark yellow or the patient urinates less frequently, fluid intake should increase. If the patient becomes light-headed with standing (orthostasis), fluid intake should also increase. In those instances the patient is unable to take in enough fluids to keep up with gastrointestinal (GI) losses, intravenous (IV) fluids may be required. These are usually given as normal saline or lactated ringers. Intravenous rehydration can also help in those instances where the athlete needs to compete while mildly dehydrated from diarrhea.

If symptoms persist for more than 2 days the patient needs to be reexamined. Microscopic stool examination and stool cultures should be performed for patients with worrisome symptoms such as fever, bloody diarrhea, recent travel history, or persistence of diarrhea beyond the expected duration of 2 days. In these patients, there is a higher likelihood of parasitic or bacterial infection. The most frequent parasitic causes are giardia and amoeba. These usually are treated with oral metronidazole. Most diarrheal illnesses due to bacteria are self-limited and mild cases should be managed conservatively. However, antibiotic therapy is occasionally required for those cases of bacterial diarrhea that produce significant symptoms such as fever, abdominal pain, or systemic illness. In these cases a fluoroquinolone, such as ciprofloxin, is usually the primary treatment.

Patients with diarrhea should be instructed to avoid certain foods such as milk products, meat, or fruit juices. These contain substances that are difficult for the body to digest and absorb following intestinal infections because of resulting damage to the lining of the gut. Once the diarrhea has resolved, the patient can slowly reintroduce these foods back into the diet, with milk and dairy products usually being the last added.

NEUROLOGY

Epilepsy

Epilepsy refers to a common neurologic condition characterized by chronic, recurrent seizures. There are many different types of seizures to which a person may be predisposed. It is common to characterize seizures as either partial or generalized. Partial seizures involve limited regions of the brain and can produce motor, sensory, autonomic, or psychic symptoms depending upon which part of the brain is affected. Simple partial seizures do not involve loss of consciousness whereas complex partial seizures result in either impairment or loss of consciousness. Generalized seizures involve widespread areas of the brain and always involve loss of consciousness. There are two major categories of generalized seizures, absence and tonic-clonic. Absence seizures, also known as "petit mal," are characterized by brief (less than 30 seconds) episodes of staring and unresponsiveness. They are most commonly seen in children. Generalized tonic-clonic seizures, "grand mal," result in loss of consciousness and uncontrolled motor activity. These are the most common type of seizure disorders and are what most lay people consider epilepsy.

Most cases of epilepsy are very treatable with a variety of anticonvulsive medications, and patients with seizure disorders are thus able to lead almost completely normal lives, which can include athletic participation. Exercise does not seem to worsen seizure control in most patients and may actually be beneficial in reducing seizure frequency. Therefore, patients who have well-controlled seizure disorders are typically not restricted in athletic participation, with a few exceptions. Epilepsy patients should be prohibited from those sports in which even a momentary loss of consciousness could cause serious or fatal injury to the athlete or others. These sports include scuba diving, water skiing, diving, rock climbing, boxing, aerial gymnastics, and auto racing. In addition, athletes should not participate in sports involving potentially lethal projectiles such as archery and riflery. Collision sports can be allowed if seizures are well controlled and activity doesn't precipitate seizure activity (7). Swimming can be allowed if the patient doesn't swim alone, and events are closely supervised. All patients with epilepsy who participate in athletics should be warned to avoid factors that predispose to increased seizure frequency, such as sleep deprivation, alcohol, or withdrawal from seizure medication. The medical staff should be aware of those athletes with a seizure history and be prepared to manage episodes should they occur.

OTOLARYNGOLOGY

Otitis Media

Otitis media, or middle ear infection, often arise as a complication of URI because of blockage of the eustachian tube that connects the middle ear to the back of the throat. The eustachian tube normally acts to equalize the pressure behind the eardrum with the atmospheric pressure, explaining why ears pop in the mountains or on a plane. When the tube gets blocked, this allows for infection to occur behind the eardrum. Acute otitis media is almost always painful. Most patients will also complain of hearing impairment ranging from actual hearing loss to excessive popping and snapping. Diagnosis is made by direct otoscopic examination of the eardrum and finding erythema and possibly fluid behind the eardrum. Although the actual benefit from antibiotic therapy is probably small in most cases, treatment is usually initiated with amoxicillin for 10 days (20). Second line antibiotics include cephalosporins, Augmentin, and trimethoprim-sulfamethoxazole. These are used in penicillin-allergic patients, treatment failures, or early recurrence. Pain relief is provided by oral analgesics such as Advil, Tylenol, or, occasionally, narcotic preparations. Warm compresses to the external ear can be helpful and ototopical analgesic drops such as Auralgan can be used if no tympanic perforation is present. In severe cases there is a risk for perforation of the eardrum, which is usually associated with relief of pain and drainage of purulent material from the ear canal. The perforation usually heals without residual problems once the infection has resolved. Chronic ear infections are often treated in children (and occasionally adults) with tubes placed through the eardrum to relieve pressure and provide drainage.

Otitis Externa

Otitis externa is a painful infection of the external ear canal and is commonly referred to as swimmer's ear. Although it can occur in any athlete, it is very common in swimmers or divers because of incomplete removal of water from the ear canal that allows for subsequent bacterial growth. The illness is usually caused by *Pseudomonas aeruginosa* but can also occasionally be fungal in origin. It typically presents with pain that is usually made worse by pulling on the external ear itself. Hearing loss occasionally occurs if the auditory canal is so swollen as to be occluded. Diagnosis is by typical history, the finding of a red, swollen ear canal on otoscopic examination (often with purulent-appearing discharge), and pain on manipulation of the external ear. The problem is usually treated by cleaning the canal thoroughly and using a combination antibiotic and steroid drops such as Cortisporin Otic Suspension. If auditory canal swelling is severe, it may be necessary to insert a cotton or commercial wick into the canal to ensure that the drops penetrate deep into the canal. When a swimmer is prone to repeated infections, silicone earplugs or the use of a one-to-one mixture of rubbing alcohol and vinegar in the ear after practice along with careful drying can help prevent recurrence.

Auricular Hematoma

Hematomas of the external ear are common among wrestlers because of the direct trauma inflicted during the course of competition. These usually present as fluctuant fluid-filled bags overlying the cartilage of the external ear, and are easy to diagnose. If left alone, they will consolidate and scar down to the well-known end result of wrestler's cauliflower ear. Although some may consider this a badge of honor, most wrestlers understandably wish to avoid this result. Auricular hematomas can present a challenge to effective treatment primarily because the wrestler usually continues to participate in his sport. This causes him to be prone to reinjuring the ear, which leads to reaccumulation of the hematoma.

Initial treatment of a hematoma usually involves drainage with a syringe. It is important to ascertain by careful palpation that there has not been any fracture of the auricular cartilage prior to aspiration. The ear should be carefully sterilized with betadyne and the hematoma aspirated with a sterile 18-gauge or larger needle. Care must be taken not to penetrate directly into the auricular cartilage as this could lead to infection of the cartilage. If the athlete is able to protect the ear adequately using a head guard, often a single aspiration is sufficient treatment. Multiple aspirations are to be avoided in order to reduce risk of infection. In patients who develop recurrences, a pressure dressing can be made using a swimmer's nose clip and gauze saturated with collodion (32). Occasionally ear, nose, and throat (ENT) referral may be required for fractured cartilage, refractory hematomas, or infections.

Nosebleeds

The management of nosebleeds (epistaxis) is a common problem among athletes due both to trauma and environmental factors, such as frequent exposure to cold dry air. Fortunately the problem is usually easily resolved. The most common cause of nosebleeds is desiccation of the nasal mucosa with resultant fragility of the capillary vessels of the nose. This is usually more of a problem during the winter when low humidity is more common. Most nosebleeds are resolved by direct pressure for several minutes by pinching the tip of the nose. It is important to remember to remove the athlete from competition until the bleeding is stopped. Occasionally it becomes necessary to pack the nose with gauze in order to achieve hemostasis. It is important to consider the possibility of nasal or basilar skull fracture in patients presenting with nosebleeds following direct trauma.

In patients with recurrent nosebleeds, daily application of petroleum jelly in the anterior nares along with nocturnal vaporizer usage can decrease frequency of bleeding episodes. Occasionally, cautery of Kisselbach's plexus on the septum becomes necessary to provide relief. This can be done in the office with silver nitrate or by an ENT specialist with electrocautery. Patients with recurrent nosebleeds should also be thoroughly evaluated to rule out hypertension, intranasal tumors, and platelet or bleeding disorders as a precipitating cause.

Dental Injury

Athletes frequently suffer oral/facial injuries because of collision or ballistic trauma. In these injuries, the teeth are frequently involved. The extent of dental injury can range from laceration of the lips, cracking or loosening of a tooth, to actual avulsion of a tooth from its socket. Proper use of mouthguards and protective facemasks in collision sports can reduce the risk of injury. In cases of oral injury, any bleeding if present should be controlled. It is important to evaluate for possible coexisting maxillary, mandibular, or nasal fracture. The oral cavity should be carefully examined for lacerations of the internal lips, gums, or tongue. Minor cuts should be managed by cleaning with hydrogen peroxide followed by a short, 3- to 5-day course of antibiotics (usually Pen G) in order to prevent infection. Owing to the excellent blood supply of the oral cavity, these wounds usually heal quickly. Deeper lacerations or those involving the vermilion border of the lips may require suturing.

Significant injury to the teeth themselves usually requires a dentist's or oral surgeon's attention. Teeth may be loosened in their sockets, cracked, chipped, or completely avulsed. Loose teeth may require bracing for stability while healing occurs. Cracked or chipped teeth can often be reconstructed with dental cement. When a tooth avulsion occurs, the tooth should be gently rinsed with sterile saline to remove loose debris if present. Great care should be taken not to touch or scrub the root. Preferably the tooth should be reinserted into its socket during transport to a dentist. If this is not possible, the tooth should be transported (in decreasing preferential order) under the patient's tongue, in a commercial transport medium, milk, or sterile saline. The sooner the patient can be examined by a dentist the better the likelihood of a successful outcome.

OPHTHALMOLOGY

Athletes are obviously prone to the same eye problems as nonathletes. In addition, athletes frequently suffer eye trauma due to fingers, projectiles, dirt, and collisions. It is important that the athletic trainers and physicians caring for athletes be familiar with techniques for the examination of the eye and management of common eye problems. In addition, it is desirable to have an ophthalmologist identified to work closely with the athletic department in order to facilitate referrals and follow-up. This chapter will deal with the most common problems encountered in the athletic population.

Stye

A stye, also known as an external hordeolum, is an inflammatory reaction of the ciliary follicles or accessory glands of the anterior lid margin. This condition usually presents as a painful, tender focal swelling on the outside of one eyelid that develops over 2 to 3 days. There is frequently formation of a central pustule as the condition progresses. In addition, there is usually some mild conjunctival inflammation as well. This problem is usually self-limited and does not require aggressive intervention in most cases. Patients should be advised to apply warm compresses to the affected eye twice daily for symptomatic relief. Antibiotic eye drops are usually not required. If the lesion fails to resolve after 1 to 2 weeks, then referral to an ophthalmologist may be necessary for surgical excision.

Chalazion

A chalazion, also known as an internal hordeolum, is an inflammation of the meibomian gland within the eyelid. This lesion is similar to a stye, but is deeper within the eyelid tissue and frequently is not visible externally. It usually presents as a painful, focal tenderness of the eyelid that develops over several days. If there is no external abnormality noted, eversion of the lid will frequently reveal a focal red mass on the underside of the eyelid against the conjunctiva. As in a stye, the condition is usually inflammatory in nature and not infectious. The patient should be instructed to use warm compresses to the eye twice daily. Antibiotic eyedrops are usually not required. Occasionally, steroid eyedrops are used for severe cases but should only be prescribed by an ophthalmologist. If the lesion fails to improve after several weeks, surgical excision may be required.

Conjunctivitis

Conjunctivitis refers to inflammation of the conjunctiva and usually presents as a red inflamed eye often with mild pain or feeling of irritation. There are several causes of conjunctivitis ranging from viral and bacterial infection, allergy, contact irritation, and systemic conditions, such as lupus or rheumatoid arthritis. By far the most common cause among young adults is viral conjunctivitis followed by allergic conjunctivitis.

Viral conjunctivitis is a self-limited infection that leaves no permanent eye damage. It is most frequently due to adenovirus, and is frequently seen in the setting of acute URI. Because the virus is extremely contagious, epidemics of pink eye frequently occur throughout a team unless athletes are educated about reducing transmission. It typically presents as a diffuse conjunctival injection and watery discharge in either one or both eyes. Patients frequently complain of matting of the eyelashes when arising in the morning and mild discomfort of the eye. Vision is usually unaffected and pain is infrequent. Physical exam reveals diffuse erythema without evidence of purulent discharge. Often there will be a tender preauricular node. Foreign bodies and corneal abrasion need to be ruled out by careful examination and fluorescein staining. Once the diagnosis of viral conjunctivitis is made, the patient is instructed to wash their hands frequently and avoid touching their eyes and sharing towels in order to reduce transmission. Antibiotic drops are not effective and should not be used in viral conjunctivitis since their application can result in allergic reactions and viral spread. Warm compresses can be used for symptomatic relief. Contact lenses should be removed while inflammation is present. The infection is self-limited and usually resolves within 5 to 7 days.

Allergic conjunctivitis is a part of a systemic reaction, involving all mucous membranes, to an allergen that is usually airborne, such as pollen. It is usually seasonal and follows the pattern of other allergy symptoms such as sneezing, nasal congestion, and asthma. It can present as the only manifestation of allergy in a patient. It usually presents as a diffuse conjunctival injection, prominent itching (which is extremely suggestive of this diagnosis), and boggy swollen conjunctiva. It always involves both eyes and any discharge if present is usually stringy and mucoid. Treatment involves use of systemic antihistamines to reduce the global allergy symptoms, and topical decongestant/ antihistamine drops such as Vasocon-A for symptomatic relief of the eyes.

Bacterial conjunctivitis is much less common than either the viral or allergic forms. It is self-limited, results in no permanent damage, and is not nearly as contagious as viral conjunctivitis. The most common pathogens are *Staphylococcus aureus, Streptococcus pneumoniae,* and *Haemophilus influenzae.* The distinguishing characteristic that usually differentiates viral from bacterial conjunctivitis is the presence of purulent discharge on physical examination. When purulent discharge is seen, it is reasonable to treat with antibiotic eyedrops in order to reduce duration of symptoms. In most patients topical sulfa is the best first-line choice because of cost considerations. In patients allergic to sulfa, aminoglycosides (gentamycin, tobramycin), quinilone (ciprofloxin, norfloxin), or a combination antibiotic can be used. Because bacterial conjunctivitis has such a low degree of contagiousness, quarantining patients is not necessary. The patient should be referred to an ophthalmologist if the patient's symptoms fail to improve within one week, significant pain or visual loss is present, there is a history of associated foreign body, or the patient uses extended wear contact lenses (because of possible *Pseudomonas aeruginosa* infection).

Subconjunctival Hemorrhage

Subconjunctival hemorrhage is a common problem seen in athletes, particularly those participating in weight training. It is caused either by direct trauma or because of increase in intrathoracic pressure such as occurs in sneezing, coughing, straining at stool, and weight lifting. The increased vascular pressure causes the weak-walled blood vessels in the conjunctiva to burst and leads to the development of a small hematoma. Less common causes include hypertension, and bleeding or platelet disorders. Presentation is an asymptomatic red blotchiness within the conjunctiva. No treatment is necessary and the lesion resolves slowly over time in the manner of other hematomas.

Corneal Abrasions

Corneal abrasions are defects in the stratum corneum of the eye and usually result from foreign bodies or direct trauma such as a finger scratch. They are exquisitely painful because of the generous innervation of the orbit. Often the patient will complain of a persistent foreign body sensation in the eye. There is frequently some decreased visual acuity, especially if the defect overlies the pupil. On examination the eye will usually be red and inflamed and the patient will find it difficult to cooperate with the evaluation secondary to pain. Installation of a topical anesthetic such as proparacaine can greatly relieve symptoms temporarily to aid in examination. The eye should be examined carefully to rule out pupillary defects or evidence of significant trauma such as hyphema or conjunctival laceration. It is extremely important to rule out a persistent foreign body in a patient with a corneal abrasion. The upper eyelid should be inverted in order to assess for a possible foreign body underneath the lid. Once these steps have been taken, the eye should be stained with fluorescein, which is an orange dye that will only stain defects of the corneal surface. When the eye is subsequently examined using a cobalt blue light, the corneal abrasion shows up as a bright green lesion.

Treatment of a corneal abrasion is usually straightforward. The corneal epithelium rapidly heals itself, usually within 24 hours. The main goal of treatment is to facilitate this healing process and provide symptomatic relief. The use of topical anesthetics, although helpful for initial evaluation, is contraindicated in the management of corneal abrasions because of the possibility of further ocular damage occurring while the eye is numb. The usual treatment consists of applying a topical antibiotic ointment such as erythromycin and patching of the eye. The patching is intended to apply enough pressure to prevent opening and closing of the eye, thus providing protection and pain relief. The antibiotic ointment is used in order to prevent secondary infection. Aspirin, acetaminophin, ibuprofen or codeine may be necessary for pain control. The patient should be scheduled for follow-up examination the next day to assess healing. Patients with large defects (particularly those overlying the pupil), evidence of significant ocular trauma, or embedded foreign bodies should be referred to an ophthalmologist for treatment.

Trauma

Athletes as a group are at risk for serious ocular trauma, particularly when participating in sports involving high-velocity projectiles such as racquet sports, baseball, and lacrosse. Basketball players are also at high risk because of elbows and fingers from competitors. The extent of injury can range from a minor self-limited corneal abrasion to global rupture and eye loss. Many of these injuries can be prevented by proper training techniques and the proper use of eye protection in sports that require them. The coaching and training staff should be familiar with these requirements and should strictly enforce compliance. Unfortunately, many eye injuries are unavoidable despite the best prevention efforts and the medical staff needs to be able to evaluate and manage these injuries when they occur.

The athlete who has suffered an eye injury should be immediately removed from participation until a thorough evaluation has been performed. Visual acuity needs to be assessed in all eye injuries. The eye should be carefully inspected to rule out pupil defects, embedded foreign bodies, globe rupture, conjunctival lacerations, or the presence of a hyphema. A hyphema refers to blood in the anterior chamber of the eye that usually will layer out underneath the pupil and over the iris. The presence of a hyphema is of great concern because of the possibility of serious injury to the posterior chamber of the eye and should never be ignored. Visual fields and fundoscopic exam should be checked to evaluate possible retinal detachment. Those patients with any significant abnormal findings should be evaluated by an ophthalmologist immediately. The patient should have an eye shield placed over the affected eye to prevent further injury to the eye. If an eye shield is not available, the bottom two inches of a paper cup can be taped over the eye. Those patients without significant abnormal findings should be carefully observed and frequently reexamined until symptoms resolve.

DERMATOLOGY

Obviously, athletes can develop all of the various dermatologic conditions to which other people are susceptible. Therefore, the team physician should be knowledgeable in the management of common skin problems such as eczema, warts, psoriasis, acne, infestations, urticaria, wounds, blisters, and skin tumors both malignant and benign. Obviously, this subject is well beyond the scope of this chapter and a dermatology textbook or atlas should be obtained as a resource for managing these problems. There are several dermatologic conditions that are important to consider in relation to sports, either because they are more common among athletes or because they can affect athletic participation.

Staphylococcal Infections

Staphylococcal (staph) infections of the skin are common and can range from minor folliculitis or small boils to furuncles or carbuncles, which can be quite extensive and require surgical drainage. Small boils with a developed ''head'' can be managed with warm soaks and will usually drain spontaneously. Systemic antibiotics for a boil will not shorten the clinical course. Larger furuncles or carbuncles that present with dermal fluctuance require drainage of the abscess with a scalpel blade in order for healing to occur. In cases with significant surrounding cellulitis, antibiotic treatment may be required. In most cases a first generation cephalosporin such as cephalexin is sufficient but dicloxicillin is recommended for severe cases. Folliculitis presents as numerous small pustules each of which involves a hair follicle. Treatment is usually with oral erythromycin or first generation cephalosporin.

Athletes with significant staph skin infections should not be allowed to participate in swimming or sports with close bodily contact such as wrestling until the infection has resolved. This is due to the possibility of infecting other athletes.

Herpetic Infections

Herpes simplex virus (HSV) is the cause of several different dermatologic conditions. Probably the best-known illness among the public is genital herpes that is most often due to the HSV-2 strain. Since genital herpes rarely affects athletic participation, it will not be discussed further. The most common herpetic lesions are probably oral/labial lesions commonly known as cold sores, most commonly because of the HSV-1 strain. In addition, wrestlers are prone by the nature of their sport to develop herpetic lesions anywhere on skin that is exposed to direct close contact with an infected wrestler during competition. This condition is known as herpes gladitorium and can present as an epidemic among team members. Herpes therefore has the potential to severely disrupt an entire team.

Herpes infections are unusual in that the affected patient may be susceptible to recurrent bouts of lesions. The initial, or primary, infection can range from completely asymptomatic to severe. Following recovery from the primary attack, the virus remains dormant within sensory ganglia within the central nervous system. It can then be reactivated during times of stress, viral URIs, sunlight exposure, local trauma, or menstruation. These subsequent attacks tend to become less frequent and severe with time. The patient will frequently feel a tingling sensation in the affected area prior to the development of the lesions, which typically present as a cluster of vesicles surrounded by an area of erythema. In most cases, the diagnosis can be made based upon the history and the appearance of the lesions. Occasionally, diagnostic testing such as Tzanck smears or HSV culture are necessary if the lesions are atypical or in an unusual location. The vesicles usually scab over and complete healing occurs over 5 to 10 days without therapy.

In order to reduce infection of others, athletes with active herpetic lesions that cannot be well covered should be told to avoid those sports that involve close bodily contact, primarily wrestling. They should not be allowed to return to active competition until the lesions are dry and healed over, which usually takes at least one week. Additional preventive measures include careful, frequent cleaning of wrestling mats with an appropriate disinfectant solution, education of wrestling coaches, athletes and athletic trainers regarding herpes lesions, and team skin checks prior to competitions.

Although treatment of active herpetic lesions with the antiviral medication acyclovir is commonly done, it is largely unproven as to exactly how effective this therapy is. The topical cream form of acyclovir is ineffective in reducing duration of illness. In studies of genital herpes, initiation of oral acyclovir 200 mg five times a day reduced the time to healing of lesions by 1 to 2 days (59). This effect is only seen if the medication is begun as early as possible, preferably when the patient feels the preliminary tingling sensation that usually heralds an attack. Studies of oral herpetic lesions are less conclusive as to benefit and most authorities do not recommend treatment of recurrent attacks because the cost involved doesn't warrant the minimal benefit. In one study, increasing the dose of acyclovir to 400 mg five times a day reduced the duration of pain by 36% and the length of time to the loss of crusts by 27%, which corresponds to 1 to 2 days' reduction in duration (69). Herpes gladiotorium is poorly studied. Since the effects of treating with acyclovir do show a definite tendency toward earlier resolution of lesions, the use of this medication may be justified in those cases in which a day or two may impact the ability of an athlete (wrestler) to compete. If treatment is decided upon, the medication should be initiated as early as possible. If the lesions have been established for more than 24 hours, then acyclovir has no effect. The medication is expensive and this frequently impacts treatment decisions.

Another related issue involves prophylaxis against future recurrences of herpes in an athlete prone to infection. Although no studies have been done on herpes gladitorium, evidence exists for the effectiveness in herpes labialis. The use of acyclovir 400 mg p.o. twice a day has been shown to reduce the incidence of lesions in oral herpes infections by 53% with only minimal side effects (61). The drawback to this approach is the expense involved. In order to prophylax a single wrestler for the duration of a five-month season, the cost would be approximately $500. This is more than most individuals or athletic departments are willing to budget. An alternative approach would be to begin prophylaxis of affected wrestlers 1 week prior to very important matches such as conference tournaments or national finals. This would tend to maximize the potential benefit while minimizing the expense.

Fungal Infections

The main fungal infections seen in athletes are ringworm (particularly common among wrestlers), athlete's foot, and jock itch. The first can have implications regarding athletic participation, whereas the other two are at best annoying and occasionally disabling.

Ringworm (also known as tinea corporis) refers to cutaneous infection of the body or face with one of a group of fungi known as dermatophytes. The dermatophytes have the ability to survive on the dead keratin of the stratum corneum, which is the outermost layer of the skin. The most common genera of infecting organisms are *Microsporum, Trichophyton,* and *Epidermophyton.* Regardless of the etiologic organism, ringworm presents in a similar fashion and responds to the same treatment regimens so exact identification is usually unnecessary. The infection usually presents as red patches of skin with a flaky scale. The lesions tend to advance in all directions and have a prominent border at the periphery of the lesion often with central clearing, which is the basis for the name ringworm. Among athletes, ringworm is most commonly seen among wrestlers because of the nature of the sport. Since the lesions are infectious, those wrestlers (or other athletes participating in mat sports or sports involving close contact) with active ringworm should be prohibited from active participation until resolution occurs. Prevention measures are similar to those observed for herpes and include early treatment, careful cleaning of wrestling mats between uses, team skin checks, and education of coaches, athletic trainers, and athletes.

Treatment of ringworm usually consists of topical antifungal creams such as clotrimazole, miconazole, or ketoconazole. The lesions usually resolve within two weeks but therapy should be continued for an additional week after resolution to reduce likelihood of recurrence. The newer antifungal agent terbinafine will often provide faster resolution but is significantly more expensive (25).

In patients with frequent recurrence or refractory infection, the use of oral antifungals such as griseofulvin or ketoconazole may be required. These drugs do have potentially significant side effects (hepatitis, headache, pruritis, gynecomastia) and should only be used in cases in which topical therapy has failed.

Athlete's foot (tinia pedis) and jock itch (tinea cruis) are related dermatophyte infections. In both cases, the infections are due to the warm, moist environments the toes and crotch afford the offending fungus, usually *Trichophyton rubrum, Trichophyton mentagrophytes, Epidermophyton floccosum,* or occasionally the yeast *Candida albicans.* Both infections are usually intensely pruritic. Athletes frequently develop these infections because of contaminated locker room floors and frequent sweating, which contributes to a favorable environment for fungal infection. Athlete's foot presents as flaking and maceration between the toes, and occasionally tender vesicles on the soles of the feet. Jock itch presents as a red scaly lesion often asymmetrically affecting both sides of the upper thighs. The outer margin is usually more inflamed and gives the appearance of an advancing border. In most cases these infections are easily managed using the same topical antifungal creams described previously. In rare instances, it may be necessary to treat severe or refractory cases with oral antifungal agents such as griseofulvin or ketoconazole (35). In addition to treatment, the patient with athlete's foot should be advised to dry between the toes carefully following showering, wear sandals in community showers, frequently change socks, alternate shoes, and to regularly use an antifungal powder. Patients with jock itch should be told not to wear wet clothing for long periods of time, to use cotton underwear instead of synthetics, to avoid tight-fitting clothing, to thoroughly dry after showering, and not to share towels or clothing with others.

Poison Ivy

Poison ivy is the common name for allergic contact dermatitis resulting from exposure to a plant belonging to the genus *Rhus.* The most common offending species in this country are poison ivy, poison oak, and poison sumac. These plants secrete an oleoresin called *urushiol* that is a potent sensitizer and in susceptible individuals results in an intense allergic dermatitis. The clinical presentation of the dermatitis depends upon the quantity of *urushiol* resin contacting the skin, the individual's susceptibility to its effects, the distribution pattern on the body, and the variation between different areas of skin in reactivity. The rash typically presents as an intensely itchy, erythematous dermatitis with overlying vesicles and blisters. The lesions are often seen in a linear distribution that occurs when the plant is drawn across the skin. The first areas to become involved usually represent those in which exposure was the most intense and the skin most susceptible. New lesions will often continue to appear over several days in areas in which there was less resin exposure or the skin was more resistant to its effects. Contrary to popular belief, once the skin and contaminated clothing are washed no further exposure occurs. The blister fluid cannot spread the inflammation to other parts of the body or other people.

Treatment of poison ivy is largely dependent upon the severity of the presentation. Small areas of mild to moderate inflammation can be managed with moderate strength topical steroid ointments such as triamcinolone 0.1%. More severe inflammation or larger areas of involvement usually require use of oral corticosteroids. The author usually prescribes prednisone 50 mg every day for 7 to 10 days. This regimen is simpler than the more traditional steroid taper and probably improves compliance. Symptomatic measures include use of oral antihistamines to control itching, soothing cool Aveeno baths, and topical calamine lotion. Preventive measures include avoidance of overgrowth, wearing long sleeves and pants when in wooded areas, and training in identification of the causative plants.

Sunburn

Sunburn is frequently seen in the spring and summer months in those athletes engaging in outdoor sports or leisure activities. Sunburn is caused by excessive exposure to the ultraviolet B (290 to 320 nm) wavelength found in sunlight and commercial tanning beds. The likelihood of developing sunburn is based on several factors; namely, the patient's skin type, the intensity of sunlight, the duration of exposure, and the presence of protective factors such as sunscreen or previous tan. Fair skinned individuals are at much higher risk of developing sunburn and need to take special precautions.

As most people know, sunburn presents as a painful erythema occasionally complicated by edema or blister formation. It typically is worse on those areas subjected to direct sun rays such as the shoulders when the patient was standing during exposure or the abdomen or back when prone. There is no effective therapy for sunburn and symptom relief is the mainstay of treatment. Aspirin can help with pain relief. Topical soothing creams such as Noxema can provide some relief. Anesthetic sprays containing lidocaine or benzocaine can also improve symptoms but occasionally compound the problem by causing an allergic reaction. The burn resolves over many days usually with subsequent peeling of the epidermis.

If the acute consequences of excessive sun exposure were the only concern, then there would be little reason for a physician to recommend against tanning and "sun-worshiping." Unfortunately, the long-term consequences of frequent excessive sun exposure are of even more con-

cern. The incidence of skin cancers has increased at an alarming rate in recent years, largely attributable to increased sun exposure. Therefore, athletes with fair skin who spend large amounts of time outdoors should be counseled regarding risks of solar damage as well as protective strategies. Exposure to the sun's most direct rays, which occur between 11 A.M. and 3 P.M., should be minimized. The use of commercial tanning beds should be discouraged as well. Protective clothing and hat use should be encouraged whenever possible. Most importantly, the use of a chemical sunscreen such as para-aminobenzoic acid (PABA) should be strongly encouraged. PABA selectively absorbs ultraviolet radiation in the wavelengths from 290 to 320 nm, which are the most damaging. A sunscreen should be chosen with a sun protection factor (SPF) of at least 15 or greater.

METABOLIC CONCERNS

Diabetes

Diabetes mellitus is a metabolic disorder characterized by the inability of the body to properly utilize the simple sugar glucose. The most frequent description of diabetes is high blood glucose levels, but this is an oversimplification of a complex physiologic derangement. Diabetes can be divided into two categories; insulin dependent (type 1) and type 2 (noninsulin dependent). The pathogenesis and treatment is very different between the two types of diabetes. Type 1 diabetes is more commonly seen among younger athletes and the management is more complicated. A brief description of type 2 diabetes will be followed by a more detailed discussion of type 1 diabetes management in the athlete.

Noninsulin dependent diabetes (NIDDM) accounts for 80% of all diabetes cases and is due to resistance of the cells of the body to the action of insulin, which is the major hormonal regulator of blood glucose. It is most commonly a disorder of older adults and usually presents after age 50, although it can occur in younger people. It is primarily due to obesity and excess calorie consumption. The mainstay of therapy in these patients is weight reduction and dietary changes, with medication being required for more severe cases. Exercise is an important component of NIDDM management as it promotes weight loss and also improves glucose control (80). In addition, frequent aerobic activity can help reduce the risk of heart disease, which diabetics are prone to develop. Anaerobic exercise such as weight lifting should be avoided because of adverse effects on the eyes, kidneys, and heart (65). It is important that a patient with type 2 diabetes be examined by a physician prior to engaging in any new exercise regimen, including consideration of an exercise stress test to evaluate the possibility of preexisting cardiac disease.

Type 1 diabetes is caused by the inability of the patient's pancreas to produce insulin, which is the major hormone responsible for glucose utilization by the cells of the body. This illness usually appears early in life and is due to destruction of the islet cells of the pancreas by what is felt to be an autoimmune process triggered by a viral infection. These patients are unable to utilize glucose at all and are subject to the development of diabetic keto-acidosis. Prior to the development of insulin treatment, these patients all died soon after diagnosis. Since insulin therapy was introduced, these patients have been able to lead active, nearly normal lives. If the patient is well motivated to monitor diet, insulin requirements, and blood glucose levels they are able to engage in athletics at the highest levels. As a general rule, no athlete should compete when their glucose is out of control (greater than 250 mg/dL) and strenuous activity should be deferred until good glycemic control is obtained.

Diet is an important component to the management of type 1 diabetes, especially when the patient engages in strenuous activity. Like all athletes, diabetics require adequate fuel for muscles to perform optimally. Unlike non-diabetics, their metabolism is not able to regulate blood sugar on its own and they must substitute careful control of food intake in relation to activity demands and insulin requirement. The standard diabetic diet is very similar to that recommended to other athletes and should consist of approximately 65% of calories from carbohydrate, 15% from protein, and 25% from fat (75). It is important that the diabetic be in the habit of eating at routine times during the day in order to coincide with peaks of insulin action. In addition, the athlete needs to time the pre-event meal properly in order to have available energy during the activity. The pre-event meal should be eaten about 3 hours before exercise and should be composed primarily of complex carbohydrates as found in pasta, grains, or rice. In addition the athlete should consume a preevent snack 30 minutes prior to activity to protect against hypoglycemia. With experience, the diabetic patient will be able to accurately predict the amount of food required for various activities. During prolonged exercise, the athlete should take frequent small snacks such as fruit or candy and these energy sources should always be available during activity. Proper hydration is also extremely important and the diabetic athlete should consume water liberally during and after activity. A postcompetition simple carbohydrate such as orange juice or candy bar should be taken immediately after exercise followed by a complex carbohydrate source such as bread, bagels, or potatoes.

The insulin-dependent diabetic needs to be able to manipulate insulin dosages in order to compensate for numerous physiologic changes because of variation in diet, activity, illness, and stress. Fortunately, a motivated patient is able with experience and medical guidance to estimate closely the insulin requirements associated with these variables. In most diabetics, the goal of therapy is tight glycemic control and this is best achieved by three or four injections of insulin daily. A longer-acting insulin is given once or twice a day to provide baseline coverage with injections of a short-acting insulin prior to meals in order to metabolize the glucose consumed in the meal. With experience, a diabetic can accurately estimate the amount of calories in a meal and administer an appropriate amount of short-acting insulin. Exercise increases glucose utilization by the body and consequently can decrease insulin requirements. As much as possible, the hypoglycemic effects of exercise should be compensated with increased food intake, but a decrease in insulin dose is also often necessary in order to prevent hypoglycemia. Again, with experience the diabetic is able to make appropriate adjustments in insulin dosages based upon the expected intensity of the activity. The athletic diabetic should have a home glucose monitor and frequently check glucose levels during the day in order to guide therapy. These results should be kept in a logbook for reference along with diet and activity in order to track insulin requirements. Initially, close consultation with the physician should be maintained while the trial and error of insulin adjustment takes place. However, with time the diabetic will develop a greater understanding of his/her metabolism than anybody else.

The two main acute problems that the diabetic can have relate to the extremes of blood glucose. Low blood sugar (hypoglycemia) occurs when there is more insulin than required, thus excessively lowering glucose levels. Mild hypoglycemia is common among all diabetics and is characterized by hunger, dizziness, and excessive sweating. When these symptoms occur, the diabetic patient should consume a quickly absorbed sugar source such as orange juice, candy, or a commercial glucose supplement. If the hypoglycemia is not corrected, the glucose levels will continue to fall until the brain (which is dependent upon glucose for energy) is unable to function properly. The patient develops resulting loss of coordination, slurred speech, and finally unconsciousness and coma. A hypoglycemic coma is a life-threatening emergency and all coaches, athletic trainers, and physicians need to be alert as to this possibility in a diabetic athlete. If the diabetic loses consciousness, a glucose gel can be placed under the tongue while waiting for appropriate help to arrive. In addition, consideration should be given to keeping a glucagon injection readily available whenever a diabetic athlete is involved in athletic participation. When given, glucagon causes increased glucose production in the liver, which can help to stabilize the patient until IV glucose can be given.

At the other end of the spectrum of acute diabetic complications is diabetic ketoacidosis. This condition occurs when insulin levels are inadequate for the proper metabolism of glucose. Without adequate insulin, the body is unable to properly utilize the glucose in the bloodstream. The glucose levels rise dramatically as a consequence. This hyperglycemia causes excessive urination (polyuria) that eventually leads to severe dehydration. The patient develops tachypnea (rapid heartbeat), nausea, dizziness, and often abdominal pain. In addition, the patient's breath will often smell fruity because of the presence of acetone. Acetone and other volatile ketone bodies are produced because of the excessive utilization of fats as an energy source during insulin absence. If untreated, the patient will deteriorate and lapse into a coma. Patients with diabetic ketoacidosis require IV fluids and insulin as treatment and should be taken to the nearest hospital for evaluation. Athletic trainers, coaches, and team physicians should keep this possibility in mind when tending to a sick diabetic athlete.

Nutrition

Probably no area of athletics, indeed modern life, is more laden with confusion, misinformation, charlatanism, and downright fraud than nutrition and its role in health and fitness. Athletes are continually bombarded by products distributed from both commercial and quasi-nutritional sources that claim to increase endurance, strength, speed, and overall athletic performance. Many athletes will take nutritional supplements on a regular basis believing they will provide a benefit during training and competition. This has led to the development of a large industry catering to (and profiteering on) the desire of the athlete to use all available means to succeed. As demonstrated by the advertising wars between competing "sports drinks" (complete with high-profile athletes extolling their virtues), the business of marketing these products is highly competitive and lucrative. Unfortunately, the actual benefit derived from most nutritional aids marketed to athletes is either minimal or nonexistent.

Athletes require several different nutritional needs from their diet, all of which can be supplied by thoughtful and varied choices of food. They need to have sufficient intake of fuel (as defined in terms of calories) to allow for the high intensity of muscle use that occurs during exercise. These calories are primarily supplied in the form of carbohydrates and fats. Athletes require adequate (as opposed to excessive) protein to build and repair muscle tissues. They must have adequate intake of vitamins and minerals. They also require proper fluid intake to prevent dehydration. Most (but not all) athletes competing in sports such as football, basketball, and soccer tend to eat heartily and will often consume twice the calories of a more sedentary person. If they are reasonably careful about eating a variety of foods, these athletes will get more than enough nutrients from their regular diet. Many sports emphasize thinness of physique in participating athletes. These sports include gymnastics, distance running, wrestling, and ice skating. In addition to potential problems with eating disorders, athletes participating in these activities usually are prone to calorie restriction and consequently need to be

TABLE 2.5. *Food group exchange system*

MILK 90–100 calories
Non-fat
  12 g carbohydrate
  8 g protein
  0 g fat
  • 1 cup skim milk, nonfat yogurt
Low-fat
  12 g carbohydrate
  8 g protein
  5 g fat
  • 1 cup 2% milk, plain low-fat yogurt
High-fat
  12 g carbohydrate
  8 g protein
  8 g fat
  • 1 cup whole milk
MEAT AND SUBSTITUTES
Lean meat 55 calories
  0 g carbohydrate
  7 g protein
  3 g fat
  • 1 oz lean beef (e.g., sirloin)
  • 1 oz lean pork (e.g., tenderloin)
  • 1 oz skinless poultry
  • 1 oz fish
Medium-fat meat 75 calories
  0 g carbohydrate
  7 g protein
  5 g fat
  • 1 oz ground beef
  • 1 oz skim/part skim mozzarella, ricotta
  • 4 oz tofu
  • 1 egg
High-fat meat 100 calories
  0 g carbohydrate
  7 g protein
  8 g fat
  • 1 oz corned beef
  • 1 oz spareribs
  • 1 oz cheese (e.g., cheddar, Swiss)
  • 1 hot dog
  • 1 Tbsp. peanut butter

BREAD/GRAINS
80 calories
15 g carbohydrate
3 g protein
0 g fat
  • 1 slice whole wheat bread
  • $\frac{1}{2}$ bagel, English muffin
  • 1 6-inch tortilla
  • $\frac{1}{2}$ cup pasta
  • 3 cups popcorn, no added butter
  • $\frac{1}{2}$ cup bran flakes
  • $\frac{1}{2}$ cup corn
  • 1 small potato
  • 2 pancakes (add 1 fat exchange)
  • 1 waffle (add 1 fat exchange)
FRUITS 60 calories
15 g carbohydrate
0 g protein
0 g fat
  • 1 small apple
  • $\frac{1}{2}$ banana
  • $\frac{1}{3}$ cantaloupe
  • $\frac{1}{2}$ cup grapefruit juice
  • 1 small orange
  • 1 cup watermelon
VEGETABLES
25 calories
5 g carbohydrate
2 g protein
0 g fat
  • $\frac{1}{2}$ cup cooked vegetables
  • 1 cup raw vegetables
  • $\frac{1}{2}$ cup vegetable juice
FAT 45 calories
0 g carbohydrate
0 g protein
5 g fat
  • 20 small peanuts
  • 1 tsp. oil
  • 1 slice bacon
  • 2 tsp. mayonnaise
  • 1 tsp. butter, margarine
  • 1 Tbsp. cream cheese
  • 2 Tbsp. sour cream

careful to pick nutrient-dense foods to ensure adequate intake. For these reasons, it is extremely important for athletes to have access to a registered dietitian to answer any questions and provide guidance in formulating a nutrition plan.

A solid, healthy athletic diet can be developed by using

TABLE 2.6. *Calculations for training diets*

Food group	Number of exchanges Calorie level					
	1500	2000	2500	3000	3500	4000
Milk	3	3	4	4	4	4
Meat	5	5	5	5	6	6
Fruit	5	6	7	9	10	12
Vegetable	3	3	3	5	6	7
Grain	7	11	16	18	20	24
Fat	2	3	5	6	8	10

Example: 3000 calorie training diet

	Carbohydrate			Protein		Fat	
Milk	4 × 12 g carbohydrate	48 g		4 × 8 g protein	32 g	4 × 0 g fat	0 g
Meat	5 × 0 g	0 g		5 × 7 g	35 g	5 × 5 g	25 g
Fruit	9 × 15 g	135 g		9 × 0 g	0 g	9 × 0 g	0 g
Vegetable	5 × 5 g	25 g		5 × 2 g	10 g	5 × 0 g	0 g
Grain	18 × 15 g	270 g		18 × 3 g	54 g	18 × 0 g	0 g
Fat	6 × 0 g	0 g		6 × 0 g	0 g	6 × 5 g	30 g
		478 g carbohydrate			131 g protein		55 g fat

478 g carbohydrate × 4 calories/gram = 1912 calories from carbohydrate
131 g protein × 4 calories/gram = 524 calories from protein
55 g fat × 9 calories/gram = 495 calories from fat

2931 total calories 1912 calories from carbohydrate/2931 total calories = 65% total calories from carbohydrate
524 calories from protein/2931 = 18% calories from protein
495 calories from fat/2931 = 17% calories from fat

some common sense and general guidelines. Table 2.5 presents the American Diabetes Association's food group exchange system, which can aid an athlete in making food choices and in defining serving sizes in a meal plan. Table 2.6 consists of a recommended athletic diet (consisting of 60% carbohydrate, 15% to 20% protein, and less than 25% fat) in terms of food exchanges from Table 2.5. The overall calorie requirement level determines the number of dietary exchanges needed daily. A rough estimate of the athlete's calorie requirements can be obtained by use of Table 2.7, which is based upon ideal body weight and activity.

Carbohydrates

Carbohydrates are the major fuel source of the body and adequate intake of this macronutrient is essential for peak athletic performance. The primary carbohydrate used by the body is glucose, which is defined as a simple monosaccharide or sugar. The other monosaccharides include fructose and galactose, which the liver is able to convert into glucose. Many simple sugars are consumed in the form of disaccharides that are combinations of two monosaccharides. These include sucrose, or table sugar, which is a combination of glucose and fructose and lactose, or milk sugar, which is a combination of galactose and glucose. Most fruits and honey consist of a combination of glucose, fructose, and sucrose. Carbohydrates are also found in long chains of simple sugars that are referred

to as complex carbohydrates. Complex carbohydrates are more commonly known as starch and are found in most breads and starchy vegetables such as potatoes and rice. Regardless of the form of carbohydrate ingested, ultimately they will either be converted into glucose for energy utilization or adipose tissue for long-term energy

TABLE 2.7. *Calculation of calorie requirements based upon ideal body weight*

Estimate of ideal body weight (IBW)
Women: 100 lb for height of 5 feet + 5 lb per inch over 5 feet
    Example: 5'6" = 100 + (5 × 6) = 130
Men: 106 lb for height of 5 feet + 6 lb per inch over 5 feet
    Example: 5'11" = 106 + (6 × 11) = 172 lb
For small frame subtract 10%; for large frame add 10%
Calculation of calorie requirement
Basal requirement = 10 Cal/lb of ideal body weight
Activity allowance
Sedentary: add 20–30% of basal requirement
Moderately active: add 50% of basal requirement
Active: add 100% or more depending upon activity (most competitive athletes are in this category)
Example: 6'1" male soccer player medium frame, very active
IBW = 106 + (6 × 13) = 184 lb with no adjustment for frame
Basal requirement = 184 × 10 = 1840 cal
Activity allowance = 100% × 1840 cal = 1840 cal
Final calorie requirement = 3680 calories

storage. The body does store some extra carbohydrate in the form of glycogen in the liver and muscle tissues. Glycogen is a very large branched complex carbohydrate storage molecule that can be readily converted back into simple glucose for energy during periods of starvation or exercise.

The ability to exercise anaerobically is directly related to the availability of glucose to the exercising muscle. At exercise levels above 60% of maximum, aerobic metabolism is unable to supply the energy requirements of the body and glucose stores are consumed. The human body has approximately 1800 calories of carbohydrate stored in various forms. The blood contains only 80 calories of glucose. Glycogen represents the bulk of glucose storage with muscle and liver glycogen containing 1400 and 320 calories respectively (14). Once these stores are exhausted, further anaerobic metabolism is impossible and the athlete must either stop or reduce the pace. It is obviously desirable to ensure maximal glycogen production in order to optimize athletic endurance.

Athletic training can increase the muscle's ability to store glycogen by 50%. However, frequent intense exercise can deplete muscle glycogen if the athlete does not consume adequate replacement carbohydrate during the recovery period. Most athletes are able to accomplish glycogen recovery from a diet consisting of 60% of calories as carbohydrate, mostly in the form of complex carbohydrate. Some marathoners or other ultra-high endurance athletes may require 70% carbohydrate from their diet. Some athletes are unable to consume enough replacement carbohydrate from their regular diet because of decreased appetite or time constraints. In these athletes a commercial high-carbohydrate drink such as GatorLode or Exceed can provide supplementation, particularly immediately after exercise when glycogen synthesis is greatest. They do not appear to offer any advantage other than convenience for most athletes, and high-glucose foods such as raisins, fruit-flavored yogurt, or applesauce can work just as well. Regardless of whether a commercial carbohydrate drink or natural snack is initially chosen, the athlete should consume a high-carbohydrate postexercise meal such as pasta, rice, or potatoes to ensure further glycogen synthesis. In addition, the athlete should be encouraged to take one rest day during a training week to help avoid exercise-induced glycogen depletion.

Many endurance athletes utilize techniques of glycogen loading prior to competing in major events. These strict dietary and exercise regimens are effective in increasing the amount of glycogen stored by the muscles, thereby increasing athletic endurance. Basically, the classic technique involves an initial week of exhaustive exertion, followed by 3 days of a low-carbohydrate diet with continued heavy exercise. This has the effect of severely depleting the muscle's glycogen reserves. Then for three days prior to competition the athlete rests while ingesting a high carbohydrate diet. The carbohydrate-starved muscles are essentially tricked into supercompensating with increased glycogen production. There have been many subsequent refinements of this technique and it has been discovered that the initial 3-day low-carbohydrate diet is unnecessary. The modified regimen in Table 2.8 can result in equal muscle glycogen stores compared to the classic regimen with decreased risk of injury or side effects from the decreased carbohydrate diet (64). Glycogen loading should not be attempted by athletes with diabetes or other metabolic disorder. The technique is not effective in increasing athletic performance in non-endurance events.

Protein

Protein is another macronutrient that is a vital component in an athletes's diet. Proteins are composed of amino acids and perform vital functions related to cellular metabolism, tissue maintenance and repair. Most athletes are concerned about protein since it is a requirement for muscle strength and growth. It needs to be reinforced that adequate protein allows for muscles to hypertrophy in response to strength training, but no amount of protein will build muscles without exercise. An astounding variety of commercial products have been developed and marketed to the athletic population with promises of increased muscle bulking and strength gains. Some tout special ratios of the various amino acids, whereas others contain extraordinarily high amounts of protein. In reality, these products offer no advantage to careful consideration of diet and are a very expensive way for the serious athlete to ingest protein.

The healthy human digestive tract is extremely efficient in digesting proteins into their constituent amino acids and then absorbing them. Therefore, products that are formulated from individual amino acids offer no advantage over naturally occurring proteins. There is no credible evidence that any artificially determined ratio of amino acids is better at building and sustaining muscle mass than the ingestion of muscle proteins themselves as found in fish, chicken, beef, or pork. The nonvegetarian athlete is easily able to obtain more than enough protein from these sources. The required protein intake recommended for athletes attempting to increase muscle size and strength is between 1.2 and 1.5 gm/kg/day (40). For

TABLE 2.8. *Modified carbohydrate loading regimen*

Day	Exercise duration (at 70% maximum exertion)	Dietary carbohydrate %
1	90 minutes	60
2	40 minutes	60
3	40 minutes	65
4	20 minutes	70
5	20 minutes	70
6	Rest	70
7	Competition	70

a 200 lb (90 kg) athlete this would amount to 135 g of dietary protein. Endurance athletes require less protein (1 g/kg/day). It is vital that the athlete consume adequate calories in the form of carbohydrate and fat to prevent excess utilization of protein as fuel.

The 3000 cal training diet as shown in Table 2.6 contains 131 g protein that comes primarily from four servings of dairy and a total of 5 oz of meat products a day. (The typical American diet contains much more than 5 oz of meat a day.) Those larger strength-training athletes such as weight lifters and football players requiring additional protein can obtain high-quality protein cheaply in dietary forms such as dry nonfat milk powder or canned tuna. For example, a cup of milk powder contains 30 g protein and a can of tuna packed in spring water contains approximately 50 g of protein with only minimal fat. Actual dietary protein intake for football players and tri-athletes has been shown to be 2 g/kg/day, which is sufficient for their needs (9,67). The commercial products may be appealing for convenience or psychological reasons, but athletes should be told that they offer no real advantage and are much more expensive than other protein sources.

The athlete following a vegetarian diet may have a difficult time obtaining enough protein without thoughtful and careful choices of foods. Lacto-vegans can utilize dairy products as a good protein source. More strict vegetarians need to emphasize high-protein sources such as beans. It is recommended that they consult with a registered dietitian to formulate a suitable meal plan.

Vitamins and Minerals

Vitamins are catalysts involved in regulating numerous biochemical reactions involved in the body's metabolism. They are involved in energy utilization, tissue maintenance, blood cell production, blood clotting, and bone formation. An adequate intake of the various vitamins is vital to health and athletic performance. Fortunately, vitamin deficiencies are rare in this country and are primarily seen in elderly, alcoholic, or other patients with limited diets. However, there is a prevalent misconception among the public (including athletes) that if a required daily intake of vitamins is good, then larger doses must provide greater benefit. This has never been demonstrated to be true for any vitamin (38). In the absence of a deficiency, vitamins do not provide energy, do not increase strength, do not prevent injuries, do not prevent illness, and do not enhance performance. Athletes should also be made aware that there are some potentially serious toxicities and side effects from taking megadoses of certain vitamins. For most athletes eating a well-balanced diet, vitamin supplementation is unnecessary and expensive. If an athlete follows a poor meal plan or ingests inadequate calories to ensure vitamin requirements, a daily multivitamin may be indicated but the athlete should see a dietitian to make proper adjustments in their diet.

Minerals are inorganic salts involved in several important metabolic processes. Like vitamins, adequate intake of these nutrients is vital to health. Minerals can be divided into two groups; major minerals and trace minerals. The major minerals are required in larger amounts and include calcium, phosphorus, magnesium, potassium, sodium, and chloride. The trace minerals are needed in very small amounts and include iron, zinc, selenium, copper, chromium, and iodine. As in vitamins, taking more minerals than the body actually requires does not provide any athletic benefit and in some cases can be detrimental. A well-rounded diet will provide adequate mineral intake and supplements are unnecessary. Two exceptions to this rule can be calcium and iron. Calcium is vital to bone and tooth formation and is found primarily in dairy foods. Some athletes may be unable to tolerate dairy products because of lactose intolerance or milk allergy. In addition, amenorrheic athletes are at increased risk of bone loss and have a higher calcium requirement. In these instances, daily calcium supplementation with calcium carbonate may be indicated. Iron is a trace mineral vital to hemoglobin production. The best source for iron is red meat. Athletes who do not eat meat may have a difficult time ingesting adequate iron from other sources. In addition, women have a higher iron requirement because of menstrual blood losses and many long distance runners will also lose significant iron through GI losses. Iron supplementation may become necessary in these instances.

Other supplements that are frequently touted as having beneficial athletic effects such as bee pollen and ginseng are not effective beyond the placebo effect the athlete may derive. There is no substitute for a good diet and no pill or potion can compensate for poor nutritional practices or improve upon good nutritional practices.

DRUGS IN ATHLETICS

Drug use among athletes can be divided into two categories, drugs of abuse and performance-enhancing drugs. Athletes experience the same pressures and problems other people have. In addition, they are expected by teammates, coaches, and fans to perform at an extremely high, consistent level regardless of injury, illness, fatigue, or mood. These facts contribute to the frequency of drug use in the athlete; either to self-medicate mood or attempt to provide a performance edge against the competition. Alcohol and drug abuse is an extremely complicated subject and can only be touched upon superficially. It is vital that the team physician have access to a qualified and interested drug counselor to assist in these problems when they are discovered. The following are brief descriptions of the most common drugs used and abused by the athletic population.

Alcohol

Alcohol is the number one drug of abuse in the United States. It should not be any surprise that it is also the most common drug problem among athletes. The effects of alcohol are well known to most people. Following a significant ingestion, there is initially a sense of euphoria and disinhibition that is followed by mental depression and stupor. Alcohol poses a danger for several reasons. The person under the influence of alcohol has impaired judgment and reaction times, placing them at risk for accidents and injury. The acutely intoxicated individual is more likely to engage in illegal activities, have violent confrontations, and attempt suicide than when sober. In addition to these more acute dangers, there can be significant long-term changes in personality, deterioration of schoolwork and athletic performance, health problems such as pancreatitis or cirrhosis, and alienation from friends and family. Alcohol abuse is therefore a potentially serious problem and should not be ignored or minimized. The coaching, athletic training, and medical staffs for an athletic team should maintain a high degree of suspicion and alertness for alcohol-related problems among team members. If an athlete is suspected of having a problem, he or she should be thoroughly evaluated and treated by an experienced clinician. The impetus for this intervention should be based upon concern for the athlete's welfare and not upon punitive reasons.

Alcohol is sometimes used by marksmen competing in riflery or archery events in order to reduce resting tremors and thereby improve sighting and aiming. This effect is offset by difficulty in concentration and eye tracking and is usually not effective and should certainly be discouraged. In a related example, archers and marksmen will frequently use the B1-blocking blood pressure medications for a similar purpose. It should be related to these athletes that this practice is banned by all relevant governing bodies including the United States Olympic Committee (USOC).

Marijuana

Marijuana (tetrahydrocannabinol) is probably the second most common drug of abuse among athletes. The drug is obtained from the plant *Cannabis sativa* and is most frequently obtained by smoking the leaves. The drug is a mild hallucinogen and leads to a feeling of increased sensory awareness, euphoria, and sedation. Heavy use can induce frank psychosis. The drug has direct adverse effects upon athletic performance by interfering with balance, muscle strength, coordination, and judgment. With frequent use, the individual will frequently experience subtle personality changes that often lead to complacency and a decreased motivation to succeed. This can have a profound impact upon the athlete's ability to maximize athletic potential and can also cause disruptions among team members. Another major concern regarding marijuana use is its well-described role as a stepping stone to use of other more dangerous drugs such as cocaine or narcotics.

Cocaine

Cocaine is an alkaloid chemical obtained from the leaves of the coca bush. It is extremely powerful and has high addictive potential after even one use. The drug, most often in the form of a white powder, is usually inhaled, "snorted," through the nose where it is absorbed across the mucous membranes. The drug acts by stimulating the central nervous system and increasing catecholamine activity. This has the effect of producing a sense of heightened awareness, increased energy, and elevated mood. The user feels an overall sense of empowerment and euphoria. However, when the effects of the drug wear off, the user almost always enters into a period of depression or letdown, which can be of equal intensity as the initial euphoria. This depression can often only be alleviated by recurrent use of the drug, and over time higher doses and more frequent use are required to get the desired effect. The user thus becomes trapped in an endless cycle and obtaining the drug often takes precedence over every other aspect of the person's life.

In addition to these potentially devastating problems, the heavy cocaine user is at risk for catastrophic cardiac problems and sudden death. The example of the death of Len Bias dramatically demonstrates this concern. The use of cocaine should therefore be thought of as a serious and potentially deadly habit. All athletes should be counseled about these dangers during preseason health evaluations and other opportunities.

Amphetamines

Amphetamines are central nervous system stimulants that are chemically related to epinephrine. When taken, they act upon the brain to increase alertness and often elevate mood. In this regard, their effects are similar to cocaine. Amphetamines are taken by some athletes to reduce fatigue, uplift mood, and to increase drive and motivation. Amphetamines are often taken to compensate for poor sleeping habits or to extend activity longer than would otherwise be tolerated. Some athletes also feel they improve performance, although this has never been demonstrated. The problem occurs when the medications are discontinued and the user "crashes" and suffers prolonged periods of depression, fatigue, and exhaustion. While taking amphetamines, the athlete may not recognize significant injuries due to the drugs' ability to mask pain. In addition, the user is at risk for cardiac arrhythmias, heat stroke, severe hypertension, and sudden death while taking amphetamines. Fortunately, these drugs are less popular now than in the past but they are still encountered in the athletic population.

Anabolic Steroids

Anabolic steroids are chemical derivatives of the male hormone testosterone. They were initially developed to provide anabolic (muscle and tissue building) effects without the androgenic (male sex characteristic) effects of natural testosterone. Since the effect of these drugs is to increase muscle bulk and strength, they have become widely misused in athletics by athletes attempting to gain an edge over the competition. It has been estimated that over 1 million athletes currently use steroids, many of high school age (76). It has also been estimated that at least 20% of athletes who routinely train in weight rooms use steroids (27). It has become commonplace at the Olympic games and other events for competitors to be disqualified for having been found to use these drugs. Since the use of these drugs is felt to represent a significant violation of the etiquette of sportsmanship, many athletes are routinely screened for their use. Unfortunately, as the ability to detect these drugs on screening urinalysis has improved, so too has the ability of athletes to disguise their drug use by various means.

Aside from the ethical concerns raised by the use of these drugs to gain unfair advantage, there are several significant medical problems that these drugs can cause. These include hepatitis, liver cancer, acne, hypertension, decreased libido, testicular atrophy, and stunted bone growth in children. In addition, these drugs can frequently cause aggressive thoughts and actions (steroid rage) that can contribute to lawlessness and personal injury. These drugs are therefore very dangerous to the individual using them and the people responsible for the training and care of athletes need to be observant for signs of their use. The strength coach is often in the best position to recognize unnatural gains in size and strength, particularly over brief time periods such as summer break. Athletes with hypertension, hepatitis, or recent onset of acne should also be assessed for steroid use.

Drug Screening

Many athletic organizations have instituted mandatory urine drug screening programs for all athletes. These include the NCAA and the International Olympic Committee (IOC). Many university and even some high school athletic programs have similar policies in place. The purpose of these programs is to ensure fairness of athletic competition, promote health among athletes, and attempt to identify those athletes in need of help due to a drug problem. Most drug screening programs involve random, unannounced urine collection that is then analyzed in a laboratory for various substances. These can include alcohol, marijuana, amphetamines, barbiturates, steroids, opiates, and cocaine. It is vital that a firm and well-understood policy be developed for cases of positive screening. The purpose of the policy should be to identify and give assistance to those athletes who require it, and should not rely on punitive measures. However, in cases of recurrent problems athletes should be aware that their athletic eligibility will be jeopardized. Regardless of how this policy is developed, it should be strictly enforced without exception for the player's importance or status on the team. There should be an identified person (usually the head athletic trainer or team physician) who is responsible for the oversight and review of the drug testing program. Recently, the Supreme Court upheld the legality of mandatory drug testing among high school athletes and this ruling will no doubt spur the development of more of these programs. A substance abuse prevention and testing model for college student athletes can be found in Chapter 1 and Appendix C.

INSECT STINGS

During the spring and summer months, athletes participating in outdoor sports are frequently stung by insects. Most of these incidents result in only local swelling and pain at the site of the sting. However, between 0.3% and 3% of insect stings will result in systemic anaphylaxis in susceptible patients. Some of these reactions have the potential to rapidly develop into life-threatening emergencies. It is estimated that around 50 to 100 people die each year in this country because of insect stings (42). It is therefore important that the medical team caring for athletes be prepared to handle these situations.

Stinging insects are members of the order Hymenoptera of the class Insecta. There are two major subgroups of stinging insects: the vespids, which include the yellow jacket, hornet, and wasp, and the apids, which include the honeybee and bumblebee. The yellow jacket is the most common cause of allergic insect stings in most parts of the United States largely because of the fact they nest in the ground and are frequently disturbed by outdoor activities. Fire ants are another frequent cause of anaphylactic reactions. The usual reaction to an insect sting is localized pain, swelling, and erythema at the sting site. This reaction usually improves over several hours and requires no treatment other than cold compresses and analgesia. The stinger, if present, should be removed by scraping it off the skin with a flat object such as the end of a credit card. During removal care should be taken not to squeeze the venom sac, which may remain attached. Although unlikely to occur, the sting site should be observed for the possible development of a secondary cellulitis and treated appropriately should this occur. If the local reaction is more extensive, the patient can be treated with oral antihistamines such as diphenhydramine at a dose of 50 mg every 6 hours. Oral prednisone can also be of benefit in extensive local reactions, usually at a dose of 40 mg a day for 2 to 3 days (58).

The presentation of full-blown anaphylactic reaction is a dramatic and often terrifying experience for the patient and those who witness it. Unfortunately, other than the patient having a prior history of anaphylaxis, there is no way to determine which athletes are at risk for anaphylaxis after an insect sting. The condition may develop in patients who have been stung many times without any problems in the past. Anaphylactic symptoms usually begin within 10 to 20 minutes following the sting, although occasionally they can occur many hours later. The most common symptoms are related to the skin and consist of generalized urticaria (hives), flushing, and angioedema (swelling). These symptoms alone can usually be managed with close observation and oral antihistamines. Life-threatening symptoms include edema of the upper airways, circulatory collapse, shock, and bronchospasm. These symptoms result in the patient showing evidence of difficulty breathing and hypotension. Any respiratory distress following an insect sting should be considered a potential medical emergency.

The treatment for anaphylaxis because of insect stings is identical to that for anaphylaxis of any other cause. The patient should be gently reassured and calmed as much as possible. Transportation to the nearest hospital, usually via rescue squad should be immediately arranged. The initial treatment for life-threatening symptoms is subcutaneous epinephrine hydrochloride in a 1:1000 dilution at a dose of 0.3 to 0.5 mL (43). This should be repeated every 10 to 15 minutes as necessary up to three doses. Intravenous epinephrine is rarely required in cases of severe hypotension, respiratory compromise, and shock. Intramuscular antihistamines such as diphenhydramine can alleviate urticaria and itching. The dose is 50 mg intramuscularly. Oxygen, if available, should be administered as well. Steroids (such as intravenous methylprednisolone followed by 2 to 3 days of oral prednisone) are often given to reduce risk of recurrence.

Athletes with a history of anaphylaxis to insect stings are at risk for recurrent reactions with subsequent stings. They should therefore be counseled to reduce risk of sting by wearing shoes, long pants, and long-sleeved shirts as much as possible outdoors. Brightly colored clothing attracts insects and should be substituted with darker clothes if possible (obviously a team's uniform color will impact

this). Patients should be provided with epinephrine for emergency use should a reaction occur. This is available in preloaded syringes (Ana-Kit or Epi-Pen) and patients can be easily taught to self-administer medication. Antihistamines should also be carried to alleviate hives and angioedema. Patients should also be considered for venom immunotherapy performed by an allergist to reduce risk of recurrence. Since it is impossible to tell which athletes may develop anaphylaxis and since many practice sites are far removed from easy medical access, it may be advisable to equip either the athletic trainer or coach with preloaded epinephrine syringes and to provide training in how to recognize and initially manage an anaphylactic reaction.

GENERAL REFERENCES

Berning JR, Steen SN, eds. *Sports nutrition for the 90's; the health professional's handbook.* Gaithersburg, MD: Aspen Publishers, 1991.

Dornbrand L, Hoole AJ, Pickard CG, eds. *Manual of clinical problems in adult ambulatory care.* 2nd ed. Boston: Little, Brown and Company, 1992.

Du Vivier A. *Atlas of clinical dermatology,* 2nd ed. London: Gower Medical Publishing, 1993.

Goroll AH, May LA, Mulley AG Jr, eds. *Primary care medicine; office evaluation and management of the adult patient,* 3rd ed, Philadelphia: J. B. Lippincott Co, 1995.

Habif TP. *Clinical dermatology,* 2nd ed. St. Louis: C.V. Mosby Co, 1990.

Kulund DN, ed. *The injured athlete,* 2nd ed. Philadelphia: J.B. Lippincott Company, 1988.

Martin H, Thrasher D. Chemical dependency and treatment of the professional athlete. In: Lawson GW, Lawson AW, eds. *Alcoholism and substance abuse in special populations.* Rockville, MD: Aspen Publishers, 1989.

Strauss RA ed. *Sports medicine,* 2nd ed. Philadelphia: WB Saunders Company, 1984.

Trobe JD. *The physicians guide to eye care.* San Francisco: American Academy of Ophthalmology, 1993.

REFERENCES

1. Ades PA. Preventing sudden death. *Phys Sportsmed* 1992;20:75.
2. American College of Physicians Task Force on Adult Immunization. Guide for adult immunization. Philadelphia: American College of Physicians, 1994.
3. American College of Sports Medicine. American College of Cardiology. 26th Bethesda Conference: Recommendations for Determining Eligibility for Competition in Athletes with Cardiovascular Abnormalities. *Med Sci Sports Exerc* 1994;26:S223.
4. American College of Sports Medicine. Position Stand. Physical activity, physical fitness, and hypertension. *Med Sci Sports Exerc* 1993;25:i.
5. Arroll B, Beaglehole R. Does physical activity lower blood pressure: a critical review of the clinical trials. *J Clin Epidemiol* 1992; 45:439.
6. Bailey RE. Diagnosis and treatment of infectious mononucleosis. *Am Fam Phys* 1994;49:879.
7. Bergfeld J, Lombardo J, Nelson M, Robinson J, Smith D, Wilkerson L. Preparticipation Physical Evaluation (PPE). American Academy of Family Physicians, American Academy of Pediatrics, American Medical Society for Sports Medicine, American Orthopaedic Society for Sports Medicine, American Osteopathic Academy of Sports Medicine, 1992.
8. Browne RJ, Gillespie CA. Sickle cell trait, a risk factor for life-threatening rhabdomyolysis? *Phys Sportsmed* 1993;21:80.

9. Burke LM, Read RSD. Diet patterns of elite Australian male triathletes. *Phys Sportsmed* 1987;15:140.

10. Centers for disease control. HIV prevalence estimates and AIDS case projections for the United States. *MMWR* 1990;39:5.

11. Center RM, Meier FA, Dalton HP. Throat cultures and rapid tests for diagnosis of group A streptococcal pharyngitis. In: Sox HC Jr, ed. *Common diagnostic tests: use and interpretation*, 2nd ed. Philadelphia: American College of Physicians, 1990:247.

12. Centor RM, Meier FA. Sore Troat. In: Dornbrand L, Hoole AJ, Pickard CG, eds. *Manual of clinical problems in adult ambulatory care*, 2nd ed. Boston: Little, Brown and Company, 1992.

13. Chalmers TC. Effects of ascorbic acid on the common cold: an evaluation of the evidence. *Am J Med* 1975;58:532.

14. Clark N. *Sports Nutrition Guidebook*. Champaign: Leisure Press, 1990.

15. Dolin R, Reichman RC, Madore HP, et al. A controlled trial of amantadine and rimantadine in the prophylaxis of influenza A infection. *N Engl J Med* 1982;307:580.

16. Dommerby H, Stangerup SE, Stangerup M, Hancke S. Hepatosplenomegaly in infectious mononucleosis, assessed by ultrasonic scanning. *J Laryngol Otol* 1986;100:573.

17. Douglas RG. Prophylaxis and treatment of influenza *N Engl J Med* 1990;332:443.

18. Drugs for asthma. *Med Lett Drugs Ther* 1995;37:1.

19. Drugs for hypertension. *Med Lett Drugs Ther* 1995;37:45.

20. Drugs for treatment of acute otitis media in children. *Med Lett Drugs Ther* 1994;36:19–21.

21. Eichner ER. ''Sports anemia'': poor terminology for a real phenomenon. *Sports Science Exchange* 1988;1:6.

22. Eichner ER. Hematuria—a diagnostic challenge. *Phys Sportsmed* 1990;18:53.

23. Eichner RA. Infection, immunity and exercise. *Phys Sportsmed* 1993;21:125.

24. Epstein SE, Maron BJ. Sudden death and the competitive athlete: perspectives in pre-participation screening studies. *J Am Coll Cardiol* 1986;7:220.

25. Evans EG, Seaman RA, James IG. Short duration therapy with terbinafine 1% cream in dermatophyte skin infections. *Br J of Derm* 1994;130:83.

26. Executive Summary: guidelines for the diagnosis and management of asthma. National asthma education program expert panel report. NIH publication no. 91-3042A, 1991.

27. Frankle MA, Cicero GJ, Payne J. Use of androgenic anabolic steroids by athletes. *JAMA* 1984;260:3441.

28. Glassock JR. Postural (orthostatic) proteinuria: no cause for concern. *N Engl J Med* 1981;305:639.

29. Goldsmith MF. When Sports and HIV share the bill, smart money goes on common sense. *JAMA* 1992;267:1311.

30. Goldszer RC, Siegel AJ. Renal abnormalities during exercise. In: Strauss RH, ed. *Sports Medicine*, 2nd ed. Philadelphia: WB Saunders, 1991:156.

31. Gonzales R, Sande M. What will it take to stop physicians from prescribing antibiotics in acute bronchitis. *Lancet* 1995;345:665.

32. Grosse SJ, Lynch JM. Treating auricular hematoma. *Phys Sportsmed* 1991;19:98.

33. Hamel R. AIDS: assessing the risk among athletes. *Phys Sportsmed* 1992;20:139.

34. Harris SS, Tanner S. Helping active women avoid anemia. *Phys Sportsmed* 1995;23:35.

35. Hoffman TJ, Schelkun PH. How I manage athlete's foot. *Phys Sportsmed* 1995;23:29.

36. Hueston WJ. Albuterol delivered by metered-dose inhalor to treat acute bronchitis. *J Fam Pract* 1994;39:437.

37. Kaplan NM, Deveraux RB, Miller HS Jr. Systemic Hypertension. Task force 4, 26th Bethesda Conference. *Med Sci Sports Exerc* 1994;26:S268.

38. Kris-Etherton PM. The facts and fallacies of nutritional supplements for athletes. *Sports Science Exchange* 1989;2:18.

39. La montagne JR, Noble GR, Quinnan GV, et al. Summary of clinical trials of inactivated influenza vaccine–1978. *Rev Infect Dis* 1983; 5:723.

40. Lemon PWR, Influence of dietary protein and total energy intake on strength improvement. *Sports Science Exchange* 1989;2.

41. Lombardo JA. Preparticipation physical evaluation. *Primary Care: Clinics in Office Practice* 1984;11:3.

42. Mackan MD. Managing the patient with anaphylaxis, mechanisms and manifestations. *Emergency Medicine* 1995;27:68.

43. Mackan MD. Managing the patient with anaphylaxis, therapeutic strategies. *Emergency Medicine* 1995;27:20.

44. Magnes SA, Henderson JM, Hunter SC. What conditions limit sports participation?. *Phys Sportsmed* 1992;20:143.

45. Maki MG, Reich RM. Infectious mononucleosis in the athlete. Diagnosis, complications, and management. *Am J Sports Med* 1982;10: 162.

46. Maron BJ, Roberts WC, McAllister HA, Rosing DR, Epstein SE. Sudden death in young athletes. *Circulation* 1980;62:218.

47. Massie B. To combat hypertension, increase activity. *Phys Sportsmed* 1992;20:89.

48. McKeag DB. Preseason physical examination for the prevention of sports injuries. *Sports Med* 1985;2:413.

49. McFadden ER, Gilbert IA. Exercise-induced asthma. *N Engl J Med* 1994;330:1364.

50. Mohr DN, Offord KP, Owen RA, et al: Asymptomatic microhematuria and urologic disease, a population based study. *JAMA* 1986; 141:350.

51. Naclerio RM. Allergic Rhinitis. *N Engl J Med* 1991;325:860.

52. 1994-95 NCAA Sports Medicine Handbook. *NCAA* 1994.

53. O'Driscoll BR, Kalra S, Wilson M, Pickering CAC, Carroll KB, Woodcock AA. Double-blind trial of steroid tapering in acute asthma. *Lancet* 1993;341:324.

54. Orr PH, Scherer K, Macdonald A, Moffatt MEK. Randomized placebo-controlled trials of antibiotics for acute bronchitis: a critical review of the literature. *J Fam Pract* 1993;36:507.

55. Peggs JF, Reinhardt RW, O'Brien JM. Proteinuria in adolescent sports physical examination. *J Fam Pract* 1986;22:80.

56. Prevention, Diagnosis, and Management of Viral Hepatitis, a guide for primary care physicians. American Medical Association, 1995.

57. Quinnan GV, Schooley R, Dolin R, Ennis FA, Gross P, Gwaltney JM. Serologic responses and systemic reactins in adults after vaccination with monovalent and trivalent influenza vaccines. *Rev Infect Dis* 1983;5:784.

58. Reisman RE. Insect stings. *N Engl J Med* 1994;331:523.

59. Reichman RC, Badger GJ, Mertz GJ, et al. Treatment of recurrent genital herpes simplex infections with oral acyclovir. *JAMA* 1984; 251:2103.

60. Rich BSE. Sudden death screening. *Med Clin North Am* 1994;78 267.

61. Rooney JF, Straus SE, Mannix ML, et al. Oral acyclovir to supress frequently recurrent herpes labilis, a double-blind placebo-controlled trial. *Annals Int Med* 1993;188:268.

62. Sears MR, Taylor DR, Print CG, et al. Regular inhaled beta-agonist treatment in bronchial asthma. *Lancet* 1990;336:1391.

63. Seltzer DG. Educating athletes on HIV disease and AIDS, the team physicians' role. *Phys Sportsmed* 1993;21:109.

64. Sherman WM, Costill DJ, Fink WJ, Miller JM. Effect of exercise-diet manipulation on muscle glycogen and its subsequent utilization during performance. *Int J Sports Med* 1981;2:114.

65. Sherman WM, Albright A. Exercise and type II diabetes. *Sports Science Exchange* 1992;4:37.

66. Sherry P. Sickle cell trait and rhabdomyolysis, case report and review of the literature. *Mil Med* 1990;155:59.

67. Short SH, Short WR. Four year study of university athlete's dietary intake. *J Am Diet Assoc* 1983;82:632.

68. Siegel AJ, Hennekens CH, Solomon HS, et al. Exercise-related hematuria, findings in a group of marathon runners. *JAMA* 1979; 241:391.

69. Spruance SL, Stewart JCB, Rowe NH, McKeough MB, Wenerstrom G, Freeman DJ. Treatment of recurrent herpes simplex labialis with oral acyclovir. *J Infect Dis* 1990;161:185.

70. Straus SE, Cohen JI, Tosato G, Meier J. NIH conference, Epstein-Barr virus infections: biology, pathogenesis, and management. *Annals Int Med* 1993;118:45.

71. Stewart JG, Ahlquist DA, McGill DB, et al. Gastrointestinal blood loss and anemia in runners. *Annals Int Med* 1984;100:843.

72. Sullivan SN. Overcoming runner's diarrhea. *Phys Sportsmed* 1992; 20:63.

73. Summary of a report on assessment of the iron nutritional status of the United States population. Expert Scientific Working Group. *Am J Clin Nutr* 1985;42:1318.
74. Sutton JM. Evaluation of hematuria in adults. *JAMA* 1990;263: 2475.
75. Taunton JE, McCargar L. Managing activity in patients who have diabetes. *Phys Sportsmed* 1995;23:41.
76. Taylor WN. *Hormonal manipulation: a new era of monstrous athletes*. Jefferson, NC: McFarland, 1985.
77. Van Camp SP. Sudden death in athletes. In: Grana WA, Lombardo JA, eds. Advances in sports medicine and fitness. Chicago: Year Book Medical Publishers, 1988:121.
78. Vehaskari VM, Rapola J. Isolated proteinuria: analysis of a school-age population. *J Pediatr* 1982;101:661.
79. Williams JW Jr, Simel DL, Roberts L, Sanga GP. Clinical evaluation for sinusitis. *Annals Int Med* 1992;117:705.
80. Zinnmann B, Vranic M. Diabetes and exercise. *Med Clin North Am* 1985;69:145.

The Injured Athlete, Third Edition,
edited by D. H. Perrin.
Lippincott–Raven Publishers, Philadelphia © 1999.

CHAPTER 3

Principles of Training

Arthur Weltman and Russell R. Pate

Successful participation in athletic activities requires preparation. Such preparation, often called training, might be described as the systematic participation in physical exercise for the purpose of improving performance in an athletic activity. The process of training can be interpreted broadly to include learning of competitive strategies, perfection of motor skills, and establishment of a proper psychological outlook. We will primarily focus here on the physical fitness aspect of athletic performance, provide guidelines for the improvement of basic fitness components in athletes, and give primary emphasis to training for improved endurance performance. In addition, however, we will also provide information on the health versus fitness benefits of regular physical activity and training.

PHYSIOLOGIC BASES OF EXERCISE

Metabolic Systems

Performing an athletic activity depends on the contraction of skeletal muscles, and the energy that fuels these contractions is provided through a complex series of chemical reactions localized in the individual skeletal muscle cells (fibers). The single immediate source of this chemical energy is adenosine triphosphate (ATP). During contraction, ATP, a high-energy phosphate compound, is hydrolyzed to adenosine diphosphate (ADP), inorganic phosphate (Pi) and energy. The breakage of ATP's terminal high-energy phosphate bond releases energy used by the muscle fiber to cause contraction. In the process of muscular contraction ATP is continually hydrolyzed to ADP + Pi + energy, and

A. Weltman: Department of Human Services, University of Virginia, Charlottesville, Virginia 22903
R. R. Pate: Department of Exercise Science, University of South Carolina, Columbia, South Carolina 29208

ADP is continually being reenergized back to ATP by phosphorylation (13).

Because only a very small concentration of ATP is maintained in the muscle fiber, sustained or repetitive muscle contractions depend on rapid resynthesis of ATP. The energy to support this resynthesis is provided by immediate, nonoxidative, and oxidative energy sources (13,26). A depiction of the energy sources used for muscular contraction as a function of duration of exercise is shown in Fig. 3.1.

Immediate Energy Sources

At the onset of muscular work ATP is rapidly used and must be continually replenished. The immediate sources of energy in the muscle are composed of three components (13). These sources are so named because they are immediately available to support muscular contraction. First, there is ATP itself. A small amount of ATP is stored within the muscle. ATP is broken down into ADP + Pi by enzymes that are generally referred to as ATPases. It is estimated that the muscle concentration of ATP is 6 mmol/kg. Assuming that a 70 kg man has 30 kg of muscle mass and ATP yields 10 kcal/mol, stored ATP can provide 1.8 kcal of total energy (13).

The second intracellular high-energy phosphate source is creatine phosphate (CP). The role of CP is critical because it provides a reservoir of phosphate bond energy that can be tapped, thereby preventing any lag in the ATP supply (CP + ADP → ATP + C). CP exists in five to six times greater concentration in resting muscle than ATP (28 mmol/kg muscle). Again, assuming that a 70 kg man has 30 kg of muscle mass and ATP yields 10 kcal/mol, stored CP can provide 8.4 kcal of total energy (13).

The third source of immediate energy in the muscle involves the enzyme called myokinase. This enzyme has the ability to generate one ATP from 2 ADPs (ADP + ADP → ATP + AMP). It is estimated that the myokinase

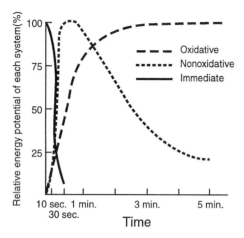

FIG. 3.1. Energy sources for muscle as a function of activity duration. The schematic presentations show the endurance of each of the major energy systems in supporting all-out work.

stimulated formation of ATP can provide 1 kcal of total energy (13).

Although ATP and CP stores that are maintained in the muscle fiber make up a critical energy reserve, at the onset of high-intensity exercise the available immediate energy sources (ATP, CP, and myokinase stimulated ATP) could, theoretically, be depleted in a few seconds. Clearly the total store of energy represented by ATP, CP, and myokinase stimulated ATP is too small (11 kcal of total energy for a 70 kg man with 30 kg of muscle) to support endurance exercise—that is, the capacity of the ATP-CP system is low. Its maximum power (rate of energy expenditure) is very high, however, and consequently the ATP-CP system is the predominant energy source for high-intensity, short-duration exercise (i.e., power activities—e.g., shot put, discus, power lifting).

Nonoxidative Energy Sources (Anaerobic Glycolysis)

Exercise of longer duration but lower intensity is supported, predominantly, by nonoxidative energy sources and metabolic pathways. This process does not require oxygen (nonoxidative), and involves the breakdown of stored muscle glycogen (muscle carbohydrate) and/or blood glucose (which must be taken up by muscle) through a sequentially arranged series of enzyme-catalyzed chemical reactions known as anaerobic glycolysis. In the skeletal muscle the concentration of free glucose is low and therefore most of the nonoxidative energy source comes from the breakdown of muscle glycogen. Glycogen is no more than a matrix of individual glucose molecules. In anaerobic glycolysis glucose is taken up into muscle from the blood and/or the stored muscle glycogen matrix is broken down. These substrates are enzymatically altered through a series of reactions so as to yield two pyruvic acid molecules. Without oxygen, pyruvic acid is converted to lactic acid. The process of glycol-

ysis releases an amount of energy from the glucose molecule sufficient to result in a net gain of two (glucose) or three (glycogen) ATP. As compared with the immediate sources of energy (ATP-CP system), the nonoxidative sources of energy (anaerobic glycolysis) result in the generation of less muscular power but greater available energy. In anaerobic glycolysis, the rate of energy production is limited by the maximum rate of the series of enzymatically stimulated chemical reactions that constitute the entire system, a rate slower than that of the ATP-CP system (which requires a single enzymatically stimulated chemical reaction). The total amount of nonoxidative energy released is limited by the amount of glycogen available (usually plentiful) and the person's maximal tolerance for the system's end-product, lactic acid (3.0 g/kg muscle). If lactic acid accumulates in the muscle, tissue acidosis and impaired functioning result, with fatigue being the outcome. Anaerobic glycolysis is a very important supplier of ATP energy during high-intensity exercise (e.g., sprinting) of moderate duration (5 seconds to 1 minute). In such forms of exercise the ability of the nonoxidative energy system (anaerobic glycolysis) to generate energy is well matched to the demands of the activity. However, it should be realized that the immediate and nonoxidative sources of energy combined only provide a small fraction of the energy available from oxidative energy sources. Intense muscular exercise lasting longer than 30 seconds cannot be sustained without the benefit of oxidative metabolism (see Fig. 3.1) (14).

Oxidative Energy Sources

Oxidative energy sources for muscle include glucose, glycogen, free fatty acids, and amino acids. Although glucose and glycogen can also serve as nonoxidative energy sources, the amount of ATP generated through oxidative mechanisms far exceeds nonoxidative generation of ATP. For example: glucose + O_2 (36 ATP + CO_2 + H_2O); glycogen + O_2 (37 ATP + CO_2 + H_2O; palmitate (a C_{16} free fatty acid) + O_2 (130 ATP + CO_2 + H_2O; alanine (an amino acid) (pyruvate, pyruvate + O_2 (15 ATP + CO_2 + H_2O.

As compared with immediate and anaerobic energy processes, aerobic metabolism is characterized by relatively low power but very high capacity. The amount of ATP energy that can be produced through prolonged aerobic metabolism (i.e., capacity) is quite large, being limited primarily by the person's store of oxidative energy sources (particularly muscle glycogen and blood glucose). Table 3.1 provides an estimate of the number of kcal available from oxidative energy sources.

In contrast, the power of the aerobic system is limited because it is restricted by the rate at which oxygen can be delivered to the active tissues by the cardiorespiratory system. The maximal aerobic power is usually expressed in terms of maximum oxygen consumption.

TABLE 3.1. *Estimation of energy available from muscle and liver glycogen, fat (adipose triglyceride), and body proteins*

	Energy equivalent (kcal)
Glycogen in muscle	480
Glycogen in liver	280
Fat (triglyceride in adipose)	141,000
Body proteins	24,000

The aerobic metabolic system is used preferentially during exercise intensities that can be sustained over time. Because the end-products of aerobic metabolism are not fatigue producing, for practical purposes, as long as the intensity of exercise does not result in fatigue-causing agents, the aerobic process may continue as long as substrate availability (i.e., muscle glycogen and/or blood glucose) is maintained.

As can be seen the immediate, nonoxidative, and oxidative energy sources are involved in energy systems that either do or do not require oxygen. The immediate energy system and the nonoxidative energy system do not require oxygen and are referred to as anaerobic. In contrast, the oxidative energy system is dependent on the presence of oxygen and is referred to as aerobic. Because of the different metabolic pathways associated with these energy systems, the capacity and power of these energy systems vary. Table 3.2 presents estimates of the maximal power and capacity of the three energy systems.

As can be seen, the power of the immediate energy system is quite high but its capacity is small compared with the oxidative energy system. Nonoxidative energy sources also generate high power (compared to oxidative energy sources) but here again its capacity is short-lived. In contrast, the oxidative energy system has high capacity but relatively low power. It should be realized that while a given exercise may rely on predominantly one source of energy, all three energy systems are always activated to some degree during exercise. This allows the three energy systems to function together to provide energy in activities ranging from all-out high-intensity and high-power performance to low-intensity sustained exercise.

Relation Between Aerobic and Anaerobic Metabolism

Some athletic activities involve forms of muscular work that derive the majority of ATP from a single metabolic process. The long jump in track and field, for example, is an activity that requires a very high rate of energy expenditure for only a few seconds, and consequently the anaerobic processes provide virtually all the required ATP. In contrast, a marathon run involves moderately intense activity sustained for several hours and energy is provided predominantly by oxidative energy sources. Many athletic activities, however, require that energy be

provided through a combination of the three energy-yielding systems. During the first few seconds of the 400-meter sprint (total duration, 40–60 seconds), for example, most energy comes through the breakdown of available ATP and CP stores. Rapidly, though, anaerobic glycolysis begins to predominate as the provider of ATP energy. Although anaerobic glycolysis continues to function at its maximum rate throughout the run, aerobic metabolism gradually increases to provide, in total, about 25% of the ATP used. Performance in the 400-meter sprint is a function of the maximal power of the three systems in combination and the capacity of the two anaerobic systems. World-class, 400-meter sprinters tend to have high anaerobic power, very high anaerobic capacity, and reasonably well-developed maximum aerobic power.

Maximal Aerobic Power

In athletic activities such as distance running and cycling, performance depends, in part, on the maximal aerobic power (VO_2 max) (13,26). The higher the VO_2 max, the greater the rate at which work may be done over extended periods and the longer the work may be done at any submaximal intensity. Thus the development of a high VO_2 max is beneficial for enhanced endurance performance.

As mentioned previously, VO_2 max is limited primarily by the maximum rate at which oxygen can be delivered to the active skeletal muscle. The cardiorespiratory system, which transports oxygen, plays a key role in supporting skeletal muscle metabolism during exercise and is comprised of four functional components: lungs and respiratory tract, heart, blood vessels, and blood. During exercise the overall system responds in such a way as to increase the rate of oxygen delivery to the active skeletal muscle, where the demand for oxygen increases markedly. Alterations in the functioning of each component contribute to this increased rate of oxygen transport.

Ventilation

As exercise begins, the rate and depth of breathing increase rapidly and substantially. Ventilation, regulated

TABLE 3.2. *Maximal power and capacity of the three energy systems*

System	Maximal power (kcal · min^{-1})	Maximal capacity (total kcal available)
Immediate energy sources (ATP + CP)	36	11.1
Nonoxidative energy sources (anaerobic glycolysis)	16	15.0
Oxidative energy sources (from muscle glycogen only)	10	480

by both neural and humoral factors, increases to a level sufficient to maintain adequate diffusion gradients across the alveolar membrane for exchange of both oxygen and carbon dioxide. At very high workloads, arterial blood is maintained at a nearly fully oxygenated level; consequently, for most persons, ventilatory function is not considered to be a factor limiting the VO_2 max. However, during extreme exercise that results in very high cardiac output, the transit time of red blood cells through the pulmonary capillary beds may decrease to a point in which a fall in arterial oxygen saturation may occur in some highly conditioned athletes (29).

Cardiac Output

The most important determinant of VO_2 max is the maximal cardiac output (Q max) (29). Cardiac output (Q), the volume of blood pumped by the heart per minute, increases rapidly at the beginning of steady state exercise but takes 2 to 3 minutes to reach a plateau. The level at which Q reaches a plateau is highly related to exercise intensity (and VO_2), and the relation between these two variables is linear up to Q max. Q max is attained at the same exercise intensity as VO_2 max and is equal to the product of maximal heart rate and maximal stroke volume. Heart rate is linearly related to exercise intensity, VO_2, and Q; maximal heart rate (HR max) is age related (HR max = 220 MS age in years) but is not related to fitness level. Stroke volume, the volume of blood pumped with each beat, is a function of heart size, venous filling pressure, ventricular volume, and myocardial contractility. Stroke volume increases with exercise and is thought to reach a maximum at workloads requiring about 50% of the VO_2 max. Maximal stroke volume increases with endurance training (as a result of increases in ventricular size, blood volume, and myocardial contractility) with little change in maximal heart rate. This results in an increased Q max, which in turn is reflected by a greater VO_2 max. Thus adaptations in myocardial function resulting in increased stroke volume represent a critical component of the body's response to endurance exercise training.

Blood Vessels

Vasomotor function supports exercise performance by redistributing the blood flow so as to increase oxygen delivery to the active skeletal muscles. Increased sympathetic tone, which occurs during exercise, results in a general vasoconstriction of blood vessels. The degree of vasoconstriction is related to the activity of the sympathetic nervous system, which in turn is related to intensity of exercise (increased intensity of exercise is associated with increased sympathetic activity). Local metabolites which accumulate at actively working muscle act to override this sympathetic vasoconstriction, resulting in a

shunting of blood to actively working muscle. During exercise, dilation of arterioles in active skeletal muscle and constriction of arterioles in inactive tissues (particularly the digestive system) may result in tripling of the blood flow to skeletal muscle. Increased blood flow is also provided to the skin during prolonged exercise, a response that facilitates dissipation of heat to the environment. In thermal neutral environments the increased blood flow to the skin does not appear to compromise endurance performance; however, in hot, humid conditions the skin may require a fraction of the cardiac output high enough to decrease significantly the fraction provided to the working muscles. With exercise, the volume of the venous system is reduced through a general vasoconstriction of venules, a response that tends to promote return of blood to the heart.

Arteriovenous Oxygen Difference

As indicated by the Fick equation, VO_2 is equal to the product of cardiac output and arteriovenous oxygen difference (a $-\bar{v}O_2$ difference). The oxygen-carrying capacity of the arterial blood is 200 mL of oxygen per liter of blood; however, under resting conditions only about 25% of this oxygen is removed by the tissues. With exercise, arteriovenous oxygen difference increases as the tissue's demand for oxygen increases. With high-intensity exercise, total body a $-\bar{v}O_2$ difference (arterial oxygen content $-$ mixed venous blood oxygen content) reaches values as high as 75% to 80% of total oxygen delivery. Skeletal muscle tissue a $-\bar{v}O_2$ difference may reach values approaching 100% of total oxygen delivery.

Arteriovenous O_2 difference reflects the ability of the skeletal muscle tissue to use, in aerobic metabolism, the oxygen offered to it by the cardiorespiratory system. Endurance exercise training causes profound adaptations in the skeletal muscle tissue: specifically, increases in mitochondrial density, myoglobin concentration, and activity of aerobic enzymes. These changes are specific to those muscles recruited during training. Collectively the adaptations contribute to an increased maximal rate of aerobic metabolism in the active muscle tissue and an increased whole body VO_2 max.

In summary, the body's physiologic response to exercise includes an increased rate of aerobic metabolism in the active skeletal muscles, a metabolic response supported by the cardiorespiratory system, which in turn increases its rate of maximal blood flow to the active muscles. Cardiac, vasomotor, and ventilatory responses contribute to an increased rate of oxygen delivery to the working muscles. The physiologic response to endurance exercise training involves both central (i.e., cardiorespiratory) and peripheral (i.e., muscle tissue) adaptations: Central adaptation is manifested as an increased maximal cardiac output (due to an increase in stroke volume) and thus increased maximal rates of blood flow and oxygen delivery to the working muscles; peripheral adaptation allows an increased rate of oxygen use at the active muscle tissue for the production of ATP energy. The outcome of these adaptations is an increase in the person's tolerance for sustained, whole-body, moderately intense exercise.

DETERMINANTS OF ENDURANCE EXERCISE PERFORMANCE

Maximal Oxygen Consumption

As mentioned previously, VO_2 max (ml/kg/minute) is one determinant of exercise endurance performance. VO_2 max reflects the maximum rate at which ATP energy may be produced aerobically. VO_2 max per se is important as a determinant of performance in activities that require maximal rates of energy expenditure for 4 to 10 minutes. In such activities the athlete is able to work at or near VO_2 max throughout the competition, and, although anaerobic sources do contribute to the total energy supply, the aerobic process is predominant, contributing 75% to 90% of the total energy expenditure.

The Blood Lactate Response to Exercise

Recently it has been suggested that parameters measured during submaximal exercise are better markers of endurance performance than is VO_2 max. In particular, the blood lactate response to incremental exercise appears to be highly related to various types of endurance performance and has been described using a variety of terms including; the lactate threshold (LT), the maximal steady state, the anaerobic threshold, the aerobic threshold, the individualized anaerobic threshold, the lactate breaking point, and the onset of blood lactate accumulation. These various blood lactate concentrations (BLC) are considered to be accurate predictors of endurance performance, indices of "submaximal fitness," and useful tools for exercise prescription. It has been suggested that training intensity be based on the VO_2 or velocity associated with one or more of these blood lactate parameters (35). An example of the blood lactate response to incremental exercise (with some of the terminology used in the literature) is shown in Fig. 3.2.

The basis for using the blood lactate response to exercise as a tool for predicting endurance performance and designing training programs comes from the large volume of research that suggests that the blood lactate response to exercise is a better indicator of endurance performance than VO_2 max. The blood lactate response to incremental exercise appears to be highly related to various types of endurance performance. It is believed that the blood lactate response to exercise and VO_2 max are determined by different factors; with VO_2 max being dependent upon cardiovascular factors such as cardiac output and stroke

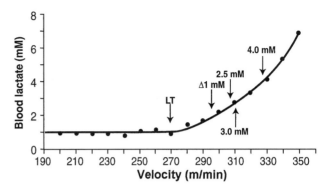

FIG. 3.2. Sample running protocol for the determination of the blood lactate response to exercise for a well-trained runner.

volume, and the blood lactate response to exercise being dependent upon peripheral factors such as muscle fiber type or the number of mitochondria. Because endurance exercise is performed at as high a percentage of VO_2 max as can be maintained over time, it is not surprising that an index of peripheral muscle function, such as blood lactate, would be a better predictor of endurance performance than VO_2 max (35).

Because the blood lactate response to exercise is a better indicator of endurance performance than VO_2 max, it is important to understand the effects of training on the various parameters of the blood lactate response to exercise. Several studies have reported a differential effect of training on the blood lactate response to exercise compared to VO_2 max. Virtually all of these studies have shown that the workload and VO_2 associated with various blood lactate parameters improve to a much greater degree with training than does VO_2 max. The available data suggest that, the blood lactate response to training adapts to a greater degree than VO_2 max, that this training adaptation is specific to the mode of training, and that changes in VO_2 max should not be the sole determinant of training adaptation. In addition, it appears that training to improve the blood lactate response to exercise is the type of training required to improve endurance performance (35).

Efficiency

Another important variable in endurance performance is efficiency (also referred to as economy). Efficiency, to the engineer, refers to the ratio of work done by a machine to energy used by it. In humans, with activities such as running or swimming, efficiency is often expressed as the rate of oxygen consumption (VO_2 in ml/kg/minute) needed to perform work at a given rate (e.g., running at 9.6 km/h [6 miles/h], or swimming at 6.75 m/minute [75 yards/minute]). Individual rates of oxygen consumption needed to work at a given pace vary, in part owing to differences in athletes' skill levels. The significance of work efficiency is seen when it is considered in combination with the VO2 max and the blood lactate response to exercise. The more efficient athlete needs a lower VO_2 at any given work rate, and therefore will work at a lower percentage of the maximal oxygen uptake at any given work rate and experience less fatigue; the athlete also will be able to work at a higher rate before reaching the lactate threshold.

Muscle Fiber Types

Physiologic variables such as VO_2 max, efficiency, and the lactate threshold all are subject to improvement through appropriate forms of training; however, each of these variables as well as potential for overall endurance performance are related to inherited, genetic factors. In recent years, studies have shown that a person's distribution of skeletal muscle fiber types is a major determinant of performance potential in certain athletic activities.

Human skeletal muscle fibers may be categorized as either fast twitch (FT) or slow twitch (ST). Fast twitch fibers are particularly well adapted for speed and power activities because they contract rapidly, possess metabolically a high glycolytic capability and generate high power relative to slow twitch fibers. These are the fibers that are well adapted to use immediate and nonoxidative energy sources. In contrast, ST fibers contract more slowly but are quite fatigue resistant because they possess a well-developed aerobic capability. Individuals vary greatly in the relative distribution of FT and ST fibers. Generally persons who inherit a high percentage of ST fibers possess greater potential for development of a high VO_2 max and a high lactate threshold, and thus greater potential for performing endurance activities. Indeed it has been shown that there is a strong direct relationship between the lactate threshold and percentage of ST fibers in competitive runners. Those who inherit a high percentage of FT fibers are better adapted to high-power activities. Performance in any athletic activity, however, is multifactorial and is not determined by any single variable. Muscle fiber type is only one variable, and it alone cannot be used to derive an accurate prediction of a person's current ability or ultimate performance potential.

PRINCIPLES OF TRAINING

Typical training programs comprise numerous specific training activities and techniques. Although selecting the proper individual activities is important, combining these activities in a complementary fashion so that the result is an optimal overall training program is crucial. Adherence to the following principles should aid coaches, athletes, athletic trainers, and team physicians in designing proper comprehensive training programs.

Overload

Perhaps the most basic principle of training is overload. Most physiologic systems can adapt to functional demands that exceed those encountered in normal, daily life. Training often systematically exposes selected physiologic systems to intensities of work or function that exceed those to which the system is already adapted. A key, however, is to avoid excessive overload because physiologic systems cannot adapt to stresses too extreme and the risk of injury is elevated.

Consistency

There is no substitute for consistency in a training program. Successful athletes, almost without exception, adhere to a training regimen with extreme regularity for several years or more. Most physiologic systems require exposure to overloading activities three times a week or more. The required frequency of training, however, depends on the season, the athlete, activity, and the specific component of fitness. Thus a particular athlete might train 12 times a week during certain stages of the year and only three times a week at other stages; he or she might participate in endurance training six times a week and resistance training (e.g., weight lifting) three times a week.

Specificity

The effects of training are highly specific to the particular physiologic system overloaded, to the particular muscle groups used, and to the particular muscle fibers performing the work. No single training technique can produce any and all desired outcomes; commercial advertising claims to that effect should be rejected.

Because athletic performance usually depends on the development of several physical fitness components, most training programs should include several training techniques and several modifications of each specific technique. The swimmer's training program, for instance, might comprise a combination of swimming activities using various strokes, intensities, and variations. In addition, the swimmer might participate in stretching exercises for flexibility and resistance exercises for muscular strength and muscular endurance. However, it should be realized that the specificity of training concept suggests that swimming performance would not be enhanced by running or bike training.

Progression

Successful training programs plan for a steady rate of progression over a long period. If an athlete is to improve over several years of participation, his or her training program must progress so that the appropriate physiologic systems continue to be overloaded. At the same time, however, too rapid an increase of the training stress may lead to overtraining, exhaustion, and impaired performance. The job of the coach or athletic trainer is to structure training programs that continue to challenge the athlete but avoid excessive overload.

Individuality

No two programs are exactly alike physiologically, and thus no two athletes should be expected to respond exactly the same to a particular training regimen. Factors such as age, gender, maturity, current fitness level, years of training, body size, body composition, and psychological characteristics should be considered by the coach in designing each athlete's training regimen. In large groups in which absolute individualization of training programs may be impractical, the coach should strive for individualization by homogeneously grouping athletes. Successful teams are composed of successful individual athletes, and the optimal training program is that which best fits the needs of each team member.

Periodization

Periodization refers to the tendency for athletic performance to vary cyclically over time. Few athletes can sustain a peak performance level for more than a few weeks, and thus training and competitive schedules should be structured so that peak performances are attained at the desired time. Intense training and competition tend to bring the athlete to his optimal performance level. The key, of course, is to avoid attaining this level too early in the competitive season. Ideally the training program should build to maximum intensity one-half to two-thirds through the season so that peak performances are achieved during championship competitions at season's end.

Plateauing

In many athletes, performance tends to improve incrementally rather than steadily and smoothly. An athlete may spend weeks, months, or even years on a performance plateau, leading to considerable frustration. If the athlete and athletic trainer are certain that the training program has progressed properly, that illness is not a factor, and that the athlete has not attained his ultimate performance potential, the athlete should persevere and maintain confidence that a substantial improvement could occur at any time.

STRESS

Stress has been defined by Hans Selye, the famous stress researcher, as the body's nonspecific response to external stressors. When the body is exposed to extreme stressors for extended periods, the so-called stress syndrome is elicited, which may lead to a stage of exhaustion typified by fatigue, illness, and injury. Coaches, athletes, trainers, and team physicians must recognize that strenuous training represents a significant stressor which, if combined with other physical or psychological stressors, may lead the athlete into a stage of exhaustion. Such exhaustion, of course, is not consistent with optimal training or performance. Stress-induced exhaustion can be prevented by designing properly individualized training programs, by carefully observing the athlete for signs of fatigue (e.g., upper respiratory illness, blood shot eyes, loss of concentration), and by reducing the training load if the athlete encounters other unavoidable stressors (e.g., examinations, personal conflicts, change of environment). Sensitive coaches and athletic trainers can prevent most stress-related illnesses in their athletes. Programs that subscribe to the "survival of the fittest" philosophy, however, can expect to lose many athletes to preventable illness and injury.

Competitive Stress

Competition is physiologically and psychologically more stressful than training, and too frequent competitions pose great risk to the athlete. Athletes who compete too frequently are particularly prone to the stress-related difficulties mentioned above. Because sporting activities vary greatly in their physical demands, drawing a generalization on the optimal frequency of competition is not possible. One may conclude, however, that the more strenuous the activity, the less frequently one should engage in competition. Contrasting examples would be golfers who compete 4 days a week over a 30- to 40-week season and marathon runners who compete at the full marathon distance only two or three times a year.

GUIDELINES FOR TRAINING THE AEROBIC SYSTEM

As discussed above, energy used in endurance exercise is provided primarily through aerobic muscle metabolism, which depends on the transport of oxygen by the cardiorespiratory system. Improvements in endurance performance are attained primarily through increases in VO_2 max and the blood lactate response to exercise (i.e., the lactate threshold). These increases are secondary to muscle metabolic and cardiorespiratory functional alternations, which can be generated through proper forms of exercise training. This section summarizes the procedures to be followed in designing training programs for improved performance of aerobic exercise.

Modes of Exercise

Numerous specific forms of exercise may be used to generate improvements in aerobic work capacity. All proper aerobic activities increase the body's rate of aerobic metabolism, increase the heart rate, and allow these increases to be sustained for extended periods. Primary aerobic activities include those that allow metabolic and cardiorespiratory functions to be increased to a particular predetermined level and maintained at that level throughout the activity. Secondary aerobic activities, which include many of the popular recreational games and sports, cause a more intermittent increase in cardiorespiratory functions and are less easily regulated in terms of work intensity. Table 3.3 presents examples of primary and secondary aerobic activity.

Primary aerobic activities generate a training effect in less time than do secondary activities and are preferred for persons with impaired heart function in whom exercise intensity must be rigorously controlled. Many persons, however, find secondary aerobic activities more enjoyable, and enjoyment, of course, can promote adherence to an exercise regimen. For a given athlete, the ideal aerobic activity is that most similar to the activity for which he or she is training (principle of specificity) and to which he or she is most likely to adhere.

Frequency

Improvements in aerobic work capacity may be generated in secondary beginners with as few as two training sessions a week. Sedentary beginners, however, improve at close to the optimal rate with three to five sessions a week (7). In some athletes, daily training sessions may be needed to maintain an already high capacity for endurance work. In activities such as distance running and swimming, many athletes train twice a day. The advantages of twice-a-day training sessions have not been clearly documented, but apparently a high frequency of training contributes to a high-exercise caloric expenditure. The continually improving world standards in endurance activities may be partly due to the increasing amount of energy expended in training by today's world class athletes. The optimal training frequency for a given athlete is a function of his or her current fitness level, the relative importance of aerobic function in the particular activity for which he or she is training, and individual tolerance for training stress.

Duration

The average person attains an acceptable level of cardiorespiratory fitness by participating in a primary aerobic activity for a duration of 20 to 30 minutes three to five times a week. Sedentary beginners may need to start with intermittent exercise (e.g., alternate walking and jogging), building gradually to 20 to 30 minutes of continuous activity. Endurance athletes, of course, may need much longer durations of exercise to attain full potential; marathon runners and swimmers, for example, often train for 2 to 3 hours. For most team sports, however, athletes who regularly participate in continuous aerobic activity for one-half hour will develop a cardiorespiratory fitness level consistent with championship caliber performance.

Intensity

Intensity and duration of exercise determine the total caloric expenditure during a training session (5,7). Similar increases in fitness may be obtained with long duration low-intensity exercise as is seen with high-intensity, shorter duration exercise (5,7). For most individuals exercise intensity that is in the low to moderate range has been recommended as long as appropriate duration is incorporated (5,7). The American College of Sports Medicine recommends that training intensity be prescribed as 50% to 85% of VO_2 max (5). This corresponds to 60% to 90% of maximum heart rate or 50% to 85% of HR reserve (5,7). In individuals with a low level of initial fitness a reduced initial intensity of exercise (40% to 50% of VO_2 max) will be sufficient to elicit a training effect (5).

HR has been used as a guide for exercise intensity based on the relatively linear relationship between HR and VO_2. The assumption that is made is that 60 to 90% of HR max corresponds to 50% to 85% of VO_2 max. However, it should be realized that maximal HR declines with age and there are large interindividual differences in maximal HR. Use of an age-predicted rather than a measured maximal heart rate will increase the degree of variability associated with HR-based exercise prescription

TABLE 3.3. *Primary and secondary aerobic activities*

Examples of primary aerobic activities
- Walking
- Jogging/running
- Hiking
- Swimming
- Rowing
- Cycling
- Cross-country skiing
  Ice-skating, In-line skating

Examples of secondary aerobic activities
- Tennis
- Soccer
- Handball
- Racquetball
- Squash
- Basketball
- Dance

(5). The two most common techniques for determining an exercise HR range for training purposes are to use: (1) a straight percentage of HR max, and (2) the HR reserve method. As mentioned, the assumption that is made is that 60% to 90% of HR max corresponds to 50% to 85% of VO_2 max. If an individual's HR max is 200 beats per minute the target HR range would be 120 (60%) to 180 (80%) beats per minute. The HR reserve method (Karvonen) is applied as follows: (1) Subtract standing resting HR from maximal HR (can be estimated by using the formula— maximal HR = 220 − age) to obtain HR reserve, (2) calculate 50% and 85% of the HR reserve, (3) add each of these values to the resting HR to obtain the target HR range. For example, for a 20-year-old with a resting HR of 50 bpm the following HR range would be calculated: (1) Max HR = 220 − 20 = 200, (2) HR reserve = 200 − 50 = 150, (3) 50% HR reserve = 75, 85% HR reserve = 128, (4) HR range = 75 + 50 = 125 bpm to 128 + 50 = 178 bpm (5).

The techniques shown above provide a lower limit for training intensity. For trained persons, a somewhat higher intensity may be appropriate for sustained, continuous training. Very high-intensity training, at heart rates approaching maximum levels, is appropriate for some endurance athletes and for athletes striving to maximize both aerobic power and anaerobic capacity. Indeed recent data suggest that a more effective technique for determining training intensity may be based on the blood lactate response to exercise, rather than on a relative percentage of maximal heart rate (i.e., HR max). The basis for using the blood lactate response to exercise as a tool for predicting endurance performance and designing training programs comes from the large volume of research that suggests that the blood lactate response to exercise is a better indicator of endurance performance than VO_2 max. The blood lactate response to incremental exercise appears to be highly related to various types of endurance performance (35). It is believed that the blood lactate response to exercise and VO_2 max are determined by different factors; with VO_2 max being dependent upon cardiovascular factors such as cardiac output and stroke volume, and the blood lactate response to exercise being dependent upon peripheral factors such as muscle fiber type or the number of mitochondria (16,23,31,37). Because endurance exercise is performed at as high a percentage of VO_2 max as can be maintained over time, it is not surprising that an index of peripheral muscle function, such as blood lactate, would be a better predictor of endurance performance than VO_2 max. Recent data support the notion that VO2 max is not the best predictor of endurance performance and that blood lactate responses to submaximal exercise are better indicators of endurance. It has been suggested that VO_2 max and blood lactate responses to exercise are determined by different mechanisms, with VO_2 max related to cardiovascular function and blood lactate responses to exercise related to adaptations that occur within the muscle. This could explain why training results in local muscular changes that are disproportionate to central cardiovascular changes, and why LT and BLC are better predictors of endurance performance than VO_2 max (35).

Because the blood lactate response to exercise is a better indicator of endurance performance than VO_2 max, it is important to understand the effects of training on the various parameters of the blood lactate response to exercise. Several studies have reported a differential effect of training on the blood lactate response to exercise compared to VO_2 max. Virtually all of these studies have shown that the blood lactate response to training adapts to a greater degree than VO_2 max, that this training adaptation is specific to the mode of training, and that changes in VO_2 max should not be the sole determinant of training adaptation. In addition, it appears that training to improve the blood lactate response to exercise is the type of training required to improve endurance performance (35).

As presented above most accepted exercise prescription techniques rely on the use of the relative percent concept, with training intensity related to a percentage of maximal heart rate (HR max), heart rate reserve (HRR), or maximal oxygen consumption (5). However, the determination of training intensities associated with various blood lactate parameters using the relative percent concept is inaccurate. When the relative percent concept was examined previously, it was shown that training intensities in the range of 50% to 85% VO_2 max and 70% to 90% HR max and HRR resulted in large individual variations in levels of metabolic stress when the ventilatory threshold was used as the criterion measure (20,24). Because of the widespread use of this relative percent concept for exercise prescription, and because of the problems associated with the use of the ventilatory threshold, we decided to examine the use of the relative percent concept for prescribing exercise training intensity and relate this to various blood lactate parameters (35). Two groups of subjects were studied, a group of trained runners (VO_2 at LT = 52.7 mL/kg/minute; VO_2 max = 63.5 mL/kg/minute) and a group of sedentary women (VO_2 at LT = 22.3 mL/kg/minute; VO_2 max = 39.1 mL/kg/minute). In both groups the relative percent concept was a poor determinant of training intensity when various levels of blood lactate were considered important for exercise prescription.

For the male runners intensities of 90% HR max and 85% HRR were required for the majority of subjects to be above LT. Even higher heart rates were required when blood lactate levels of 2.0 mM, 2.5 mM, and 4.0 mM were examined. It was concluded that exercise prescription techniques that use the relative percent concept don't work well for male runners if training intensity is based on blood lactate levels. If LT is used then male runners would need to incorporate exercise at a minimum of 90% HR max, 85% HRR, or 90% VO_2 max as part of their training regimen. For 2.5 mM, 95% of HR max and HRR would be required. If 4.0 mM is used then intensities in excess of 95% HR max, HRR, or VO_2 max would be required for the majority of male runners to be training above 4.0 mM.

It could be argued that the relative percent method of exercise prescription was not designed for competitive athletes. However, similar results were observed when sedentary women were examined. For sedentary women, heart rates of 75% HR max and 55% HRR were required for the majority of women to be above LT. Even higher heart rates were necessary when blood lactate concentrations of 2.0 mM, 2.5 mM, and 4.0 mM were used (for 4.0 mM heart rates in excess of 95% HR max and HRR were required). Here again, for sedentary women the use of standard exercise prescription techniques, based on the relative percent concept, does not appear to be applicable when exercise is prescribed based on blood lactate concentrations.

A recent suggestion for the noninvasive determination of the blood lactate response to exercise has focused on the use of ratings of perceived exertion (RPE) (35). Ratings of perceived exertion are being used to prescribe exercise intensity, as well as to evaluate and monitor the level of physical activity during clinical exercise, during occupational tasks and during exercise training. The Borg scales for RPE (10,27) are presented in Tables 3.4 and 3.5.

There are a number of recent studies that have shown that a strong relationship exists between RPE and the blood lactate response to exercise. This relationship does not appear to be affected by gender, training state, type of exercise, specificity of training, or intensity of training (35).

We have examined several of these relationships in our laboratory. Seip et al. (30) examined the relationship between training state, the blood lactate response to exercise, and RPE. As expected, the trained runners ran at faster velocities, and had higher heart rates, oxygen uptake values, and ventilation levels at the lactate threshold and blood lactate concentrations of 2.0, 2.5, and 4.0 mM, than did the untrained subjects. However, in spite of these differences in physiology between individuals of differing training state, no differences were found for ratings of

TABLE 3.4. *Borg's ratings of perceived exertion scale*

6	No exertion at all
7	
8	Extremely light
9	Very light
10	
11	Light
12	
13	Somewhat hard
14	
15	Hard (heavy)
16	
17	Very hard
18	
19	Extremely hard
20	Maximal exertion

From Borg G. *An introduction to Borg's RPE-scale.* Ithaca, NY: Mouvement Publications, 1985. Copyright 1985 by Gunnar Borg. Reprinted by permission.

TABLE 3.5. *Category-ratio scale of perceived exertion*

0	Nothing at all	
0.5	Very, very weak	Just noticeable
1	Very weak	
2	Weak	Light
3	Moderate	
4	Somewhat strong	
5	Strong	Heavy
6		
7	Very strong	
8		
9		
10	Very, very strong	Almost max
*	Maximal	

A category-ratio perceived exertion scale: relationship to blood and muscle lactates and heart rate by Noble BJ, Borg GAV, Jacobs I, Ceci R, Kaiser P. *Medicine and science in sports and exercise.* **15**(6):523. Copyright 1981 by Gunnar Borg. Reprinted by permission of copyright holder.

perceived exertion. Independent of training state, the velocity at LT was associated with an RPE value of 11, an RPE of 14 was associated with a blood lactate level of 2.0 mM, 2.5 mM blood lactate concentration was related to an RPE of 14.5, and an RPE of 16.5 was related to 4.0 mM blood lactate.

Another study from our laboratory examined the effects of exercise mode on the relationship between RPE and blood lactate concentration (22). Although treadmill running resulted in higher heart rates and oxygen uptake values at the lactate threshold and blood lactate concentrations of 2.0, 2.5, and 4.0 mM, than did cycling, in both modes of exercise the velocity/power output at LT was associated with an RPE value of 10 to 11, a RPE of 13 to 14 was associated with a blood lactate level of 2.0 mM, 2.5 mM blood lactate concentration was related to a RPE of 14 to 14.5, and a RPE of 16 to 16.5 was related to 4.0 mM blood lactate.

A third study from our laboratory examined the effects of specificity of training on the relationship between the blood lactate response to exercise and RPE (12). In spite of the fact that the group that trained running improved LT to a much greater degree running compared to cycling, and in spite of the fact that the group that trained cycling only improved the LT during cycling, there were no differences in the RPE at LT. This was true independent of whether training was done running or cycling, whether testing was done on the cycle or the treadmill, or whether the evaluation was performed before or after training. In all cases the lactate threshold was associated with a RPE of about 10 to 11.

Another study from our laboratory examined the effects of training intensity on the relationship between the blood lactate response to exercise and RPE (21). Once again, in spite of a large differential training response in the women who trained above the LT compared to those women who trained at LT, no differences were observed between groups or over time for RPE values at the LT and BLC of 2.0 mM, 2.5 mM, and 4.0 mM. LT was associated with an RPE value of 11 to 12, an RPE of about 14 was associated with a blood lactate level of 2.0 mM, 2.5 mM blood lactate concentration was related to an RPE of 14 to 15, and an RPE of 16 to 17 was related to 4.0 mM blood lactate.

A recent study from our laboratory (33), examined whether the relationship between RPE, LT, and BLC (determined with an incremental protocol using 3-minute stages) remained constant during duration more typically seen with training (i.e., 30 minutes). Nine males (age = 24.7 ± 3.8 years) completed a continuous, incremental, level running treadmill protocol to determine the RPE (11.6, 14.9, 16.8, 18.9), VO_2 (3.2, 3.7, 3.9, 4.2 L/minute) and velocity (V) (168, 196, 215, 227 m/minute) at LT, BLC of 2.5 and 4.0 mM and peak. Subjects also completed three 30-minute runs at the V associated with the LT and BLC of 2.5 and 4.0 mM, with RPE, BLC and VO_2 measured every 5 minutes. The data revealed that during the 30-minute runs no significant differences existed between RPE, VO_2, and BLC from minute 10 to minute 30 and the associated RPE, VO_2, and BLC observed during the incremental protocol. For each individual subject a regression equation was generated from results obtained during the incremental protocol, in which BLC was predicted from RPE. The RPE values obtained during the 30-minute runs were used to predict BLC and the measured BLC was used to validate the use of RPE as a predictor of BLC. Correlations from this analysis ranged from r = 0.79 to r = 0.98 with total error (TE) ranging from 0.6 to 1.3 mM. Results of this study suggest that the use of RPE for prescribing exercise intensity is physiologically valid and has particular utility for exercise prescription in which the goal is to exercise at the LT or a given BLC.

The latest RPE/blood lactate study from our lab (34) examined whether RPE observed during an incremental (response) protocol could be used to produce target blood [HLa] of 2.5 mM and 4.0 mM during a 30-minute treadmill run at a constant RPE. RPE (15.3, 17.6, 19.1), oxygen uptake (VO_2) (3.31, 3.96, 4.00 L/minute), velocity (V) (198, 218, 223 m/minute), and heart rate (HR) (179, 185, 190 bpm) at blood [HLa] of 2.5 mM and 4.0 mM, and peak were determined for nine subjects (5 males, 4 females) during incremental exercise. Subjects then completed two 30-minute runs at the RPE corresponding to blood [HLa] of 2.5 mM (RPE 2.5 mM) and 4.0 mM (RPE 4.0 mM) measured during the incremental protocol. For both 30-minute runs, VO_2 was not different from VO_2 corresponding to either 2.5 or 4.0 mM blood [HLa] during the incremental test. During the 30-minute run at RPE 2.5 mM: (a) only during minute 25 to 30 was the blood [HLa] significantly different than 2.5 mM (3.2 + 0.6 mM, P < 0.05), (b) for the first 20 minutes HR was significantly lower than the HR at 2.5 mM during the incremental protocol, and (c) V did not differ from V at 2.5 mM during the incremental protocol. During the 30-minute run at RPE 4.0 mM: (a) blood [HLa] was not significantly

different from 4.0 mM, (b) HR at every time point was significantly lower than HR 4.0 mM during the incremental protocol, and (c) V was decreased over time by an average of 24.6 m/minute (P < 0.05). Because RPE from the response protocol was able to produce a blood [HLa] close to the criterion value during each 30-minute run, we conclude that RPE is a valid tool for prescribing exercise intensities corresponding to blood [HLa] of 2.5 mM and 4.0 mM.

The above data suggest that there is a consistent link (although not necessarily cause and effect) between the blood lactate response to exercise and ratings of perceived exertion. This relationship appears to be stable, independent of a number of factors including gender, training state, type of exercise, specificity of training, and intensity of training. Therefore, if an exercise prescription is based on the LT or BLC (at least up until 30 minutes of exercise and perhaps longer), RPE should be an effective tool. If LT is a desired training intensity then the individual should exercise at an RPE of 11 to 12, a RPE of 14 to 15 should be used to produce a BLC of 2.5, and a RPE of 16 to 17 should be appropriate to produce a BLC of 4.0 mM.

SPECIFIC TRAINING TECHNIQUES

Primary aerobic activities may be used in several specific ways. Of these aerobic activities, running has spawned the greatest range of training techniques, and these methods are discussed below. Many of the techniques described are easily adapted for use by swimmers and cyclists.

Continuous Activity

Perhaps the most commonly used aerobic training technique is continuous activity. With such activity, the heart rate or RPE is increased to a predetermined level and maintained at that level for the duration of the training session. The guidelines presented in the previous section apply most directly to continuous training. The intensity of continuous activity may be varied from one training session to the next. The bulk of the training for endurance activities should consist of continuous activity of moderate intensity (60% to 90% maximum heart rate or an RPE associated with a given blood lactate concentration, 12 to 16) and relatively long duration, so-called long, slow-distance training. The endurance athlete will benefit, however, from occasional bouts of higher intensity continuous training (greater than 90% of maximum heart rate or an RPE greater than 16) of moderate duration.

Interval Training

Interval training involves alternating periods of very intense work with periods of active recovery. Interval training is usually done in a controlled environment (e.g., a track) in which the duration of work and recovery periods may be accurately timed. Interval training offers the benefit of allowing the athlete to perform, in total, a considerable volume of very high-intensity exercise in a single training session. An endurance swimmer, for instance, might perform 20 repetitions of a 50-meter sprint with 30 seconds of recovery between each sprint; altogether the swimmer will have covered 1000 meters at very high intensity. All approaches to interval training require that the following variables be designated in advance: duration and intensity of the work interval, duration and intensity of the recovery period, and the number of repetitions. Intensity of exercise may be designated in terms of heart rate. During the work interval, heart rate should increase to 75% or more of the maximum heart rate; during recovery it should fall to about 60% of the maximum heart rate.

Repetition Training

Repetition training differs from interval training only in intensity of exercise during the work and recovery phases. The work phase of repetition training should be almost exhaustive and the recovery phase, almost complete. For instance, in a given repetition training session, an 800-meter runner might perform two 600-meter runs at race-pace with a full recovery intervening between the two.

Fartlek Running

Fartlek running involves a combination of techniques such that continuous, interval, and repetition training are used in a single session. Fartlek is a Swedish term meaning ''speed play'' and denotes that the various intensities of work are selected by the athlete on an unstructured basis. A typical Fartlek running session might involve an hour of continuous running during which the athlete runs, in random order, several fast sprints, interval runs, and repetition runs. Fartlek training may be conducted in an attractive environment (e.g., park or golf course) and thus may be a relatively enjoyable means for the athlete to participate in high-intensity exercise.

Circuit Training, Parcours

Circuit training provides a combination of training techniques and is particularly well adapted for groups. The individual athlete rotates through a series of stations and at each performs a different exercise. Circuit routines may include activities to improve muscular strength, muscular endurance, flexibility, and other fitness components. The training session can involve an alternation between continuous aerobic training and a series of strength and flexibility exercises.

A recently popularized modification of the circuit train-

ing concept is the parcours. A parcours is, essentially, a graded jogging trail along which exercise stations have been erected. The participant jogs from station to station, performing a different calisthenic exercise at each stop. Often attractive signs and suitable permanent equipment are provided at each exercise station.

In summary, the energy for sustained muscular work is provided through the process of aerobic metabolism. Performance of aerobic exercise depends on the cardiorespiratory system, which provides the active skeletal muscles with needed oxygen. One determinant of athletic performance in endurance activities is maximal oxygen uptake; however, more recently the lactate threshold has been shown to affect the rate at which work is done for extended periods.

Training programs should be designed in accordance with established principles of training. In training the aerobic system, research indicates that if a primary aerobic activity is used, 20 to 30 minutes of continuous activity three times a week at about 60% to 90% of maximum heart rate or at an RPE of 12 to 16 will result in the desired training effect.

Basic principles of exercise training are similar for everyone. But because each subgroup of the population possesses certain unique characteristics and needs, training programs should be tailored so as to optimize the benefits for the specific participant group. The following sections provide guidelines for the design of exercise training programs for several specific populations, including special training problems encountered by competitive athletes.

FITNESS PROGRAMS FOR ADULT BEGINNERS

Regular physical activity has long been recognized as an important component of a healthy lifestyle. Recent evidence has reinforced this concept as regular physical activity has been linked with a wide array of physical and mental health benefits (28). However, in spite of the overwhelming evidence about the benefits of regular physical activity, millions of adult Americans remain essentially sedentary. Recently the Centers for Disease Control and the American College of Sports Medicine presented a recommendation for physical activity and public health (28). The information that follows provides highlights of this special communication. The focus of the recommendation was on physical activity and the health benefits associated with regular physical activity. Physical activity was defined as ''any bodily movement produced by skeletal muscles that results in energy expenditure.'' Physical activity is closely related to, but distinct from, exercise and physical fitness. Exercise is a subset of physical activity defined as ''planned, structured, and repetitive bodily movement done to improve or maintain one or more components of physical fitness.'' Physical fitness is ''a set of attributes that people have or achieve that relates to the ability to perform physical activity.''

RELATIONSHIP BETWEEN PHYSICAL ACTIVITY AND HEALTH

Cross-sectional epidemiologic studies as well as controlled experiments have demonstrated that physically active adults develop and maintain higher levels of physical fitness than their sedentary counterparts. Most epidemiologic data support the notion that there is a protective effect between physical activity and developing risk for a variety of chronic diseases. These include coronary heart disease, hypertension, noninsulin-dependent diabetes mellitus, osteoporosis, colon cancer, and anxiety and depression (28).

In contrast, other studies have shown that low levels of regular vigorous physical activity and low levels of physical fitness are associated with increased all-cause mortality (25,28). It is estimated that as many as 250,000 deaths per year (12% of all deaths) can be attributed to a lack of regular physical activity. Fortunately, an increase in vigorous physical activity, even after years of sedentary behavior, is associated with a decreased risk of mortality (28).

There are also data reported from training studies that indicate that exercise training improves health-related factors including a more favorable blood lipid profile, lower resting blood pressure in borderline hypertensives, improved body composition (lower percent body fat and a reduction in intraabdominal visceral fat), improved glucose tolerance and insulin sensitivity, increased bone density (or a reduction in the rate of decline in bone), improved immune function, and improved psychological function (28).

Physical activity recommendations have been made in Healthy People 2000. One goal is to "increase to at least 30 percent the proportion of people aged 6 and older who engage regularly, preferably daily, in light to moderate physical activity for at least 30 minutes per day." However, only about 22% of adults are active at this level recommended for health benefits, 54% are somewhat active but don't meet this objective, and 24% or more are completely sedentary (28).

Participation in regular physical activity gradually increased during the 1960s, 1970s, and early 1980s, but seems to have plateaued in recent years (28). A lack of time is the most commonly cited barrier to participation in physical activity and injury is a common reason for stopping regular activity (28).

PHYSICAL ACTIVITY RECOMMENDATION FOR ADULTS

The CDC and ACSM argue that "the current low participation rate in regular physical activity may be due in part to the misperception of many people that to reap health benefits they must engage in vigorous, continuous exercise" (28). They suggest that the available scientific evidence clearly demonstrates that regular, moderate-intensity (defined as 3 to 6 METs or 4.7 kcal/minute) provides substantial health benefits. Based on the scientific literature the expert panel made the following recommendation: Every U.S. adult should accumulate 30 minutes or more of moderate-intensity on most, preferably all, days of the week.

This recommendation emphasizes the benefits of moderate-intensity exercise and of physical activity that can be accumulated in short bouts during the day (rather than one long bout). Adults who expend 200 calories per day in moderate physical activity can expect many of the health benefits of exercise. The unique aspects of this new recommendation are that (1) the health benefits of moderate-intensity physical activity are emphasized, and (2) accumulation of physical activity in intermittent, short bouts is considered an appropriate approach to achieving the activity goal (28). The health benefits of physical activity appear to be related to the total amount of activity performed, measured as either caloric expenditure or minutes of exercise.

In contrast, a recent study on exercise intensity and longevity in men indicated that although there was a graded inverse relationship between total physical activity and mortality, participation in vigorous activities (more than six METs) but not nonvigorous activities (less than six METs) were associated with longevity (25). These findings suggest that exercise prescription designed to improve physical fitness (i.e., include vigorous activity) is more beneficial than simply increasing physical activity for reducing all-cause mortality. However, it should be realized that the findings of this study only applied to mortality. Although nonvigorous exercise was not related to a reduction in mortality, even modest exercise has been shown to benefit other aspects of health (28). Thus, while increased physical activity, which includes vigorous exercise, may be optimal, it is clear that even nonvigorous exercise is preferable to being sedentary.

Although a large number of adults begin exercising each year, many do not become habitual exercisers. Many drop out owing to failure to improve fitness, exercise-related injuries, or fatigue and muscle soreness after overtraining. Much of the attrition from personal fitness programs can be ascribed to improper training programs; the information that follows is intended to provide the knowledge needed to prescribe proper exercise programs for adult beginners.

Objectives and Potential Benefits

Physical fitness is the ability to perform daily tasks with vigor and alertness, without undue fatigue, and with ample energy to enjoy leisure-time pursuits and to meet unforeseen emergencies. This suggests that a person is physically fit if he can readily cope with the physical demands presented by his preferred lifestyle and selected environment. Of course, in our modern technological society, the lifestyle of the typical adult presents few physical challenges. Thus it might seem that the average American would have no need to maintain a high level of physical fitness. Mounting evidence, however, suggests the opposite—that modern man needs, more than ever, to be concerned about his physical activity habits.

Research and clinical evidence strongly suggests that several of the more frequently observed chronic diseases are related to physical inactivity (28). Sedentary living is itself a risk factor for developing (coronary heart disease) CHD, and some studies have indicated that exercise may ameliorate other CHD risk factors, such as elevated blood lipid concentrations and hypertension. Obesity, a risk factor for CHD, hypertension, and diabetes, is clearly linked to low levels of habitual physical activity and, in most patients, is responsive to exercise therapy. Lower back pain, one of the most frequently reported health problems, is most typically due to inflexibility of the lower back-hamstring region and weakness of the abdominal musculature. An accepted conservative treatment for lower back pain is exercise.

Although regular exercise may aid in the prevention and treatment of certain disease processes, it also contributes profoundly to positive health or ''wellness.'' Most sedentary persons who initiate proper exercise programs report feeling better and more ''energetic'' within a few weeks. Although this effect may be at least partially psychological, a convincing physiologic explanation can be presented. With training, as a person's physical working capacity improves (increases in the LT and/or VO_2 max), the percentage of his maximum working capacity required by any submaximal level of exertion decreases. Because fatigue is highly related to the blood lactate response to exercise and percentage of VO_2 max required by physical activities, the fitter person will experience less fatigue in response to standard physical work situations. Greater enjoyment of activities that require strenuous exertion results, as does less fatigue during long duration, low-intensity activity (e.g., occupational endeavors).

The objectives of adult physical fitness programs should focus primarily on the health-related fitness components, including cardiorespiratory fitness, body composition, flexibility, and strength. Proper programs can, and should, be structured so as to develop and maintain an acceptable level of fitness in each of the health-related components. Although the designation of any specific fitness level as ''acceptable'' must be somewhat arbitrary and based on the goals of the individual, fitness levels that seem to be consistent with the avoidance of associated health problems and with maintenance of an acceptable physical working capacity may be identified.

Risks and Safety Procedures

Although regular exercise is associated with improved health and a reduction in risk of various diseases and all cause mortality, it should be realized that physical activity increases the risk of musculoskeletal injury and life-threatening events such as cardiac arrest (ACSM). Fortunately, the incidence of these events is low. In apparently healthy adults the acute event rate has been reported to be 1 per 187,500 person-hours of exercise with a death rate for male joggers of 1 per 396,000 man hours of jogging (5). The incidence of cardiac arrest is 1 episode per year for every 18,000 healthy men, but appears to be lower for men with higher levels of regular physical activity.

Therefore, for a small percentage of adults, the risks associated with regular exercise outweigh the potential benefits. Consequently, those persons must be identified before initiation of a training program. Males younger than 40 years of age and females younger than 50 years of age with no history of cardiovascular disease and who show fewer than two CHD risk factors (family history, current cigarette smoking, hypertension—blood pressure greater than 140/90, hypercholesterolemia—serum cholesterol greater than 200 mg/dL or 5.2 mmol/L, diabetes mellitus, sedentary lifestyle) may safely start both moderate and vigorous exercise programs without a medical examination (5). Males younger than 40 years of age and females younger than 50 years of age with two or more risk factors but no symptoms of cardiovascular disease may start a moderate exercise program without a medical examination or clinical exercise test (5); however, if vigorous exercise is desired, or if symptoms of cardiovascular disease are present (symptoms include pain, discomfort in the neck, chest, jaw, arms, or other areas that may be ischemic in nature; shortness of breath at rest or with mild exertion; dizziness or syncope; orthopnea or paroxysmal nocturnal dyspnea; ankle edema; palpitations or tachycardia; intermittent claudication; known heart murmur; unusual fatigue or shortness of breath with usual activities), or if known disease (cardiac, pulmonary, or metabolic) is present, then both a medical examination and clinical exercise test are recommended prior to initiating an exercise program. For asymptomatic males older than 40 years of age and females older than 50 years of age moderate exercise programs can be initiated without a medical examination or clinical exercise test, but initiation of vigorous exercise should be preceded by a medical examination and a clinical exercise test (5). Older adults who have two or more risk factors, have symptoms, and/or have known disease should have a medical examination and a clinical exercise test prior to initiating any form of regular exercise (moderate or intense) (5).

Among properly screened persons, the risks associated with regular exercise are minimal. As mentioned above, serious cardiovascular complications during exercise are exceedingly rare. Indeed, for most of the population, regular exercise is no more dangerous than any other normal activity of daily life. Some physical activities, such as jogging, involve risk of musculoskeletal injury. Mostly, these injuries can be prevented through use of proper equipment and training procedures; a small fraction of adults do, however, encounter considerable difficulties with running activities and should be encouraged to try non–weight-bearing activities such as cycling.

Principles of Adult Fitness Programs

The principles of training outlined previously apply to adult fitness programs. Research has shown that an acceptable level of cardiorespiratory fitness can be developed through participation in a primary aerobic activity three to five times a week for 20 to 60 minutes of continuous activity (5). Intensity of exercise should be such as to elevate the heart rate to about 60% to 90% of maximum, or if perception of effort is used, the exercise should be perceived as hard. Greater frequencies, durations, and intensities of activities may be safely used by already trained participants; such training will lead to further enhancement of cardiorespiratory fitness. However, in order to minimize the risk of overuse injuries when frequency of exercise is increased, hard exercise bouts should be alternated with easy exercise bouts (or the mode of exercise should be varied from day to day).

All the basic tenets of training apply to adult exercisers, but two principles are of particular significance. The principle of progression is important for sedentary adults who seek to attain higher levels of fitness. Such persons must be convinced to begin with a very light dose of exercise and then to increase the weekly quantity of exercise very gradually. Many orthopaedic injuries experienced by beginning adult exercisers are caused by a training load that increases too rapidly. Also, exercise regimens that begin at too high an intensity contribute to the high rate of recidivism in adult beginners. High-intensity exercise may contribute to muscle soreness, overuse injuries, and long-term fatigue, all of which lead to lack of adherence to an exercise regimen.

Also of profound importance in adult fitness programs is individuality. Training programs for adults must be individualized according to the age, sex, current fitness level, health status, and interests of the participant. The principles of exercise prescribed above contribute to individualization by adjusting the intensity of activity to the current fitness level. Further, exercise programs should be designed so as to optimize the chances of adherence. Personal preference should carry great weight in selecting the mode of activity. The participant's health status may dictate the mode and intensity of exercise: Patients with heart disease should not exercise at intensities so high as to elicit symptoms (e.g., angina pectoris, ischemic electrocardiographic changes), and exercisers with orthopaedic limitations may need to use non–weight-bearing or specially modified activities.

Stretching and Strengthening Programs

While focusing on cardiorespiratory fitness, adult fitness programs should include activities that contribute to development and maintenance of adequate muscular strength and flexibility.

Musculoskeletal Flexibility

It is important that individuals maintain an adequate range of motion in all joints. This will help to ensure optimal musculoskeletal function (5). It is particularly important that the flexibility is maintained in the lower back and in the posterior thigh areas. This should help to decrease the risk of chronic low back pain (5). It is particularly important that individuals maintain flexibility as they age, as lack of flexibility is prevalent in older persons and is associated with reduced ability to perform activities of daily living (5).

Of the different types of stretching techniques (e.g., static, ballistic, and proprioceptive neuromuscular facilitation, PNF), static stretching is recommended. Static stretching involves slowly stretching a muscle to the point of mild discomfort and holding the stretch for 10 to 30 seconds. The risk of injury is low, it requires little time and assistance, and has been shown to be effective (5). Ballistic stretching uses bouncing movements to produce muscle stretch. This type of stretching can cause muscle soreness or injury if the momentum created by the bouncing movement (and hence the forces generated) are too great (2). PNF requires a partner and involves a combination of alternating contraction and relaxation of both agonist and antagonist muscles. This method has been shown to be effective, but is associated with some degree of muscle soreness (5).

Stretching exercises can be used to maintain and/or improve range of motion in a joint. The American College of Sports Medicine recommendations for achieving and maintaining flexibility are presented in Table 3.6.

More information about specific stretches can be found in the ACSM Fitness Book (4).

Muscular Fitness

Every activity requires a certain amount of muscular strength and muscular endurance. The ability to maintain an adequate amount of muscular strength and endurance allows the individual to perform activities of daily living and other activities with less physiologic stress. The physiologic stress involved with lifting is proportional to the percentage of maximal strength involved.

The American College of Sports Medicine suggests

TABLE 3.6. *ASCM flexibility recommendations*

• Frequency:	At least 3 days/week
• Intensity:	To a position of mild discomfort
• Duration:	10–30 seconds for each stretch
• Repetitions:	3–5 for each stretch
• Type:	Static, with a major emphasis on the lower back and thigh area

From ref. 5 with permission.

that resistance training of sufficient intensity to develop and maintain muscular fitness and fat-free mass be an essential part of any adult fitness program (5). In addition to the development and maintenance of muscular strength and muscle mass, strength training has been shown to increase bone mass (or to slow the rate of the age-associated decrease in bone mineral content) and connective tissue. These benefits have particular importance for individuals as they age because of the age-associated decrease in bone mineral content. Other health-related benefits of strength training include small improvements in cardiorespiratory fitness, reductions in body fat, small reductions in blood pressure, improved glucose tolerance, and improved blood lipid and lipoprotein profiles.

The resistance training guidelines recommended by the American College of Sports Medicine for the apparently healthy adult are shown in Table 3.7.

Weight Control Through Exercise

Regular exercise contributes importantly to the maintenance of an acceptable body weight. Body composition, the percentage of total body weight that is fat tissue, is significantly correlated with habitual physical activity levels in all age and sex categories. Moderate obesity can be effectively treated by increasing the daily caloric expenditure through exercise and ingestion of a sensible diet. For most persons, such an approach to weight loss is preferable to dieting alone because it leads to a loss that is almost entirely fat

TABLE 3.8. *ASCM weight loss recommendations*

- Provides intake of not lower than 1200 kcal/day for normal adults and ensures a proper blend of foods to meet nutritional requirements*
- Includes foods acceptable to the dieter in terms of sociocultural background, usual habits, taste, costs, and ease in acquisition and preparation.
- Provides a negative caloric balance (not to exceed 500–1000 kcal/day), resulting in gradual weight loss without metabolic derangements, such as ketosis
- Results in maximal weight loss of 1 kg/week
- Includes the use of behavior modification techniques to identify and eliminate diet habits that contribute to malnutrition
- Includes an exercise program that promotes a daily caloric expenditure of 300 or more kcal. For many participants, this may be best accomplished with low intensity, long duration exercise, such as walking
- Provides that new eating and physical activity habits can be continued for life in order to maintain the achieved lower body weight

From ref. 5 with permission.
* Note: this requirement may not be appropriate for children, older individuals, and athletes.

tissue, whereas dieting alone results in a substantial loss in lean tissue. Moderate exercise combined with mild caloric restriction is most effective because the resultant weight loss is relatively rapid and the regimen involves the adoption of habits that are quite tolerable.

Exercise programs adopted for the purpose of weight loss should adhere to all principles previously discussed. The primary focus, however, should be on expenditure of calories. Thus total amount of work done rather than intensity of activity should be emphasized. In obese adults, intensity of exercise can be reduced so that duration can be increased substantially. For example, an obese person might be instructed to walk for 40 minutes at an intensity that elicits 50% of maximum heart rate. However, it should be realized that recent data suggest that high-intensity exercise is associated with an increased reliance on fat as a substrate during recovery from exercise (14). This suggests that obese individuals may benefit from high-intensity exercise provided that they can tolerate the activity from an orthopaedic standpoint. The participants should also attempt to burn additional calories whenever possible—by climbing stairs, mowing a lawn, or walking to work, for instance.

Obesity predisposes the adult exerciser to orthopaedic difficulties and may require adoption of non–weight-bearing activities. Because obesity is a risk factor for hypertension, diabetes, and CHD, overweight persons should be carefully screened before initiation of exercise programs. It should be realized that although most individuals are concerned about absolute amounts of body fat, the regional distribution of body fat is a more powerful predictor of risk of developing disease. Individuals with elevated abdominal fat and in particular intraabdominal visceral fat have the highest risk of developing cardiovas-

TABLE 3.7. *ASCM resistance-training guidelines for healthy adults*

- Perform a minimum of 8–10 separate exercises that train the major muscle groups
  A primary goal of the program should be to develop total body strength in a relatively time-efficient manner. Programs lasting longer than 1 hour per session are associated with higher dropout rates.
- Perform one set of 8–12 repetitions of these exercises to the point of volitional fatigue
- Perform these exercises at least 2 days/week
  While more frequent training and additional sets or combinations of sets and repetitions elicit larger strength gains, the additional improvement is relatively small
- Adhere as closely as possible to the specific techniques for performing a given exercise
- Perform every exercise through a full range of motion
- Perform both the lifting (concentric phase) and lowering (eccentric phase) portion of the resistance exercises in a controlled manner
- Maintain a normal breathing pattern, since breath-holding can induce excessive increases in blood pressure
- If possible, exercise with a training partner who can provide feedback, assistance, and motivation

From ref. 5 with permission.

cular disease, Type II diabetes, hyperlipidemia, and hypertension (11).

In recent years, numerous exercise and weight-control programs have been promoted through the print and broadcast media. Although some of these programs are consistent with the established principles of exercise physiology, many widely advertised programs are not only ineffective but also unsafe. Before adopting or recommending any "prepackaged" exercise routine, one should evaluate a program for its consistency with the principles discussed earlier in this chapter, such as overload, consistency, specificity, and progression. Programs that offer "overnight" results, recommend crash diets, or promise maximum benefits with minimum effort should be viewed skeptically. Other programs are of excellent quality and have benefited many thousands of adult exercisers. The American College of Sports Medicine (5) suggests that a desirable weight-loss program should meet the criteria in Table 3.8.

PROGRAMS FOR THE ELDERLY

Aging is a term often used to describe the biologic, psychologic, and sociologic changes that occur in persons over time. In biology, aging has come to be associated with a gradual decline in the body's functional capacities and a reduction in the system's resistance to stress and disease. Age-related functional changes may, at least in part, be due to genetically coded phenomena, but some biologic effects of aging may be due to disease processes as yet unidentified. In addition, much of the age-related decline in physiologic functioning results not from aging per se but from the sedentary lifestyle that has come to be associated with advanced age in our society. This section provides insight into the relation between aging and exercise habits as well as information on the design of fitness programs for older persons.

Physiology of Aging

Cross-sectional observations of physiologic variables reveal that many exercise-related functions decline gradually with increasing chronologic age, a decline that begins at about 30 years of age. These changes, however, while consistently observed in American society, may not be normal. Habitual physical activity often begins a gradual decline in early adulthood, and thus age-related reductions in many physiologic variables may be abnormal and reflective of the hypokinesis that is endemic in the older adult population of the United States.

Cardiovascular Fitness

Aging is associated with marked reductions in cardiovascular functional capacity. Maximum heart rate declines at the rate of about 1 beat a year (maximum heart rate = 220 − age. Maximal oxygen consumption declines between 0.4 and 0.5 mL/kg/minute each year in adults. However, the rate of decline is related to the activity patterns of individuals. Sedentary men and women have a nearly twofold faster rate in decline in VO_2 max as they age. Recent research has indicated that if individuals maintain relatively constant training and body composition over time they have less decline in VO_2 max with aging (0.25 mL/kg/minute per year). Because of a lower maximum heart rate, maximum cardiac output also decreases with age. A reduction in stroke volume is also observed with aging and may account for as much as 50% of the reduction in VO_2 max with age (26). Pathologic conditions such as hypertension, CHD, and peripheral vascular disease are very common in the elderly and may combine with decreased functional capacities to reduce exercise tolerance.

The degree to which decrements in cardiovascular function are a direct result of aging as opposed to a lack of habitual physical activity has not been determined. However, it has been suggested that a sedentary lifestyle may cause losses in functional capacity that are as great as the effects of aging (26). Furthermore, among healthy elderly individuals, exercise training can enhance the heart's systolic and diastolic properties and increase aerobic capacity to the same relative degree as in younger adults (26).

Pulmonary Function

Both static and dynamic pulmonary functions decline with age. Under resting conditions, vital capacity is reduced and residual volume is increased, perhaps because of decreased thoracic wall compliance. Pulmonary diffusing capacity is reduced under both resting and exercise conditions. However it appears that training may offset some of the decline in pulmonary function associated with aging. For example, older endurance athletes have higher vital capacity, total lung capacity, residual volume, maximal voluntary ventilation, forced expiratory volume and forced vital capacity (FEV1.0 and FEV1.0/FVC) than sedentary age-matched control subjects (26).

Muscle Function

The body's skeletal muscle tissues reflect the aging process through decreases in muscle mass, muscular strength, and muscular endurance. The highest strength levels for men and women are generally observed between the ages of 20 to 30, at the time when the muscle cross-sectional area is the greatest. Between the ages of 25 to 80 a 40% to 50% reduction in muscle mass is observed. This is due to motor unit losses and muscle fiber atrophy. In addition to the progressive neuromotor processes that occur with aging, a reduction in muscle strength can also be related to a decrease in the daily

TABLE 3.9. *Summary results of studies investigating the relationship between physical activity or physical fitness and selected chronic diseases or conditions 1963–1993*

Disease or condition	Number of studies	Trends across activity or fitness categories and strength of evidence[a]
All-cause mortality	>10	↓↓↓
Coronary artery disease	>10	↓↓↓
Hypertension	5–10	↓↓
Obesity	>10	↓↓
Stroke	5–10	↓
Peripheral vascular disease	<5	→
Cancer		
Colon	>10	↓↓
Rectum	>10	→
Stomach	<5	→
Breast	<5	↓
Prostate	5–10	↓
Lung	<5	↓
Pancreas	<5	→
Noninsulin-dependent diabetes	<5	↓↓
Osteoarthritis	<5	→
Osteoporosis	5–10	↓↓
Functional capability	5–10	↓↓

From ref. 9 with permission.

[a] →, No apparent difference in disease rates across activity or fitness categories; ↓, some evidence of reduced disease rates across activity or fitness categories; ↓↓, good evidence of reduced disease rates across activity or fitness categories, control of potential confounders, good methods, some evidence of biological mechanisms; ↓↓↓, excellent evidence of reduced disease rates across activity or fitness categories, good control of potential confounders, excellent methods, extensive evidence of biological mechanisms, relationship is considered causal.

level of muscle loading. In older individuals resistance training facilitates protein synthesis and retention and blunts the loss of muscle mass and strength seen with aging (26).

Objectives of Exercise Programs

The objectives of exercise programs for the elderly must be established in accordance with the individual participant's age, fitness level, and health status. Each of these factors varies widely within the older population; thus one should never consider the elderly as being one homogeneous group. Although it is always important that adult fitness programs be individualized, individualization with the elderly is critical.

Nonetheless, the general goals of fitness programs for older persons are the same as those for younger adults. The focus should be on health-related fitness components: cardiorespiratory endurance, body composition, flexibility, and muscular strength and endurance. Reduced joint mobility, often secondary to arthritis, is a debilitating malady for many elderly persons, and exercise routines may be devised to aid in retention of adequate levels of static and dynamic flexibility in key joints. Accidents are a major cause of injury and death in the elderly population, and many of these tragedies can be linked to inadequate muscular strength. A strength deficiency impairs the ability to control the body weight (e.g., stair climbing) and to handle external objects (e.g., carrying a bag of groceries). Properly designed and graded resistance exercises can promote maintenance of acceptable levels of muscular strength.

Perhaps the most critical factor in the elderly person's ability to function independently in society is the ability to move without assistance. Clearly, older people who maintain good levels of cardiorespiratory fitness and acceptable body composition are more likely to retain the ability to move independently longer than those who become obese or who allow their muscular and cardiorespiratory systems to degenerate. As mentioned previously, the cardiorespiratory system of the older person is trainable, and good levels of aerobic fitness may be attained. Likewise, regular exercise may lead to a loss of fat and maintenance of an acceptable percentage of body fat.

Effects of Habitual Physical Activity or Physical Fitness on Selected Chronic Diseases or Conditions

As has been stated previously the majority of research in the literature suggests that the maintenance of a physically active lifestyle with aging is associated with a dramatic reduction in risk of many diseases. Table 3.9 summarizes the findings of over 30 years of research relating physical activity and fitness to disease risk (9).

EXERCISE TESTING

According to the American College of Sports Medicine "the rationale for exercise testing within an elderly population is similar to that of any adult population. Several key points deserve mention. First, knowledge of the effects of the aging process on variables measured during exercise testing is critical to the safe and effective performance of exercise testing in the elderly"(5) (Table 3.10). As reviewed previously such changes include:

"Physiological aging does not occur uniformly across the population; therefore it is not wise to define 'elderly' by any specific chronological age or set of ages. Individuals of the same age can and will differ drastically in their physiological status and response to an exercise stimulus. Third, it is difficult to distinguish effects due to deconditioning, age-related decline, and disease. Fourth, while aging is inevitable, both the pace and potential reversibility of this process may be amenable to intervention. And finally, the possibility that an active or latent disease process may be present in the subject must always be considered"(5). Medical clearance is advised for older adults

TABLE 3.10. *Effects of aging on variable measures during exercise training in the elderly*

• Resting heart rate	Little or no change
• Maximal heart rate	Decreases
• Maximal cardiac output	Decreases
• Resting and exercise BP	Increases
• Maximal oxygen uptake	Decreases
• Residual volume	Decreases
• Vital capacity	Decreases
• Reaction time	Increases
• Muscular strength	Decreases
• Bone mass	Decreases
• Flexibility	Decreases
• Fat-free body mass	Decreases
• Percent body fat	Increases
• Glucose tolerance	Decreases
• Recovery time	Increases

From ref. 5 with permission.

prior to maximal exercise testing or their participation in vigorous exercise.

According to the American College of Sports Medicine ''various test protocols utilizing a variety of modalities have been used for testing the elderly population. In addition, many protocols have been developed for those who are highly deconditioned or physically limited. As aging increases the adaptation time to a given workload and VO₂ max declines with age, an optimal protocol combines a prolonged warm-up and adaptation period with a low initial exercise intensity. However, no ideal protocol exists for all older adults. Other factors to be considered when selecting an exercise testing protocol for older adults are presented'' in Table 3.11 (5).

Although no specific exercise test termination criteria are necessary for the elderly population, the attainment of a lower VO₂ max coupled with the increased prevalence of cardiovascular, metabolic, and orthopaedic problems in the elderly leads to the reality that the test may

TABLE 3.11. *Factors to consider when selecting an exercise testing protocol for older adults*

Characteristic	Suggested test modification
Low VO₂ max	Start at low intensity (2–3 METs)
More time to attain a steady state	Long warm-up (>3 min), small increments in work rate (0.5–1.0 MET per stage), longer stages
Increased fatigability	Reduce total test time (ideally 8–12 min)
Increased need to monitor ECG, BP, and HR	Cycle ergometer preferred
Poor balance	Cycle ergometer preferred
Poor ambulatory ability	Increase treadmill grade rather than speed
Poor neuromuscular coordination	Increase amount of practice, may require more than one test

From ref. 5 with permission.

need to be terminated earlier (either volitionally or due to achievement of established criteria) (5).

EXERCISE PRESCRIPTION

The general principles of exercise prescription apply to individuals of all ages. However, the wide range of health and fitness levels observed among older adults make generic exercise prescription more difficult (5).

Aerobic Training

Table 3.12 presents the American College of Sports Medicine recommendations regarding the type, intensity, duration, and frequency of exercise for the elderly.

Resistance Training

As mentioned, recent research findings suggest that resistance training can improve muscular fitness (muscular

TABLE 3.12. *ACSM exercise recommendations for the elderly*

Mode
- The exercise modality should be one that does not impose significant orthopedic stress
- The activity should be accessible, convenient, and enjoyable to the participant—all factors directly related to exercise adherence
- Consider walking, stationary cycling, water exercise, swimming, or machine-based stair climbing

Intensity
- Intensity must be sufficient to stress (overload) the cardiovascular, pulmonary, and musculoskeletal systems without overtaxing them
- High variability exists for maximal heart rates in persons over 65 years of age; thus, it is always better to use a measured maximal heart rate (HRmax) rather than age-predicted HRmax whenever possible
- For similar reasons, the HR reserve method is recommended for establishing a training HR in older individuals, rather than a straight percentage of HRmax
- The recommended intensity for older adults is 50%–70% of HR reserve
- Since many older persons suffer from a variety of medical conditions, a conservative approach to prescribing aerobic exercise is initially warranted

Duration
- During the initial stages of an exercise program, some older adults may have difficulty sustaining aerobic exercise for 20 minutes; one viable option may be to perform the exercise in several 10-minute bouts throughout the day
- To avoid injury and ensure safety, older individuals should initially increase exercise duration rather than intensity

Frequency
- Alternate between days that involve primarily weight-bearing and nonweight-bearing exercise

From ref. 5 with permission.

strength and muscular endurance) in older adults. Resistance training may enable elderly individuals to perform activities of daily living with greater ease and counteract muscle weakness and frailty in very old persons. Some minimal level of muscular fitness is critical for individuals to retain their independence. The American College of Sports Medicine (5) guidelines with respect to the intensity, frequency, and duration of resistance training are presented in Table 3.13.

ACSM also recommends several common sense guidelines pertaining to resistance training for older adults that should be followed (Table 3.14) (5).

Flexibility

An adequate range of motion in all of the joints of the body is important to maintaining an acceptable level of musculoskeletal function in older adults. It is generally agreed that maintaining adequate levels of flexibility will enhance an individual's functional capabilities (e.g., bending and twisting) and reduce injury potential (e.g., risk of muscle strains and low back problems)—particularly for the aged. A sound stretching program should be included as part of each exercise session for older adults (ACSM). The American College of Sports Medicine recommendations for development and maintenance of flexibility in older adults is presented in Table 3.15.

Sample Programs

In recent years, exercise programs for the elderly have become commonplace; consequently several standardized programs have been developed and implemented both commercially and through nonprofit agencies. The best of these programs have several characteristics in common (Table 3.16).

TABLE 3.13. *ACSM resistance training recommendations*

Intensity
- Perform one set of 8–10 exercises that train all the major muscle groups (e.g., gluteals, quadriceps, hamstrings, pectorals, latissimus dorsi, deltoids, and abdominals). Each set should involve 8–12 repetitions that elicit a perceived exertion rating of 12–13 (somewhat hard)

Frequency
- Resistance training should be performed at least twice a week, with at least 48 hours of rest between sessions

Duration
- Sessions lasting longer than 60 minutes may have a detrimental effect on exercise adherence. Adherence to the guidelines set forth in this chapter should permit individuals to complete total body resistance training sessions within 20–30 minutes

From ref. 5 with permission.

TABLE 3.14. *ASCM resistance training recommendations for the elderly*

- The major goal of the resistance training program is to develop sufficient muscular fitness to enhance an individual's ability to live a physically independent lifestyle
- The first several resistance training sessions should be closely supervised and monitored by trained personnel who are sensitive to the special needs and capabilities of the elderly
- Begin (the first 8 weeks) with minimal resistance to allow for adaptations of the connective tissue elements
- Teach proper training techniques for all of the exercises to be used in the program
- Instruct older participants to maintain their normal breathing pattern while exercising
- As a training effect occurs, achieve an overload initially by increasing the number of repetitions, and then by increasing the resistance
- Never use a resistance that is so heavy that the exerciser cannot perform at least 8 repetitions
- Stress that all exercises should be performed in a manner in which the speed is controlled (no ballistic movements should be allowed)
- Perform the exercises in a range of motion that is within a ''pain free arc'' (i.e., the maximum range of motion that does not elicit pain or discomfort)
- Perform multi-joint exercises (as opposed to single-joint exercises)
- Given a choice, use machines to resistance train, as opposed to free weights (machines require less skill to use, protect the back by stabilizing the user's body position, and allow the user to start with lower resistances, to increase by smaller increments, and to more easily control the exercise range of motion)
- Don't overtrain. Two strength-training sessions per week are the minimum number required to produce possible physiological adaptations; depending on the circumstances, more sessions may be neither desirable nor productive
- Never permit arthritic participants to participate in strength-training exercises during active periods of pain or inflammation
- Engage in a year-round resistance training program on a regular basis
- When returning from a lay-off, start with resistances <50% of the intensity at which the patient had been previously training, then gradually increase the resistance

From ref. 5 with permission.

THE FEMALE ATHLETE

An analysis of existing world record performances in various sporting activities indicates that women have not achieved the same peaks of athletic performance as have men. On the basis of world records in 1991, the female world record holder:

- ran 6.4% slower in the 100 m dash and 11.0% slower in the 1500-meter run
- jumped 14.3% lower in the high jump
- swam 8.4% slower in the 400-meter free-style swim (38)

TABLE 3.15. *ASCM flexibility recommendations for the elderly*

Intensity
- Exercises should incorporate slow movement, followed by a static stretch that is sustained for 10–30 seconds
- Exercises should be prescribed for every major joint (hip, back, shoulder, knee, upper trunk, and neck regions) in the body
- 3–5 repetitions of each exercise should be performed
- The degree of stretch achieved should not cause pain, but rather mild discomfort

Frequency
- Stretching exercises should be performed at least three times a week (preferably daily) and should be included as an integral part of the warm-up and cool-down exercises
- Devoting an entire exercise session to flexibility may be particularly appropriate for deconditioned older adults who are beginning an exercise program

Duration
- The stretching phase of an exercise session should last approximately 15–30 minutes
    Several guidelines pertaining to stretching by older adults should be followed.
- Always precede stretching exercises with some type of warm-up activity to increase circulation and internal body temperature
- Stretch smoothly and never bounce
- Do not stretch a joint beyond its pain-free range of motion
- Gradually ease into a stretch, and hold it only as long as it feels comfortable (10–30 sec)

From ref. 5 with permission.

At issue, of course, is whether the observed sex differences in athletic performance are due to genetically determined biological factors or to environmental factors such as training and societal attitudes. Available data suggest that some combination of genetic and environmental factors account for these differences. Certainly society has not been totally supportive of the female athlete, and training programs for women have, in many instances, been less vigorous than those for men. In addition, a smaller percentage of women than of men have chosen to participate in athletics, and thus the process of selection has been less demanding among the women. Nonetheless, available physiologic data indicate that certain genetically determined traits do limit exercise performance in women as a group.

Characteristics

The smaller stature of the female athlete has several ramifications. Obviously, performance is adversely affected in those activities in which height and body mass determine performance. In addition, the smaller body mass of the woman is composed of less lean tissue than that of the man; lower lean body mass dictates lower muscular strength because the strength of a muscle, independent of sex, is highly correlated with its gross size (cross-sectional area). A woman's lower strength-to-body-weight ratio is disadvantageous in activities that involve lifting or rapid propulsion of the body mass. The sex differences in vertical jumping and sprinting ability may be primarily due to this strength and body weight factor.

A high(er) percentage of body fat is a detriment to performance in nearly all athletic activities that involve movement of the body mass. This is particularly evident in endurance activities, such as distance running, because "excess" fat tissue adds to the mass that must be moved but does not contribute to the energy for the performance of work. The suggestion that women may actually be at an advantage in long duration activities since, in such activities, free fatty acids are an important raw material for aerobic metabolism belies an inadequate understanding of exercise biochemistry, overlooking the knowledge that use of free fatty acid is dependent not on the magnitude of the body fat store but rather on the activity of the enzymes of fat metabolism. Thus a woman's higher percentage of body fat tends to affect performance adversely in most athletic activities and accounts for many of the observed differences between men and women in sports.

Women tend to have decrements in cardiovascular function when compared with men of similar competitive standing. Heart size, stroke volume, and maximum cardiac output are smaller in women than in men even when differences in body size are controlled. In addition, hemoglobin concentration is substantially lower in women than in men (14 g Hb/100 mL blood vs. 16 g Hb/100 mL blood), and this represents a limiting factor in a woman's oxygen transport capacity. Indeed, the differences between men and women in endurance performance may largely be accounted for by differences in hemoglobin concentration and body composition.

In addition to differences in body composition and car-

TABLE 3.16. *Characteristics of exercise programs for the elderly*

- All activities begin at a low level of intensity and build gradually to suitable maintenance of fitness.
- Activities are incorporated that deal with cardiorespiratory fitness, flexibility, and muscular strength, including flexibility, and strength exercises for all major muscle groups and joints. The total caloric expenditure involved in each exercise session is high enough to contribute to optimal improvement of the body composition.
- Designated activities can easily be scaled to the fitness level and health status of each participant.
- The program is easily adapted for use in a wide range of physical settings (e.g., home, senior citizen centers, church halls).
- The program is organized and presented in a manner that promotes enjoyment and long-term adherence. Often, background music and rhythmic activities are provided.

From ref. 5 with permission.

diovascular function, women tend to be weaker than men largely due to their lower absolute amount of muscle mass. Women also tend to have smaller muscle fiber cross-sectional area (with smaller fiber areas for both ST and FT fibers). However, available data suggest that the functional capacities of skeletal muscle are similar in the two sexes as long as muscle mass is not a factor. Muscular strength, expressed per square centimeter of muscle cross-sectional area, is similar in men and women. Maximal oxygen consumption, expressed as milliliters of oxygen consumed per kilogram of lean body weight, is only slightly lower in women than in men, a small difference probably due to cardiovascular, not muscle metabolic, limitations. Thus, by inference, skeletal muscle enzyme systems probably are developed about equally in female and male athletes. Likewise, no sex differences are observed in neuromuscular coordination and motor learning ability as long as muscular strength is not a significant factor in the physical skill being performed.

Trainability

At one time women were thought to be less trainable than men, that is, less improvement should be expected in women than in men in response to a training program. Available data now indicate that this premise is false. Training studies have shown that, if exposed to exercise of similar frequency, intensity, and duration, women exhibit percentages of improvement similar to those observed in men.

Until recently, heavy resistance training for strength improvement had been rare in female athletes. Misconceptions on trainability and fear of developing masculine characteristics kept many women away from strength training. These reservations are gradually being laid to rest by controlled research studies that have shown women do increase muscular strength through resistance training and do so without developing the heavy musculature of men. Apparently most of a woman's strength gain occurs through neuromuscular adaptations rather than through hypertrophy of skeletal muscle fibers. Lack of hypertrophy in women may be accounted for by lower levels of testosterone, which may be an obligatory intermediate in the anabolic process of hypertrophy.

Cardiorespiratory functions in women seem to be as responsive to aerobic training as do those in men. Although the absolute pretraining and posttraining levels of women are lower than those of men, the percentage of improvement tends to be similar. Of course, proper training in women results in attainment of cardiorespiratory capacities that substantially exceed those of sedentary men.

Exercise and Menstruation

The relation between exercise habits and menstruation may be studied from two perspectives: first, if exercise performance is affected in any way by the menstrual cycle. Available data have reported equivocal results. Some studies have reported that phase of the menstrual cycle does affect exercise performance whereas the majority of studies have reported that the menstrual cycle phase has no effect on performance (38). Studies in which measures of performance-related physiologic variables have been repeated in the various stages of the menstrual cycle have failed to observe any consistent relationships. This conclusion is based, of course, on group findings. A particular athlete may be affected positively or negatively by the physiologic changes that accompany the stages of a menstrual cycle. From existing data it can be suggested that performance in some women can be affected by phase of the menstrual cycle, but that most women are not affected (38).

Second, interest has been expressed in the possible effects of training on menstruation. In recent years several published studies have suggested that the incidence of menstrual dysfunction, such as amenorrhea and oligomenorrhea, is higher in athletes than in nonathletes. Some investigators have concluded that athletes involved in very heavy training or endurance activities are particularly prone to secondary amenorrhea. At present, the causes of so-called athletic amenorrhea have not been identified but several factors have been associated with exercise-induced menstrual dysfunction. These include:

- Prior history of menstrual dysfunction
- Stress
- Energy drain associated with high quantity and intensity of exercise
- Low body weight and body fat
- Inadequate nutrition and/or disordered eating
- Hormonal alterations

At present the underlying cause of secondary amenorrhea related to exercise is not known.

Regardless of the underlying mechanism for exercise-induced amenorrhea the associated reduction in estradiol has been related to diminished bone mineral density. It has been reported that amenorrheic female athletes have bone mineral density at the lumbar spine that is markedly reduced. Although the long-term effects of this diminished bone mineral content have not been determined there is increasing concern that these young women may be at increased risk for osteoporosis later in life (17–19,32).

Eating Disorders

Eating disorders have gained much attention in recent years. This is a disorder that is reported primarily in women with men accounting for less than 10% of the total cases. Although the prevalence of eating disorders is not established, in part due to the secretive nature of the disorder, it has been suggested that in some activities the prevalence may be as high as 50% for elite female athletes (38). Activities that have been associated with the greatest risk include: sports and activities in which success is based in part on appearance (e.g., gymnastics, diving, figure skating, body building, ballet); endurance sports; and sports in which athletes must compete in a given weight class. The two main clinical syndromes associated with disordered eating are anorexia nervosa and bulimia nervosa.

Anorexia nervosa is a disorder that is characterized by a refusal to maintain more than the minimal body weight, a distorted body image, an intense fear of fatness or gaining weight, and amenorrhea. Bulimia nervosa is a disorder characterized by recurrent episodes of binge eating, a feeling of lack of control during these binges, and purging behavior including self-induced vomiting, use of laxatives and diuretic use (38).

Eating disorders are generally considered to be addictive behaviors and are difficult to diagnose and treat. Although there are several inventories available that were designed to diagnose disordered eating (EDI—Eating Disorders Inventory and EAT—Eating Attitudes Test), these inventories have low diagnostic abilities. This is thought to be related to the secretive nature of the disorders. The NCAA has provided a list of warning signs for eating disorders (Table 3.17).

Female Athlete Triad

Recently it has been reported that there is a relationship between disordered eating, secondary amenorrhea, and reduced bone mineral content in female athletes. This has been referred to as the female athlete triad.

Exercise and Pregnancy

Beliefs about exercise during pregnancy have changed markedly in recent years among both physicians and the public. At one time, pregnant athletes and fitness exercis-

TABLE 3.17. *NCAA warning signs for eating disorders*

Warning Signs for Anorexia Nervosa
1. Dramatic loss in weight
2. A preoccupation with food, weight, and calories
3. Wearing baggy or layered clothes
4. Relentless, excessive exercise
5. Mood swings
6. Avoiding food-related social activities

Warning Signs for Bulimia Nervosa
1. A noticeable weight loss or gain
2. Excessive concern about weight
3. Bathroom visits after meals
4. Depressive moods
5. Strict dieting followed by eating binges
6. Increasing criticism of one's body

From ref. 38 with permission.

TABLE 3.18. *Four physiological risks to the fetus associated with exercise during pregnancy*

1. An acute risk associated with reduced blood flow to the uterus as blood is diverted to the actively working muscle resulting in fetal hypoxia.
2. Fetal hyperthermia as a result of an increase in maternal core temperature during prolonged exercise or during exercise in unfavorable environmental conditions.
3. Reduced carbohydrate availability to the fetus as more carbohydrate is used by the actively working muscle.
4. The possibility of miscarriage and/or an alteration in the final outcome of pregnancy.

From ref. 38 with permission.

ers were advised to quit training for the duration of the pregnancy. This was based on the belief that exercise during pregnancy might increase risk to the fetus (Table 3.18). However, although exercise during pregnancy can have associated risks, it has been suggested that the benefits far outweigh the risks (Table 3.19).

However, it should be recognized that a pregnant woman should not initiate an exercise program without coordinating the exercise program with her obstetrician. The American College of Obstetricians and Gynecologists have established guidelines for exercise prescription in pregnancy, reasons to discontinue exercise during pregnancy, and contraindication to exercise during pregnancy (3,5) (Table 3.20).

Nutritional Considerations

Although most athletes are physically fit, their performance can be compromised if their diets are not nutritionally sound. During low-intensity exercise much of the energy required to sustain exercise is provided by the oxidation of free fatty acids. As exercise intensity increases plasma fatty acid utilization does not increase and additional energy is obtained by increased utilization of muscle glycogen, blood glucose, and intramuscular triglycerides. At higher intensity exercise muscle glycogen utilization and some additional increase in blood glucose utilization provides the majority of fuel. Muscle glycogen depletion as well as hypoglycemia have both been associ-

TABLE 3.19. *Benefits during pregnancy associated with exercise*

1. Increased energy level
2. Reduced cardiovascular stress
3. Prevention of excessive weight gain
4. Facilitation of labor
5. Faster recovery from labor
6. Promotion of good posture
7. Prevention of low back pain
8. Prevention of gestational diabetes
9. Improved mood state and body image
10. Fewer fetal complications of a difficult labor

From ref. 38 with permission.

TABLE 3.20. *American College of Obstetricians and Gynecologists (ACOG) recommendations for exercise in pregnancy and postpartum*

General Considerations

1. During pregnancy, women can continue to exercise and derive health benefits even from mild to moderate exercise routines. Regular exercise (at least 3 times/week) is preferable to intermittent activity.
2. Women should avoid exercise in the supine position after the first trimester. Such a position is associated with decreased cardiac output in most pregnant women. Because the remaining cardiac output will be preferentially distributed away from splanchnic beds (including the uterus) during vigorous exercise, such regimens are best avoided during pregnancy. Prolonged periods of motionless standing should also be avoided.
3. Women should be aware of the decreased oxygen available for aerobic exercise during pregnancy. They should be encouraged to modify the intensity of their exercise according to maternal symptoms. Pregnant women should stop exercising when fatigued and not exercise to exhaustion. Weight-bearing exercises may under some circumstances be continued at intensities similar to those prior to pregnancy throughout pregnancy. Nonweight-bearing exercises, such as cycling or swimming, will minimize the risk of injury and facilitate the continuation of exercise during pregnancy.
4. Morphologic changes in pregnancy should serve as a relative contraindication to types of exercise in which loss of balance could be detrimental to maternal or fetal well-being, especially in the third trimester. Further, any type of exercise involving the potential for even mild abdominal trauma should be avoided.
5. Pregnancy requires an additional 300 kcal/day in order to maintain metabolic homeostasis. Thus, women who exercise during pregnancy should be particularly careful to ensure an adequate diet.
6. Pregnant women who exercise in the first trimester should augment heat dissipation by ensuring adequate hydration, appropriate clothing, and optimal environmental surroundings during exercise.
7. Many of the physiological and morphological changes of pregnancy persist 4–6 weeks postpartum. Thus, prepregnancy exercise routines should be resumed gradually based upon a woman's physical capability.

Reasons to Discontinue Exercise and Seek Medical Advice During Pregnancy

1. Any signs of bloody discharge from the vagina
2. Any "gush" of fluid from the vagina (premature rupture of membranes)
3. Sudden swelling of the ankles, hands, or face
4. Persistent, severe headaches and/or visual disturbance; unexplained spell of faintness or dizziness
5. Swelling, pain, and redness in the calf of one leg (phlebitis)
6. Elevation of pulse rate or blood pressure that persists after exercise
7. Excessive fatigue, palpitations, chest pain
8. Persistent contractions (>6–8/hour) that may suggest onset of premature labor
9. Unexplained abdominal pain
10. Insufficient weight gain (<1.0 kg/month during last two trimesters)

Contraindications for Exercising During Pregnancy

1. Pregnancy-induced hypertension
2. Preterm rupture of membrane
3. Preterm labor during the prior or current pregnancy
4. Incompetent cervix
5. Persistent second to third trimester bleeding
6. Intrauterine growth retardation

From refs. 3 and 5 with permission.

ated with fatigue. When the ingestion of dietary carbohydrate is optimal, muscle glycogen resynthesis can occur within 24 to 48 hours (depending on the type of activity). In order for muscle glycogen resynthesis to occur in a rapid time frame it is important for the endurance athlete to consume 50 g carbohydrate every 2 hours, beginning soon after exercise, and ingest 7 to 9 g/kg of body weight in 24 hours. Foods with a high glycemic index will promote enhanced muscle glycogen restoration if consumed soon after exercise (15). For most athletes a nutritionally sound diet is recommended (70% carbohydrate, 20% fat, 10% protein) with the most important factor determining the daily caloric requirement being the daily level of physical activity (6,26).

TRAINING IN CHILDREN

Sports programs for children have assumed a high profile in American society since World War II. Organized programs for boys in baseball, football, and basketball have been available for many years. But recently we have seen large increases in participation in swimming, soccer, gymnastics, and track and field, among others. These expanded opportunities for sports participation are found in both community and school settings. Whereas the typical school system in the 1940s offered interscholastic athletic programs only in a few sports and only for secondary level boys, today many schools offer a wide range of sports activities for both boys and girls beginning at the elementary or middle school level. Clearly, sports programs for children have grown dramatically, and no plateau is yet in sight.

As the number of youthful participants in sports has increased, so has the intensity of their participation. Many of the training and competitive programs to which children are exposed are far more intense than those designed for mature adults only a few years ago. It is not uncommon, for instance, for a young gymnast to train for 3 hours a day year-round, for a child track star to run 50 to 70 miles a week, or for a youthful football player to undergo a preseason weight-training program. The intensity of athletic training programs and the competitive level in youth sports have risen in parallel, but the side effects and long-term outcomes of high-intensity training and competition in children may not always be positive. Discussed in this section are goals for youth exercise and sports programs, physiologic trainability of children, proper training techniques for youngsters, and trends in the fields of physical education and physical fitness programming for children.

Purposes of Training Programs

Sports and exercise programs for children come in many different forms. Although the specific purposes of these programs vary according to specific circumstances, certain general goals should provide the philosophical basis for all exercise and sports programs for children. These goals should be considered by all persons who serve in leadership roles in youth exercise and sports programs. Such programs should do the following:

Provide a positive experience in exercise for all children. Exercise and sports activity should be conducted in a supportive, enjoyable environment that engenders positive feelings toward exercise, sports, and physical fitness.

Provide exposure to sports activities and training procedures. The child's sports experiences should serve to provide knowledge of, and basic skill in, a range of sporting activities and exercise-training procedures. Acquiring such knowledge and skills is a valuable aspect of acculturation in modern American society.

Aid in the development of acceptable levels of health-related physical fitness. Youngsters should participate in activities that promote maintenance or development of good cardiorespiratory fitness, body composition, muscular strength, and flexibility.

Promote acquisition of basic movement skills. Later success and enjoyable participation in sports activities depend on early development of fundamental movement patterns, such as throwing, catching, striking, running, and jumping. Youth exercise and sports programs should attend to these basic skills.

Expose children to a wide range of lifetime fitness and recreational activities. Studies show that few of the popular competitive sports for youngsters are engaged in by adults. Thus the child's experiences should include exposure to those activities that have potential lifelong usefulness and benefit.

Provide special remedial fitness and instructional programs for youngsters who manifest fitness or movement deficiencies. Intervention programs in the areas of physical fitness and movement skills are most likely to be successful if they start early in life. Youngsters with low fitness or who fail to develop normal motor functions should be provided with appropriate special corrective programming.

Promote enhanced athletic performance. Many youth sports programs, although focusing exclusively on this goal, fail to achieve it because of improper teaching techniques. Properly designed training and instructional programs should result in improved performance in children, and such improvements may have important, positive side effects.

No single exercise or sports program is likely to attain all these objectives. The child's total exercise and sports experience should, however, lead to accomplishment of the stated goals. Thus the youngster's movement experiences at home and in school sports, physical education, and community-based activities, in toto, provide a well-rounded and positive lead-up to an adult life characterized by vigor and enjoyable participation in physical activities.

Limits to Performance

A child's body is subject to the same primary laws of physics and chemistry that determine the movement capabilities of an adult. Basically, then, the mechanical and physiologic principles of human movement apply equally across the entire age range. Although the basic principles may be the same, a child's maximal performance capacities differ markedly from those of older brothers and sisters, and these differences are important in the design of sports and exercise programs for children.

A child becomes an adult through the process of growth and development. Growth, the gradual increase in body size that occurs during the first 15 to 20 years of life, results in marked increases in physical performance abilities. Many anatomic characteristics (e.g., limb lengths, muscle mass, heart volume) can be accurately predicted from height. Likewise, numerous functional variables, such as strength, maximal cardiac output, and VO_2 max (liters/minute), are determined largely by gross body size. In many respects, then, the performance capacity of a child is a function of body size.

In addition, developmental processes independent of variations in body size profoundly affect the functional capacities of a child. For example, increases in certain muscle enzyme activities, hemoglobin concentration, and work efficiency accompany the aging process and serve to expand the physical working capacity at a rate exceeding that predicted from changes in size alone. In addition, muscle strength is known to be lower in younger children even when variations in body size are controlled. Thus a child's states of growth and development are powerful determinants of physical performance capabilities, and these factors should weigh heavily in the design of exercise programs for children (8).

Trainability

A fundamental American belief is that hard work pays off. Thus we tend to accept as axiomatic the concept that physical training results in improved performance. For children, however, this may not always be true. As mentioned above, the primary determining factors of a child's functional capacity are size and developmental state. Although a child's physical activity habits affect performance capacities, these effects may be manifested only at the extremes of physical activity range—that is, youngsters who are very sedentary tend to show physical fitness deficiencies, and youngsters who are extremely active manifest higher movement capacities. It is not clear whether moderate doses of exercise generate significant physiologic adaptations in the typical youngster. Some studies of the effects of endurance training in children have reported significant gains in VO_2 max and related variables; these changes, however, have been observed only with very intense and long-term training programs. Other studies have reported that children manifest little or no change in VO_2 max when exposed to training programs that would be expected to yield improved performance in adults. This apparent lack of responsiveness to training may indicate that the habitual physical activity level of the average child is already quite high, since mean VO_2 max values in children approximate 50 mL/kg/minute, a value considered quite good in adults.

A well-established principle of exercise physiology is that trainability is a function of initial fitness level. A moderate dose of physical exercise may not provide a significant stimulus to the child's developmental processes, which may already be proceeding at maximal rates.

Recent evidence suggests that children can safely participate in properly designed and monitored strength-training programs (36). The American College of Sports Medicine (5) offers suggestions for developing strength-training programs for children (Table 3.21).

Remember that exercise safety for children should always be of primary concern.

Responses to other forms of physical training largely have been unexplored in children. Some studies have shown that beneficial body composition changes occur with proper exercise programs.

Training Techniques

Given the dearth of training studies conducted with young subjects, extensive, specific guidelines for training procedures in children cannot be provided. In general, experience indicates that the same basic principles and techniques of training apply to both children and adults. This section emphasizes possible modifications of basic training principles that may be needed when working with youngsters.

Epiphyseal Injuries

The growth plates of the long bones are, of course, active in children. Until the plates ossify, they remain in

TABLE 3.21. *ASCM strength-training recommendations for children*

- No matter how big, strong, or mature a young man or woman appears, remember that he/she is physiologically immature
- Teach proper training techniques for all exercise movements involved in the program and proper breathing techniques
- Stress that exercises should be performed in a manner in which the speed is controlled, avoiding ballistic movements
- Under no circumstances should a weight be used that allows less than eight repetitions to be completed per set
- As a training effect occurs, achieve an overload by first increasing the number of repetitions and then by increasing the absolute resistance
- Perform 1 to 2 sets of 8 to 10 different exercises, ensuring that all of the major muscle groups are included
- Limit strength-training sessions to twice per week and encourage children and adolescents to seek other forms of physical activity
- Perform full-range, multi-joint exercises
- Do not overload the skeletal and joint structures with maximal weights
- All strength-training activities should be closely supervised and monitored by appropriately trained personnel

From ref. 5 with permission.

a cartilaginous state that leaves them vulnerable to traumatic injury and prone to overuse. The vulnerability of the growth plates requires that training programs for children avoid activities that could traumatize these structures. Youngsters should avoid the following forms of physical activity:

- Falling, leaping, or landing in the straight leg position.
- Repeated throwing movements that apply excessive stress to the shoulder and elbow joints (e.g., excessive throwing in baseball or throwing implements whose weight is disproportionate to the youngster's strength).
- Extremely long-duration exercise that involves weight bearing (e.g., marathon running).
- Weight training with very heavy resistance.

Sexual Maturation

Some scientific evidence suggests that heavy training may delay the onset of puberty in girls. Whether this effect, if real, is harmful in the long term is unclear, but coaches, athletic trainers, and physicians should be aware that delayed menarche and late development of secondary sex characteristics may result from heavy training in young girls.

Psychological Burnout

Heavy training and high-pressure competition in youngsters may lead to a loss of interest in sports and exercise. Training programs for children should emphasize enjoyment, wide variation of training techniques, short competitive seasons, moderate numbers of competitions, and frequent breaks from training and competition. For most youths, early specialization in a single sport and year-round training are contraindicated by the high risks of psychological and perhaps physiologic burnout.

External Rewards

Most children are naturally drawn to sports, games, and exercise; thus, intrinsic motivation is usually more than sufficient to sustain a child's interest in competitive and recreational sports activities. Unfortunately, many current sports programs for children seem to assume the opposite—that numerous and elaborate external rewards (e.g., trophies, uniforms) are needed. Evidence suggests that such external rewards not only are unnecessary but actually have the effect of decreasing the intrinsic motivation that initially existed. The ultimate consequence for many youngsters is failure to participate in exercise when external rewards are missing or removed, as they ultimately will be for most persons. External rewards should be used sparingly, and the highest priority should be placed on rewarding participation rather than competitive success.

Physical Fitness

Nearly everyone agrees that promotion of physical fitness in children is a worthy goal. Few have agreed, however, on how this goal can best be achieved. Indeed, there is considerable disagreement in professional circles about the basic definition of youth fitness.

Perhaps the most traditional approach to fitness programming for children has been to emphasize motor fitness, a broad concept encompassing a wide range of physical fitness components (e.g., movement abilities). Usually included under motor fitness are muscular strength, muscular endurance, cardiorespiratory endurance, speed, flexibility, power, agility, coordination, and balance. The concept of motor fitness is embodied in the American Alliance for Health, Physical Education, Recreation and Dance (AAHPERD) Youth Fitness Test, which, since the 1950s, has been the dominant test of physical fitness in American schools and which is currently the basis for the Presidential Fitness awards offered

TABLE 3.23. *Health-related physical fitness components*

Fitness component	Health factor
Cardiorespiratory endurance	Coronary heart disease risk
	Physical working capacity
Body composition	Diabetes
	Hypertension
	Coronary heart disease
Lower back/hamstring flexibility	Lower back pain
Strength of abdominal muscles	Lower back pain

through the President's Council on Physical Fitness in Sports. The AAHPERD Youth Fitness Test (1) includes the test items in Table 3.22.

An exclusive focus on motor fitness can precipitate certain problems. One problem is that many of the motor fitness components are heavily dependent on genetically determined factors. Thus it seems inappropriate to encourage youngsters to improve in areas in which training has little impact (e.g., speed, anaerobic power). Moreover, motor fitness, although important for the athlete, includes several components that have little import for the typical person. Consequently, emphasizing motor fitness may result in a muddled, inappropriate definition of physical fitness. In response to these perceived problems, the concept of health-related physical fitness came into wide acceptance in the late 1970s (Table 3.23). Health-related physical fitness is, by definition, narrower than motor fitness and includes only those fitness components significantly related to some aspect of physical health. Typically included in the health fitness category are cardiorespiratory endurance, body composition, strength and endurance of the abdominal musculature, and flexibility of the lower back and hamstring region. Each of these components of fitness has been found to play a significant role in disease prevention or health promotion.

Health-related physical fitness, long recognized as important for adults, is now receiving great attention with children, a trend manifested by the development and implementation of the AAHPERD Health-Related Physical Fitness Test (2) (Table 3.24).

In the future, motor fitness and health-related fitness should receive balanced emphasis in fitness and exercise programs for children. Motor fitness should be presented, evaluated, and interpreted for what it is: a determinant of overall physical ability particularly important in the athletic context. Health-related physical fitness should be

TABLE 3.22. *AAHPERD youth fitness test*

- 50-yard dash
- Agility run
- One-minute timed sit-up test
- Pull-ups or flexed-arm hang
- Standing long jump
- 600-yard walk/run or optional distance run

From ref. 1 with permission.

TABLE 3.24. *AAHPERD health-related physical fitness test*

- Mile or 9-minute distance run
- Triceps and subscapular skinfolds
- One-minute timed sit-up test
- Sit-and-reach test of flexibility

From ref. 2 with permission.

presented as an important determinant of physical health, a matter that should concern everyone in our society.

SPECIAL PROBLEMS OF COMPETITIVE ATHLETES

Sports medicine is rapidly being recognized as a distinct medical specialty. One reason why sports medicine has emerged as a discipline is that athletes often pose medical questions totally unique to the sports environment. This section hopes to address at least a few problems of competitive athletes.

Long-Term Planning of Training Programs

At one time, training for athletic competition was primarily a seasonal activity. Football players, for instance, trained from August to November, basketball players from October to February, and track athletes from March to June. Now, attainment of championship performances requires that athletes, even at the high school level, train year-round. Further, if an athlete is to continue to improve over several years, the training and competitive program must progress in an orderly fashion from one year to the next. These factors suggest that the coach, athletic trainer, and athlete must participate in long-term planning; no longer is it sufficient simply to plan from day to day or game to game.

Long-term planning should involve setting realistic short-, medium-, and long-term goals. Coaches should establish general competitive and training plans for each athlete on at least a yearly and seasonal basis and, in selected situations, for several years in advance. Long-term plans should include goals for training loads, training techniques, physical fitness measures, skill performance, and competitive achievements. Shorter-term goals (i.e., seasonal) should be established in each of these areas and should be quite specific. Monthly and weekly plans must be highly specific and individualized.

Staleness

One major reason for developing long-term training plans is to avoid staleness or overtraining. Staleness might be defined as an unexplained drop-off in performance, usually associated with overexposure to highly stressful training and competitive activities. Training plans should incorporate adequate periods of rest and other activities, mainly for psychological reasons but also for physiologic ones. Each athlete possesses a certain tolerance for sustained heavy training and competition. If this tolerance is exceeded, the athlete may lapse into physical exhaustion and psychological depression, circumstances that can be avoided by providing adequate rest periods on a weekly, seasonal, and yearly basis, by designing training programs that involve a variety of activities and environments, and by avoiding an excessive number of competitions.

If an athlete does show signs of staleness (e.g., reduced performance, illness, lack of attention, irritability), the best prescription is either reduced training or total rest. In severe cases of staleness, athletes may need a complete rest and change of environment. Under no circumstances should athletes who are stale increase their training dose. Further competition is not recommended until signs of staleness reverse.

Peaking

A major aim of the competitive athlete is attainment of optimal performances in championship competitions. This so-called "peaking" may be brought about by long-term planning and adherence to the training principle of periodization. Numerous factors combine to bring an athlete to peak performance levels, including training techniques, competitive schedule, psychological outlook, and diet. As the athlete approaches championship competitions, the training should increase in intensity but decrease in total load. Thus, as the swimmer's season progresses, the training might emphasize shorter, faster interval swims rather than total yardage.

Competitions tend to bring an athlete to peak performance; however, too many competitions may cause staleness. The optimal number and rate of competitions are quite specific to the sport and to the individual athlete. The athlete should enter championship competitions with an eager, optimistic outlook and be well rested. Before major competition in endurance activities, 2 to 3 days of significantly reduced training are recommended. During these final days before a championship, the athlete's diet should emphasize carbohydrates so as to fill the body's store of muscle glycogen. Perhaps the most important keys to successful peaking are attempting to peak only once a season and sustaining a peak for no more than a few weeks. Too many coaches and athletes meet with failure in championships because of attempts to peak too often or to sustain a peak too long.

Pacing

In long-duration endurance activities, one of the keys to performance is proper pacing. Research has indicated that even-pacing, perhaps with a "kick" at the end, is most effective and efficient. In moderate-duration activities, even-pacing prevents the premature accumulation of lactic acid, which is associated with fatigue. In very long-duration events, even-pacing ensures that muscle glycogen will not be depleted earlier than necessary. Novice competitors often tend to begin races at paces significantly faster than can be sustained for the entire distance, and this always has an adverse effect on performance.

Hitting the Wall

"Hitting the wall," a term popularized by marathon runners, refers to the sudden onset of fatigue and depression that may be encountered in later stages of very long-duration exercise. This phenomenon is probably due to depletion of muscle glycogen and blood glucose and thus may be avoided or delayed through proper training, pacing, and nutritional practices. Highly trained athletes seldom report "hitting the wall," which suggests that experience and training adaptations may prevent the problem. Even-pacing, a high-carbohydrate diet for 48 hours before competition, and ingestion of a dilute sugar solution during competition should help the endurance athlete to avoid "the wall."

REFERENCES

1. American Alliance for Health, Physical Education, Recreation, and Dance. *Youth fitness test.* Washington, DC: The Alliance, 1976.
2. American Alliance for Health, Physical Education, Recreation, and Dance. *Health-related fitness test.* Washington, DC: The Alliance, 1980.
3. American College of Obstetricians and Gynecologists. *Exercise during pregnancy and the postpartum period.* Technical Bulletin #189. Washington, DC: ACOG, 1994.
4. American College of Sports Medicine. *ACSM's fitness book.* Champaign, IL: Human Kinetics, 1992.
5. American College of Sports Medicine. *ACSM's guidelines for exercise testing and prescription.* Baltimore: Williams & Wilkins, 1995.
6. American College of Sports Medicine. Position stand: exercise and fluid replacement. *Med Sci Sports Exerc* 1996;28:i–vii.
7. American College of Sports Medicine. Position stand: the recommended quantity and quality of exercise for developing and maintaining cardiorespiratory and muscular fitness and flexibility in healthy adults. *Med Sci Sports Exerc* 1998;30:975–991.
8. Bar-Or O. *Pediatric sports medcine for the practicioner: from physiologic principles to clinical adaptations.* New York: Springer-Verlag, 1983.
9. Blair SN. Physical activity, fitness and health. *Res Q Exerc Sports* 1993;64:365.
10. Borg GAV. Perceived exertion as an indicator of somatic stress. *Scand J Rehabil Med* 1970;2:92–98.
11. Bouchard C, Despres JP, Mauriege P. Genetic and nongenetic determinants of regional fat distribution. *Endocrine Reviews* 1993;14:72–93.
12. Boutcher SH, Seip RL, Hetzler RK, Pierce EF, Snead D, Weltman A. The effects of specificity of training on rating of perceived exertion at the lactate threshold. *Eur J Appl Physiol* 1989;59:365–369.
13. Brooks GA, Fahey TD, White TP. *Exercise physiology: human bioenergetics and its applications.* Mountain View, CA: Mayfield, 1996.
14. Brooks GA, Mercier J. The balance of carbohydrate and lipid utilization during exercise: the "crossover" concept. *J Appl Physiol* 1994;76:2253–2261.
15. Coyle EF. Substrate utilization during exercise in active people. *Am J Clin Nutr* 1995;61(suppl):968S–979S.
16. Denis C, Fouque R, Poty P, Geyssant A, Lacour JR. Effects of 40 weeks of endurance training on the anaerobic threshold. *Int J Sports Med* 1982;3:208–214.
17. Drinkwater BL, Bruemmer B, Chesnut III CH. Menstrual history as a determinant of current bone density in young athletes. *JAMA* 1990;263:545–548.
18. Drinkwater BL, Nilson K, Chesnut III CH, Bremner WJ, Shainholtz S, Southworth MB. Bone mineral content of amenorrheic and eumenorrheic athletes. *N Engl J Med* 1984;311:277–281.
19. Drinkwater BL, Nilson K, Ott S, Chesnut III CH. Bone mineral density after resumption of menses in amenorrheic athletes. *N Engl J Med* 1986;256:380–382.
20. Dwyer J, Bybee R. Heart rate indices of the anaerobic threshold. *Med Sci Sports Exerc* 1983;15:72–76.
21. Haskvitz EM, Seip RL, Weltman JY, Rogol AD, Weltman A. The effect of training intensity on rating of perceived exertion. *Med Sci Sports Exerc* 1992;13:377–383.
22. Hetzler RK, Seip RL, Boutcher SH, Pierce E, Snead D, Weltman A. Effect of exercise modality on ratings of perceived exertion at various lactate concentrations. *Med Sci Sports Exerc* 1991;23:88–92.
23. Hurley BF, Hagberg JM, Allen WK, et al. Effect of training on blood lactate levels during submaximal exercise. *J Appl Physiol REEP* 1984;56:1260–1264.
24. Katch V, Weltman A, Sady S, Freedson P. Validity of the relative percent concept for equating training intensity. *Eur J Appl Physiol* 1978;39:219–227.
25. Lee IM, Hsieh CC, Paffenbarger RS. Exercise intensity and longevity in men: the Harvard alumni health study. *JAMA* 1995;273:1179–1184.
26. McArdle WD, Katch FI, Katch VL. *Exercise physiology: energy, nutrition, and human performance.* Baltimore: Williams & Wilkins, 1996.
27. Noble BJ, Borg GAV, Jacobs I, Ceci R, Kaiser P. A category-ratio perceived exertion scale: relationship to blood and muscle lactates and heart rate. *Med Sci Sports Exerc* 1983;15:523–528.
28. Pate RR, Pratt M, Blair SN, et al. Physical activity and public health: a recommendation from the Centers for Disease Control and Prevention and the American College of Sports Medicine. *JAMA* 1995;273:402–407.
29. Rowell LB. *Human circulation: regulation during physical stress.* New York: Oxford University Press, 1986.
30. Seip RL, Snead D, Pierce E, Stein A, Weltman A. Perceptual responses and blood lactate concentration: effect of training state. *Med Sci Sports Exerc* 1991;23:80–87.
31. Sjodin B, Jacobs I, Svendenhag J. Changes in the onset of blood lactate accumulation (OBLA) and muscle enzymes after training at OBLA. *Eur J Appl Physiol* 1982;49:45–57.
32. Snead DB, Weltman A, Weltman JY, et al. Reproductive hormones and bone mineral density in women runners. *J Appl Physiol* 1992;72:2149–2156.
33. Steed JC, Gaesser GA, Weltman A. Rating of perceived exertion and blood lactate concentration during submaximal running. *Med Sci Sports Exerc* 1994;26:797–803.
34. Stoudemire NM, Wideman L, Pass KA, McGinnes CL, Gaesser GA, Weltman A. The validity of regulating blood lactate concentration by ratings of perceived exertion. *Med Sci Sport Exerc* 1996;28:490–495.
35. Weltman A. *The blood lactate response to exercise.* Champaign, IL: Human Kinetics, 1995.
36. Weltman A, Janney C, Rians CB, et al. The effects of hydraulic resistance strength training in pre-pubertal males. *Med Sci Sports Exerc* 1986;18:629–638.
37. Weltman A, Seip RL, Snead D, et al. Exercise training at and above the lactate threshold in previously untrained women. *Int J Sports Med* 1992;13:257–263.
38. Wilmore JH, Costill DL. *Physiology of sport and exercise.* Champaign, IL: Human Kinetics, 1994.

The Injured Athlete, Third Edition,
edited by D. H. Perrin.
Lippincott–Raven Publishers, Philadelphia © 1999.

CHAPTER 4

Designing Strength and Conditioning Programs

Martin A. Fees and Anthony Decker

OVERVIEW

Into the early 1980s athletes relied primarily on preseason practice to get themselves physically ready for in-season competition. Only elite or professional athletes utilized formal strength and conditioning programs. Today, that has changed dramatically. Leaders in the strength and conditioning profession such as Boyd Epley, Louis Riecke, and Clyde Emerich and researchers Michael Stone and William Kraemer have changed the way athletes now prepare for in-season competition. These pioneers have formalized year-round training specific to each sport. In addition, the influence from professionals in related fields such as biomechanics, psychology, physiology, and nutrition has enhanced the training of contemporary athletes.

It is for these reasons the strength and conditioning profession has grown to include its own national organization (National Strength and Conditioning Association, see Appendix A: Sports Medicine Organizations) and employ coaches from the professional, collegiate, high school, and private sectors. The field has become highly visible and science plays as much of a role as brute strength. Today's athletes are bigger, stronger, and faster than those of 25 years ago. Much of this has to do with the broad acceptance and understanding that, to be competitive, athletes must train on a regular basis throughout the year.

The health care professional must have a clear understanding of the design and administration of a well-organized strength and conditioning program. The major objective of any program should be injury prevention. Secondary objectives include performance enhancement and team camaraderie. The program should consist of warm-up, resistance, and plyometric training. Each segment of the program should have a specific purpose, placement, and outcome.

Warm-Up

The warm-up is defined as a series of activities with a desired outcome of mentally and physically preparing the athlete for practice or competition. This series of activities includes light physical activity, static, dynamic, and sport-specific flexibility and abdominal/lumbar strengthening. Two extremely important but underrated areas are addressed in the warm-up.

First, flexibility is a key component to injury prevention and performance. An example would be improved hamstring flexibility decreasing the risk of hamstring strains. In addition, improved hamstring flexibility leads to increased stride length. Speed is developed through two components: stride rate and stride length (5). Therefore, one component of improving speed has been addressed. Second, abdominal/trunk strength provides the critical link between transferring power from the lower extremity to the upper extremity. If an athlete is extremely powerful in the upper and lower extremity, but weak in the trunk, then the transfer of power will be ineffectual. The abdominal/trunk musculature is a crucial link that shouldn't be overlooked.

The warm-up should be tailored for the athlete's sport or activity and performed on a consistent basis. Many injuries occur because athletes inconsistently warm up. If the athlete doesn't have time to warm up, then he doesn't have time to complete his/her program. Listed below is

M. A. Fees: Joyner Sportsmedicine Institute, Inc., Gettysburg, Pennsylvania 17325

A. Decker: Department of Athletics, University of Delaware, Newark, Delaware 19716

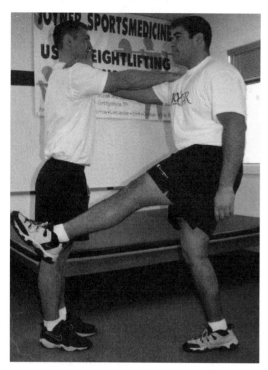

FIG. 4.1. Dynamic stretching through hip flexion range of motion.

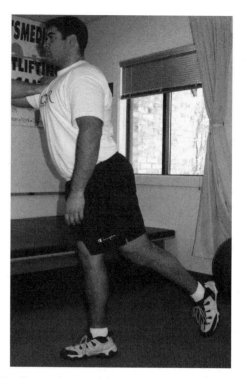

FIG. 4.2. Dynamic stretching through hip extension range of motion.

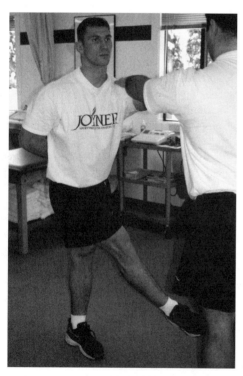

FIG. 4.3. Dynamic stretching through hip adduction range of motion.

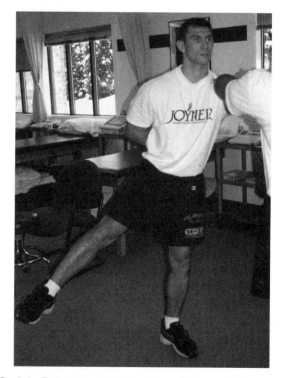

FIG. 4.4. Dynamic stretching through hip abduction range of motion.

a general model for warm-up and example exercises, which can be adapted to any sport.

Warm-Up Model

Light physical activity should be extensive enough to raise the core temperature, but not fatigue the neuromuscular system. A classic mistake is athletes completing a long run (more than 20 minutes) before doing their strength training or plyometrics. Example warm-up activities include half-mile run, 3 to 5 minutes of jump rope, 5 to 7 minutes on the stair stepper (10 minutes stationary bike or 5 minutes on upper-body ergometer (specifically for upper extremity sessions).

Simple static stretches are used to improve range of motion. These stretches are traditionally held for 15 to 30 seconds. These stretches should be done lightly and briefly at this point in the session. *Greater time* should be devoted during the *cool-down for static stretching*. *Brief* hamstring, hip flexor, adductor, and gastroc/soleus stretches are good examples.

Dynamic stretching involves rhythmic movement through the available range of motion. These stretches prepare the musculature for the ballistic motion in all sports. The movements are rhythmic in nature and kept in a comfortable range of motion. Two examples are presented in Figs. 4.1 to 4.4. The first demonstrates a dy-

TABLE 4.1. *Warm-up and cool-down guidelines for the abdomen and trunk*

- Nonresisted exercises should be done in the early phase with emphasis placed on warm-up
- Low volume should be done during warm-up phase to prevent fatigue before core movements
- Resisted drills should be completed during the cool-down
- Emphasis of motion should be on transverse (rotational) and sagittal plane (flexion/extension)

namic stretch for the hip flexors, rectus femoris, and hamstrings. In the example one athlete stabilizes the upper body by holding onto a partner. The athlete is shown swinging the lower extremity in a pendulum type manner through hip flexion and extension (Figs. 4.1 and 4.2). The second example is identical except the athlete is swinging through hip adduction and abduction (Figs. 4.3 and 4.4). These exercises can be done in 30 to 60 repetition sets with one to two sets per body part adequate.

Sport-specific stretching is defined by the coach or health professional associated with the team. The exercises are customized to stress the specific muscles involved in the sport. Also, these exercises can be tailored to the strength program. An example is one partner guiding an athlete through the proper back squat technique. The partner controls the motion with his hands in order to stretch the proper musculature (Fig. 4.5). Additional examples include: shoulder stretches for throwing athletes, hurdles stretches for track athletes, and goalie stretches in ice hockey.

Abdominal/trunk strengthening exercises at this time serve two purposes. They warm up this often-injured area before practice or competitive activity. In addition, this area is so critical to strength and power development the added work is needed. These exercises should be done in warm-up and cool-down according to the guidelines presented in Table 4.1. A sample workout is presented in Box 1.

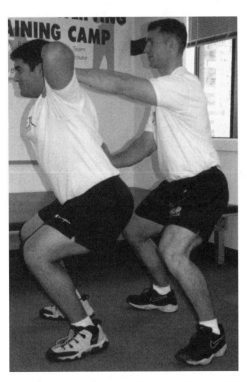

FIG. 4.5. Sport-specific stretching guiding athlete into proper back squat position.

BOX 1:
A Sample Pre- and Postworkout Program

Preworkout
Bridging 2 × 15, crunches 2 × 15, prone hip extension off hyperextension rack 2 × 12
Postworkout
Resisted hyperextensions off hyperextension bench 2 × 15 (15–25 lb), side-to-side ball toss (plyoball 6–10 lb) 3 × 12, and twisting crunches holding 10 lb plyoball

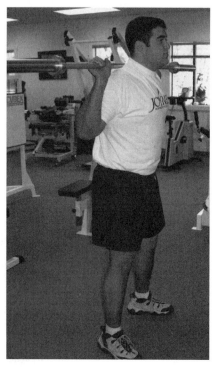

FIG. 4.6. Back squat—Starting position.

- Feet are placed at hip width with the toes turned slightly outward
- The lumbar region should maintain a normal lumbar lordosis
- Bar rests high on the trapezius below the spinous process of C-7
- Hand placement is slightly wider than shoulder width
- Scapula are retracted to support the upper spine
- The head should remain neutral with the focal point straight ahead
- Inhale at the start of the movement

Strength

In its simplest form strength can be defined as the ability to produce force (11). However, strength must be operationally defined within each individual strength and conditioning program. Consequently, an athlete's strength is directly related to the method and evaluation technique employed by the strength and conditioning professional. An example would be measuring strength on an isokinetic dynamometer versus free weights. The issue of strength is critical when assessing the exercises that are applied to any program. In general, exercises can be divided into strength and power movements. Exercises in the strength category are usually done in a slow and controlled fashion with the ultimate goal of enhancing basic strength. Figures 4.6–4.30 describe the more common strength exercises (referred to as *core* exercises) utilized in training programs. A checklist for each exercise, including technique

and common errors in each activity, is present in Boxes 1 to 10.

Power

Power is defined as work per unit time (14). Time is the critical factor that differentiates power from strength movements. These terms are often used interchangeably, but should be carefully separated. The confusion may have started with the sport, powerlifting. The sport consists of three lifts: bench press, back squat, and deadlift. These lifts are strength movements, but the sport is called powerlifting. Therefore, athletes assumed these lifts enhanced power. Increasing strength is a factor in attaining enhanced power, but specific power movements must be trained. The power exercises require strength and speed to be completed. These exercises are complicated and take thorough teaching and constant coaching for them to be incorporated safely into a training program. Health

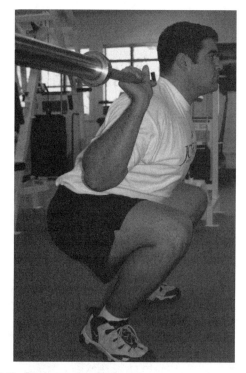

FIG. 4.7. Back squat—Descent.

- Heels should be flat with the pressure felt in the posterior aspect of the longitudinal arch throughout the movement
- The descent should be initiated with the hips sitting back
- Torso angle should remain as vertical as possible. Less than 30 degrees of trunk flexion is ideal
- Knees should remain behind the toes and in line with the ankle
- In the bottom position the top of the thigh should be parallel to the floor

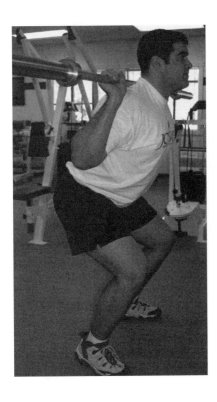

BOX 2:
Back Squat—Common Errors

- Hips or shoulder do not ascend in unison
- Heels rise off the floor either during the descent or ascent placing the foot pressure to far anterior
- The cervical region is hyperextended, placing undo stress on the soft tissue
- The knees come forward over the toes or adduct during the ascent
- The scapula protracts, causing a kyphotic posture in the upper spine
- The athlete is unable to maintain the proper lordosis during any part of the movement
- Uneven leg pressure during the lift (shifting to one side). Particularly common status post-knee injury or surgery
- Improper breathing technique. Performing Valsalva maneuver during exercise
- Bouncing in the bottom position

FIG. 4.8. Back squat—Ascent.

- Hips and shoulders should rise at the same rate
- Exhale throughout the ascent
- Pressure should be felt in the back of the arch of the foot
- Finish in starting position

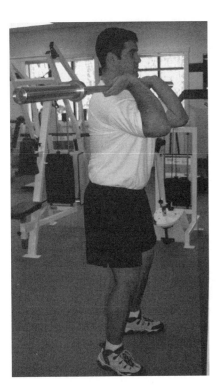

FIG. 4.9. Front squat—Starting position.

- Feet are positioned at hip width with the toes turned slightly outward
- The lumbar region should maintain a normal lordosis
- Bar rests across the chest on top of the upper pectoralis, clavicle, and anterior deltoid
- Grip is shoulder width apart with thumbs just adjacent to the middle deltoid
- Elbows are high in front (almost parallel to the floor)
- Chest is expanded to provide a platform for the bar
- The head should remain neutral with the focal point straight ahead

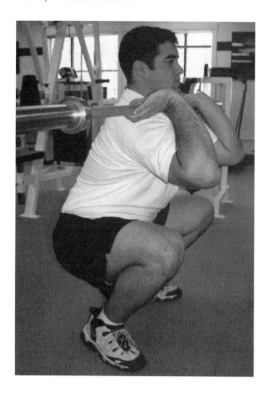

FIG. 4.10. Front squat—Descent.

- Heels should be flat with the pressure felt in the posterior aspect of the longitudinal throughout the movement
- The descent should be initiated with the hips sitting back
- Torso will be slightly more upright than the back squat. Less than 20 degrees is ideal
- Knees should remain behind the toes and in line with the ankle
- In the bottom position the top of the thigh should be parallel to the floor

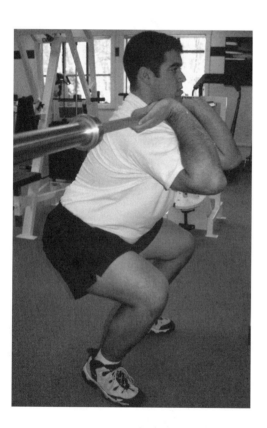

BOX 3:
Front Squat—Common Errors

- Same as back squat with the following additions:
- Elbows drop during the lift leading to a kyphotic back position
- Bar slides forward and downward on the chest causing the centers of gravity to move anteriorly

---

FIG. 4.11. Front squat—Ascent.

- Hips and shoulders should rise at the same rate (elbows remain high throughout the ascent)
- Pressure should be felt in the back of the arch of the foot
- Finish in starting position

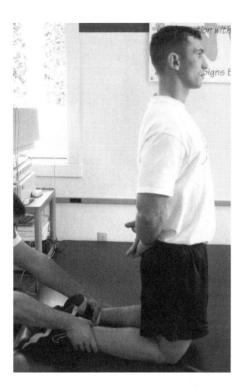

FIG. 4.12. Partner hamstring—Starting position.

• Athlete kneels on padded surface with ankle stabilized by partner
• Torso is rigid with hands behind the back
• Head in neutral

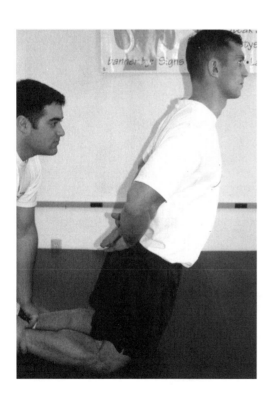

FIG. 4.13. Partner hamstring—Descent.

• Lower upper body toward ground in slow controlled manner
• Torso stays rigid
• Axis of motion occurs at the knee

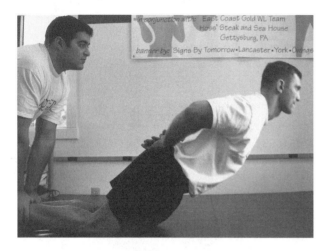

FIG. 4.14. Partner hamstring—Finish.

• Continue to lower toward ground until muscle failure
• Either have additional partner catch athlete or put hands out front to control last part of descent

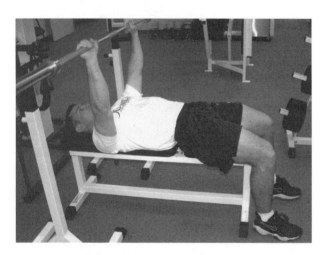

FIG. 4.15. Bench press—Starting position.

• Feet flat on the floor and knees bent to 90 degrees
• Buttocks, shoulders, and head are centered and in contact with the bench
• Shoulder or sport specific grip width

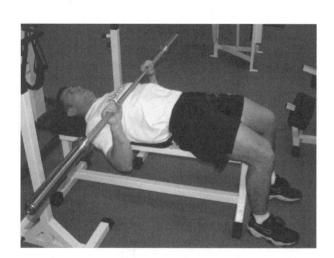

FIG. 4.16. Bench press—Descent.

• Shoulders should retract before beginning the descent phase
• Elbows are rotated slightly inward to prevent bar from drifting toward neck
• Inhale before descent of the bar
• Bar should be lowered in a controlled pace
• Touch the bar to the highest point on the chest usually slightly above the nipple

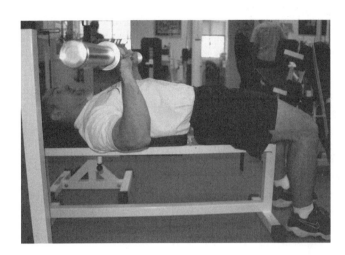

BOX 5:
Bench Press—Common Errors

- Feet do not remain in contact with floor
- Bouncing the bar off the chest
- Shoulders and buttocks not centered
- Buttocks coming off the bench thus creating excessive lumbar lordosis
- Uneven grip
- Arms rising at different rates
- Head lifting off the bench into excessive cervical flexion

FIG. 4.17. Bench press—Ascent.

- Exhale during pressing motion
- Bar should be pressed back toward the upper chest in a slightly arched pattern

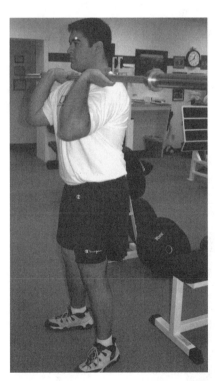

FIG. 4.18. Front shoulder press—Starting position.

- Feet placement hip width apart or slightly wider
- Normal lumbar lordosis
- Grip width same as the front squat (commonly called the clean grip)
- Elbows slightly inferior to the deltoid and just anterior of the body
- Chest elevated and expanded
- Chin tucked slightly backward for clear bar path

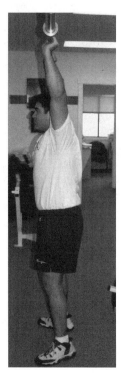

FIG. 4.19. Front shoulder press—Finish position.

- Head and shoulders shift under the bar at the completion of the lift
- Bar pressed and finished overhead and in line with the centers of gravity (ears, shoulders, greater trochanter)
- Exhale during pressing motion and inhale while returning bar to starting position

BOX 6:
Front Shoulder Press—Common Errors

- Feet too wide or too narrow
- Excessive lumbar extension or flexion during pressing motion
- Elbows drop before pressing the bar
- Finished pressing motion not aligned with centers of gravity (ears, shoulders, greater trochanter)
- Grip too wide placing excessive stress on the shoulder joint
- Improper breathing

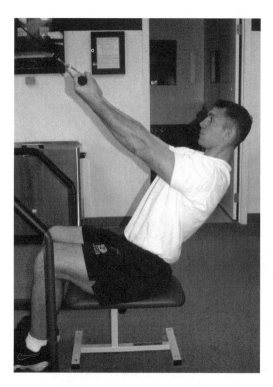

FIG. 4.20. Front latissimus pull-down—Starting position.

- Feet flat and contacting the floor
- Shoulder width or sport specific grip
- Trunk angle is 30 degrees to 45 degrees of extension
- Head neutral (focal point straight ahead)

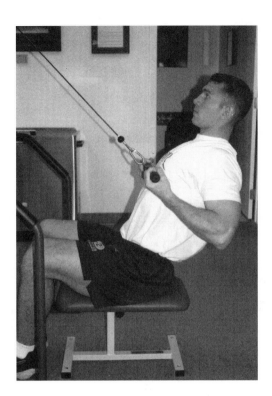

> **BOX 7:**
> **Front Lattisimus Pull-Down—Common Errors**
>
> - Improper breathing
> - Feet not maintaining contact with floor
> - Rocking or swinging of the upper extremity during the pulling motion
> - Shoulders not retracted during initiation of the movement
> - Improper trunk angle
> - Scapula not remaining retracted during the descent

FIG. 4.21. Front latissimus pull-down—Chest position.

- Shoulders retract before beginning the descent of the bar
- Initiate movement by retracting the scapula
- Inhale before initiating the pulling motion
- Bring bar down to touch the highest point on the chest above the xiphoid process
- No bouncing or rocking of the upper body during the movement
- Inhale while returning the bar to starting position

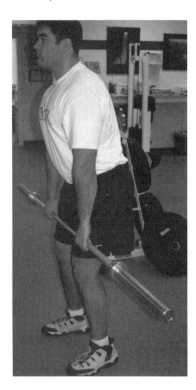

FIG. 4.22. Romanian deadlift—Starting position.

- Feet are placed at hip width or slightly narrower
- Knees are slightly flexed (10 degrees to 15 degrees)
- Back maintains normal lumbar lordosis
- Shoulders retracted
- Holding the bar at waist level with clean grip

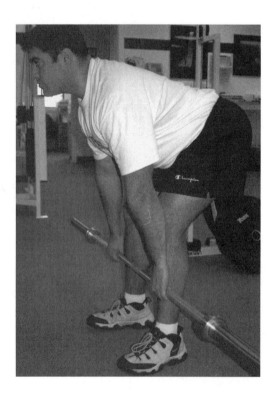

FIG. 4.23. Romanian deadlift—Descent.

- Bar is lowered toward the ground while maintaining lumbar lordosis
- Axis of motion occurs at the hips
- Hips remain at their starting height
- Weight is shifted toward the heels for greater hamstring involvement
- Torso should not drop more than a few degrees parallel to the floor

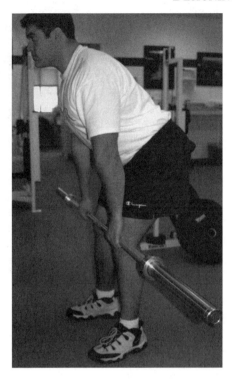

BOX 8:
Romanian Deadlift—Common Errors

- Feet placed too wide at the start of the lift
- Knees extend during the descent of the bar
- Bar drifts away from the body
- Weight shifts toward the balls of the feet
- Hips drop and knee flexion increases during the descent
- Kyphotic posture throughout the movement

FIG. 4.24. Romanian deadlift—Ascent.

- Inhale while lowering the bar and exhale during ascent of bar
- Maintain bar close to shins and thighs
- Maintain slight knee flexion
- Return to starting position

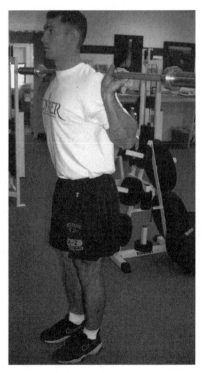

BOX 9:
Lunges—Common Errors

Same as squatting with these additions:
- Stride leg crosses toward the midline thus causing loss of balance
- Increased trunk flexion and extension throughout the exercise
- Ipsilateral knee crashes to the floor during the bottom of the movement
- Knee flexion on stride leg greater than 90 degrees, therefore causing increased patellofemoral joint forces.
- Platform elevated too high causing excessive pressure about the knee joint
- Foot not firmly planted on the platform (unstable base)

FIG. 4.25. Lunge—Starting position.

- Feet are positioned at hip width with the toes turned slightly outward
- The lumbar region should maintain a normal lumbar lordosis
- Bar rests high on the trapezius below the spinous process of C-7
- Hand placement is slightly wider than shoulder width
- Scapula are retracted to lock the upper spine
- The head should remain neutral (focal point straight ahead)

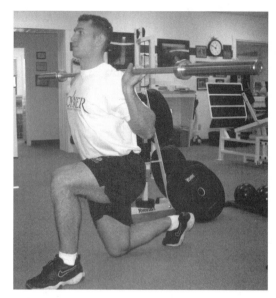

FIG. 4.26. Lunge—Descent.

- Step forward with one foot
- Knees should remain behind the toes and in line with the ankle (torso angle should remain 0 to 10 degrees)
- In the bottom position the top of the thigh should be parallel to the floor and at a 90-degree angle to the tibia
- Ipsilateral knee should gently touch on the ground

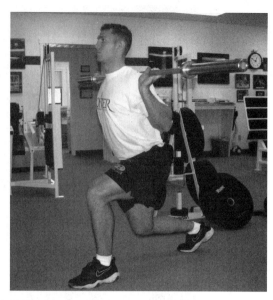

FIG. 4.27. Lunge—Ascent.

- Push off foot in quick, but controlled manner
- Hips and shoulders should ascend in unison
- Pressure should be felt in the back of the longitudinal arch during push off
- Finish in starting position

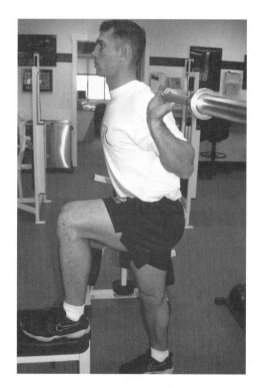

FIG. 4.28. Step-up—Starting position.

- Feet are positioned at hip width with the toes turned slightly outward
- The lumbar region should maintain a normal lumbar lordosis
- Bar rests high on the trapezius below the spinous process of C-7
- Hand placement is slightly wider than shoulder width
- Scapula are retracted to lock the upper spine
- The head should remain neutral (focal point straight ahead)
- One foot placed on stable platform bring the hip and knee into 90 degrees of flexion
- Ipsilateral lower extremity remains in contact with the floor and knee in full extension

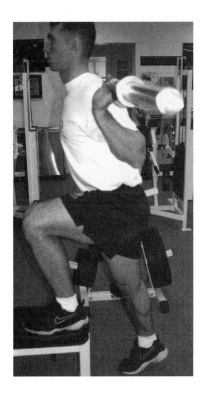

FIG. 4.29. Step-up—Initiation of movement.

- Lower extremity in contact with the ground initiates movement with plantar flexion of the ankle. The knee remains extended and provides no force
- Simultaneously, the lower extremity on the platform initiates motion with hip and knee extension

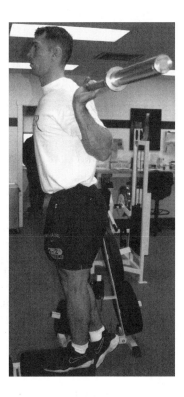

BOX 10:
Step-Ups—Common Errors

Same as squatting with these additions:
- Use of knee extension by lower extremity in contact with the floor to initiate movement
- Increased trunk flexion and extension throughout the exercise
- Rapidly descending back to starting position
- Foot not firmly planted on the platform (unstable base)

FIG. 4.30. Step-up—Ascent.

- Hip and knee extension continue until full range of motion is completed
- Hips and shoulders should ascend in unison
- Important to return to starting position with slow controlled motion

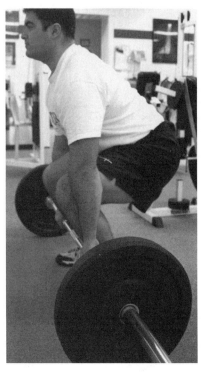

FIG. 4.31. Power clean—Starting position.

- Grip slightly wider than shoulder width
- Feet are hip width apart and knees flexed between 60 degrees and 90 degrees
- Hips remain elevated and the shoulders should be anterior to the bar
- Back maintains normal lumbar lordosis
- Arms are straight and relaxed with elbows turned outward and in line with the bar
- Weight is distributed in the middle of the foot while the toes can still be wiggled

care professionals teaching power movements should, at minimum, be a certified strength and conditioning specialist. Additional certifications to support teaching power techniques would be Club Coach and Senior Coach Certification through the United States Weightlifting Association. Figures 4.31–4.38 list the more common power movements (core exercises) with a technique list and description of common errors for each exercise given in Boxes 11–13.

Summary

The section on technique provides the reader with information to follow for basic strength and power movements. This section does not certify or qualify the reader to coach and teach these exercises. Teaching and coaching of these exercises takes time and experience. Remember that technique development is no different than developing skills for a specific sport. Safety and proper biomechanics must be applied to each exercise.

PROGRAM DESIGN

Definitions

Program design is defined as a systematic schedule with consideration of repetition (Box 14), intensity, and exercise leading to a specific outcome. This program is completed in a predetermined period of time. Program design can be divided into basic, intermediate, and advanced. The fundamental differences between these categories are relative to the variations in repetition, intensity, and exercise. Three examples of various basic programs include DeLorme's progressive resistance exercise, Nautilus Training, and Knight's DAPRE technique. This list is not inclusive, but provides a sampling of basic program design. Each program is summarized below.

DeLorme's Progressive Resistance Exercise

The program (2) is based on completing three sets of ten repetitions for each exercise as seen in Table 4.2. If all repetitions are completed an additional 5% is added to each set during the next training session.

Nautilus Program

This program (12) is based on performing four to six exercises for the lower extremity and six to eight exercises for the upper extremity. Total exercises per session shouldn't exceed 12. The athlete selects a weight that will allow completion of 8 to 12 repetitions in a controlled and steady form. If less than eight repetitions are performed, the resistance is too heavy, therefore decrease the weight. If 12 or more repetitions are performed, the resistance is too light, therefore increase the weight. Once a satisfactory weight is established, exercise in a controlled fashion until no more repetitions are possible. After the athlete is capable of 12 repetitions during one session, the weight should be increased by approximately 5%.

Knight's DAPRE (Daily Adjustable Progressive Resistance Exercise) Program

This program (2) is based on completing four sets of exercises as seen in Table 4.3. The novice strength-

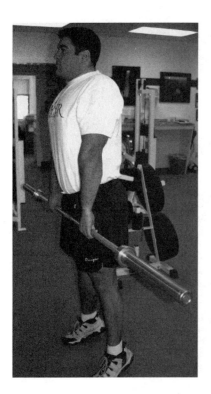

FIG. 4.32. Power clean—Pulling sequence.

- Initiate slow pulling motion off the floor with the legs and hips
- Trunk angle remains constant with isometric contraction of the lower back
- As the bar approaches the upper third of thigh, begin explosive pulling motion initiated by the hips
- Weight shifting toward the balls of the feet
- The athlete completes an explosive jumping motion with the arms remaining straight and relaxed
- At the completion of the jumping motion the athlete produces an aggressive shrug (arms still straight)
- At the completion of the shrug the body is pulled under the bar
- The bar remains close to the body

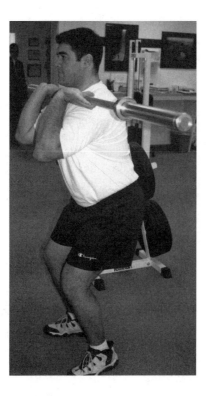

BOX 11:
Power Clean—Common Errors

- Elbows bend too early before the completion of the explosive jump and shrug
- Feet start too wide
- Shoulders drift behind the bar at the start of the lift
- Head does not remain neutral
- Jumping motion not completed
- Bar swings away from the body during the pull phase
- Improper weight distribution of the feet during the lift
- Back does not maintain normal lumbar lordosis
- Feet shuffle too wide when catching the bar
- Athlete finishes in a poor front squat posture (see technique)
- Movement is initiated by excessive trunk extension instead of knee extension and hip extension

---

FIG. 4.33. Power clean—Finishing position.

- The feet shuffle as the bar is caught into a 1/4 squat position
- Upon catching the weight the athlete should end up in a 1/4 front squat position (see technique)
- Vertical displacement of the body is emphasized to keep the bar and body close together

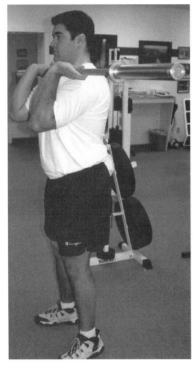

FIG. 4.34. Push press—Starting position.

• Same as front shoulder press

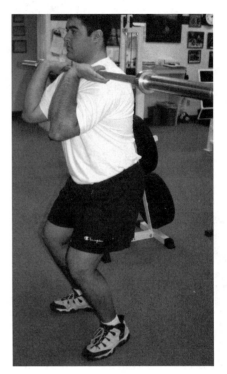

FIG. 4.35. Push press—Dipping motion.

• Knees flex in a controlled, but quick motion about 4 to 6 inches
• Feet remain flat during the knee flexion and hips remain directly under the torso
• The knees extend driving the bar overhead
• Simultaneously the arms press the bar overhead

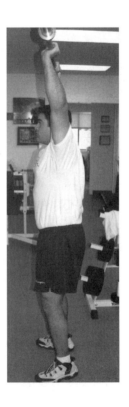

BOX 12:
Push Press—Common Errors

• Same as front shoulder press with these additions
• Heels rise during the dip
• Body does not completely extend during the drive phase
• Elbows drop during the dip and hips do not remain directly under the torso
• Bar does not finish in line with the center of gravity

FIG. 4.36. Push press—Finishing position.

• Bar finishes in line with centers of gravity (ears, shoulders, greater trochanter)
• Arms finish in an extended position
• Lower bar to starting position

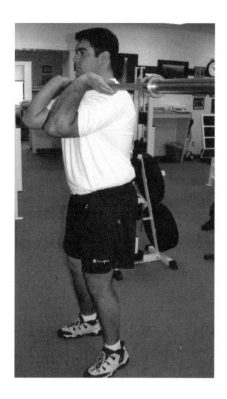

FIG. 4.37. Power jerk—Starting position.

• Same as push press

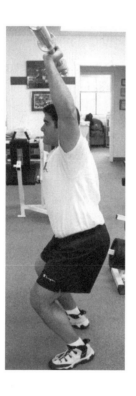

BOX 13:
Power Jerk—Common Errors
Same as push press and front shoulder press with these additions:

• Feet shuffle too wide during the catch phase
• Athlete does not dip under the bar
• Athlete hops forward or backward during the drive and catch phase

FIG. 4.38. Power jerk finishing position.

• The initial phase is the same as the push press with the dipping motion and driving the bar overhead
• Upon completion of the drive the athlete will flex the knees and hips and finish in a 1/4 squat position
• Feet will shuffle into a squat foot position at hip width or slightly wider
• Return to starting position with bar aligned properly

training athlete should be introduced to resistance training utilizing a basic program. This provides several advantages to the novice. First, the program is very simple to follow; therefore the athlete can be independent in the weight room. Second, the progressive nature of these programs allows the athlete constant improvement, which is a motivating factor to continue weight training. Third, the programs start with a minimal number of sets; therefore the total time will not overwhelm the novice strength athlete. There is one major disadvantage with all basic programs. The lack of variation in repetitions and intensity provides only brief stimulus to the muscle. Therefore, strength gains are made rapidly in the beginning of the program, but this lack of variation leads to a decrease in muscle stimulation commonly referred to as plateauing (stagnation in the weight being lifted). Therefore, when implementing these programs improvements can be expected to occur quickly, but reach a physiologic plateau within 3 to 6 months.

In the previous section, variations in repetition and intensity were discussed, but a second area of program design is the exercise schedule. Two areas to consider would include exercise selection and exercise order. Exercise selection can be divided into multi-joint and single-joint exercises. Multi-joint exercises present several advantages, which include targets several muscle groups per exercise, generally more sport specific and performed in a functional closed-chain position. Disadvantages are that the athlete must take time to learn a new skill and the exercises require spotting (supervision while performing activity for safety). Examples of multi-joint exercises include back squat, bench press, front shoulder press, and lunges. Single-joint exercises have one advantage, which is the ability to isolate a specific muscle group. The disadvantages are that they are less functional or sport specific, are performed in open chained position, and only target one muscle group per exercise. Examples of single-joint exercises include leg extensions, biceps curls, and seated calf raises. Exercise selection for strength training should incorporate both multi-joint and single-joint exercises. The activi-

TABLE 4.2. *DeLorme's progressive resistance exercise program*

First set—1 × 10 at 50% of 10 RM
Second set—1 × 10 at 75% of 10 RM
Third set—1 × 10 at 100% of 10 RM

ties should predominantly consist of multi-joint exercises and a few selected single-joint exercises. The novice strength athlete should be exposed to eight to ten exercises per session. This number allows proper physiologic development, but does not psychologically overwhelm the athlete. In addition, exercise selection for the novice athlete should consist of strength exercises as previously described in the chapter. The emphasis of basic program design is establishing a strength base and *proper technique*. Power exercises, as previously described, should be developed with the advanced program design.

Exercise order is developed after the exercise selection has been made. Several rules will simplify the ordering of exercises. First, multi-joint exercises should precede the single-joint exercises. Second, pressing activities (bench press, front shoulder press) can be alternated with pulling (front lat pull down, seated rows) and leg activities (squats, lunges). This allows the muscle groups involved in pressing (chest, anterior deltoid, triceps) to rest while performing pulling or leg activities that stress the latissimus dorsi, posterior deltoid, or quadriceps. Third, place the exercises that are most important and/or the athlete has the most difficulty completing in the beginning of the session. This allows the athlete to concentrate on the most important or their weakest exercises in the beginning of the session while the neuromuscular system is not fatigued.

The final factor to consider with basic program design is frequency. The typical program can be completed every other day. These schedules usually follow a Monday, Wednesday, and Friday or Tuesday, Thursday, and Saturday model. This allows the athlete to have a full

---

BOX 14:
Program Design Definitions

Intensity: Average weight per exercise used during resistance training
Repetition maximum: The maximum number of repetitions completed for a specific exercise. Repetition maximum can range from 12 to 1. Usually abbreviated (RM)

TABLE 4.3. *Knight's DAPRE program*

Determine the initial working weight (6 RM)
First Set—10 repetitions at 50% of the 6 RM
Second Set—6 reps at 75% of the 6 RM
Third Set—As many reps as possible with the full 6 RM
Use Table 4.5 to adjust weight for the fourth set
Fourth Set—As many reps as possible with the adjusted weight from previous table
The number of reps completed in the fourth set is used to determine the working weight for the next day

TABLE 4.4. *Example of a strength program for a novice high school wrestler*

First 4 weeks—technique emphasis

Back squat	—2 sets of 10 repetitions
Bench press	—2 sets of 10 repetitions
Front lat pull down	—2 sets of 10 repetitions
Front shoulder press	—2 sets of 10 repetitions
Seated rows	—2 sets of 10 repetitions
Dumbbell bench press	—2 sets of 10 repetitions
Dumbbell rows	—2 sets of 10 repetitions
Triceps extensions	—2 sets of 10 repetitions
Biceps curls	—2 sets of 10 repetitions

Second 4 weeks—DeLorme's progressive resistance exercise

Back squat	—3 sets of 10 repetitions
Bench press	—3 sets of 10 repetitions
Front lat pull down	—3 sets of 10 repetitions
Front shoulder press	—3 sets of 10 repetitions
Seated rows	—3 sets of 10 repetitions
Dumbbell bench press	—3 sets of 10 repetitions
Dumbbell rows	—3 sets of 10 repetitions
Triceps dips	—3 sets of 10 repetitions
Dumbbell curls	—3 sets of 10 repetitions

At the end of the second 4 weeks complete 6 RM for each lift.

Third 4 weeks—DAPRE

Back squat	—DAPRE
Bench press	—DAPRE
Front lat pull down	—DAPRE
Front shoulder press	—DAPRE
Seated rows	—DAPRE
Dumbbell bench press	—DAPRE
Dumbbell rows	—DAPRE

TABLE 4.5. *DAPRE Weight Adjustment*

# of Reps during Set 3	Adjustment to working weight for Set 4	Adjustment to working weight for next day
0–2	Decrease weight by 5–10 lbs and repeat set	Decrease weight by 5–10 lbs
3–4	Decrease weight by 0–5 lbs	Keep weight the same
5–7	Keep weight the same	Increase by 5–10 lbs
8–12	Increase weight by 5–10 lbs	Increase weight by 5–15 lbs
13+ reps	Increase weight by 10–15 lbs	Increase weight by 10–20 lbs

a week schedule prevents the danger of overtraining. As the athlete progresses from a novice to advanced, then additional days of training can be incorporated. This will be discussed in the advanced program design section.

Development of a typical strength program for a novice high school wrestler is presented in Table 4.4. The program time frame is 4 weeks. During the first 4 weeks the athlete will perform two sets of ten repetitions for the exercises listed in Table 4.4. The emphasis at this time should be technical. The athlete should be monitored for proper technique and posture during weight training. If the athlete develops correct technique at this early stage, then their technique will remain proper throughout their career. The athlete should be encouraged to choose a weight that allows smooth controlled motion and the completion of all the repetitions. After the 4 weeks, the athlete can complete a ten repetition maximum (RM) for each of the multi-joint exercises. If they don't achieve exactly ten repetitions, a 10 RM can be calculated from the conversion chart below. The second 4 weeks can be completed using DeLorme's progressive resistance exercise program (see Table 4.2 for basic program design).

day recovery before returning to the weight room. The novice athlete needs this day of recovery in order to promote recovery from the microtrauma incurred during the weight training session. In addition, the novice athlete's muscle and connective tissue aren't well adapted to the rigors of an organized weight-training program leaving them susceptible to overtraining. The three days

TABLE 4.6. *Sample intermediate program for bench press*

	Day 1	Day 2	Day 3
Week 1	5 × 3 × 80% (L)	5 × 4 × 80% (H)	5 × 3 × 80% (L)
Week 2	5 × 5 × 80% (H)	5 × 3 × 80% (L)	4 × 4 × 85% (H)
Week 3	5 × 3 × 80% (L)	3 × 3 × 90% (H)	5 × 3 × 80% (L)
Week 4	2 × 2 × 95% (H)	5 × 3 × 80% (L)	Max

H, heavy day; L, light day; Max, new repetition maximum.
Each workout should be preceded by warm-up sets of 5 reps at 50%, 60%, and 70%.

Intermediate Program Design

Intermediate program design involves the development of a heavy/lightweight training schedule. The basic premise utilizes alternating heavy and light days in order to increase volume and intensity. In addition, these schedules begin to allow the athlete to predict specific days when strength levels are peaking. The difference between a heavy and light day is based on changes in intensity. The athlete follows a predetermined schedule of alternating intensities, then gradually tapers to produce a new maximum. This type of program presents increased variation in exercise and intensity and a smooth transition into advanced program design and periodization. A sample program is listed in Table 4.6.

ADVANCED PROGRAM DESIGN

Advanced program design implements additional exercises and variations in intensity and repetitions. The addition of power exercises and plyometrics into a program provides the key ingredients needed by the athlete to develop explosiveness and speed. Several factors should be considered before starting into more advanced programs.

First, the general order of exercises should be as follows. Sport-specific drills and plyometrics (e.g., medicine ball chest pass for offensive lineman in football) should be completed in the beginning of the training session. This allows the correct neuromuscular pattern to be engrained and development of the proper stretch shortening cycle without alteration from fatigue. Second, the power movements such as power clean, push press, push jerk should be executed while the muscles and nervous system are in a state of limited fatigue. This is secondary to the high degree of coordination and skill required by these exercises. Local muscle fatigue may alter technique placing the athlete at risk for injury and not allow the development of proper intensity. Third, multi-joint strength exercises such as back squats, bench press, and lunges should be performed after the power movements. The neuromuscular system is in a state of limited fatigue, but is excited from the power movements. Therefore, technique can be maintained and the excitatory state of the nervous system elevates the performance. Fourth, the isolated single-joint movements and rehabilitation exercises such as leg extensions, rotator cuff exercises, and bicep curls are performed after the neuromuscular system is fatigued. These exercises are specific and don't require the metabolic effort or skill of the previous exercises.

Muscle imbalance is another consideration that can be prevented with the following guidelines. Each workout should include a leg movement, press movement, and at least two pulling movements. Muscle balance is very important to minimizing the risks of straining muscles. The agonist and antagonist muscle groups operate in appropriate ratios. These ratios should be developed along with proper posture to reduce the risk of shoulder, lumbar, and hamstring injuries. A general recommendation to maintain balance is a press-to-pull ratio of 1:2.

Once the exercise order and selection have been made, then variation in repetition and intensity should be addressed. As previously discussed basic program design provides a physiologic stimulus for 3 to 6 months, after which improvement is significantly decreased. Therefore, variation in repetition and intensity is needed to provide the stimulus for continuous strength and power gains. This concept is termed periodization.

Periodization

Recently, advanced writing of strength and conditioning programs has developed from the model of periodization. Based on yearly, monthly, and weekly training cycles, periodization has been shown to be superior in attaining strength and power gains over extended periods of time. Although various interpretations exist, a general consensus exists for the basic format. This basic format can be individualized based on the needs of the sport and the athlete.

General Interpretation

In its simplest form, periodization programs are written on multiple-week cycles each designed to progress toward new peaks at the end of a training period. These training periods are divided into preparation, strength, strength/power, and maintenance or peaking (3,10,15).

The first phase is called preparation. The goals of the preparation phase are seen in Table 4.7. In order to achieve these goals this phase consists of low weight (intensity) and high volume (number of total reps) activity. Intensity varies from 60% to 70% of the predetermined 1 RM with the number of reps in each set ranging from eight to twelve. The only variation from this repeti-

TABLE 4.7. *Goals of the periodization preparation phase*

1. Increase lean body mass
2. Increase lactate threshold
3. Stress technical mastery with exercises
4. Physically and psychologically prepare for more intense activity in the next phases

TABLE 4.8. *Goals of the periodization strength phase*

1. Increase utilization of type II fibers
2. Increase recruitment of larger motor units
3. Increase synchronization of movement
4. Continue to refine exercise technique
5. Gradual transition into power and speed movements

TABLE 4.10. *Goals of the periodization peaking/ maintenance phase*

Peaking
  1. Attain physiological and biomechanical peak
  2. Maximize number of large motor units recruited
Maintenance
  1. Maintain physiological and biomechanical peak for designated season

tion scheme is associated with the power exercises. The power exercises are restricted to less than four repetitions per set. The lower number of repetitions limits the fatigue in the neuromuscular system allowing the athlete to complete the exercise with proper intensity and technique. Therefore, to get the desired volume additional sets must be added to the power exercises. Rest periods are kept short, less than one minute, in order to stimulate muscle hypertrophy and short-term endurance. The number of sets for the core lifts are four to five and sets for accessory movements is two to three. The preparation phase can last from 4 to 8 weeks.

The second part of the periodization cycle is the strength phase. The goals of the strength phase are seen in Table 4.8. At this time volume drops to five to seven reps per set and the intensity gradually increases to 70% to 80% of the predetermined 1 RM. This increasing intensity and decreasing volume promote recruitment and utilization of larger motor units and fast-twitch fibers, hence increased strength output. The only exercises that will employ less than five to seven reps are the power movements. During the strength phase, two to three reps per set should be utilized for power exercises. Two additional changes denote the strength phase, the choice of exercise begins to get more specific, and the number of accessory movements begins to decrease. The basic strength phase is usually 3 to 6 weeks in duration.

The third part of the periodization cycle is the strength/power phase with the emphasis beginning to change from strength to power and speed. The goals of the strength/power phase are seen in Table 4.9. During this phase volume begins to dramatically decrease as intensity continues to increase. The phase utilizes three to four reps

per set for core movements while the intensity climbs to 80% to 90%. The power exercises utilize two to three reps per set. The choice of exercises during this phase continues to be more specific as emphasis is placed primarily on core movements. This phase usually lasts 2 to 4 weeks.

The periodization cycle ends with the peaking/maintenance phase. The goals of the peaking/maintenance phase are listed in Table 4.10. The peaking phase usually lasts no more than 2 weeks as intensity is at its highest and volume at its lowest. Reps per set are one to three for core lifts, one to two for power movements, and the intensity increases to 90% and above for the predetermined 1 RM. Table 4.11 presents a sample program for the periodization model.

Wave Model

As athletes mature and become more experienced, training programs should also provide greater challenges in order to stimulate continued physical adaptation. The wave model takes the general periodization

TABLE 4.9. *Goals of the periodization strength/power phase*

1. Increase recruitment of the largest motor units
2. Finish transition to functional power and speed-oriented movement patterns
3. Decrease inhibition of Golgi tendon organs
4. Increase utilization of stretch-shortening cycle activities

TABLE 4.11. *Sample program for the periodization model*

Week(s)	Intensity	Reps	Sets	Exercise
1–4	60%–70%	4	6	Power clean
1–4	60%–70%	5–6	5–6	Back squat
1–4	60%–70%	8–12	3–5	Bench press
5–7	70%–80%	3–4	6–8	Power clean
5–7	70%–80%	4–5	5–7	Back squat
5–7	70%–80%	5–7	4–5	Bench press
8–9	80%–90%	2–3	8–10	Power clean
8–9	80%–90%	3–4	8–10	Back squat
8–9	80%–90%	3–4	6–8	Bench press
10–11	90%+	1–2	10–12	Power clean
10–11	90%+	1–2	10–12	Back squat
10–11	90%+	1–2	10–12	Bench press
12 (taper)	75%–80%	2–3	5–8	Power clean
12 (taper)	75%–85%	3–4	5–8	Back squat
12 (taper)	75%–85%	3–4	4–5	Bench press
13 (test)	Establish new RM			

TABLE 4.12. *Sample program for the wave model*

Week(s)	Intensity	Reps	Sets	Exercise
1	65%	4	6	Power clean
	65%	5	5–6	Back squat
	65%	8–10	3–5	Bench press
2	75%	3–4	8–9	Power clean
	75%	4–5	6–8	Back squat
	75%	5–7	5–6	Bench press
3	70%	3–4	6–8	Power clean
	70%	3–4	5–6	Back squat
	70%	6–8	4–5	Bench press
4	80%	2–3	8–10	Power clean
	80%	3–4	8–9	Back squat
	80%	5–6	5–6	Bench press

BOX 15:
Checklist for Calculating Volume and Intensity

- 1 to 2 press-to-pull ratio
- Speed and explosive movements early in the workout and before slower movements
- No more than 35 reps per exercise per workout for strength movements
- No more than 25 reps per exercise per workout for speed movements
- No more than 25% of workout should come from one exercise
- Hamstring strength at least 65% of quadricep strength
- Core and complicated exercises early in workout when fresh
- Minimum of ten reps per exercise to have a training effect
- Planned recovery and restoration (i.e., taper weeks, proper physiological modalities
- 0–50 reps per workout (light day/maintenance)
- 50–100 reps per workout (moderate workout)
- 100–150 reps per workout (heavy workout)
- 150+ reps per workout (huge workout)

---

principles and alters the variety of repetitions and intensity on a weekly basis. Instead of relying on multiple-weeks training sessions (mesocycles), the wave principle is designed around weekly progressions called microcycles (9). The wave model alternates a light week with a progressively heavier week. This includes not only intensity, but volume as well. This format is continued for 13 weeks. During the 13-week training session, goals should be set to reach 80% of the predetermined 1 RM by week 4, 90% of the predetermined 1 RM by week 8, and establish a new 1 RM at week 12. The thirteenth week is used as a week to taper in preparation for the upcoming event or season. The intensity of the taper week is executed at 75% to 85% of the predetermined 1 RM and sessions are performed only 2 to 3 days during that week. This enables the athlete to handle higher volume with higher intensity throughout the 13-week plan. Novice athletes should probably avoid this format until they can safely handle the excessive demands. If two or three of these 13-week cycles are incorporated in succession, then this period is termed a macrocycle. Table 4.12 presents a

sample program of the wave model. (This sample shows the first 4 weeks of the program.)

Stair Model

Another advanced program design is the stair theory, which likewise utilizes weekly training cycles (9). The stair model is a 13-week program whereas weeks 1, 2, and 3 are progressively heavier with the light week not coming until week 4. This progression is repeated three times with each 4-week section progressively increasing in intensity. During the 12-week training session, goals should be set to reach 80% of the predetermined 1 RM by week 3, 90% of the predetermined 1 RM by week 7, and 100% of the predetermined 1 RM at week 11. Unlike the wave model in which week 12 is a peak and week 13 is a taper week, the stair model reverses these concluding sessions. Therefore, the athlete tapers in week 12 and establishes new maximums in week 13. The premise of tapering in week 12 is to allow for the neuromuscular system to recuperate; consequently the athlete is well rested prior to establishing new maximums. Table 4.13 presents a sample program of the first 4 weeks of the stair model.

TABLE 4.13. *Sample program for the stair model*

Weeks	Intensity	Reps	Sets	Exercise
1	70%	4	6–7	Power clean
	70%	5–6	5–6	Back squat
	70%	8	3–4	Bench press
2	75%	3	8–9	Power clean
	75%	4–5	6–8	Back squat
	75%	5–7	5–7	Bench press
3	80%	2–3	10–12	Power clean
	80%	3–4	8–10	Back squat
	80%	3–4	8–10	Bench press
4	75%	3	6–8	Power clean
	75%	3–4	4–5	Back squat
	75%	4–5	4–4	Bench press

BOX 16:
Safety Precautions and Exercise Modifications

- Avoid behind the neck lat pull-down for any athletes. Potential brachial plexus injuries and stretching of the glenohumeral ligaments (14).
- Avoid behind the neck press for any athletes. Potential stretching of the glenohumeral ligaments.
- Avoid relaxing shoulders at the end of shoulder shrugs. Potential stress on inferior glenohumeral ligaments.
- Avoid excessively wide grip (greater than two times shoulder width) on the bench press with athletes. Potentially increases stress on the rotator cuff and long head of the biceps tendon.
- Avoid exercises that promote excessive flexion (i.e., stiff-legged deadlifts). Maintain lumbar extension during pulling activities (e.g., seated rows). Potential microtraumatic changes with repetitively resisted flexion.
- Avoid excessive lumbar extension during exercises. Increased stress on the pars interarticularis.
- All shoulder-pressing motions should be done in a standing position. Seated shoulder-press motions develop significant intradisk pressure in the lumbar region.
- Utilize a weight-training belt when lifting weights that are greater than 75% of 1 RM. Use no belt under 75% of 1 RM. The belt should be used to provide support during heavier exercises to increase intrathecal pressure. It shouldn't be overutilized, particularly in those lifts in which the back is supported (e.g., bench press, leg press).
- Avoid placing a board or extra weights under the heel during back or front squats. Increased knee flexion angle yields increased patellofemoral joint forces.
- Bench press: Improve scapular stability for athletes with shoulder pathology by adding concentric and eccentric protraction after each set of bench press. This is accomplished by locking the arms and protracting shoulders with weighted bar.
- Lat pull-down: To avoid impingement have athletes complete seated lat pull downs with trunk in 30 degrees of extension and utilize an underhand grip (hand in supination).
- Shoulder press: If the athlete must complete behind the neck press for a sport specific movement, then lower bar to only ear level.
- Power clean high pull: To avoid repetitive trauma to the distal clavicle have the athlete high-pull the power clean, but not rack the bar.

BOX 17:
"Plyometric training is like chocolate. A little tastes good, but too much can make you sick."

—Unknown

Checks and Balances

Regardless of which system is utilized, it is important to be able to review the workouts to ensure a safe and adaptable program (personal communication, Johnny Parker, 1995). The checklist presented in Box 15 will allow professionals to quickly evaluate their program. This checklist is commonly used for calculating volume and intensity for the core (primary) exercises (i.e., power cleans, squats, snatches, jerks).

Summary

The top priority in designing a program is to establish safe training routines. Just as important is the timely application in which different level programs are incorporated. Athletes should always be introduced to basic programs and should progress safely and in a well-timed manner. Strength and power development is a process of evolution. Well-planned and implemented programs allow for application of a training stimulus to safely enhance the development of the athlete. Keep in mind

BOX 18:
Guidelines for Plyometric Routines

- Develop a proper strength base (minimum 3–6 months)
- Limit sessions. Only two to three times each week is needed
- Workout duration should be no more than 45 minutes including warm-up and cool-down
- Combine with agility and speed work
- Progress volume (termed foot contacts) in slow manner
- Use firm, but cushioned shoe
- Complete on proper surface. Tartan track, grass or wooden basketball court is acceptable. Concrete and macadam are unacceptable

TABLE 4.14. *Low intensity plyometric workout*

General warm-up followed by specific warm-up
Flexibility including static, dynamic, and sport specific
Box jumps 8–10 sets with 10 reps per set
Sprint drills 8 sets × 30-yard dash
Cool-down
Flexibility including static, dynamic, and sport specific

BOX 19:
Strength Assessment Criteria for Plyometric Training

- Complete 10 strict single leg step-ups with thigh parallel to the floor emphasizing controlled eccentric phase (refer to proper step technique in beginning of chapter)
- 10 single leg squats in 15 seconds. Each squat is completed when the top of the thigh is parallel to the floor. The starting position and parallel position are shown in Figures 4.39 and 4.40
- Equal bilateral circumferential measurement of thigh girth at 3-inch and 6-inch mark above knee

---

that many interpretations can be applied to the above examples. Finally, thorough warm-up, flexibility, trunk exercises, and cool-down should be a major part of all programs written.

EXERCISE SAFETY AND EXERCISE MODIFICATION FOR THE INJURED ATHLETE

The health care professional must possess the knowledge to progress an athlete from the training room back onto the field. It is critical to possess the proper knowledge for safety and modification of exercises in the weight room for several reasons. First, the athlete may be able to continue weight training the uninjured extremity or extremities during the rehabilitation process. Second, atrophy of the injured body part may warrant a return to the weight room in order to prepare for a return to sport. Third, continued weight training may provide an active attachment to the team and bolster the athlete psychologically. The checklists in Box 16 provide safety considerations and exercise modifications for the injured athlete (7,16). These should be carefully considered for not only macrotraumatic injuries, but also microtraumatic changes that occur in sport.

Plyometrics

Coaches in the Soviet Union originated plyometric training during the late 1950s and early 1960s. The Soviet coaches, particularly Yuri Veroshanski, concep-

tualized an activity that could bridge the gap between strength training and high-speed athletic activities. The exercises were developed for a coach to easily organize and administer in a progressive manner. These exercises came to the attention of American coaches in the early 1970s and have moved to the forefront of training programs with athletes attempting to improve speed and power.

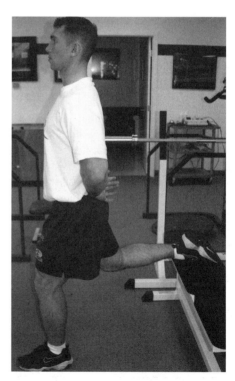

FIG. 4.39. Single leg squat—Starting position.

TABLE 4.15. *High-intensity plyometric workout*

by specific warm-up
ynamic, and sport specific
dles 5 sets with 8 reps per foot

d dash
r tubing 6 sets of 20 to 30 yd.

ynamic, and sport specific

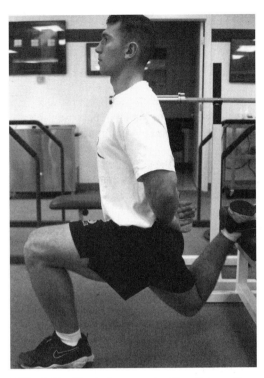

FIG. 4.40. Single leg squat—Parallel position.

Plyometrics are very beneficial in a well-designed training program. They enhance an athlete's power and explosiveness by training the stretch-shortening cycle. However, these exercises can be extremely injurious and detrimental to performance if administered inappropriately.

Many programs use plyometrics to enhance explosive training. However, caution should be taken when developing programs. Several guidelines should be considered in program design and implementation (13).

Plyometrics are divided into different categories with varying degrees of intensity (Box 17 and 18). As the intensity increases with each drill the volume should subsequently drop to provide for a safe training session. With low-intensity programs, sets and reps should be kept to ten each (ten sets maximum, ten reps per set). Moderate intensity plyometric exercise sets should be kept at less than eight with no more than eight to ten reps in each set. High intensity drills are therefore kept at less than six sets with no more than eight reps in each set. And finally, with very high intensity plyometric routines the sets are kept to no more than three to four with each set having only five to six reps.

Tables 4.14 and 4.15 provide a low-intensity and high-intensity plyometric workout.

As with resistance training, technique plays a significant role in successful utilization of plyometric exercises. Posture, balance, and minimal contact time between the athlete and ground are critical to enhancing the training effect. This rapid change from eccentric to concentric muscular contraction is what ultimately leads to the desired training effect of developing muscular power. Speed is also an essential ingredient with this type program.

TABLE 4.16. *Rehabilitation progression using a plyometric program*

Quick hops—A distance of ten feet is marked on the proper surface. The athlete is instructed not to concentrate on horizontal or vertical distance. The objective of this exercise is to quickly complete short (4–6 inches), low (1–2 inches in the air) hops. The goal is to teach proper foot contact technique and controlled body movements. Similar to jumping rope, but much quicker.

Box jumps—A solid bench or plyobox of 12 inches is placed on the proper surface. The athlete is instructed to jump onto the box. Two important cues are stressed. The athlete starts with a quick, continuous movement at the knees and hips to facilitate the stretch reflex while jumping onto the box. This motion at the knees should be no greater than an athlete attempting to rebound a basketball. Second, the athlete is instructed to land softly on the box emphasizing the eccentric action of the lower extremity.

Double leg hops (limited distance)—A distance of 15 feet is marked on the proper surface. The athlete is instructed to complete standard repetitive broad jumps. The athlete is also cued to spend minimal time in contact with the ground during the jumps. The plyometric intensity is controlled by telling the athlete to complete the designated distance (15 ft) in no more than 6 jumps and no less than 4 jumps. Therefore, their average distance per jump is restricted to between 2–3 feet.

Single leg quick hops—Same as the above description, but using single leg. The distance is decreased to 3 feet.

Single leg hops (limited distance)—Same as the double leg hops using a single leg. Distance is decreased to 8 feet and limitation in jumping is between 6 and 8 jumps.

Power skips—The athlete starts with basic skipping movement. After they have demonstrated good technique a distance of 25 feet is measured. The athlete increases the intensity of the arm swing and drive off their legs. The athlete is initially limited to completing the distance in 6–8 power skips.

TABLE 4.17. *Beginning sample plyometric program at the start of rehab session*

General warm-up followed by specific warm-up
Quick hops—2 sets of 10 feet (not added to total foot contacts)
Box jumps—2 × 10
Double leg hops—2 × 6
Quick hops (single leg)—2 sets of 10 feet (not added to total foot contacts)
Single leg hops—2 × 6
Total foot contacts—44

TABLE 4.18. *Advanced sample plyometric program at the start of rehab session*

General warm-up followed by specific warm-up
Quick hops—3 sets of 10 feet (not added to total foot contacts)
Box jumps—4 × 10
Double leg hops—4 × 4 (increased distance per jump)
Quick hops (single leg)—3 sets of 10 feet (not added to total foot contacts)
Single leg hops—4 × 4 (increased distance per jump)
Power skips—3 × 8
Total foot contacts—96

Slow movements and delayed contact time between the ground should be avoided. Any health care professional interested in developing the technical aspect of plyometric training should consult additional texts specific to this area (4,13).

Plyometrics in Rehabilitation

Introducing plyometrics into rehabilitation must be done in a progressive manner. Professionals must have the knowledge of proper strength criteria, correct exercise technique, and varying intensities of plyometric exercise.

Establishing a plyometric program during rehabilitation requires the athlete to meet certain strength criteria. Chu developed strength assessment criteria for plyometric training (4). The criteria for a normal athletic population included completing a back squat with 1.5 times their body weight and completing five repetitions in 5 seconds with 60% of their 1 RM in the back squat. These criteria may be difficult to assess or attain with the injured athlete. In addition, these criteria were set for a normal, healthy athlete to start into a standard plyometric program, not a rehabilitation plyometric program. Therefore, other strength criteria may be established for plyometrics within the rehabilitation setting.

These criteria can be assessed quickly and require only the athlete's body weight for resistance and a tape measure (6) (Box 19). The rationale for equal circumferential measurements considers that a plyometric program primarily stimulates the neural system. If the athlete has not reached maximum hypertrophy from rehabilitation, more time should be spent in the preparation phase. Completion of these criteria establishes that the athlete is capable of starting and benefiting from a plyometric program.

The general development for an athlete using plyometrics in rehabilitation follows the principles of functional progressions. The athlete should be started on bilateral lower intensity plyometrics, then progress to bilateral moderate intensity plyometrics. If these activities are completed without any difficulty, then the athlete is progressed to unilateral low-intensity plyometrics. The final progression involves unilateral moderate intensity plyometrics. This will ensure the athlete safe and beneficial plyometric rehabilitation. Table 4.16, presenting a sample progression, is listed below with descriptions of each activity.

The intensities of these exercises are gradually progressed through increasing the distance (single-leg hops, double-leg hops, and power skips) and increasing box height. These increases are moved up in small increments. The distance for the individual hops may be increased by 6 to 12 inches per session, while increasing the box height by 6 inches every 1 to 2 weeks.

The volume of plyometric exercises is referred to as foot contacts. This format is applicable in the rehabilitation setting. The volume is calculated by counting the total number of times the foot/feet contact the ground. This number is progressed throughout the rehabilitation. Two sample programs and total foot contacts are listed in Tables 4.17 and 4.18.

In summary, plyometrics can play an integral part of the rehabilitation process providing functional training and testing. The athletic therapist must be very knowledgeable in exercise technique and intensity in order to benefit the athlete with this type of training.

SUMMARY AND CONCLUSIONS

This chapter outlines the basic format that any allied health professional can use to organize, design, and implement a strength and conditioning program. Critical issues include development of proper technique, slow steady progression in program design, and proper expansion into power exercises. The reader is advised to pursue books and courses on this topic to ensure safe and progressive program development.

REFERENCES

1. Amundsen LR, ed. *Muscle strength testing*, 1st ed. New York: Churchill Livingstone, 1991.
2. Arnheim D. *Modern principles of athletic training*. St. Louis: Times Mirror/Mosby College Publishing, 1989.
3. Bompa T. *Theory and methodology of training*. Dubuque, IA: Kendall/Hunt Publishing Company, 1990.
4. Chu D. *Jumping into plyometrics*. Champaign, IL: Leisure Press, 1992.
5. Dintiman G, Ward B. *Sport speed*. Champaign, IL: Leisure Press, 1988.
6. Fees MA. Plyometrics in rehabilitation. *Athletic Therapy Today* 1996;3:26–28.
7. Fees MA, Decker TA, Snyder-Mackler L, Axe M. Upper extremity

exercise modifications for the injured athlete. *Am J Sportsmed* 1998; 26:1998.

8. Jones L. *USWA coaching accreditation course. Club coach manual.* Colorado Springs: US Weightlifting Association, 1991.

9. Jones L. *USWA coaching accreditation course. Senior coach manual.* Colorado Springs: United States Weightlifting Association, 1992.

10. Komi PV, ed. *Strength and power in sport*, 1st ed. Oxford: Blackwell Science, 1991.

11. Lambrinides T. Strength: what is it? *American Fitness Quarterly* Oct; 1991:18–20.

12. Pearl B, Moran G. *Getting stronger weight training for men and women.* Bolinas, CA: Shelter Publications, 1986.

13. Radcliffe J, Farentinos R. *Plyometrics. Explosive power training.* Champaign, IL: Human Kinetics Publishers, 1985.

14. Shea JM. Acute quadriplegia following the use of progressive resistance exercise machinery. *Phys Sports Med* 1986; 14:120–124.

15. Stone MH, O'Bryant HS. *Weight training: a scientific approach.* Edina, MN: Burgess International Group, 1987.

16. Zatsiorsky VM. *Science and practice of strength training.* Champaign, IL: Human Kinetics, 1995.

The Injured Athlete, Third Edition,
edited by D. H. Perrin.
Lippincott–Raven Publishers, Philadelphia © 1999.

CHAPTER 5

Principles of Therapeutic Exercise

David H. Perrin and Joe H. Gieck

Rehabilitation of the injured athlete is a process that involves the team physician, the sport rehabilitation specialist, and most importantly, the athlete. The team physician can do only so much; the remainder, in the form of rehabilitation, must be done by the athlete with guidance from the athletic trainer or other sport rehabilitation specialist. The athlete must not simply be provided a list of exercises and sent away. The optimal effects are achieved when the athletic trainer shows concern and gives individual attention to the athlete from the time of injury to his or her return to practice and competition.

Each injury to an athlete has both a physical and emotional component, and emotional conflicts may confound the rehabilitation process. As such, the athlete must be both physiologically and psychologically rehabilitated. Athletes often pass through a series of emotions following injury. At first, the athlete may not accept the diagnosis. ''It can't happen to me'' is a typical response. He or she then becomes angry, and frequently reacts, ''Why did this happen to me?'' This anger may be vented on the athletic trainer. The athletic trainer should listen and avoid being offended, because anger cannot be matched with anger. If the athletic trainer were to react defensively, the clinician-athlete relationship would be strained, making successful rehabilitation a trying experience. Later the athlete may express the sentiment that ''I'll never be able to play again.'' However, in the final and desirable phase, the athlete decides to accept the injury and to overcome its effects.

Initially, the athlete may be skeptical of the recommendations of the athletic trainer. In this scenario, repetition, patience, and reinforcement are important. The athletic trainer should seek to guide the athlete into the final acceptance phase as rapidly as possible, and this guidance will help to heal the athlete's shattered sense of worth. The athletic trainer should be nonjudgmental, show empathy, concern and understanding, and provide encouragement. Lack of interest and beratement result in mutual

frustration and paranoia for the athlete. If the athletic trainer fails to be positive, the athlete may never emerge from one of the first three phases of injury, and thus never attain complete rehabilitation.

Every athletic injury is unique, and the reaction of every athlete to an injury varies as well (Fig. 5.1). As such, the athletic trainer should be cautious about predicting length of disability and projecting a definitive time line for return to competition.

GOAL SETTING

Following injury, the athlete is apprehensive and anxious about return to play. The athlete must be an active participant in goal setting because it increases his or her involvement in the rehabilitative process. Responsibility for the athlete's progress is then shifted from the team physician and athletic trainer to the athlete. The medical staff thus assumes the supervisory role within the rehabilitative process.

The immediate goal is functional activity within the limits of pain-free exercise—it may be simply to complete a straight leg-raise exercise. Short-term goals must be constantly reinforced to the athlete to maintain his or her motivation and to provide the emotional rewards of attaining success in each phase of the rehabilitation program.

EFFECTS OF EXERCISE AFTER INJURY

After injury, hemarthrosis in the area changes to adhesions in and around muscles, tendons, and ligaments, binding these soft tissue structures to bony structures and obliterating the otherwise normal smooth gliding surfaces of joints. Active exercise increases blood flow to injured areas and mechanically stretches and softens fibrous scar tissue, resulting in regained range of motion, strength, and endurance. The adverse effects of immobilization and

D. H. Perrin and J. H. Gieck: Curry School of Education, University of Virginia, Charlottesville, Virginia 22903

the benefits of mobilization on muscles, ligaments, tendons, and joints are well known (1,2,11,21).

Functional inactivity from immobility causes joint stiffness. Lymphatic and venous stasis lead to articular surface breakdown as the joint is without synovial lubrication. The resultant edema from compromised circulation allows adhesions to form from the serofibrinous fluid leading to decreased tendon, muscle, and ligamentous strength, as well as possible osteoporosis.

Functional activity improves blood flow, relieving stasis and resultant edema. The more prolonged and strenuous the exercise within pain-free limits, the greater are the after-effects of exercise. The cast/brace concept is an especially valuable concept because exercise is permitted within the physiologic range of motion. As strength and range of motion are regained concurrently, the capacity for strong functional activity within the new range is simultaneously restored. Joint motion regained passively cannot be used with sufficient strength in a newly gained range. Early active exercise is not always possible because of injury, yet early passive motion is preferable to inactivity, since early passive motion increases the strength of ligaments and tendons by encouraging collagen alignment in a normal sequential pattern.

Resistance exercise as tolerated further reduces adhesions. Fibroblasts become oriented along lines of stress

TABLE 5.1. *Signs of the inflammatory response*

Heat	Loss of motion
Redness	Swelling
Pain	Malfunction
Crepitation	Atrophy

with collagen laid down along these lines instead of a disorganized alignment as seen in fibrous scars. Thus Wolff's law of tissue reacting to the stress placed upon it is implemented.

The body's response to overuse can produce inflammation. The histamine response to such abuse reverses the osmotic process and results in the signs presented in Table 5.1.

Acutely the skin is warm and moist as contrasted to dry, smooth, shiny skin in chronic inflammation. With inflammation, rest is required to allow recovery from overuse.

Muscular strength is important in preventing the degenerative process in loose joints by controlling excess motion. However, early excessive weight-bearing exercises can lead to early degenerative changes, especially after prolonged immobilization or a state of non-weight-bearing mobilization. As such, early exercise must be within the pain-free range of motion. Vigorous lower extremity weight-bearing exercise should be used cautiously with acute injury.

REHABILITATION OBJECTIVES

The objectives of rehabilitation are to regain range of motion, strength, proprioception, muscular endurance, power, cardiovascular endurance, speed, agility, and sport-specific skills. The rehabilitation process comprises many steps, and each one must be successfully completed— pain free— before the athlete returns to competition. Criteria for return are established for each injury in terms of the functional skills and abilities the athlete will need to regain before returning to his or her sport. The athlete may return only when near-normal strength, flexibility, proprioception, speed, power, endurance, and agility have been regained. To facilitate attainment of concrete goals, the athlete must accept the criteria for return to competition presented in Table 5.2. Adherence to these criteria for return to activity will reduce the likelihood of reinjury.

The decision to return an athlete to competition requires consensus among the team physician, athletic trainer, coach, and athlete. The athlete must be involved in this decision so that maximum performance can be achieved; otherwise, he or she may lack confidence and aggressiveness, which will result in sub-par performances and possible reinjury. It is advisable to delay return to competition if the athlete is not completely confident with this decision. Reinforcement of his or her preinjury athletic successes will facilitate recovery of the athlete's confidence.

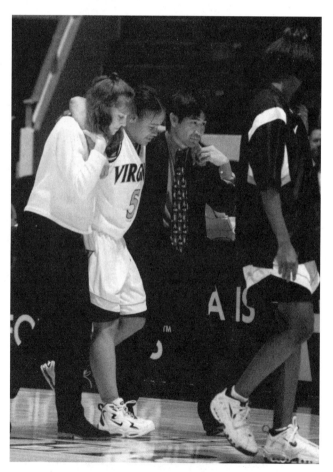

FIG. 5.1. Acute athletic injury.

TABLE 5.2. *Criteria for return to competition following athletic injury*

- Full pain-free range of motion of the injured part
- Preinjury strength and power in comparison to the uninjured side
- Preinjury muscular endurance in comparison to the uninjured side
- Preinjury levels of cardiovascular fitness and endurance
- Preinjury levels of speed and agility for lower extremity injuries according to the following tests:
  - running full speed straight ahead without limp
  - 90 degree cuts to the left and right from full speed without a limp
  - full carioca without a limp
  - figure of eight running with acceleration and deceleration around pylons without a limp
  - one-leg timed hops for 30 sec equal to uninjured side
  - long jump and vertical jump equal to uninjured side
- Preinjury size of muscular mass in comparison to the uninjured side
- Reabsorption of acute edema
- Ability to perform all exercises free of pain
- Ability to dynamically control joint instability
- Return to preinjury levels of pain threshold
- Cerebromuscular rehabilitation complete
- Ability to perform tests appropriate to physical demands of the sport
- Presence of a strong desire to return to competition
- 80% to 90% attainment of above during the season

The process of healing and rehabilitation takes time. It is not unusual for an athlete with a mild or moderate injury to lose up to three weeks from competition, even when following an appropriate rehabilitation regimen. Reinjury and possible early joint deterioration may result with an athlete's premature return to competition. Furthermore, if rehabilitative procedures are inadequate, the likelihood of reinjury is greater. This is often the case with the athlete who experiences recurrence of the same injury over the course of a sport season. Reinjury most often occurs if the athlete skips some of the criteria for return.

EXERCISE

Exercise is the ultimate modality. Cold, heat, and other modalities are useful in facilitating pain-free exercise, but alone are inadequate in the successful rehabilitation of an athlete. The application and correct timing of rehabilitative exercises are essential to the rehabilitation process. For example, an athlete who has failed to comply with a rehabilitation program or who has been performing painful exercises may very well require extra time to return to competition (Fig. 5.2A).

Exercise should begin the day following injury, especially with injuries of mild or moderate severity. In this manner loss of strength can be retarded and normal motion regained as soon as possible. Exercise should progress in a pain-free manner from the onset of injury to complete recovery (see Fig. 5.2B). The enthusiasm of most athletes to quickly return to competition can result

in a rehabilitation program that exceeds the body's normal physiologic limits. This scenario often results in a peak-and-valley progression as the athlete exceeds pain-free limits (see Fig. 5.2C). Although some exercises may produce some discomfort, a key element is that the athlete should experience no undue pain or swelling the day following the exercise routine. The application of ice may be useful in preventing this residual discomfort following rehabilitative exercises.

The goal of all rehabilitation programs is for the athlete to exercise just below the point of pain (see Fig. 5.2B) and without antalgic gait in the case of lower extremity injury. The philosophy of no pain, no gain is extremely inappropriate in acute rehabilitation. There is no gain with pain in acute rehabilitation. Even a minor limp or exercise through a painful arc can retard return to competition. A cane or crutches should be used until gait is normal (Fig. 5.3). The athlete should bear weight as much as possible without pain and within physiologic limits. A cane or single crutch is used on the side opposite of the injury to simulate normal gait mechanics.

STRENGTH

The foundation of a rehabilitation program begins with the strength and flexibility phase (see Fig. 5.2D). It is important that exercises addressing strength and flexibility occur simultaneously. Full range of motion should not be a prerequisite for strengthening exercises, as strength can actually help improve flexibility. For example, hamstring strength can increase knee flexion in the injured knee.

Strength is the capacity to do work against resistance. Strength of muscular and connective tissue are the first lines of defense in providing joint stability.

A certain amount of neural learning takes place in early phases of rehabilitation. The athlete who can lift 50 pounds with the quadriceps and the next day after a mild medial collateral ligament sprain can lift only 5 pounds has not lost this strength. Pain and effusion from soft tissue injury causes a reflex inhibition of strength to prevent further injury by limiting the athlete's functional activity. The return of strength must thus be relearned. This is accomplished by using pain-free resistive exercise performed in multiple sets of usually ten repetitions per set (Fig. 5.4). In general, an outside stimulus of at least a 70% overload is recommended for strength gains. Hypertrophy normally accompanies strength gains but not in a linear fashion.

Three to eight sets of 10 repetitions are commonly used. As the athlete begins to plateau using multiple sets, a program modified from the original DeLorme system may be established (Table 5.3).

In this program, the athlete's ten-repetition maximum (10 RM) is determined by the maximal amount that can be lifted through a complete range of motion ten times.

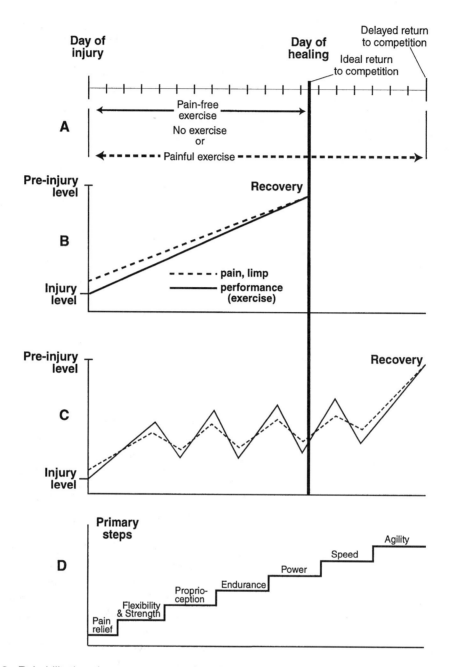

FIG. 5.2. Rehabilitation time sequence and performance. If the athlete has pain during flexibility exercise, vary the degree of motion. If there is pain with strength and power exercise, vary the repetitions and resistance. If there is pain with endurance or speed exercises, vary the distance or duration. If there is pain with agility drills, vary the quickness and duration. The athlete must rehabilitate to the pre-injury level or higher or to the same level as the uninjured side.

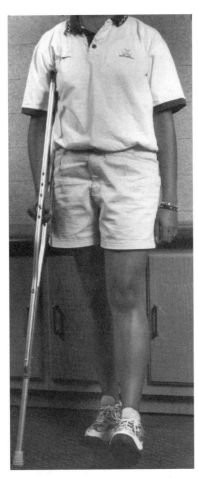

FIG. 5.3. One-crutch gait.

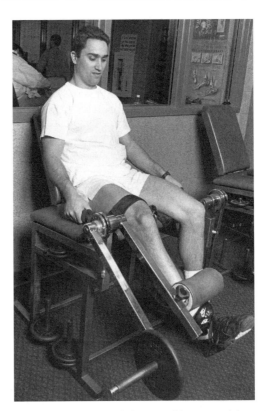

FIG. 5.4. Strengthening of the quadriceps and hamstring muscles with a commercially available resistance device, such as an N-K table. (From ref. 18, with permission.)

Forty repetitions are then performed according to the protocol illustrated in Table 5.3. Initially, the athlete will not be able to perform the last set of ten repetitions. When the athlete can perform the fourth set, the 40 repetitions are recalculated with the weight of the fourth set now becoming the third set. This is a less complicated model of the DAPRE system (8).

Repetitions and sets are changed as the athlete peaks with a certain routine. He or she may begin with eight sets of ten repetitions, progress to four sets of ten, peak out, switch back to eight sets of ten, and so forth. Care should be taken to prevent overtraining and muscle fatigue. As strength progresses, exercises are performed three times weekly and a muscular endurance routine on alternate days. Using the knee as an example, Table 5.4 illustrates a rehabilitation progression that addresses both strength and endurance.

Proprioceptive Neuromuscular Facilitation

Proprioceptive neuromuscular facilitation (PNF) can also be a useful adjunct for restoration of strength, range of motion, and neuromuscular control. This technique uses proprioceptive, cutaneous, and auditory input through diagonal movement patterns of the head and neck, trunk, and extremities. According to Knott and Voss (9), PNF incorporates methods of promoting or hastening the response of the neuromuscular mechanism through stimulation of the proprioceptors.

Isometric Resistance

Isometric resistance is the exercise of choice early in rehabilitation, especially when joint movement may be limited or contraindicated. Increases in strength resulting from isometric exercise are limited to a 20-degree range of motion around the position of exercise. Therefore, several isometrics within the available range of motion are indicated.

Initially, the athlete needs to contract at only 40% to 50% of maximal effort for a few seconds to gain strength. As strength returns, however, a more forceful contraction is needed to produce further increases in strength. These maximal contractions should be held for a duration of 6 seconds.

TABLE 5.3. *Early progression of resistive exercise*

Ten repetitions at 1/2 of 10 repetition maximum
Ten repetitions at 3/4 of 10 repetition maximum
Ten repetitions at 10 repetition maximum
Ten repetitions at 10 repetition maximum RM + 5 lbs

TABLE 5.4. *Knee rehabilitation progression addressing muscular strength and endurance*

Monday—Wednesday—Friday
a. Eight sets of 10 repetitions, knee extension to 5% of body weight, then progress to line work of 4 sets of 10 repetitions illustrated below
b. Progress to next line when 4 sets of 10 repetitions can be performed with no compromise in exercise technique
c. The goal is to be able to lift more with the injured leg than with the uninjured leg

	1st Set 10 reps	2nd Set 10 reps	3rd Set 10 reps	4th Set 10 reps
1.	5 lbs	7 1/2 lbs	10 lbs	15 lbs
2.	7 1/2	11 1/4	15	20
3.	10	15	20	25
4.	12 1/2	18 3/4	25	30
5.	15	22 1/2	30	35
6.	17 1/2	26 1/4	35	40
7.	20	30	40	45
8.	22 1/2	33 3/4	45	50
9.	25	37 1/2	50	55
10.	27 1/2	41 1/2	55	60

Tuesday–Thursday
One set of 200 continuous repetitions with appropriate weight

From the isometric exercise, a slow pain-free pattern should be used to develop a good base for which neural learning can occur.

Isotonic exercise with free weights is started as soon as possible to address the deficiencies left by isometric exercise. In regular strength training, repetitions are usually done with maximum weight. In rehabilitation, however, the athlete should go through a full range of motion with submaximal weight to prevent the edema and soreness that would develop with three sets of maximum lifts. The part to be exercised should be isolated to prevent accessory input from other muscles. Momentum and inertia should be minimized by performing the exercises slowly during the early phases.

WEIGHT-BEARING AND NON-WEIGHT-BEARING EXERCISE

At this point, the strengthening program should incorporate a combination of weight-bearing and nonweight-bearing exercises, sometimes referred to as closed (or functional) and open chain exercises, respectively. Weight-bearing exercises require muscular cocontraction at multiple joints, which can be advantageous in reducing joint shearing forces and in attaining a more functional progression through rehabilitation. However, weight-bearing exercises also permit compensation of weak muscle groups by stronger muscles (3,6,7,10) (Fig. 5.5). For example, the step exercise can be performed by the hip extensors and the gastrocnemius with a weak quadriceps. Non-weight-bearing exercises enable isolation of specific

muscle groups and are useful in preventing the avoidance patterns that can result from weight-bearing exercise. It is important to establish a foundation of strength in the extremity before the functional exercise program is initiated.

The value of a combination of weight-bearing and non-weight-bearing exercise for the lower extremity is obvious. However, recent evidence suggests that a combination of both types of exercise is useful for rehabilitation of the upper extremity as well. For example, weight-bearing exercise for the shoulder can facilitate development of strength of the muscles acting on the scapula (proximal stablizers), which is essential to the complete rehabilitation of the upper extremity.

Early in the rehabilitation program, strength increases are optimized from daily work efforts. However, as the increases in strength begin to peak, the weight training program should be performed on an every-other-day basis. A minimum of three sets of repetitions are needed for optimal gains in strength and muscle size. The repetitions should be performed slowly with a two or three count through a range of pain-free motion. A four count should also be used while returning the weight to the starting position.

Eccentric Contraction

Eccentric contraction is an essential component of virtually every athletic activity. Eccentric loading is especially important in overuse injuries and those in which deceleration is needed. The hamstrings and the rotator

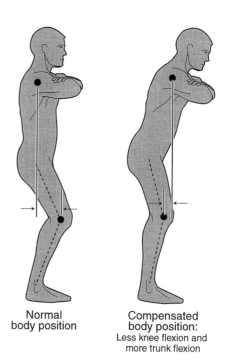

Normal body position

Compensated body position: Less knee flexion and more trunk flexion

FIG. 5.5. Compensation for a weak knee extensor muscle group by forward flexion of the trunk to activate the hip extensors.

cuff are two examples in which added eccentric work is needed to achieve functional return. Accordingly, the rehabilitation program should use exercise equipment that includes both a concentric and eccentric component of resistance.

ISOKINETIC DYNAMOMETRY

The accurate assessment of human muscle performance has been the objective of exercise scientists and rehabilitation therapists for many decades (17). Exercise scientists interested in comparing the effects of various strength and conditioning programs seek the accurate measurement of muscular force. Practitioners of rehabilitation medicine attempt to document the efficacy of therapeutic exercise in restoring preinjury levels of strength in patients recovering from injury to the musculoskeletal system. Athletic trainers and sports physical therapists emphasize prevention of injury through identification of underlying deficits in strength and in bilateral and reciprocal muscle group strength relationships. Underscoring the objective of each of these professionals is the valid and reliable quantification of the human muscles' capacity to produce force.

The capacity of a human muscle to produce force may be assessed through either a static or dynamic contraction. Static (isometric) assessment reveals the amount of tension a muscle can generate against a resistance permitting no observable joint movement. Dynamic (isotonic) strength refers to the application of force through all or part of a joint's available range of motion. Dynamic strength may be assessed via a concentric (shortening) or eccentric (lengthening) mode of contraction.

Isokinetic devices govern the rate of angular movement to a preset velocity, allowing an individual to exert as great or little force as they can generate at a given position and velocity. In other words, the force produced by the muscle is met with an equal counterforce so that the angular rate of limb movement remains constant. Isokinetic resistance has several advantages over other exercise modalities. One advantage is that a muscle group may be exercised to its maximum potential throughout a joint's entire range of available motion. For example, at the midrange of joint motion in which a muscle is at its optimum length-tension relationship for the binding of actin and myosin and has its greatest mechanical advantage, the isokinetic dynamometer will maintain its preset velocity and thus more force will be produced. Conversely, at the extremes of joint motion in which a muscle is at a physiologic and mechanical disadvantage, the dynamometer will still maintain its preset velocity, but less force will be produced. Since there is no fixed resistance to move through the weakest point in a given arc of motion (as with isotonic exercise), isokinetic exercise facilitates a maximum voluntary force to be produced throughout the entire range of motion.

Isokinetic dynamometry enables the rapid and reliable

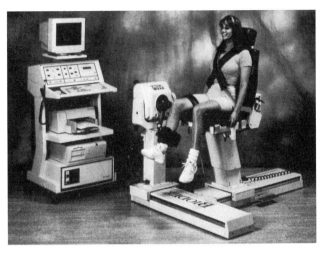

FIG. 5.6. Biodex System 3 isokinetic dynamometer.

quantification of force or torque (Fig. 5.6). If the force and distance of a given muscle contraction are known, the amount of tension produced by the muscle may be expressed as work. If the quantity of time required to produce work is known, the ability of the muscle to generate power may be determined. Research has shown the predictability of work and power from peak torque is good in both the knee and shoulder (19,22). However, the neuromuscular demands of some activities on upper extremity torque, work, and power within a single muscle group has not been adequately elucidated in the scientific literature. Moreover, the return of peak torque in a rehabilitating muscle may not necessarily be closely related to the work and power capabilities of that same muscle. As such, the ability to quantify torque, work, and power may be useful in both the laboratory and clinical settings.

Isokinetic instruments have the ability to express the muscular effort produced by a specific exercise repetition as a "curve" or "tracing" via an analog signal sent from the dynamometer. Isokinetic resistance accommodates to the amount of force generated by a given muscle group. The combined length-tension relationship and overall effectiveness of a muscle contraction is greatest through the midrange of a joint's available range of motion and is less near both the beginning and end of that motion. The isokinetic torque curve reflects these variations in capacity to generate force as a muscle contracts throughout a joint's range of motion.

Several factors contribute to production of a normal, smooth, and coordinated isokinetic torque curve. The muscle group and joint being tested must be free from pain or injury. An isokinetic dynamometer accommodates to pain by essentially disengaging when the patient produces less force. Pain originating from a muscle-tendon unit or from sources within an articulation crossed by a muscle group will frequently result in artifacts within the torque curve. Of special interest to a variety of clinicians has been the difficulty involved with replicating these artifacts from one curve to another when indeed the muscle group or joint in question is free from pain. The implication of this clinical observation is that perhaps visualization of inconsistent torque curves is useful in identifying a malingering athlete or workman's compensation patient. However, since this phenomenon has not been adequately elucidated in the scientific literature, caution should be exercised when drawing such impressions based on an isokinetic torque curve.

It has also been suggested that pathology within a muscle-tendon unit and/or bony articulation frequently manifests itself with characteristic artifacts within an isokinetic torque curve. For example, isokinetic testing of the anterior cruciate ligament deficient knee with a distally positioned resistance pad is thought to result in a bimodal (two peaks) torque curve. The mechanism for this characteristic curve is purportedly related to the anterior translation that occurs at the proximal tibia as the quadriceps muscle group begins to contract (first peak). In the absence of an intact anterior cruciate ligament, other soft tissue structures about the knee subsequently "catch" the anterior translation of the tibia (second peak). Some clinicians also claim the ability to predict a variety of other joint or muscle maladies from torque curves, including chondromalcia patella, a subluxing patella, and even a knee plica syndrome. Since little or no scientific evidence exists to validate this practice, clinicians are advised to confine their interpretation of the isokinetic torque curve to a muscle's capacity to produce torque, work, and power.

The profile obtained from an isokinetic evaluation may be used to predict susceptibility to injury in a healthy individual, to monitor an injured patient's progress through a rehabilitation program, or to determine readiness to return to activities of either daily living or athletic participation at the conclusion of a therapeutic exercise program. Depending on instrument capabilities, interpretation of an isokinetic evaluation usually involves a careful analysis of an individual's ability to generate torque, power, or work. Torque may be assessed as either a peak or average value. Peak torque is often obtained from the highest point of one of several isokinetic torque curves. However, since several isokinetic contractions are necessary to obtain a true peak value, the average of the peak points from several consecutive torque curves (average peak torque) may be a better indicator of the maximum performance of a given muscle group. The primary advantage of using peak values of torque is that muscle performance can be assessed when full and complete range of joint motion may be restricted.

Average torque is measured from the complete tracing of one or several consecutive isokinetic curves. The primary advantage of this value is that artifacts, which might occur in the torque curve from deceleration of the limb and lever arm, have a less dramatic effect on an average value than on a measure of peak torque or force. However, since this measure is obtained from the complete isoki-

netic curve, care must be taken to ensure that the range of motion tested is consistent between injured and uninjured sides, and within the injured side in subsequent evaluations throughout a rehabilitation program.

Underscoring the value of an isokinetic evaluation, however, is the need to evaluate all components involved with rehabilitation of injury to the musculoskeletal system. In particular, strength, flexibility, proprioception, functional ability, and psychologic status are all essential to returning to one's occupation or athletic endeavor (14,25).

FLEXIBILITY

Flexibility goes hand in hand as a rehabilitation foundation along with strength (see Fig. 5.2), and residual deficits in flexibility can predispose athletes to reinjury (24). Joint degeneration can be retarded if the athlete regains strength and flexibility while recovering function. Slow static stretching (23), proprioceptive neuromuscular facilitation, and joint mobilization techniques (20) are methods that may be used to help gain flexibility and joint mobility. The goal is a normal joint, not a hypermobile one. A corresponding gain in strength provides joint stability so that a normal range of motion may be achieved without producing abnormal motion. An increase in strength will facilitate range of motion; by the same token, an increase in motion needs an accompanying increase in strength within the newly gained range. The full range of functional motion is necessary for the successful return of the athlete. A warm-up prior to flexibility techniques will facilitate efficient flexibility exercises.

PROPRIOCEPTION

Proprioception has been defined as a specialized variation of the sensory modality of touch that involves the sensation of joint movement (kinesthesia) and joint position sense (12). Trauma to tissues that contain mechanoreceptors, such as those found in joint ligament and capsule, muscle, and skin can disrupt normal neuromuscular path-

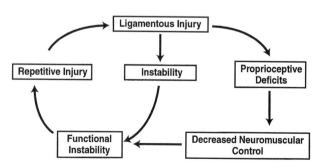

FIG. 5.7. Functional stability paradigm depicting progression of functional instability. (From ref. 13 with permission.)

ways and result in proprioceptive deficits. This disruption in neural feedback to the central nervous system can result in the progressive functional joint instability illustrated in Fig. 5.7. To offset this progressive decline in function, the mechanoreceptors responsible for unconscious neuromuscular control must be retrained in order for the athlete to regain normal function and dynamic joint stability.

TABLE 5.5. *Progression of exercises leading to restoration of function and return to sport*

Phase 1.	Step-ups—4″	60 times daily
	Walk	30 minutes M, W, F
	Swim	30 minutes T, H, S
Phase 2.	Step-ups—8″	60 times daily
	Walk rapidly	30 minutes M, H
	Bike	30 minutes T, F
	Swim	30 minutes W, S
Phase 3.	Step-ups—12″	60 times daily
	Walk, jog (stairs)	30 minutes M, H
	Bike	30 minutes T, F
	Swim	30 minutes W, S
	Begin alternating versa climber and bike	
	Begin 1/2 squats	3 sets of 10 M, W, F
	Alternating leg press	3 sets of 10 T, H, S
Phase 4.	Step-ups 18″	60 times daily
	Jog (20% BW in water)	30 minutes M, W, F
	Bike	30 minutes T, H, S
	Swim (optional)	
	Begin alternating bike, versa climber, circuit	
Phase 5.	Jog, run, cut	30–45 minutes M, W, F
	Swim (optional)	
	Bike	30 minutes T, H, S
Phase 6.	Cross country	M, W, F
	Bike	T, H, S
	(25% BW in water)	
	Straight-ahead, full-speed running daily	
Phase 7.	Full-speed cutting activities daily	
	Bike	3 times per week
	Plyometrics	2 times BW with squat
Phase 8.	Return to sport	

Proprioception Progression (3 times 30″)
1. Eyes open—flat, soft surface
   a. balance
   b. lean forward, back
   c. bend down, touch floor
   d. toe raises
   e. tube opposite leg
   f. balance-board training
2. Eyes closed—flat, soft surface
   repeat a–e
3. Eyes open—trampoline surface
   repeat a–e
4. Eyes closed—trampoline surface
   repeat a–e
5. Cable column—hip, both legs
   a. flexion
   b. extension
   c. abduction
   d. adduction
   e. 45 degrees

Exercise should be performed with no pain or limping and should be preceded and followed with static stretching. Ice should be applied for 30 minutes for pain or swelling.

For the lower extremity, bilateral balance training is initiated, then advanced to unilateral balance with eyes closed. This is performed first on a hard surface for three sets of 30 seconds (Table 5.5).

The degree of difficulty is increased with weight shifting and by switching to a soft surface. As balance improves the athlete is switched to an unstable platform. Pool exercises are appropriate for proprioception at this time as well. As the athlete progresses, faster speed and functional activities are incorporated with power, speed and agility work.

Injury to the upper extremity can also result in proprioceptive deficits (15), and so the same exercise principles apply. The loss of proprioception is easily demonstrated by having the athlete attempt to perform directed activities with the shoulder in abduction and external rotation with eyes closed. The athlete progresses as with the lower extremity by balancing on both hands from a kneeling position and shifting body weight in multiple directions. The use of early pool exercises aids in regaining proprioception. From here unilateral balance on an unstable surface such as a wobble board or ball is useful. A partner can apply manual resistance to increase the difficulty of the exercise. Partner rhythmic stabilization to the arm while in a supine position and bouncing a basketball off a wall in an overhead position are other effective drills. Finally, incorporating rapid speed functional activities as in power, speed, and agility are used. A cable pulley machine or weighted balls on a rebounder unit are good adjuncts at this time.

ENDURANCE

The rehabilitation should incorporate activities that enhance muscular endurance. A less obvious goal should be the maintenance of cardiovascular endurance. A complete rehabilitation program returns the injured body part to preinjury levels and returns an athlete who possesses the cardiovascular status necessary for the demands of high-level physical activity. In implementing endurance exercises the athlete's sport should be taken into consideration. Excessive endurance exercise negatively affects power that is important in some sports.

Muscular

Rehabilitation for muscular endurance should not be neglected, although it takes time and can be monotonous. Endurance training may be done during the intermediate phases of rehabilitation in the intervals between strength exercises. Strength training and endurance training can complement each other by incorporating strength training 3 days a week and endurance training in between. Repetitions of 20 to 30 are in the endurance range. A 30-minute a day low-load endurance exercise program will enhance bone, ligament, and connective tissue strength and is recommended to facilitate successful return to function.

Cardiovascular

An injured athlete should strive to have better cardiovascular endurance upon return to competition than was present at the time of injury. One of the goals of cardiovascular endurance is to delay fatigue, which can result in reinjury to the athlete. A 35% to 50% effort is required for endurance training to be effective. A pulse rate above 120 must be sustained for at least 20 minutes to achieve a training effect. This should be accomplished according to the specific demands of the sport. For example, running long distance doesn't contribute to the efficiency of a football player or a field hockey goalie. Probably the most effective means of functional sport training is the circuit training whereby the athlete trains from a pulse rate of 120 at rest to 180—according to the individual demands of the sport. Elite athletes need a 95% heart rate training effect to increase and maintain their reserves.

Endurance exercise overtraining results in breakdown of tissue and a decrease of power as in vertical jumps. For this reason the athlete should not exceed a 10% increase in endurance training a week. Additional principles related to cardiovascular training can be found in Chapter 3.

POWER

Perhaps the most neglected phase of rehabilitation is that of power. Often the athlete works on strength and flexibility, begins endurance, and then a functional phase in the absence of power training. An athlete must regain power before returning to competition as this is a significant functional component. If training occurs only with slow repetitions, the athlete will regain strength but will not be ready for the rapid bursts of energy necessary for competition. The athlete should start high-speed power training as soon as strength is adequately developed. A 50% effort is required to establish the power phase. There is a crossover effect in maximal oxygen uptake (VO2 max) and strength as well as is seen in a circuit training program. A classic example of the importance of power is seen in the athlete who is post-anterior cruciate ligament reconstructed. Rapid gains are seen early followed by slower gains in the functional stages of rehabilitation that occur later.

Circuit training is often used in power training. A weekly one-repetition maximum (1-RM) is first determined for each exercise. Then, the athlete trains three times a week with three sets of 30-second repetitions with one-half of this 1-RM, with 20 seconds rest between sets. These sets are done explosively with proper technique. Usually 8 to 12 exercises comprise the circuit. The circuit

weights are adjusted once per week as determined by another 1-RM lift by the athlete.

Plyometrics, a rapid eccentric contraction followed by a quick concentric motion, is another effective training technique (4). Lower extremity exercises consist of double and single leg hops, vertical jumps, bounding, box and depth jumping. Upper extremity exercises can include pushups with a clap, using a weighted ball against a rebounder, and medicine ball routines.

It is important to remember that power and especially the plyometric phase is toward the terminal phase of rehabilitation. Plyometrics should not begin until the athlete has participated in at least 8 to 12 weeks of supervised strength training. For the lower extremity, the athlete should be able to squat twice his or her body weight before embarking on plyometrics. Care should be taken not to overload and break down the athlete. For this reason, a 2- to 4-day interval between plyometrics should be observed. Also, with the addition of plyometrics some activities should be eliminated.

SPEED

Speed is one of the final phases of returning to functional activity after lower extremity injury. Speed training occurs with a maximal effort over a short period of time, usually for 6 to 10 seconds. Proper mechanics of running consist of a relaxed and erect posture, high knee activity with straight-ahead arm swing. Work on starts will improve speed more than that in full stride. A 10% improvement in strength may be possible with proper mechanics, technique and training. Increasing stride length, frequency, flexibility, and strength all are contributors.

Bench steps with weights, plyometrics, and weight control will also assist in the development of speed. Downhill running on a 5% to 10% grade emphasizes stride frequency and length. Although the 40-yard sprint is often used to gauge speed, a 20-yard sprint may be a better predictor. The full return of speed is especially critical to the athlete who requires speed of movement in comparison to other positions.

AGILITY AND COORDINATION

Agility and coordination are the final phase in the rehabilitation process. Agility is the ability to change direction without the loss of motion while maintaining proper body control. In essence, this phase necessitates return of timing for the athlete. The athlete learns to make cuts rather than to round corners, which is essential to regaining preinjury levels of quickness and confidence in performance of sport-specific skills. During this phase confidence is restored and the athlete can visualize successful return to competition. Activities such as racquetball, squash, running obstacle courses, and basketball can aid in this development. These activities incorporate all of the previous phases of the rehabilitation process: strength, flexibility, proprioception, endurance, power, and speed.

EXERCISE PROGRESSIONS FOR LOWER EXTREMITY INJURY (EPLEI)

The exercise progressions for the lower extremity should consist of a series of short-term goals. For example, the first goal should be to walk comfortably with crutches, then later to do low step-ups (see Table 5.5). With successful achievement of short-term goals, the athlete sees improvement and develops confidence in the ability to recover from injury. The athlete should first warm up and stretch, and then perform the entire rehabilitation routine. After exercising, stretching should be repeated, and if pain or swelling is present, ice should be applied for 20 minutes. As the goal levels increase, the exercises become more demanding. By the time the athlete reaches goal 8, he or she should be ready to return to full athletic participation.

Isodynamics, exercise in which there is equal resistance throughout the range of motion as illustrated by exercise in the water, can also be useful in facilitating the progression to weight-bearing exercise during rehabilitation. For example, exercise in water at the level of the shoulders necessitates bearing of approximately 25% of body weight. Progression to water exercise at waist level bears approximately 50% of the body's weight. Table 5.6 suggests pool exercises for rehabilitation of lower extremity injuries.

Aquatic therapy has several important qualities that make it a natural for rehabilitation. Less pain, muscle spasm, soft tissue swell, joint swelling, and less overall soreness have been observed as compared to land exercise. The principles of hydrostatic pressure, buoyancy, viscosity and turbulence, and water temperature are all important properties. Hydrostatic pressure is increased with the depth of water (5). Thus, edema reduction is aided with the use of exercise while immersed in water.

The upward forces of buoyancy aid in assisting joint motion and help in unloading weight on the lower extremity as previously mentioned (16). Turbulence and viscosity aid in resisting motion by varying the flow of current against the body part (5). The temperature of the water plays a role in rehabilitation as well. Water temperature above skin temperature with an exercise routine adds heat to the body whereas lower temperature may aid in edema reduction when combined with exercise and hydrostatic pressure. For the general athletic population, temperatures of 72 to 82 degrees are recommended during rehabilitation activities.

Aquatic therapy can facilitate the return of strength, flexibility, proprioception, endurance, power, speed, and agility without undue muscle fatigue (Fig. 5.8). Patients

TABLE 5.6. *Pool exercises for rehabilitation of the lower extremity*

Exercise	Water depth
Walk	Shoulders to waist
10 laps, down and backwards, carioca	
Front-back kick	Waist
30 reps, rest, 30 reps	
Flutter kick	Supine
2 min, rest, 2 min	
Scissors	Supine
35 reps, rest, 35 reps	
High steps	Shoulders to waist
8 laps	
Walk-run	Shoulders to waist
10 laps	
Tucks	6 feet
10, rest, 20	
Sitting kick	N/A
1 min, rest, 1 min	
Body lifts	8–10 feet
15	
Squats	Waist
15, rest, 15	

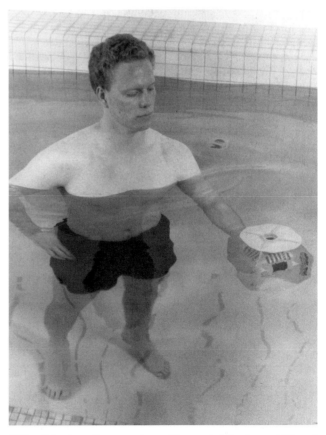

FIG. 5.8. Aquatic exercise with a paddle for additional resistance.

are able to begin exercise earlier, with anterior cruciate ligament reconstructions and rotator cuff repairs being notable examples. For example, gait training can often be resumed one week after ACL surgery provided good healing is occurring.

REHABILITATION PROGRESSIONS

Rehabilitation progressions for specific body areas and for specific injuries can be found in Chapters 9 to 16. However, all rehabilitation progressions follow essentially the same format, and progress through initial, intermediate, and advanced stages.

The initial stage includes the acute phase and usually encompasses the time when ice is used. The athlete can usually leave the initial stage and enter the intermediate stage when the five criteria for using heat have been attained (Table 5.7).

The intermediate stage might also be called the preparticipation stage. The advanced stage is a participation level stage during which the athlete can return to practice.

When to Move to the Next Stage

In each stage, the exercises increase in intensity as if there were an initial, intermediate, and advanced level within each stage. When the athlete reaches the advanced level within a stage, he or she is ready to move to the initial level of the next stage. The art of rehabilitation is knowing when the athlete is ready to move to the next stage. In general, pain is the best criterion to use for progression through rehabilitation. Table 5.8 provides guidelines for progression through rehabilitation.

TABLE 5.7. *Criteria for switching from cold to heat*

- Edema has stabilized
- There is almost a full range of motion
- The range of motion is pain free
- There is no hyperemia at the injury site
- Progress with ice has plateaued

TABLE 5.8. *Rehabilitation progression*

Symptoms day after exercise	Exercise
Increased pain, soreness, edema	Decrease exercise level
No change in pain, soreness, edema	Maintain exercise level
Decreased pain, soreness, edema	Increase exercise level

TABLE 5.9. *Window of opportunity during rehabilitation*

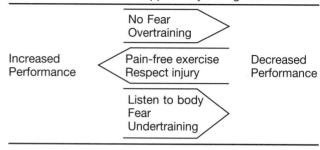

There is a window of opportunity in rehabilitation during which optimal results can be achieved (Table 5.9). To undertrain or overtrain retards return to activity. Awareness of this principle is the art of rehabilitation. To overdo sets back the athlete and prevents progression of the rehabilitation process. Conversely, to undertrain prevents the most rapid progression to return to athletic participation.

ATHLETIC TAPING AS AN ADJUNCT TO RETURN

The application of athletic tape can provide a useful adjunct to exercise and return to play during rehabilitation (18). Athletic tape can provide support to unstable joints through limitation of excessive or abnormal movement. Perhaps more important is the role of tape in enhancing proprioceptive feedback, which can signal the central nervous system to an impending movement that will exceed normal ranges of joint movement. Tape can also be used to support injuries to the muscle-tendon unit and to secure protective pads, dressings, and splints. At no time should the application of tape replace exercise, a point that needs to be continually reinforced to the rehabilitating athlete.

Nonelastic and Elastic Tape

Nonelastic tape should be used when optimal joint support is needed. The support provided by applying nonelastic white tape to the inversion sprained ankle is the most common example (Fig. 5.9). However, nonelastic tape can also be used when greater freedom of movement is needed, such as at the elbow (Fig. 5.10) and thumb (Fig. 5.11).

Elastic tape and wraps tend to be more appropriate for providing support to body parts that require greater freedom of movement, or when it is necessary to completely encircle a major muscle group such as the adductors, quadriceps, or hamstrings (Fig. 5.12). Elastic wraps are also especially useful to apply compression following acute injury, alone or in combination with ice (Fig. 5.13).

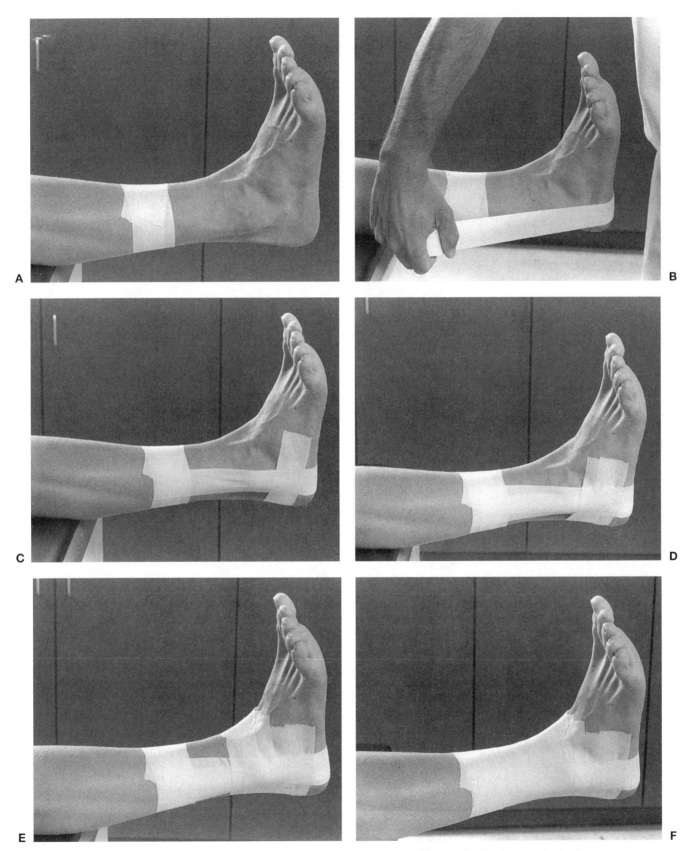

FIG. 5.9. The closed basket weave taping procedure. (From ref. 18, with permission.)

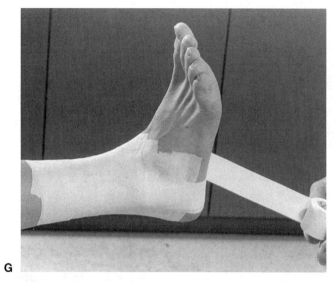

G

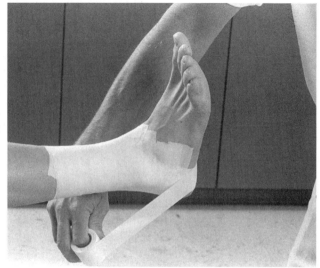

H

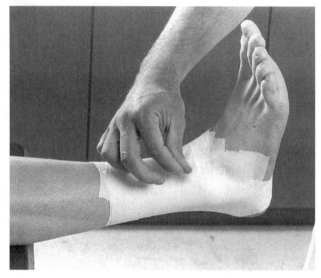

I

FIG. 5.9. *Continued.*

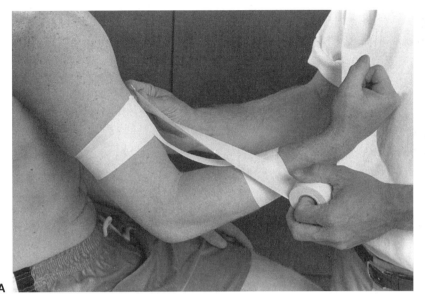

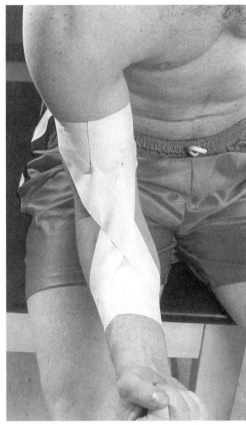

FIG. 5.10. Elbow hyperextension taping procedure. (From ref. 18 with permission.)

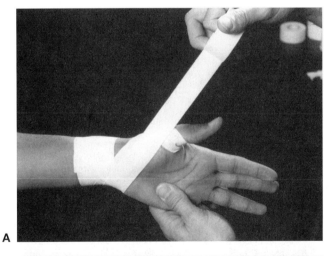

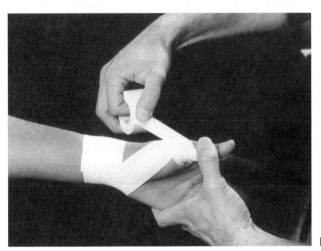

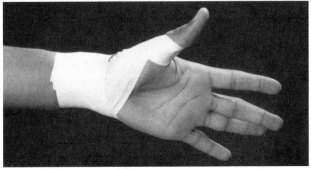

FIG. 5.11. Figure-eight taping procedure to support the thumb's metacarpophalangeal joint. (From ref. 18, with permission.)

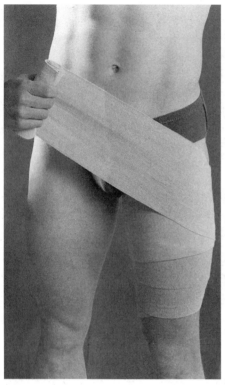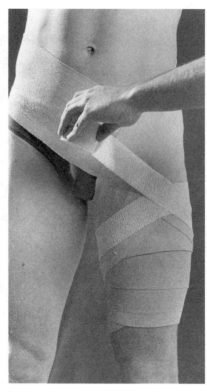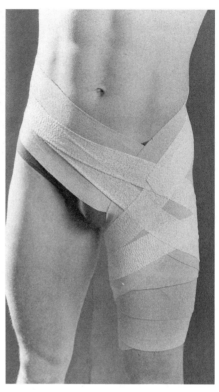

A,B

C

FIG. 5.12. A hip spica with elastic wrap to support a strain of the adductor muscles. (From ref. 18, with permission.)

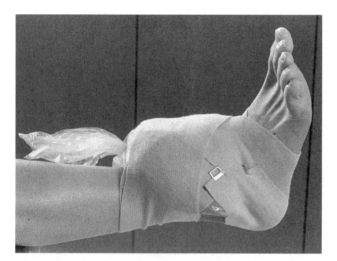

FIG. 5.13. Elastic wrap to secure an ice bag to the ankle. (From ref. 18, with permission.)

REFERENCES

1. Akeson WH, Amiel D, Abel MF, Garfin SR, Woo SL-Y. Effects of immobilization on joints. *Clin Orthop Rel Res* 1987;219:28–37.
2. Amiel D, Woo SL-Y, Harwood FL, Akeson WH. The effect of immobilization on collagen turnover in connective tissue: a biochemical-biomechanical correlation. *Acta Orthop Scand* 1982;53:325–332.
3. Berchuck M, Andriacchi TP, Bah BR, Reedier B. Gait adaptations by patients who have a deficient anterior cruciate ligament. *J Bone Joint Surg* 1990;72A:871–877.
4. Chu DA. *Jumping into plyometrics*. Champaign, IL: Human Kinetics, 1992.
5. Duffield MH. *Exercise in water*, 2nd ed. London: Bailliere Tindall, 1976.
6. Ernst GP. Lower extremity kinetics following anterior cruciate ligament reconstruction. Doctoral Dissertation, University of Virginia, 1997.
7. Gauffin H, Tropp H. Altered movement and muscular activation patterns during the one-legged jump in patients with an old anterior cruciate ligament rupture. *Am J Sports Med* 1992;20:182–192.
8. Knight KL. Knee rehabilitation using a daily adjustable progressive resistance exercise technique. *Am J Sports Med* 1970;7:336–337.
9. Knott M, Voss DE. *Proprioceptive neuromuscular facilitation*. New York, NY: Harper & Row, 1968.
10. Kowalk DL, Duncan JA, McCue FC, Vaughan CL. Anterior cruciate ligament reconstruction and knee dynamics during stair climbing. *Med Sci Sports Exer* 1997;29:1406–1413.
11. Lehto MUK, Jarvinen MJ. Muscle injuries, their healing process and treatment. *Ann Chir Gyan* 1991;80:102–108.
12. Lephart SM, Pincivero DM, Giraldo JL, Fu FH. The role of proprioception in the management and rehabilitation of athletic injuries. *Am J Sports Med* 1997;25:130–137.
13. Lephart SM, Henry TJ. The physiological basis for open and closed kinetic chain rehabilitation for the upper extremity. *J Sport Rehabil* 1996;5:71–87.
14. Lephart SM, Perrin DH, Fu F, Gieck JH, McCue FC, Irrgang JJ. Relationship between selected physical characteristics and functional capacity in the anterior cruciate insufficient athlete. *J Orthop Sports Phys Ther* 1992;16:174–181.
15. Lephart SM, Warner JP, Borsa PA, et al. Proprioception of the shoulder in normal, unstable, and post-surgical individuals. *J Shoulder Elbow Surg* 1994;3:371–380.
16. Levin S. Aquatic therapy. *Phys Sportsmed* 1991;19(10):119–126.
17. Perrin DH. *Isokinetic exercise and assessment*. Champaign, IL: Human Kinetics, 1993.

18. Perrin DH. *Athletic taping and bracing.* Champaign, IL: Human Kinetics, 1995.
19. Perrin DH, Tis LL, Hellwig EV, Shenk BS. Relationship between isokinetic average force, peak force, average torque, and peak torque of the shoulder internal and external rotator muscle groups. *Isokin Ex Sci* 1993;3:85–87.
20. Quillen WS, Gieck JH. Manual therapy: mobilization of the motion-restricted knee. *Athl Training* 1988;23:123–130.
21. Tipton CM, Matthes RD, Maynard JA, Carey RA. The influence of physical activity on ligaments and tendons. *Med Sci Sports* 1975; 7:165–175.
22. Tis LL, Perrin DH. Relationship between isokinetic average force, average torque, peak force, and peak torque of the knee extensor and flexor musculature. *Isokin Ex Sci* 1994;4:150–152.
23. Webright WG, Randolph BJ, Perrin DH. Comparison of modified neural slump and static stretch techniques on hamstring flexibility. *J Orthop Sports Phys Therap* 1997;26:7–13.
24. Worrell TW, Perrin DH, Gansneder BM, Gieck JH. Comparison of isokinetic strength and flexibility measures between hamstring injured and non-injured athletes. *J Orthop Sports Phys Therap* 1991; 13:118–125.
25. Worrell TW, Perrin DH. Hamstring muscle injury: the role of strength, flexibility, warm-up, and fatigue. *J Orthop Sports Phys Therap* 1992;16:12–18.

The Injured Athlete, Third Edition,
edited by D. H. Perrin.
Lippincott–Raven Publishers, Philadelphia © 1999.

CHAPTER 6

Therapeutic Modalities in the Rehabilitation of Athletic Injuries

Susan Foreman and Ethan N. Saliba

Minimizing the time lost to injury is a major goal for sports medicine professionals. Various physical agents are available to the athletic trainer or physical therapist, which create an optimum environment for injury healing while reducing pain and discomfort. Modalities include forms of heat, cold, light, water, electricity, massage, and any mechanical means. These agents are used in an effort to promote healing during rehabilitation.

Early intervention with physical agents helps to limit the pain-spasm cycle by minimizing the inflammatory response (69). As the injury matures, the progression of the modalities can augment circulation and the transfer of nutrients, which enhances the healing process (46,47,69). A reduction in the inflammatory effects allows better tolerance to the ultimate modality— rehabilitative exercise (51). The early application of exercise minimizes the degree of deconditioning, therefore rehabilitation can be accomplished more quickly allowing the athlete to return to activity more expediently. The sports medicine practitioner's goal, therefore, is to minimize the inflammatory response, augment the healing environment, and incorporate timely therapeutic exercise.

EFFECTS OF INJURY

The sports medicine clinician should have a good understanding of the physiologic consequences of tissue injury and how the intervention with modalities can affect the inflammatory process. Inflammation occurs to some degree whenever tissue is crushed, stretched, or torn and occurs cyclically with overuse injuries. The series of vascular and cellular events stabilize the injury and evoke

the healing response (69,76,108,139). Inflammation cannot be stopped, and the final result is often the formation of fibrous tissue and scar, which can be deleterious to normal function (48). The effects of inflammation: redness, pain, heat, and swelling, however, can be minimized with effective intervention.

Cellular responses occur immediately following acute injury. Cellular death causes the release of histamine, which induces a series of vascular changes (69,108). Vasodilation of local blood vessels with formation of edema and pain are the major consequences of the inflammatory response. Hemorrhage from damaged, dilated vessels adds additional trauma to the injured area. Local circulation is disrupted and the vessels are no longer able to meet the tissues' oxygen demand. Further cellular damage and death results from these secondary hypoxic conditions. Heat and redness are also signs of inflammation and are the result of increased blood flow and increased metabolic activity in the injured area (108).

In addition to histamine, bradykinins and prostaglandins are synthesized at the area of trauma when cells are damaged. These chemical mediators increase local swelling and pain. There is an increase in capillary permeability, which results in an imbalance of the osmotic pressures within the tissues (46,76). Plasma proteins, colloids, and water flow into interstitial spaces from normal vessels, leading to edema production in the area.

Within 12 hours, white blood cells begin to migrate to the traumatized area (139,145). Neutrophils arrive first and release active proteolytic enzymes into the injured area. The enzymes help to isolate the area so that infectious material does not become systemic, but these enzymes can become toxic to joint structures, which can cause degenerative changes with prolonged inflammation (108). The neutrophils are then phagocytized by the macrophages along with the cellular debris, fibrin, and red

S. Foreman and E. N. Saliba: Department of Athletics, University of Virginia, Charlottesville, Virginia 22903

blood cells. The amount of tissue damage and the extent of the inflammatory cascade in the area determines the healing time.

Muscle spasm is induced in the body's effort to splint damaged tissues to prevent further trauma. The chemical mediators released from inflammatory process, as well as pressure from swelling and spasm, stimulate pain fibers and contribute to the pain–spasm cycle (45). Inflammatory conditions involving joints with pain and effusion may result in inhibition of muscular contraction which results in atrophy (88).

The early inflammatory sequence of events lasts for 1 to 3 days (47,69). Fibroblasts, which are the connective tissue cells, proliferate. Collagen is also laid down, which is the main supporting protein of connective tissue (45,47,48). Capillary buds then begin to appear as the process begins to shift toward regeneration and repair. Granulation tissue fills the collagen matrix. Reepithelialization begins and by the fifth day a loose mesh of fibrous connective tissue complete with vascularity is generated.

During the second week following injury, fibroblasts proliferate further as collagen is oriented along normal stress lines if proper therapeutic exercise with graded stress has begun (51). With immobilization or a lack of exercise, an excess of collagen is produced which causes the structures to stick together in a bramble-bush effect (45,145). There is more scarring and the fibrous connective tissue becomes devascularized. Exercise within pain-free limits causes a reduction in edema and an increase in the tensile strength of scar tissue that promotes function. Too vigorous exercise or premature return to sports at this stage of healing can rupture vulnerable collagen tissue and reinstigate an inflammatory process.

Fibroblast proliferation slows by the end of the first month (69,145). The fibrous tissue continues to mature and remodel for up to one year following the injury. The athlete is able to return to competition when there is no edema, full range of motion, equal strength compared to the contralateral extremity, and the athlete has dynamic control of any instability. Finally, the athlete should be successful in a gradual progression of function.

Treatment of Injury

Ice

Cryotherapy is the most effect modality for the management of acute athletic injuries and postoperative conditions (8,59,62,66,77). When applied acutely, especially in conjunction with compression and elevation, ice can greatly reduce the severity of an injury by controlling the inflammatory process (78,140). Inflammation cannot be stopped and is necessary to allow the mechanisms for healing and repair to occur, however, the by-products of inflammation such as swelling and pain can cause further debilitation. Ice delays or minimizes swelling and decreases pain and muscle spasm, thus limiting the magnitude of injury. Lowering tissue temperature causes a local vasoconstriction, reduces capillary permeability due to the lessened effect of chemical mediators and makes the blood more viscous (136). Ho and associates recorded a 26% reduction in blood flow to the knee when an ice pack was applied for 20 minutes (64).

The exact mechanism in which ice dulls peripheral pain is not known (25,37). However, lowering tissue temperature interferes locally with nerve impulses and decreases nerve conduction velocity (102). Ice relieves spasm by decreasing muscle activity, muscle spindle firing, and acetylcholine levels so that ischemia due to constant muscle contraction is prevented (6). Ice limits the magnitude of tissue damage by lowering the metabolism of adjacent uninjured cells. By decreasing the cellular demand for oxygen, cells are put into partial hibernation, which increases their survival rate while local circulation is disrupted (64,78).

Initial treatment of an injury follows the acronym ICE (ice, compression, and elevation) (Fig. 6.1). The injured part should also be protected from painful stimuli. Ice may be applied as soon as possible after the injury for 20 to 30 minutes to allow good penetration. The athlete may then shower before receiving another 20-minute treatment of ICE. If a fracture is suspected, an ice pack can be left in place until x-rays are taken. Although it is not possible to prevent all hematomas because of frank bleeding, ice helps minimize swelling so that a better fitting cast may be applied. Ice may then be used for 20 minutes each hour as necessary or for 30 to 60 minutes over a cast (71). Ice can also be applied over a compression bandage postoperatively to manage pain and swelling, but longer durations of application are necessary (25,62).

There are many ways to apply ice, including ice wraps, ice packs, ice slush, or a cold whirlpool. Additionally, there are commercially available units that circulate cold water or antifreeze with a mechanical pump. Elastic wraps can be kept in ice water so that the cold, wet ice wrap can be applied initially since a dry bandage acts as an insulator. An ice pack should be applied over the cold wrap (10,66).

Chipped or crushed ice conforms better than cubes and is generally more comfortable and more effective. The ice should be put in a plastic bag to prevent dripping. There should be minimal air in the bag since this reduces the conformity of the ice pack and acts as an insulator. The ice bag should be left in place over the injured area for 15 to 30 minutes, depending on the depth of tissue injured (10). Deeper injuries, such as to a belly muscle, require longer application times whereas superficial injuries can be treated in less time.

Chemical ice packs are expensive and can be used only once. They are handy when used in first aid kits because

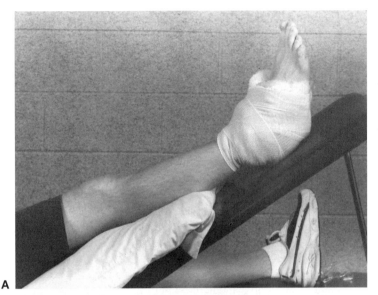

A

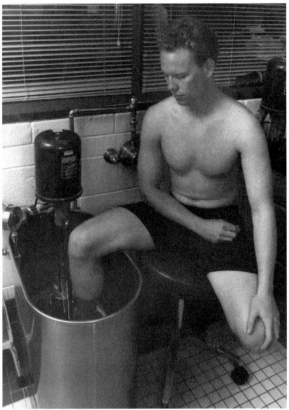

B

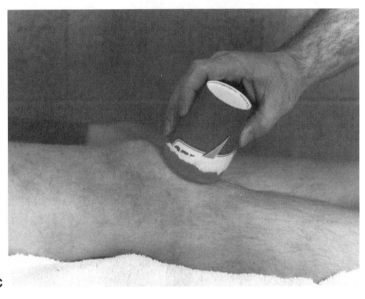

C

FIG. 6.1. Ice, compression, elevation. **A:** An ice pack should be wrapped with a compression bandage over the injured part as soon as possible after an injury. The extremity should be elevated above the level of the heart and left in this position for 15–30 minutes, depending on the depth of the injured structures. **B:** Cold submersion. **C:** Ice massage.

they do not have to be kept cold. Chemical ice packs have two separate chemicals that produce an endothermic reaction when combined, causing a cold temperature. Care should be taken, however, not to puncture the outer bag because the chemicals can be caustic to the skin.

Synthetic gel packs stay below freezing for up to 2 hours depending on the temperature of the freezer. They usually remain flexible and conform to the injured area well and are convenient when using cold therapy on a regular basis and when chipped ice is not available. These reusable frozen gel packs can be dangerous, however, because they can cause frostbite to the skin. A moist towel should be used as an interface so that the gel pack is not applied directly to the skin. A dry interface may not be sufficient in reducing tissue temperature (9).

Ethyl chloride, fluoromethane, and other cold sprays provide an expensive mechanism for temporary anaesthesia. These sprays also have environmental implications

on the ozone layer and should be used prudently. A cold spray may temporarily relieve the pain from a hard blow by superficially cooling the skin, but cold sprays do little to control internal bleeding (102).

Ice submersion baths are made by mixing chips or flakes of ice in water to produce a temperature of 13°C to 18°C (55°F to 65°F). Because it is impossible to combine an ice bath with elevation, the extremity can be wrapped with a single layer of wet elastic wrap to provide some compression during the treatment. The submersion method, however, provides circumferential cooling. Temperatures should stay within the recommended range since lower temperatures are noxious and can promote swelling by creating a mild histamine response (102).

An inexpensive method of ice application for localized areas of injury is the ice massage (16). Water is frozen in a styrofoam cup and then stroked over the injured area using gentle pressure. The area to be treated should be less than 3 times the surface area of the ice to allow effective cooling (144). The treatment should take about 7 to 15 minutes, making the ice massage a convenient but messy method of ice application.

The indications for the use of ice are numerous in an athletic population. In addition to reducing the pain and swelling of acute injuries, ice can be used with therapeutic exercise throughout rehabilitation (59). Ice reduces pain and spasm so that active range of motion can be increased. Ice can also be used to reduce postexercise inflammation. Ice should be used cautiously when applied over superficial nerves such as the ulnar or peroneal nerves. Permanent injury to these nerves has been documented with cryotherapy (28,63,85).

Compression

A cold, wet elastic wrap provides compression to help control hemorrhage mechanically, and the combination of ice and compression has been shown to be more effective in controlling edema than ice alone (119,138). Following an initial ICE treatment, a dry compression or elastic wrap should be applied to control edema formation (1). Elastic wraps are most effective on uniform body parts because the wrap will not compress hollow areas, such as the area surrounding the ankle malleoli. To enhance compression in soft tissues, a felt horseshoe or pad should be placed in these areas. Care should be taken not to strangle tissues, which would impede circulation. The wrap should be applied with even pressure from distal to proximal and the clinician should educate the athlete to loosen the wrap if there is a sensation of pulsing or pain. The athlete should be told to wear the wrap at all times.

Intermittent compression serves as a valuable adjunct to cold in reducing edema (1,11,26,113) (Fig. 6.2). Although most intermittent compression units use air in a vinyl-encased bladder that surrounds the extremity, some units combine a refrigerant fluid with the pressure to provide simultaneous cryotherapy. The pressure within the sleeve is alternately applied and released to force edema from the limb. Active motion should be done during the rest phase to take advantage of the effects of muscle pumping on edema reduction (93). Generally the pressure in an intermittent compression device should not exceed the diastolic blood pressure and the clinician should reduce the pressure if the athlete perceives pain, paresthesia, or the pulse.

Whenever a compression wrap or an intermittent compression unit is used, the limb should be elevated. Elevation above the level of the heart decreases blood flow to the limb and enhances venous return. An elevation block should support the entire limb, rather than placing pillows under the distal part, which can place stress on joint structures. The athlete should be encouraged to elevate the injured extremity as often as possible in his or her daily routine. Table 6.1 presents the technique of applying a compression wrap.

Contrast Therapy

Contrast treatments of hot and cold may begin when the athlete's progress with ice has plateaued, edema has stabilized, and there is no hyperemia or heat in the injured area. Contrast treatments are proposed to provide an alternating effect of vasodilation-vasoconstriction effect that helps mobilize edema (97). There is an increased sensory effect that decreases pain and allows greater pain-free range of motion. The active motion, which is optional, also contributes to edema resorption (126). Contrast therapy also provides a conservative progression to heat therapy for subacute injuries. Contrast therapy is more common in sports medicine environments because early athletic participation and activity can cause a reactive inflammatory process that can be exacerbated by using heat alone. Contrast therapy, even with a 4:1 ratio of hot to cold, does not significantly increase temperature at depths of 1 cm (96).

Treatment begins when the ankle, for example, is placed in a warm tub or whirlpool of 39°C (102°F), followed by a session in cold water of 13° to 18°C (55° to 65°F). Times of treatment begin with 2 minutes in warm water and 2 minutes in cold water with subacute injuries. If the athlete is tolerating heat without increasing discomfort or edema, the heat sessions can increase to 4 minutes, alternating with 1 minute in cold. All treatments typically end in the cold whirlpool since the athlete should be performing therapeutic and functional exercise in addition to the hydrotherapy that increases the tissue temperature. Contrast treatments may be repeated several times daily. Contrast treatments are most commonly applied to distal extremity joint injuries. Hot pack/cold pack applications are impractical, but can be used if durations are extended, for example 5 minutes/5 minutes.

Heat

Heat is used during rehabilitation to both prepare the athlete for exercise and to increase flexibility when combined with a stretch (Fig. 6.3). Superficial heat provides a mild inflammatory action and should not be used with acute injuries (59,126). Both ice and heat are analgesic agents and both can reduce muscle spasm when used at the appropriate time during rehabilitation. Heat is often preferred by the athlete because of its sedating properties, but ice is more effective when the athlete complains of pain versus tightness in the injured area.

Physiologically, superficial heat induces a vasodilation effect from a sensory reflex which increases blood flow (58). This vasodilation can be beneficial since there is an

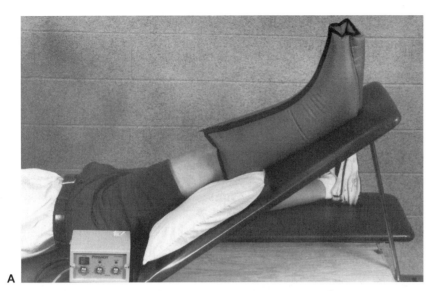

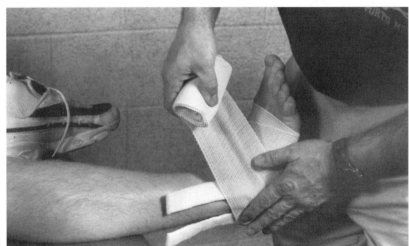

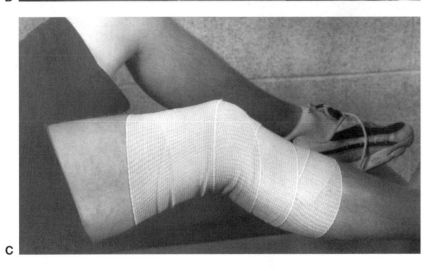

FIG. 6.2. Compression. **A:** Pneumatic compression is used to further prevent and treat edema. The part should be elevated in a comfortable position above the level of the heart. Active motion within pain-free range should be performed in the "rest" phase to encourage lymphatic action. **B:** A dry compression bandage should be placed over the injured part after the ice treatment. Felt can be placed around bony prominences or over a contused part to emphasize compression in irregular areas. **C:** Compression wrap applied to the knee.

TABLE 6.1. *Steps in applying a compression wrap*

1. Apply distal to proximal, overlapping by 1/2 of the wrap's width.
2. Maintain even compression without strangulation. This is often accomplished by wrapping at a spiraling angle rather than wrapping circumferentially.
3. Avoid wrinkles and "windows" which are non-wrapped areas.
4. Educate the athlete on loosening the wrap if there is a pulsing sensation, pain or discoloration in the nails. The athlete should also be told to continue elevation.

influx of oxygen and nutrients to the injured area while waste products and metabolites are carried away. Superficial heat is most effective when combined with exercise. Heat increases the extensibility of connective tissue, but changes in range of motion can only be achieved when the tissue is stretched while the temperature is increased (82). It is also proposed that increases in intramuscular temperatures can decrease the chance of muscle injury (101,130).

There are many methods of applying superficial heat including whirlpools, hot packs, heating pads, and paraffin wax. All have a depth of penetration of about 1 cm, depending on the thickness of the layer of subcutaneous tissue which tends to insulate (13). Treatment times vary with the structure to be treated, but it generally takes about 20 minutes for the tissues to reach therapeutic temperatures. Superficial areas such as the hands do not require as long a treatment.

When using whirlpool treatments, the water temperature may range from 37° to 45°C (98° to 110°F) depending on the amount of surface area submerged. There is less ability to cool the body when large areas are heated, so

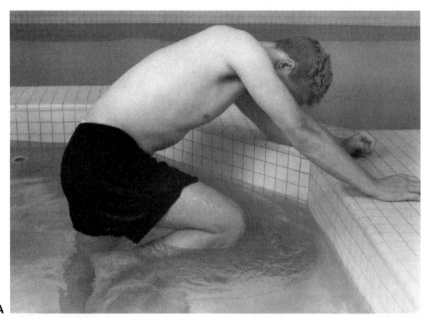

A

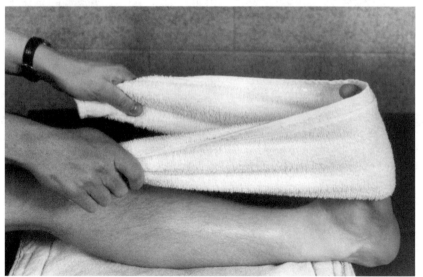

B

FIG. 6.3. Superficial heat. **A:** Warm whirlpool: allows active range of motion during the heat treatment and can be adapted for the treatment of large areas. **B:** Hot packs: position so that the athlete perceives a comfortable stretch.

lower temperatures should be used with jacuzzi or whole-body submersion.

Heat packs are segmented canvas bags filled with a hydrophilic silica gel. These packs are stored in a water-filled stainless steel container at temperatures of 140° to 190°F and then wrapped in towels for use (55,59,126). The number of towel layers determines the temperature of treatment delivered to the athlete. Waterproof electrical heating pads are also useful, but the athlete should only use these pads for 20 minutes at a time. There is a more rapid rise to therapeutic temperatures when moist heating pads are used, but dry heat can be used with similar results (132).

Electrical Principles

Often a clinician can recognize the capability of an electrical modality by the manufacturer's name or by what the sales representative states the unit is capable of doing. The better the clinician can understand and recognize the effects of current parameters on biologic tissues, the more appropriately the equipment can be used, and with greater versatility. It is difficult to address all the concepts and terms relevant to the area of electrotherapy, but the following is an attempt to clarify some of the confusion.

Neurophysiology

A thorough understanding of muscle physiology and neurophysiology is helpful when addressing the effect of electrical stimulation on a biologic system. Whenever the nervous system is intact and an electrical current is applied, the muscular response is through the nerve. The basic unit of the peripheral nervous system is the neuron, with its dendrites and axons (57) (see Fig. 6.4). Neurons make up an extensive network of relay systems that conduct both sensory information (afferent fibers) from the periphery to the spinal cord and motor stimulation (efferent fibers) from the spinal cord to the muscles. The dendrites take in information from other neurons and receptors, and the axons direct the stimulation to other neurons, muscles, or the spinal cord, depending on their type. Nerve fibers are classified as either myelinated or nonmyelinated, depending on the presence of a phospholipid-insulating membrane, the myelin sheath. Myelinated fibers carry their impulses faster, since the impulse is transmitted from node to node (interruptions in the membrane). Larger diameter fibers tend to have more myelination and therefore transmit an impulse faster than smaller, less myelinated fibers.

Nerve fibers are also classified by their function: pain, sensory or motor (57,80,111,134). The largest nerve fibers

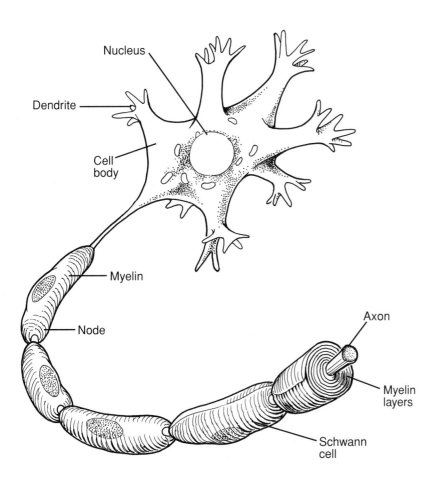

FIG. 6.4. Neuron.

are the "A" fibers, which are the fastest-conducting motor and sensory nerve fibers. This group is subdivided into A alpha, A beta, A gamma, and A delta, depending on their size. These larger nerve fibers have a low capacitance and are the most quickly stimulated (Table 6.2).

The "B" fibers are smaller myelinated fibers and are generally the efferent fibers of the autonomic nervous system. These fibers are not usually associated with direct responses of electrical stimulation, but may act indirectly as an important link between some of the physiologic effects of electrical stimulation (80). The "C" fibers are unmyelinated and include the efferent postganglionic fibers of the sympathetic nervous system and the smallest afferent peripheral nerves, which are usually associated with pain. The C fibers are the slowest in conduction and take more stimulation to elicit a response. Because the A and C fibers have sensory components, they play the largest role in both pain and pain control. Many of the pain control theories and electrical stimulation protocols utilize the properties of these nerve fibers to produce their response.

An excitable membrane such as a nerve or muscle has an active transport system of sodium and potassium, as well as an electrical gradient of other ions to create a membrane resting potential or voltage. If the hormonal, thermal, chemical, mechanical, or electrical stimulation is great enough, there is a change in the membrane's permeability that results in the depolarization of the tissue (57,111). When the threshold level is surpassed by this stimulation, an action potential results that can lead to a sensory or motor response, depending on the fiber stimulated. This response can occur naturally or can be induced through some exogenous application of a stimulus, such as electricity. The current applied to biologic tissues causes an ion migration, which induces a current to be generated inside the body (111).

The biologic effects of electrical stimulation are physiologic, thermal, and physiochemical (80,111). The specific effect is influenced by the type of electric current used and its parameters. The physiologic effects refer to the changes on membrane potentials and their subsequent action potentials. Inducing these physiologic effects is usually the primary goal with electrical stimulation since the result is either a sensory or motor response. The thermal response occurs as electric energy is converted to heat. However, the average current of most electric stimulators used in physical medicine is too low to cause a substantial temperature change. Diathermies, which use high-frequency radio waves, create their thermal effects in this manner. The physiochemical response is usually associated with galvanic or direct currents (DC) and is also the result of the higher average current delivered. These currents enable the clinician to utilize polarity effects of the positive and negative electrodes, which determines the ion flux and electrophoretic effect in the tissues.

Electrophysiology

Several factors affect the flow of current through the body, including tissue impedance, electrode size and placement, and the current stimulation parameters. The current parameters include waveform, amplitude (intensity), phase duration, rate of rise of the leading edge of the pulse, frequency, and duty cycles (52,80,111,134,143). Impedance includes resistance to the flow of current and follows Ohm's Law:

$$\text{Voltage} = \text{Current} \times \text{Resistance (V = IR)}$$

For a given voltage, the more resistance that is met, the less current is delivered to the tissues. The body does not have uniform conductivity because of varying amounts of tissue resistance. This resistance is strongly affected by the tissue's water content. Tissues with high water content, such as blood or muscle, have less resistance than does fat or bone, and therefore conduct the current much more easily.

Another factor that affects tissue impedance is the capacitance of the tissues (4,52). Capacitance is the ability to store and separate charge. The larger the capacitance of a tissue, the longer the current must flow in one direction (either positive or negative) before the fiber discharges. The larger nerve fibers, such as the A beta sensory nerves, have lower capacitance than the nonmyelinated C pain fibers. This means that large nerve fibers are more responsive to a stimulus than the smaller nerve fibers such as the C fibers (63). The tissue with the largest

TABLE 6.2. *Nerve fiber classification*

Nerve	Diameter (μm)	Speed (m/sec)	Function
A alpha (α)	13–22	70–120	Motor neuron
A beta (β)	8–13	40–70	Light touch, proprioception
A gamma (γ)	4–8	15–40	Pressure, muscle spindle
A delta (δ)	1–4	5–15	Pain, crude touch, temperature
B	1–3	3–14	Preganglionic autonomic
C	0.1–1	0.2–2	Unmelinated fibers—pain, temperature, postganglionic autonomic

Data from ref. 111.

capacitance of all excitable tissue is the muscle membrane. It requires a very long phase duration (several milliseconds) to exceed the capability of the membrane to store that charge and elicit a response. Since a nerve has a lower capacitance than the muscle membrane, an electrically stimulated muscle contraction will occur via stimulation of the nerve if the nervous system is intact (4,52,63). Because different-sized nerve fibers, each with their own functions, have different capacitances, modulating the electrical currents can alter which fibers are recruited. The clinician can therefore target specific tissues to elicit the desired effects.

The electrode size and orientation also affects the flow of current through the body. The electrodes and their placement ultimately affect the current density and therefore the degree of response that occurs (55). Current density is the amount of current delivered per unit of surface area. Unequal sized electrodes result in a greater current density under the smaller electrode (4,80). The smaller electrode is classically called the active electrode for that reason. The electrode termed the dispersive is appropriately named, since this electrode spreads the same amount of current as its smaller counterpart over a larger area, resulting in a less stimulating effect (4).

The distance between electrodes influences which tissues are affected and the depth of stimulation. When the electrodes are placed close together, the current flows more superficially. As the electrodes are spread apart, the current can spread and reach the deeper fibers, although the current density is still greater in more superficial tissues immediately under the electrodes (4,55) (Fig. 6.5).

Within the stimulus parameters, the waveform describes the configuration of the pulses of the electrical current. Very strict definitions have been assigned to waveforms such as alternating current (AC) and direct current (DC) to provide consistent terminology within physical medicine and to minimize confusion when communicating with other professions (Fig. 6.6). There are two major classifications of waveforms: monophasic and biphasic. DC and AC currents can be categorized as monophasic and biphasic respectively, but DC and AC currents have no interruption between each pulse and continue indefinitely (5,110). Monophasic currents have uniquely positive and negative electrodes whereas biphasic currents shift polarity continually and each electrode has identical effects if the waveform is symmetrical. Polar effects to the tissues are minimized or eliminated with a biphasic current.

Modulation of the waveform within the unit produces pulsatile currents that have temporary interruptions between each pulse (5). Pulsatile currents have various shapes, phase durations (usually short), and interpulse spacings. The space between each pulse eliminates the normal inverse relationship between frequency and wavelength as with AC. This allows the clinician to independently control the number of pulses per second (frequency) and the phase duration of pulsatile currents (Fig. 6.7).

Other parameters that need to be considered and are often manipulated by the clinician are the phase duration, amplitude, and the pulse frequency. The duration is the time to complete one phase of a pulse and, as discussed previously, affects the type of fiber recruited (52,143) (Fig. 6.8). The amplitude refers to the intensity or magnitude of the current (Fig. 6.9). The peak current is the maximum amplitude of the current at any point during the pulse without regard to its duration. A high peak current has a greater depth of penetration, which allows

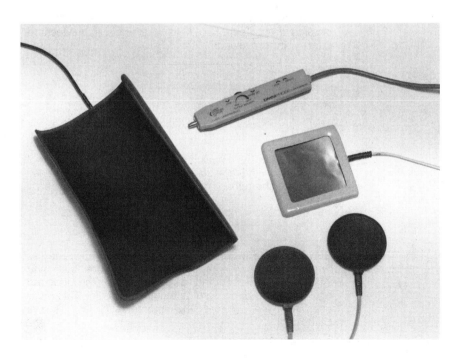

FIG. 6.5. Current density. All stimulators require at least two electrodes to complete the circuit. If the electrodes vary in size, the current density is highest in the smaller electrode.

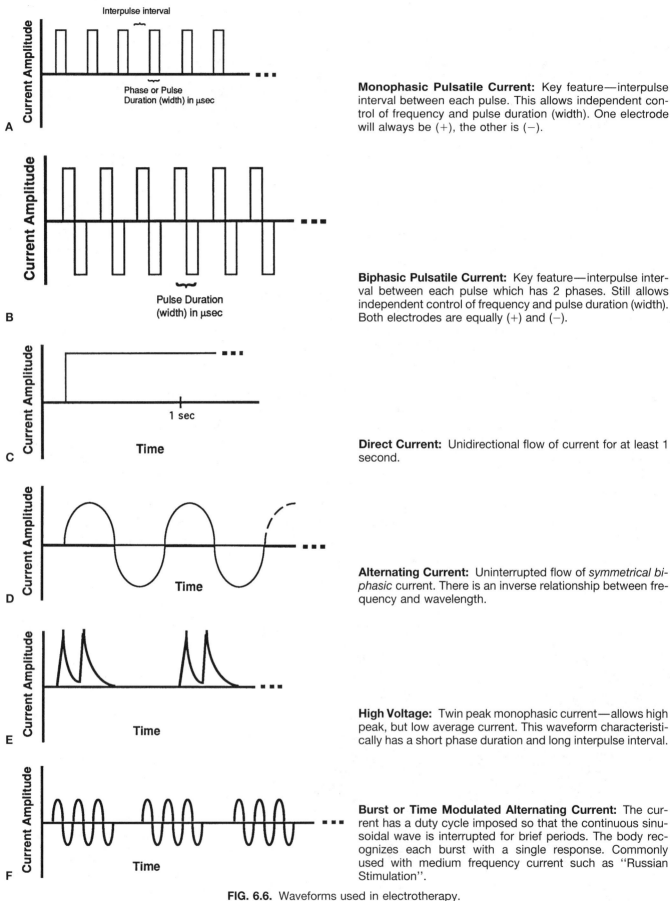

Monophasic Pulsatile Current: Key feature—interpulse interval between each pulse. This allows independent control of frequency and pulse duration (width). One electrode will always be (+), the other is (−).

Biphasic Pulsatile Current: Key feature—interpulse interval between each pulse which has 2 phases. Still allows independent control of frequency and pulse duration (width). Both electrodes are equally (+) and (−).

Direct Current: Unidirectional flow of current for at least 1 second.

Alternating Current: Uninterrupted flow of *symmetrical biphasic* current. There is an inverse relationship between frequency and wavelength.

High Voltage: Twin peak monophasic current—allows high peak, but low average current. This waveform characteristically has a short phase duration and long interpulse interval.

Burst or Time Modulated Alternating Current: The current has a duty cycle imposed so that the continuous sinusoidal wave is interrupted for brief periods. The body recognizes each burst with a single response. Commonly used with medium frequency current such as "Russian Stimulation".

FIG. 6.6. Waveforms used in electrotherapy.

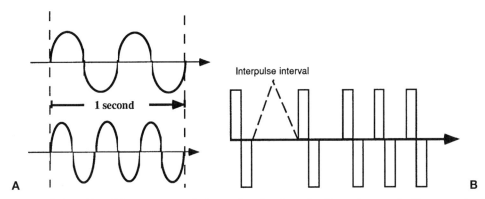

FIG. 6.7. Relationship of frequency and phase duration in pulsatile and nonpulsatile currents. **A:** In the electromagnetic spectrum and in AC currents, there is no interruption in the sinusoidal waveform and the frequency is inversely proportional to the wavelength. **B:** In pulsatile currents, there is an interruption in the current with an interpulse interval. Therefore, the clinician may manipulate the frequency (pps), phase duration, and intensity independently.

more fibers to be recruited. Average current, however, refers to the amount of current supplied over a period of time, which takes into consideration both the peak amplitude as well as the phase duration (4). Depending on the waveform, it is possible to have a high peak but low average current, which is a characteristic of a high voltage stimulator. The average current ultimately determines the physiochemical response of a tissue and, if too high, can damage tissue. Often, the average current is lowered to a safer level by modifying the waveform or parameters, specifically the phase duration.

The phase duration and amplitude are related when determining whether a specific nerve fiber can be targeted using the parameters available on an electrical stimulator (4). Because of the capacitance of each nerve fiber type, there is a limiting phase duration that must be exceeded to cause an action potential. However, when a waveform has a long phase duration, small increases in amplitude cause a stronger sensory or motor reaction. The relationship between the amplitude and phase duration is called the strength-duration curve (98) (Fig. 6.10).

The frequency of the stimulation is the number of pulses generated per second (pps or Hertz) (Table 6.3). The frequency affects the number of action potentials elicited during the stimulation. Although the same number of fibers are recruited, a higher frequency causes them to fire at a more rapid pace, which ultimately increases the tension generated. Nerve membranes must repolarize, however, after discharging. There is an absolute refractory period in which the resting membrane potential is reinstated and another action potential cannot be elicited during this time. The absolute refractory period is ultimately the rate limiting factor of the number of impulses that can be generated by a nerve.

The rate of rise of the leading edge of the pulse is a parameter that is incorporated into a waveform, but it will also affect the type of nerve targeted. The rate of rise references the time it takes to get from zero to maximal

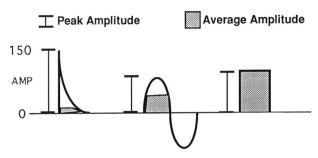

FIG. 6.9. Amplitude of current. The amplitude or the magnitude of the current can be expressed by either its peak current or average current value. Peak amplitude is associated with the depth of penetration and the physiologic effects of electrical stimulation. The higher the amplitude of the current, the greater the depth of penetration, therefore, the greater the number of fibers stimulated. The average intensity is associated with the thermal and physiochemical effects of stimulation on biologic tissues. Peak current is the measure from the isoelectric line (zero) to the maximum positive or negative point without regard to the time duration that the pulse is maintained.

Phase Duration

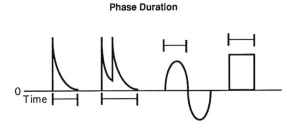

FIG. 6.8. Phase duration. The phase duration refers to the time duration that the current flows in one direction before an interruption (monophasic) or before changing phases (biphasic). The phase duration should be long enough to overcome the capacitance of the nerve or muscle membrane so that an action potential may occur.

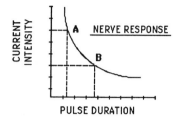

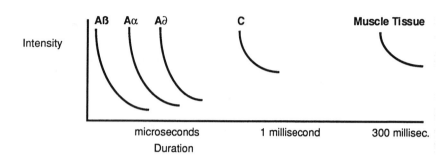

A) Short duration requires a higher intensity for the nerve response.
B) Longer duration allows lower intensity for the same nerve response.

FIG. 6.10. Strength duration curve. The strength duration curve shows that for a given intensity, changing the duration of the pulse directly affects the strength of the response. If the duration decreases, the strength of the stimulus must increase to elicit the same response. Tissue impedance, which includes the resistance, capacitance, and inductance qualities of the tissue, also relies on adequate pulse duration to respond. Tissue capacitance, which is the ability of a tissue to hold a charge before discharging, varies within and between types of tissues. The higher the capacitance of a tissue, a longer pulse duration necessary to elicit a response (it holds more charge).

amplitude within each pulse (5) (Fig. 6.11). Fast rates of rise times are necessary, especially with low capacitance tissues such as large motor nerves. The low capacitance membrane cannot store charge and quickly accommodates to a stimulus. These nerves can dissipate the charge from a pulse with slow rates of rise times, and the ion flux needed to alter the voltage to exceed threshold is never reached. Sensory nerves that carry light touch, for example, have low capacitance and easily accommodate. This explains how a person is aware of clothing when it is first put on, but there is accommodation to this minimal stimulus and the person no longer pays attention to the sensation at the skin. Generally, tissues with low capacitance accommodate to a stimulus easily whereas high capacitance tissues, because they store the charge, do not accommodate or dissipate the charge readily.

When determining whether there will be a physiologic response within the tissues, three important factors within each pulse of an electric current must be considered. First, the stimulus must be of adequate amplitude to reach the threshold level of excitatory tissues. Second, the rate of voltage change (rate of rise of the leading edge of the

pulse) must be rapid enough so that tissue accommodation cannot take place. Third, the length of stimulus or phase duration must be long enough to overcome the capacitance of the tissue to allow an action potential. The Law of Dubois–Reymond addresses these three factors (52) (Table 6.4).

The final parameter of electric stimulation to discuss is the duty cycle. Duty cycles can be imposed by the clinician to interrupt the current periodically for several seconds. This on-off time creates a rest time that is variable on most units. Pulses can also be incorporated into duty cycles inherently in the machine, which creates envelopes or packages of pulses. These duty cycles interrupt the current at specific intervals so that the manufacturer

Rate of Rise of the Leading Edge of the Pulse
(Time to peak amplitude)

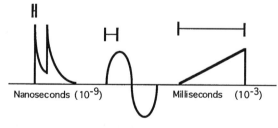

FIG. 6.11. Rate of rise of leading edge of pulse. If a stimulus is applied too gradually, the membrane has the ability to diffuse the ion flux (which brings about a response) so that it will not result in an action potential. This is termed accommodation. Tissues with lower capacitance (nerve) accommodate much more rapidly than the high capacitance (muscle) tissues. A stimulus of adequate intensity and duration to elicit a response is necessary, but the onset of the stimulus must also be rapid enough or no action potential will result.

TABLE 6.3. *Frequency*

The classical delineations of current frequencies are low, medium, and high:
- Low frequency is 1000 Hertz (cycles per second) and below (e.g., TENS units, high voltage, neuromuscular stimulators)
- Medium frequency is 1,000–100,000 Hertz (e.g., interferential, "Russian stimulators")
- High frequency is greater than 100,000 Hertz (e.g., diathermy)

TABLE 6.4. *Law of DuBois Reymond*

1. Each phase of a pulse must have adequate intensity to reach threshold.
2. The phase duration must be long enough to exceed the capacitance of the tissue.
3. The onset of the current or the rate of rise of the leading edge of the phase must be fast enough to reduce accommodation.

can produce time modulated AC currents, otherwise known as "Burst Mode" (5). The carrier frequency is usually an AC current and is interrupted at regular intervals often in the millisecond range. Interruptions are generally imperceptible but enables the clinician to take advantage of the characteristics of the carrier frequency. The classical Russian stimulators utilize this method to modulate medium frequency sinusoidal waves into bursts of 10 milliseconds-on and 10 milliseconds-off (79). The duty cycle reduces the high average current of the sinusoidal wave because the off time lowers the net average current that is delivered, making this a safer modality. The duty cycle also modulates the net frequency of medium frequency generators to physiologically active frequencies.

Electrical Stimulation

There are numerous types of electrical stimulators available with various parameter controls. It is difficult to appreciate the nuances of different stimulators and waveforms available. Various manufacturers have modified the current and the packaging of the current parameters to create a multitude of units, each purporting to elicit unique results attained only by their machine. The stimulators can be categorized into different groups according to their specific applications or unique features. All electrical stimulators are transcutaneous electrical nerve stimulators (TENS) because the stimulation will occur through the nerve if the nerve is intact (4,52). High voltage, interferential, and microcurrent stimulators are examples of TENS units that are generally used for pain relief. Another category is the neuromuscular stimulator that has unique uses such as reducing muscle atrophy (98,110). Finally, DC generators have the capacity to induce physiochemical responses and allow the clinician to perform iontophoresis, which utilizes electrical current to drive medications in their ion forms. DC current is also used to stimulate denervated muscles directly.

Transcutaneous Electrical Nerve Stimulation

Transcutaneous electrical nerve stimulation (TENS) is often used to describe the category of stimulators that are used for the purpose of relieving pain. TENS units are often versatile in their parameters and often allow the clinician freedom to manipulate the phase duration, frequency, amplitude and duty cycle (4,52,75). TENS is much more than the small portable device that attaches to the patient's belt. High voltage stimulators, interferential units, microcurrent, and some low voltage stimulators are examples of TENS units that can be used for pain relief. Although any type of electric stimulator that crosses the skin to excite the nerve is considered to be TENS, there are other uses of these stimulators including edema reduction, wound healing, and muscle stimulation.

Variations of TENS can be achieved by adjusting the current parameters. The proposed mechanisms of pain modulation appropriate for each type of electric stimulation will be discussed. Because therapy with electric stimulation treats the symptoms of an ailment and generally not the cause, proper evaluation of the etiology of the injury and rectification of the cause is important. Modalities are often considered to mask symptoms, so management of the condition with any modality while the patient maintains an active lifestyle often brings about ethical scrutiny. It is often difficult to convince an injured athlete to accept the ideal healing conditions needed to eliminate the problem, which often includes rest. The modalities discussed in this chapter provide a noninvasive method of pain relief, but it is our belief that they will not enable the athlete to tolerate activity beyond a significant stress level. The modality is not used during competition and the athlete must be in a competitive state before activity is allowed. Ideally, the pain modulation allows the athlete to perform therapeutic exercise that will contribute to the alleviation of the problem.

Electrode placement and preparation are important (100). As with all electrical stimulation, the skin should be clean and inspected for any abrasions to ensure good conduction. If carbon-rubber electrodes are being used, sufficient gel should be applied to cover the entire surface of the electrode. Disposable electrodes with preapplied gel and adhesive are expensive but convenient and effective. Excessive gel increases the size of the conductive surface and therefore should not extend beyond the size of the electrodes. Most clinical stimulators use metal electrodes that are covered with rubber. Because of the higher usage, these electrodes can be applied with a saturated sponge or gauze as a conductive interface. This method keeps costs of electrode upkeep at a minimum.

Electrode placement is generally applied over the painful site, but can also include dermatomes, myotomes, trigger-acupuncture points, peripheral nerve trunks, or spinal root levels (Fig. 6.12). The desired response—sensory or motor—should be perceived in the painful region. Two or four electrodes can be used and their placement is readjusted if the desired response does not occur. The skin and electrodes should be inspected with each use in the clinic and daily when the patient or athlete is using the device at home. Tape and adhesives, as well

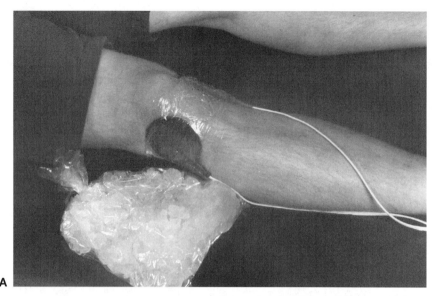

A

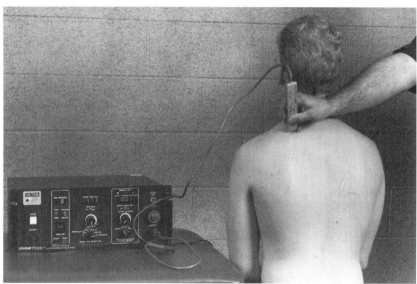

B

FIG. 6.12. Electrode placements vary depending on the goal of the treatment. For example, pain relief or muscle contraction, on either side of the patellar tendon, allows simultaneous ice treatment and the electrical stimulation to treat tendinitis. The ice pack should be placed under the strap to secure both the electrodes and ice. **A:** Surrounding a painful area. **B:** Point stimulators allow focal stimulation over acupuncture points.

as certain types of electrical currents, can cause skin irritation especially with continuous use.

If a portable unit is used, the athlete should be instructed in the operation of the unit because adjustments in parameters, namely amplitude, will be necessary over time. Parameters such as frequency and phase duration should be preset before the unit is used and depend on the goal of the treatment (52). The athlete is to note how long it takes for pain relief to occur. A response to sensory level stimulation should be noticed within the first 10 to 15 minutes of the treatment. If there is no reduction in the symptoms, either parameter or electrode adjustments should be made. Once relief occurs, the athlete should keep the unit on for 1 hour. After 1 hour, the unit should be turned off and the length of pain relief monitored. This process is continued as often as necessary to maintain as pain free a state as possible.

TREATMENT OF PAIN

Pain is a multifaceted component of every musculoskeletal injury. Acute pain has the purpose of alerting the athlete of the injury and preventing further damage that could be caused by further activity (116,118). Pain and swelling, which are indicative of tissue reaction, are often the guidelines for rehabilitation progression. Pain with a purpose should not be eliminated with anaesthetics. However, pain that prevents therapeutic exercise or continues beyond its purpose is deleterious to rehabilitation. The pain-spasm cycle presents an example of pain that can impair progress. Therapeutic modalities including TENS and ice are intended to *reduce* pain, but do not eliminate pain or alter sensory function.

Pain is a complex entity that involves the understanding of neuroanatomy and neurophysiology as well as pharmacology. For the purposes of this chapter, a brief overview of some of the pain modulation theories will be presented with parameters of electric stimulation that may invoke these physiologic responses. Contraindications of electrical stimulation are included in Table 6.5.

Sensory TENS

In the most basic mechanism of pain control, pain is modified at the spinal level such as in Melzack and Wall's gate theory (88). The key to this mechanism of pain relief is sensory stimulation that ultimately decreases the transmission of pain fibers at the spinal cord synapse (89). TENS is used to stimulate large diameter sensory afferent fibers (A beta). Since these fibers are large and have a lower capacitance than A delta or C fibers (pain), they are easily stimulated with a current of short phase durations and relatively low intensities.

When A beta fibers are selectively stimulated, an area in the dorsal horn of the spinal cord known as the substantia gelatinosa is active (52,86). This area causes interneurons to inhibit the synapse of pain fibers that carry the transmission to the brain where the pain is localized. Neurohormonal substances such as enkephalin and dynorphin are released at the interneurons of the spinal cord and sensory nerves. These substances have characteristics of endogenous opioids, which are powerful analgesics. Enkephalin, however, has a relatively short half-life (45 seconds to 2 minutes), which causes pain relief to be short-lived (123). Often the pain relief is diminished as the stimulation ceases (89).

The application of the sensory level of pain modulation requires that the stimulation parameters selectively recruit the A beta fibers; therefore amplitude levels should be below the motor threshold and the athlete should perceive a comfortable tingling sensation. The parameters of the unit should be preset and the amplitude of the current adjusted once the electrodes are in place. The phase duration should be short so that the possibility of recruiting pain fibers with their higher capacitance is minimized. Generally the phase duration is less than 200 microseconds and is ideally between 60 to 100 microseconds (4,20). If the phase duration is too short, there may be

TABLE 6.5. *The contraindications of electrical stimulation rarely involve the athlete, but include the following*

- Patients with demand pacemakers
- Over the carotid sinus in the neck
- During pregnancy—although this has become an accepted method of pain modulation, the electrical activity will interfere with monitors
- Over the chest when there are cardiac problems
- Any type of cerebral vascular disorder
- Over eyes or mucosal membranes

From refs. 55 and 56.

TABLE 6.6. *Parameters for TENS used for pain modulation*

Subsensory:
  Phase duration: Varies—can be galvanic or pulsed
  Pulse rate: Varies
  Amplitude: Low: subsensory—less than 999 μamps
Sensory:
  Phase duration: Less than 100 microseconds
  Pulse rate: 60–120 pulses per second (pps)
  Amplitude: Low: submotor
Motor:
  Phase duration: Wide: 200–300 microseconds
  Pulse rate: Low: 2–4 pulses per second (pps)
  Amplitude: Strong, visible contractions should be elicited but should not cause pain
Noxious:
  Phase duration: Longer than 1 millisecond (target C Fibers)
  Pulse rate: 100–150 pps or low: 2–7 pps (low rate allows combination of motor and noxious)
  Amplitude: As high as tolerated
Nerve block:
  Phase duration: Very short—usually dependent on frequency (because of AC current)
  Pulse rate: 1000–5000 Hz
  Amplitude: Strong sensory and increase with accommodation

no perception of stimulation at all, even with high intensities. The frequency should produce a constant stimulation with no perception of pulses. Frequencies greater than 50 pps are necessary and there are several recommended ranges to target specific neurohormonal responses at the spinal cord. Generally 60 to 100 pps is effective, although research is still needed to indicate which frequency causes the longest lasting pain modification (52,55,98).

Once these parameters are set, the amplitude should be a strong, comfortable stimulation with no muscle contraction. Because of the fast accommodation of A beta fibers, adjustments may be necessary in phase duration and/or amplitude over time. Some units attempt to deter accommodation by continually modulating the amplitude, duration, or pulse frequency or any combination of these parameters over the length of the treatment. Generally, the changes will oscillate 20% above and below the preset levels, which would minimize gross changes in the treatment goals. Treatment durations can be indefinite, but generally last from 20 minutes to 1 hour at a session. In acute injuries, sensory TENS and cold combined produce significant analgesic effects compared to either modality alone (37). This type of TENS can be administered immediately after an injury since there is no disruption in clot formation and it has been effective in treating postoperative pain when sterile electrodes are placed around the incision during surgery (49,129) (Table 6.6).

Motor TENS

The motor theory of pain modification involves much more complex neurophysiologic mechanisms, including descending pain modulation (20). This implies that pain impulses have reached cognitive areas of the brain and other cerebral centers that have emotional and endocrine functions. When a strong, rhythmic stimulation of A delta fibers at or near the pain site is induced, several areas of the brain that have analgesic neurohormonal influences are activated. Specifically, the hypothalamus influences the pituitary gland to release beta lipotropin, a precursor to the endogenous opiate endorphin. Endorphin is a powerful analgesic with a half-life of up to 4 hours, creating a longer-lasting pain relief (123). Clinical trials comparing sensory and motor TENS, however, have had difficulty demonstrating increases in blood plasma beta endorphin despite improvements in pain levels (35,70).

In order to stimulate A delta fibers, a motor response is desired (123). Although motor fibers are large diameter, fast fibers, they are deeper structures than sensory nerves and therefore require a greater stimulus to be recruited electrically. A rhythmic motor response or muscle contraction is a good indication that A delta (fast pain) fibers are being stimulated as well. Because this method of pain modification utilizes strong motor contractions, it is often not recommended for acute injuries. This method should be used only after acute bleeding has stopped and the injury can safely tolerate the agitation of strong rhythmic muscle contractions.

The application of motor TENS is similar to sensory TENS with respect to electrode set-up, although motor points or acupuncture points are often targeted in addition to pain sites (86,98). The electrodes need to be secured adequately to prevent slippage during the treatment. The parameters will induce sensory stimulation first, but the amplitude should induce strong muscle contractions to ensure that A delta fibers are recruited. The phase duration should be long enough to overcome the capacitance of A delta fibers, therefore the phase duration should be over 200 microseconds (4,36). Often, a phase duration of 200 to 300 microseconds is used. The pulse frequency should be low so that individual contractions can be seen and felt. Frequencies of less than 10 pps is necessary and 2 to 4 pps is recommended (23). The amplitude should again invoke strong, well-tolerated rhythmic contractions. Treatment durations last from 15 to 30 minutes and can be repeated several times a day. This method of pain modulation will take longer to achieve pain relief, but the decrease in pain is generally longer lasting because the half-life of beta endorphin is approximately 4 hours. This method of pain modulation has been shown to be effective in treating numerous painful conditions such as muscle spasms or subacute muscle injuries (36,84) (see Table 6.6).

Noxious TENS

A similarly complicated mechanism of pain control that also involves descending inhibition is the noxious pain theory. This theory implies that pain is used to treat pain and is sometimes referred to as hyperstimulation analgesia (123). This method is often reserved for pain that is difficult to manage such as myofascial pain syndromes, sympathetically mediated pain, or with overuse injuries that should not be treated with pharmacologic interventions because of continued activity levels. Muscle spasms are also effectively treated with noxious TENS and Paris et al. found that second degree ankle sprains had significantly greater range of motion and were released from therapy sooner than subjects who had standard treatment (103).

Inhibition of pain with noxious level TENS occurs primarily through the Raphe nucleus and the periaqueductal gray matter (PAG) of the brain, which produces serotonin and enkephalin (7). These neurohormones inhibit the transmission of pain impulses in the dorsal horn of the spinal cord. Pain relief generally lasts 4 to 6 hours (89).

This method of pain modulation requires the activation of C fibers, which are small, unmyelinated pain fibers. They have a high capacitance and are difficult or impossible to stimulate with traditional electric stimulators. Most units have a much lower limit on the phase duration, which provides an important safety device that minimizes average current. To stimulate C fibers, a phase duration of a minimum of 1 millisecond is needed; most electric stimulators have a maximum of 300 to 500 microseconds (microsecond = 1/1,000,000 second vs. millisecond = 1/1,000 second) (20). The long phase duration required for noxious TENS causes physiochemical responses under the electrodes (55,4). To minimize this response and the potential for skin irritation, noxious TENS is usually delivered with a point stimulator. Point stimulators allow the treatment of acupuncture, motor and trigger points that correspond to the painful region (86). Some point stimulators are equipped with an ohmmeter that measures skin resistance, which help the clinician locate potential sites for stimulation. Areas of relatively low skin resistance correlate to acupuncture, trigger, and motor points.

The parameters of noxious TENS require a long phase duration (over 1 millisecond) and high amplitude. Stimulation should be within tolerable pain limits and is often compared to a "bee sting" sensation. The frequency can be either continuous (60 to 100 pps) or low (2 to 4 pps), which may take advantage of the motor TENS effects as well. The clinician must inform the athlete that the stimulation will be painful, although the amplitude can be modified at any time during the stimulation. Using a point stimulator, the amplitude should be increased gradually, with feedback from the athlete. Since the application of a current will decrease skin resistance, there may be an increase in the perception of the stimulation. Current flow is therefore increased with the same applied voltage (Ohm's law). It is imperative that the athlete trust the clinician because of the painful nature of the treatment. Each point should be treated for at least 30 seconds and it is generally recommended to treat 8 to 12 points depending on the area of pathology (see Table 6.6).

Nerve Block TENS

The application of medium frequency currents (1,000 to 100,000 Hz) can result in a disruption of the normal action potential transmission along a nerve. The refractory periods following an action potential dictate the ultimate frequency of impulses on an excitable membrane. When there is stimulation at a higher frequency than the membrane can respond to, the resting membrane potential is altered. The result is that the membrane's voltage is constantly changing at a subthreshold level, making it more difficult for the fiber to generate an action potential (14). The activity of the sodium-potassium pump increases in an attempt to stabilize the membrane and return it to the resting level. When a frequency of electrical stimulation is applied above 1,000 Hz, there is an inability for the membrane to respond normally and an action-potential failure results. The action potential failure is also called Wedenski inhibition and occurs with the application of medium frequency currents such as with interferential and Russian stimulation, which is also known as time-modulated AC current (98).

The action potential failure is a localized response that frequently occurs between the electrodes and lasts only as long as the stimulation is being applied. There is a decrease in all sensory input in the treated area, including pain. This method is not commonly used for pain management because it requires a machine that is capable of delivering a medium frequency, which usually is associated with high average currents. Also the pain relief and sensory modification are short-lived and can be accomplished similarly with other techniques.

Subsensory TENS

The subsensory mode of pain modulation with electrical stimulating devices is often associated with microcurrent stimulators (MENS) or low-intensity stimulators (LIS) (5). The intensities used in LIS are limited to a maximum of 999 amps which is much lower than traditional stimulators (68,121). Numerous waveforms and parameters have been suggested to enhance the subtle effects on healing that these stimulators are purported to have. Variations in polarity, frequencies and phase duration however, make comparisons of clinical trials difficult.

Theories that are used to explain the positive effects of LIS are based on the ''current of injury,'' which is a measurable charge emitted from an injury site (22,68). This charge may be responsible for the chemotactic attraction of leukocytes during the inflammatory phase. By delivering a low amplitude charge to the area, the chemotactic influence is potentiated, which may result in faster

healing (105). The tissue healing is responsible for the decrease in pain when using this modality. There have been numerous empirical statements regarding the efficacy of this treatment, however, more research is needed to clarify the parameters needed to produce effective results.

Virtually any stimulator can be used for LIS by leaving the amplitude so low that there is no perception of energy. However, to reproduce results, the unit should be able to register these low outputs. High voltage stimulators can be used for this purpose especially since they utilize a monopolar waveform and deliver microcurrent amperage. Many of the effects of microcurrent have been addressed using high voltage stimulators.

Other Uses for Electric Stimulation

Electric stimulation can be used for purposes other than pain relief. There have been studies to support the use of electric stimulation for edema reduction, muscle spasm reduction, and muscle reeducation. Some types of stimulators have specific features that make them more effective in these treatments than other types of units. Iontophoresis and denervated muscle stimulation are other examples of clinical uses of electrical stimulation, but require units with direct current (DC). These treatments cannot be performed with traditional TENS units.

Edema Reduction

It has been proposed that electrical stimulation can be used for edema reduction (56,90). Most of the research involves the use of the high voltage stimulator, although some of the principles of edema reduction by electrical stimulation, such as muscle pumping, can be achieved with other types of stimulators as well. High voltage stimulation has been shown to significantly reduce edema (56,90).

However, conflicting results with other types of stimulators and parameters can be found in the literature (27,94). Cosgrove et al. found no significant difference in edema reduction when either monophasic or biphasic current was used at a submotor amplitude (27).

The high voltage units are monophasic, which means that each electrode has its specific polarity. Although there is minimal physiochemical response with high voltage units because of the very short phase duration, there is a possibility for an electrophoretic effect (98). Cathodal treatment (negative electrode) delivered in an immersion technique at 120 pps with an intensity of 10% less than required to elicit a minimal muscle contraction have been recommended for edema reduction (91). The treatment should be at least 30 minutes in duration and should be repeated several times a day (131). Although some studies have shown a decrease in edema, others have found that the effect of high voltage stimulation on edema has been minimal and was usually equated with some of the subsensory effects of electrical stimulation. Clinical research is difficult to perform because there are so many variables that are impossible to control and may contribute to edema resorption. For example, injuries may result in varying degrees of bleeding and exudate even when the force applied is the same. Activity, immobilization, and elevation also affect edema and vary even with laboratory animals. Additionally, nutrition and hydration can be confounding variables that make the subtle effects of electric stimulation difficult to measure, especially when there are so many different parameters available.

As the acute injury begins to resolve and active motion is well tolerated, electric stimulation can be used to encourage edema resorption by augmenting the muscle-pumping effect. The exudate with its large particles can only be resorbed through the lymphatic system, which is a passive mechanism (99). Active muscle contractions create pressure differentials which encourage venous return and lymphatic flow (135). Electrical stimulation can be applied to either produce a twitching response or alternating contractions to propagate the fluid movement. The effectiveness of this technique is similar to the results seen with active range of motion, but the pain modification associated with TENS can make the treatment more comfortable and therefore, more effective.

When treating edema, the athlete should have the extremity elevated with the electrodes applied to the surface of the muscle. Motor points are ideal sites for stimulation. The phase duration should be adequate to produce a contraction; usually over 150 seconds. For a twitch response, the frequency should be two to four pulses per second, for a sustained contraction, the frequency should be tetanus, which is 30 to 50 pulses per second. The amplitude should be high enough to give a comfortable contraction of the muscles. When using the sustained contraction, the antagonistic muscle group can be stimulated reciprocally, which causes the extremity to move through a range of motion. A duty cycle of 1:3 gives the muscles adequate rest for the purposes of edema reduction and further enhances the muscle pumping effect (2). Generally, a 20- to 30-minute treatment is given and can be repeated several times a day.

Muscle Spasm Reduction

Muscle spasms are a common and painful consequence of an injury. Muscle spasms in the paraspinal often cause more disability and pain than the initial sprain, strain, or bruise. The muscles go into spasm in an attempt to splint or self-immobilize the area to prevent further injury. However, a vicious cycle develops when the sustained contractions impede blood flow to the muscle and metabolites accumulate, causing more pain due to ischemia and chemical agitation of free nerve endings. Therefore, it is advantageous to minimize spasm so that controlled activity and rehabilitation can begin (67).

Many of the protocols for muscle spasm reduction are identical to those for pain modulation with the pretense that if pain is diminished, spasm will be decreased as well and the cycle will be broken (115,116). Another theory is to attempt to fatigue the muscle, which would cause subsequent relaxation. Since electrically produced muscle contraction will cause a synchronous contraction of all stimulated motor units, the motor units may relax when the stimulation is off (143). A duty cycle is imposed to allow reciprocal periods of contraction and relaxation. There are numerous suggested techniques such as 10 seconds on and 10 seconds off, but there is little research to substantiate an ideal parameter set-up. Continuous muscle twitches as in the motor pain modulation theory also may cause relaxation of the muscle because this technique also synchronizes muscle contractions in addition to evoking the descending tract pain modulation.

General parameters utilized would be a phase duration adequate to produce muscle contraction, usually over 150 seconds. The frequency should be high enough to produce tetany, which is 30 to 50 pulses per second, although higher frequencies can also be used (52). The amplitude should be high enough to achieve a comfortable contraction. When utilizing a pain modulation theory, the suggested parameters for the desired technique should be used (Table 6.7).

Muscle Reeducation

Neuromuscular stimulators (NMES) in sports medicine are primarily used to improve contractility and flexibility or to reduce atrophy in the injured area while healing is taking place (38,95,107,120,122,125). These units are directed toward stimulating muscles with an intact nervous system and act to reeducate the muscles after trauma. If peripheral nerve damage has occurred, the muscle membrane has to be stimulated directly (EMS) to achieve a contraction; therefore, most neuromuscular stimulators cannot be used for this purpose.

Following an injury, there is an inhibition of the muscles surrounding the injured site (24,107). The athlete often has difficulty generating a significant and consistent contraction of these muscles. An electrically induced contraction can help teach the athlete how to overcome the

TABLE 6.7. *Modality options for muscle spasm reduction*

- Pain modification parameters (sensory, motor, noxious)
- Electrical stimulation to fatigue muscles (strong motor with minimal rest)
- Electrical stimulation to coordinate contraction so that relaxation may occur (strong motor with duty cycle to allow relaxation of muscles)

inhibition so that atrophy is minimized and function can return earlier. The electrically produced contraction gives the athlete proprioceptive feedback so that he or she can learn how to contract the muscle without the stimulation. Neuromuscular stimulation improves the magnitude of the contraction especially when a voluntary contraction is superimposed with the exogenous contraction (32,34,95). This improves the force generation of the muscle, especially in the early phases of rehabilitation.

Some researchers suggest that neuromuscular stimulation can improve strength (79,115,133). In these cases, it is necessary to electrically contract the muscle at a higher intensity than is possible volitionally. For example, if the athlete can lift 20 pounds with his biceps, he would need to lift 25 pounds with the electrical stimulation to achieve greater strength gains than with lifting the weight under his own power alone (31). This amplitude of electrical stimulation is often uncomfortable and usually intolerable. Manufacturers of electrical stimulation devices have utilized numerous waveforms and classes of currents to produce more comfortable stimulation (122,137). Most researchers advise combining a voluntary contraction superimposed with the electrically induced contraction to achieve the strongest contraction (106).

Many of the current parameters for muscle stimulation are similar to those used for pain management and these units can often be used interchangeably.

Constant stimulation of the TENS units, however, causes muscular fatigue (79). To prevent fatigue and maximize force generation, a duty cycle (on-off) mode in the current delivery should be made available. There is much controversy in the literature as to the types of training programs and current parameters needed to optimize the results of a neuromuscular stimulator.

Many types of units claim similar results. Portable units enable the patient to continue treatment independently throughout the day, although the stronger clinical models are usually more effective. The portable units are very useful when the athlete is immobilized. Windows can be cut into a cast over motor points and the electrical stimulation can be applied to unused muscles to reduce atrophy (52).

Neuromuscular stimulators can be used to isolate specific muscles that cannot be isolated and strengthened volitionally. For instance, with patellofemoral problems, the vastus medialis muscle is emphasized during quadriceps stimulation to aid in patella tracking changes (25). Rehabilitation problems such as inhibition can also be overcome in this manner. When the athlete can volitionally exercise the muscle, these units can be used to increase the effectiveness of the contraction by superimposing the electrical contraction.

Several factors make the electrically induced contraction different from the volitional contraction (107):

1. When the muscle is stimulated electrically, all motor units fire in synchrony.

2. There is no inhibitory reaction with the electrically induced contraction. Normally, the Golgi tendon organs (GTO) at the musculotendinous insertion react to a potentially threatening contraction by reflexively relaxing the muscle. There is GTO activity with electric stimulation, but the inhibition or relaxation does not occur. Absence of this protective reflex allows the potential for a stronger contraction, but increases the possibility of injury.

3. Larger nerve fibers are recruited first with electric stimulation, which is the opposite of what the body would preferentially do (117). Larger nerve fibers are associated with fast twitch fibers which fatigue easily because of their demand on glycolytic function. Muscle stores of phosphocreatine require time to be regenerated following a contraction (79). This dictates the rest time that is necessary with neuromuscular stimulation compared to voluntary exercise.

4. The frequency of the nerve fiber firing is also affected by electric stimulation. Muscle tetany normally occurs when a nerve fires at a frequency between 30 and 50 pulses per second. Electric stimulators often operate at higher frequencies than those needed to achieve tetany, which causes fatigue more rapidly.

These factors provide the benefits of neuromuscular stimulation, but should be considered in application, especially with more powerful machines. Electric stimulation superimposed with a volitional contraction can create a very strong contraction. The uninhibited contraction can cause joint jamming to occur. This problem arises when the knee, for example, attempts to prevent hyperextension because of the strong quadriceps stimulation. Joint jamming can be prevented by blocking terminal extension mechanically so that pressure is removed from the joint.

The "Russian" stimulator is one of the more popular classifications of neuromuscular stimulators available. These units were modeled after the Russian design that was purported to result in significant strength gains in world-class athletes. Studies performed in the United States using this type of unit have found strength gains in a normal population, but its efficacy is no greater than that of volitional exercise (34,95). Treatment of atrophied muscles has resulted in 10% to 20% gains in strength, but these figures are consistent with the results of other electric stimulators that cause vigorous contractions (34).

The classic Russian parameters utilize a medium frequency generator with a sinusoidal waveform with a frequency of 2,500 Hz. The current is internally modulated into bursts of 10 msec on and 10 msec off. This modulation results in 50 bursts per second, which is consistent with a strong tetanic contraction. The contemporary term for Russian stimulation is "time modulated AC." The medium frequency potentially allows a deeper penetration of the stimulation and utilizes Wedenski's inhibition or an action potential failure at the cutaneous level to achieve

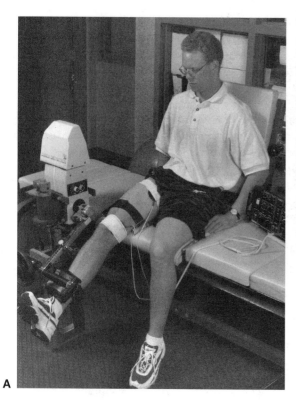

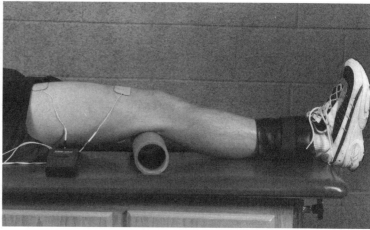

FIG. 6.13. Neuromuscular stimulation to the quadriceps in an isokinetic unit that blocks the range of motion **(A)**, and with a portable neuromuscular electric stimulator (NMES) unit **(B)**.

a more comfortable stimulation. These units have a relatively high average current compared to most TENS models. The high average current is effective for stimulation of large muscle groups, but can be potentially dangerous when applied over the thorax.

Classically, Russian stimulation applies the stimulation for 15 seconds and has a 50-second rest phase between contractions. The on-time allows for a ramping of the amplitude and reaches the maximal set intensity in 3 to 5 seconds. The ramping prevents startling the athlete with a sudden strong current, and allows 10 seconds for the strong contraction. These parameters were found to optimize the recovery time between contractions and allow consistently strong contractions for the treatment (32). Because of the intensity and fatigue, only 10 to 15 contractions are suggested per session.

TABLE 6.8. *Stimulation protocol for the quadriceps muscle that may be used after a knee injury or surgical procedure*

1. The treatment protocol is explained to the athlete who is encouraged to increase the current amplitude according to his or her tolerance. The contraction should be as strong as possible and the athlete is encouraged to superimpose a volitional contraction in conjunction with the stimulation.
2. One electrode is placed over the femoral nerve in the femoral triangle and the other electrode is placed over the distal quadriceps proximal to the patella. The distal electrode can be placed over the motor point of the vastus medialis obliquus if patella tracking is a concern. The athlete should be positioned so that there is resistance or blocking of terminal extension to prevent joint jamming and damage to articular structures.
3. Treatment parameters are adjusted and vary according to the type of unit used:
   - Frequency: preset with Russian parameters, otherwise 30–50 Hz for tetany.
   - Phase duration: preset with Russian parameters, otherwise 200–300 μsec (which is high) to achieve a strong contraction.
   - Duty cycle: 15 seconds on/50 seconds off in the early phases of treatment, gradually increase to a 1:3 ratio to accommodate the training effects.
   - Ramp time: generally 3–5 seconds. When ramping up and down, add more time on so that there is still at least 10 seconds at the maximal amplitude.
   - Amplitude: adjusted and increased to a strong tolerable contraction. Make sure there is no adjustment in amplitude when the unit is in the "off" phase.
4. The treatment durations vary according to the type of neuromuscular stimulator being used. The stronger clinical models may require only 10–15 contractions daily. The home portable units should be used up to three times a day for up to an hour because the intensity of the contraction is not as high.

From refs. 55 and 112.

Various protocols are purported to be the most effective in strengthening isolated muscles. The parameter considerations, as with most TENS units, include amplitude, phase duration, pulse frequency, and duty cycle. One of the most important considerations with neuromuscular stimulation is the rest phase. These units create a tetanic contraction that is often combined with a volitional contraction. If there is not an adequate rest phase, the muscle fatigues too quickly for strengthening to occur. On-off ratios should allow a rest phase of three to five times the on-time to prevent fatigue, especially as the training program begins. As the stimulation program progresses, the duty cycle can change from a 1:5 to a 1:3 or 1:1 on-off cycle. Figure 6.13 illustrates the neuromuscular technique for the quadriceps and Table 6.8 lists the stimulation protocol.

Iontophoresis

A galvanic current or direct current (DC) is monophasic and flows for an indefinite duration, usually in excess of 1 second (4). There are significant polarity and physiochemical responses from DC. If enough average current is supplied, a significant electrophoretic response can occur. Under the positive electrode, an acidic reaction occurs, along with a tissue-hardening effect and diminished nerve-tissue irritability. At the negative electrode there is an alkaline reaction, a tissue-softening effect and an increase in nerve-tissue irritability. In addition to these local polarity effects, there is a driving effect of ions under the electrodes.

A DC or galvanic current is required for iontophoresis, which is the driving of ions using electricity. Iontophoresis is a noninvasive procedure in which a medication can be administered into a local region using an electric current with a high average current. The electrophoretic principle that like charges repel and unlike charges attract is used with iontophoresis. The electrolytes of similar charge are repelled from the source by applying an electrical current of the same polarity as the medication. In this manner, the ions of certain pharmacologic agents can be driven into the body (73). Although iontophoresis has been used for many years, problems such as poor electrodes, determining drug dosage, unsafe electrical instrumentation, and inconvenience have made its reliability questionable. There are some commercial units that specifically are manufactured for iontophoresis, which have made the treatment more consistent and easier.

Commercial iontophoresis units are compact galvanic generators. The clinician is able to administer the recommended medications into specialized electrodes that are provided by the manufacturer. A small dispersive electrode is also included. The electrodes containing the medications minimize error and poor technique, making the procedure more consistent. Developments have been made in buffering certain medications to prevent polarity changes with the application of current. Guidelines are also available to provide the clinician with a better indication of the dosage by manipulating the time and amplitude of current when using the same volume and solution of medication.

Animal studies have found that iontophoresis is an effective means of delivering the chemicals into the subcutaneous tissues (73). Compared to injection, the advantages of using iontophoresis are that it is a noninvasive means of administering medication so there is less chance of infection. A carrier fluid is not needed with the medication so there is less tissue tension and pain from the volume expansion when iontophoresis is used.

Caution should be used with iontophoresis because of the high average current necessary for the treatment. Iontophoresis should not be done over abraded skin, anaesthetic areas, near metal implants, or when there is sensitivity to medications. Prescriptions should be obtained for the medications used.

Conditions that are treated with iontophoresis include epicondylitis, tendinitis, bursitis, fasciitis, arthritis, and myofascial trigger points. Hypertrophic scars and heterotopic ossifications can be treated with iontophoresis as well. Each condition has its recommended medication, polarity, and dosage guidelines for both concentration of medication and electrical stimulation. Figure 6.14 illustrates the technique for iontophoresis and Table 6.9 lists the application guidelines.

When a commercial iontophoresis unit is not available, the treatment application is similar, but the electrodes are prepared differently. The dispersive electrode should be twice the size of the active electrode. The electrode pads should be clean since any ions present on their surface can affect the treatment. The active electrode should be saturated with the solution. Solution strength is generally 1% or less since higher concentrations have been found to be less efficacious (29). A submersion technique can be used in which the extremity is placed in a bath of medicinal solution. The desired polarity should be checked before the application of current.

The electric parameters that vary are the current amplitude and length of treatment. The amplitude is generally suggested to be at least 0.5 to 1 mAmp per square centimeter of electrode surface area. This amplitude may need to be adjusted gradually and patient comfort should always be the guideline. Treatments usually last 20 to 30 minutes depending on the amplitude achieved during treatment. When terminating the treatment, slowly reduce the amplitude. The remaining solution should be rinsed off and the skin inspected. An erythematic patch may be present under the electrodes, but this is normal and should resolve (73). Iontophoresis can be administered up to three times per week.

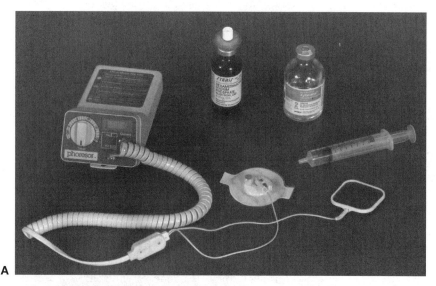

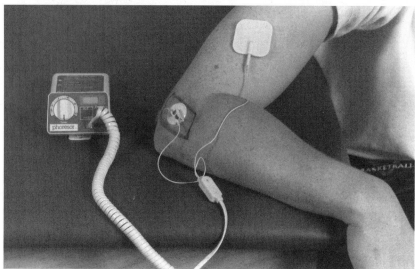

FIG. 6.14. A: Phoresor with injectable bladder electrodes to hold mediation. **B:** Application of dexamethasone iontophoresis.

Stimulation of Denervated Muscles

There are few applications for the stimulation of denervated muscles in the athletic population. Occasionally, peripheral nerve damage results and the atrophic re-

TABLE 6.9. *Iontophoresis application guidelines*

1. The procedure is explained to the athlete.
2. Treatment surface is cleaned.
3. The medications are placed in the active electrode which is placed over the treatment site.
4. The dispersive electrode is applied, usually proximally.
5. The unit is turned on (phase duration and frequency are not applicable because of the DC waveform).
6. Always using patient comfort as a guideline, the current is increased 1 mAmp per minute up to 4–5 mAmp.
7. Following treatment, the skin is inspected and the electrodes are disposed of.

From refs. 113, 114, and 115.

sponses of the muscles may be reduced with direct current stimulation. A DC current is the only stimulator available that has a phase duration long enough to overcome the capacitance of the muscle membrane directly to allow depolarization. Muscle membrane depolarization usually requires a phase duration of at least 300 milliseconds.

Stimulation of denervated muscles is controversial since it does not promote the regeneration of nerve tissue. Some references have indicated that stimulation inhibits the regrowth of peripheral nerve fibers (124). The goal of treatment is to maintain the actin and myosin structure of the muscle tissue and to prevent fibrotic changes within the muscle. Passive range of motion should also be done to prevent restrictions in joints.

The application of denervated muscle stimulation requires the use of a point stimulator and dispersive electrode. The point stimulator allows concentration of the current near motor point locations and reduces the physiochemical responses around the area. The amplitude should evoke a muscle twitch and should be adjusted at each motor point treated. A denervated muscle is not able to sustain a contraction because this would require successive pulses, which is impossible with the galvanic waveform because the phase duration is so long. The clinician should allow 2 to 5 seconds of rest between contractions to allow the membrane to stabilize. The number of contractions or twitches at each motor point is limited by fatigue. If the quality of contraction diminishes, the treatment should be stopped. Generally each point is stimulated eight to ten times. Because of the controversy associated with the effectiveness of denervated muscle stimulation, treatments should not exceed three times per week.

SPECIFIC CATEGORIES OF STIMULATORS

High Voltage Stimulators

High voltage stimulators are classified by having two distinct specifications: they must be able to transmit a voltage in excess of 100 V and they must use a twin-peaked monophasic current. The 100 V delineation is an arbitrarily set value that demarcates high and low voltage units (3). The major claims of this type of unit are that the high voltage allows deeper penetration of the energy and that the short phase duration of the twin peaks does not allow the capacitance of smaller sensory fibers (A delta or C fibers) to be stimulated, resulting in greater comfort (2). Since the stimulator is monophasic, there is a polarity difference in the electrodes, allowing the clinician to choose a positive or negative electrode for the treatment area. However, since the phase duration is so short, there are minimal physiochemical changes under the electrodes. High voltage units are used clinically for pain control, edema reduction, tissue healing, and muscle spasm reduction (91). Muscle reeducation can be done with high voltage units if the stimulator allows a rest cycle.

The voltage amplitude available with most high voltage machines ranges from 0 to 500 V (3). The amplitude, as with most electrical stimulators, is determined by patient comfort and to meet the desired objective of the treatment (sensory or motor response). One of the features of the high voltage machine is that although the voltage is high, there is a low average current. It is therefore a very safe modality. The twin-peaked waveform allows the high peak, but low average current. The decay of the pulse occurs almost immediately, and the second pulse begins before the first peak reaches the isoelectric line. The duration of both peaks together varies with each manufacturer, but is generally between 50 and 120 microseconds. The phase duration is not adjustable by the clinician, which ensures the safety of the unit.

Many claims have been made as to the relevance of the polarity control of high voltage units, although the low average current minimizes any ion flux or physiochemical response. However, during healing, the wound emits a charge potential depending on the stage of healing (23). This potential is believed to be reinforced by applying the polarity of a like charge, either positive or negative from the stimulator. This process promotes a stronger physiologic response, which may enhance healing and edema reduction. However, the electrophoretic effect with this type of unit is negligible, especially with short treatment durations. The net ion flux across the membrane is minimal and is self-limiting (98). The short phase durations cause only a minor shift in ion migration, and with the interpulse interval the membrane can neutralize any change in the normal ion status. Iontophoresis cannot be performed with this unit because no net ion flux occurs (73). Several studies have addressed the possibility of edema reduction with high voltage with inconclusive results (27,91,94,131).

The frequency range offered by most high voltage units is from 2 to 120 pulses per second. The frequency adjustment allows the incorporation of either sensory or motor TENS principles when pain tolerance is the goal. The variation in frequencies also allows the clinician to optimize parameters for either muscle pumping or muscle reeducation.

Electrode placement for high voltage often utilizes the monopolar technique (2) (Fig. 6.15). This procedure uses one or more active electrodes and a larger dispersive electrode. The active electrodes are smaller in size and concentrate the current and therefore the level of stimulation. As the name implies, the dispersive electrode spreads the same amount of current over a larger surface area, causing a minimum, if any, sensory perception under the dispersive electrode. The active electrodes are placed over the treatment site, and the dispersive electrode is placed on a site distant to the treatment area. Since the distance between electrodes is increased with the monopolar method, there is potentially a deeper penetration of the current.

The bipolar technique, which uses equal-sized electrodes over the same treatment area, can also be used with high voltage. The larger electrode is replaced by a smaller one, although the cord must be plugged into the dispersive socket in the unit. Otherwise the circuit is not complete.

A key feature of the high voltage unit is its ability to be used with appendage submersion treatments. Submersion is a preferred method of treatment for acute ankle injuries because it provides circumferential cooling and sensory TENS for irregular surfaces. Even though the extremity is in a dependent position, the submersion method allows an active range of motion during the treatment. The active electrodes are placed in the cold water bath (55° to 65° F), and a 20- to 30-minute treatment is applied. The treatment is followed by other modalities

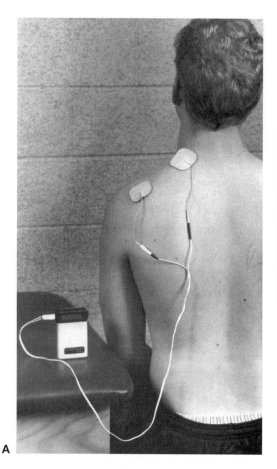

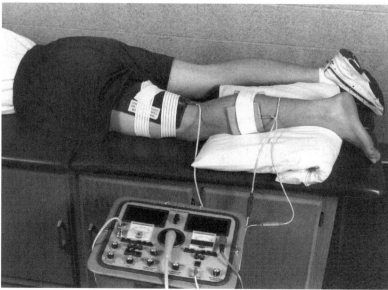

FIG. 6.15. Monopolar setup vs. bipolar electrode placement. **A:** *Monopolar technique:* The utilization of two (or more) differently sized electrodes with a dispersive pad placed distant to the treatment site. This is commonly used with high voltage. **B:** *Bipolar technique:* Two equal sized electrodes are used on the same treatment surface. Can be used with monophasic or biphasic waveforms. With a monophasic current, one lead will be positive whereas the other is negative. These may be designated as red and black respectively.

A

and exercise, as indicated for the condition. The treatment can be repeated several times throughout the day (91).

Interferential

Interferential stimulation is another form of TENS used for pain relief, increased circulation, and for muscle stimulation (33) (Fig. 6.16). This unit simultaneously applies two medium-frequency currents to allow deeper penetration of the stimulation. Higher-frequency currents overcome some of the skin impedance encountered by low-frequency currents. However, unless the currents are modulated, there is minimal or no response in the tissues (33). Low-frequency currents within the range of 1 to 100 Hz have a physiologic response but create more surface resistance. In theory, to overcome some of the resistance, yet still provide a stimulation that allows sensory or motor response, two different medium-frequency (within the range of 1,000 to 10,000 Hz) sinusoidal wave currents are applied. Their waveforms are superimposed on each other, which causes interference. Interference creates points of augmentation and attenuation of the phases where peaks and valleys are added together. The interference results in the modulation of a beat mode with a

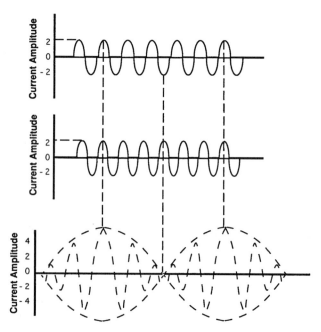

FIG. 6.16. Interferential current.

frequency that ranges from 1 to 100 beats per second, which is well within the conventional low-frequency range.

The carrier frequencies of an interferential unit typically range from 4,000 to 5,000 Hz, which allows a stronger perception at a lower amplitude and deeper stimulation. The medium-frequency carrier currents reduce skin impedance but also shorten the phase duration because they are sinusoidal waves, allowing more comfort. The medium frequency-currents used with interferential units can cause a cutaneous nerve inhibition as with the action-potential block mode of TENS (60).

The frequency of the beats can vary by changing one of the two carrier frequencies. The beat frequency, not the carrier frequencies, affects the tissues, and changes in this parameter alter the stimulation responses. The number of muscle twitches is greater as the beat frequency increases, until a tetanic contraction is attained. Some units have a feature that constantly changes the frequency of one of the carrier currents while the other remains constant. This mode is a sweep frequency that causes a rhythmic change throughout a range of frequencies. The purpose of the rhythmic mode is to reduce accommodation. Because the stimulation continuously changes, the body cannot adapt to it. The sweep frequency provides a more effective stimulation in this manner.

Some models include a rotating vector system that periodically changes the orientation of the electrical field 45 degrees to further reduce accommodation. The efficacy of this modification has not been substantiated.

The beat frequency is selected according to the condition to be treated. A frequency of 60 to 100 beats per second (bps) is used for sensory TENS, 50 to 60 bps for muscle contraction, and 2 to 4 bps for motor TENS.

Four electrodes should be used for an interferential treatment, two for each carrier current. The electrodes of each current are placed diagonally over the treatment site. The area to be treated should be surrounded by the electrodes if it is an extremity or joint. The electrodes should be placed all on one surface if the treatment area is large, such as the low back. Some interferential units also offer suction electrodes in which a mild vacuum is created under the electrode to allow it to stick to the body part. The electrodes produce a convenient method of application because they do not have to be strapped down, and they stay in place throughout the treatment.

The passage of current through the tissues does not occur linearly between the electrodes but creates an electric field. This field is purported to be shaped in a cloverleaf pattern situated three-dimensionally between the electrodes. If the conductivity of the tissues were uniform, this perfectly formed electric field would occur with the maximal current concentration in the central region between the electrodes. However, differences in the tissue impedance affect the location of the electric field and the degree of superposition of currents. Therefore, the concentration of current is not always centralized. To maximize the probability of properly placed electrodes and subsequent electric fields, adjust the electrodes so that maximal intensity is perceived in the painful region.

Interferential stimulation can be used with other modalities. Although it is sometimes difficult with the suction electrodes, ice or heat can be used in conjunction with the stimulation. Treatment durations are dictated by the goal of treatment: pain relief, muscle reeducation, muscle spasm reduction. Interferential units have been shown to reduce pain and edema posttraumatically (65).

Contraindications to using interferential stimulators are the same for any other form of TENS, but caution should be taken when using interferential machines in the proximity of diathermy units. Amplitude surges have been documented when there is simultaneous use of these types of machines in the same treatment area.

Ultrasound

Ultrasound is the application of high-frequency sound waves beyond human audible perception. Although ultrasound is used diagnostically for various medical purposes, it has become an important therapeutic modality in physical medicine. The high-frequency sound waves emitted from early underwater sonar were found to have an effect on the biologic tissues of marine life. The uses of ultrasound then began to be researched extensively in Europe (52). Therapeutic application of ultrasound on soft tissues began in the United States in the 1950s and is now purportedly the most effective deep-heating modality in the physical therapy realm (21,81).

Ultrasound is very effective in providing heat to soft tissues because it operates with a minimal increase in superficial temperature. The mechanical energy causes ultrasound to also have nonthermal effects, which have been explored through research on tissue healing (43,44). The clinical uses of ultrasound are numerous in a sports medicine environment. Thermal effects can increase tissue extensibility, which can increase range of motion when combined with a stretch or be used to treat muscle spasm. Nonthermal effects can relieve pain, affect inflammation, and may affect collagen production and alignment.

Frequency

Unlike most other modalities that operate in the electromagnetic spectrum, ultrasound uses mechanical energy that is part of the acoustic spectrum. The frequency of ultrasound is above the audible ranges for humans, which is normally 15 Hz to 20,000 Hz. Therapeutic ultrasound operates at the frequencies of approximately one megahertz (1 MHz : mega = million) or up to 3 MHz. State of the art synthetic crystals can be manufactured to provide

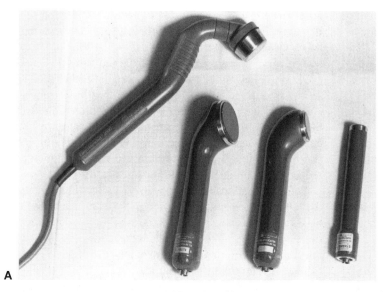

A

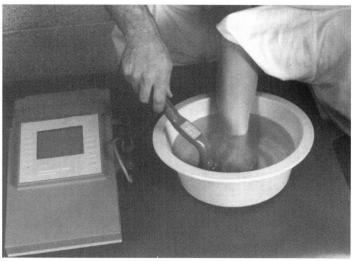

FIG. 6.17. Choosing ultrasound transducer size. **A:** Examples of transducer sizes. **B:** Transducer size should be approximately two to three times the size of the treatment area. Some units have interchangeable sound heads to allow the clinician more versatility. **C:** If surface contact cannot be maintained during the treatment, indirect or underwater ultrasound should be performed. The body part should be submerged in skin temperature, degassed water, and the sound head should be kept about 1 inch away from the body part. The intensity of the ultrasound should be increased by 0.5 W/cm² and the transducer should be kept moving throughout the treatment.

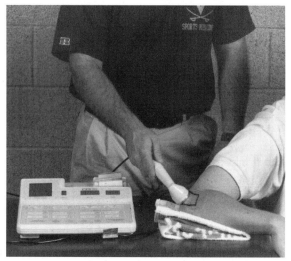

B

C

almost any resonating frequency, but either 1 or 3 MHz is most often used because there is little research to substantiate the effectiveness of other frequencies in physical medicine. Having two available frequencies gives the clinician the option of choosing the frequency that is best suited for the tissue to be treated.

There is an inverse relationship between the frequency of ultrasound and the depth of penetration into the soft tissue. A 1-MHz ultrasound will dissipate 50% of its energy at a depth of 5 cm into soft tissue, while a 3-MHz unit will dissipate 50% of its energy at 1 cm depth (42). There are some modifications in the depth of penetration with either frequency because tissues are not homogeneous. Tissues with a high protein content like muscle and nerve, for example, absorb more ultrasound energy, resulting in less penetration. The depth of penetration is determined by frequency, not by intensity of the ultrasound. The half-value thickness is used to describe the depth of penetration in which one half of the intensity has been absorbed (21,42). Generally, superficial tissues

such as the hand or patellar tendon are treated with 3-MHz ultrasound, and deeper structures, such as the quadriceps muscle, are treated with 1 MHz. Since ultrasound cannot penetrate through bone, there is less of a chance of periosteal irritation with 3-Mz ultrasound. A general rule of thumb is that if the target tissue is over 1 inch deep, the 1-MHz frequency should be used. If the target tissue is more superficial than 1 inch, 3 MHz should be used.

Equipment

The components of an ultrasound unit consist of an electrical generator, an oscillating circuit with a duty cycle selector, a coaxial cable, and the sound head or transducer (52). The unit contains a timer that regulates the duration of the treatment and a power meter to provide information about the total watts (power) and the watts per square centimeter (intensity) that the unit is generating.

Ultrasound is produced by the machine through the conversion of electrical energy to sound energy, which occurs by the reverse piezoelectric effect (146). The piezoelectric effect, as observed by the Curies in the late 1800s, is the production of an electrical charge with deformation of a crystal. A reverse piezoelectric effect is the opposite—the production of mechanical deformations of a crystal by the introduction of an electrical current. The compression and expansion of the crystal result in a vibrational activity that ultimately creates the ultrasound. Each crystal has an inherent resonating frequency depending on its composition, diameter, and width. This resonating frequency occurs when the crystal's deformation and subsequent vibration is at a maximum for a given amount and rate of energy applied. Some crystals are capable of resonating at frequencies of both 1 and 3 MHz, eliminating the need to change transducers when changing frequencies (21). These units are more expensive but are more convenient and practical.

Two factors that must be considered when referencing the transducer are the effective radiating area (ERA) and the beam nonuniformity ratio (BNR). These address the output characteristics of the crystals and can affect treatment parameters.

The ERA describes the surface area of the crystal that is emitting significant mechanical energy and is always smaller than the actual size of the crystal. The ERA is calculated by scanning the sound head 5 mm away from the radiating surface and measuring the areas that emit at least 5% of the maximal power output anywhere over the surface of the transducer. Any area that produces this minimal amount of energy is considered in the ERA (21,52). Transducers whose ERAs are close to the actual size of the transducer are generally better quality crystals and provide a more consistent treatment.

The clinician should be aware of the ERA when determining the dosage of ultrasound treatment. Intensity is determined by taking the total watts delivered divided by the ERA and is measured in watts per square centimeters.

Total Power (watts)

$$\text{Intensity} = \text{ERA (cm}^2) = \text{watts/cm}^2 \ (I = W/\text{ERA})$$

The ERA also determines the size of the area that can effectively be treated. When treating large surface areas, the energy is dispersed over a broad area, which causes a decreased response. It is generally suggested to treat each area that is no larger than two to three times the size of the transducer for 5 minutes. Larger areas can be divided into treatment fields , and each one treated for the appropriate duration (19,21). This method does not provide an effective thermal treatment for larger areas, such as the paraspinal, because one subfield may cool before exercise is initiated. Diathermy may be the modal-

---

TABLE 6.10. *Duty cycles for ultrasound*

Calculation of duty cycle is the percentage of time that the ultrasound is "on" compared to the total time. For example, if the ultrasound is on for 2 milliseconds and off for 8 milliseconds, the duty cycle is:

$$\frac{2 \text{ msec}}{2 \text{ msec} + 8 \text{ msec}} = 20\%$$

The following is a generalization of ultrasound duty cycles used clinically:
- 20%—wound healing
- 50%—nonthermal effects
- 100%—thermal effects

---

ity of choice for providing deep heat to larger surface areas.

Beam nonuniformity ratio (BNR) is another measure of the consistency and quality of the crystal. Ultrasound energy is not consistent as it is emitted from the sound head. The meter displays the average intensity delivered (watts/cm^2), but there may be regions that are delivering much higher intensities in the beam (21,146). The BNR is the ratio of the highest intensity found in the ultrasound beam compared to the average intensity indicated on the power meter. A BNR of 6:1 indicates that intensities of 6.0 W/cm^2 can be found in the near-field region when the intensity is set at 1.0 W/cm^2. The lower the BNR, the better, although a BNR of 6:1 is generally considered to be acceptable. The higher the BNR, the greater the chance for hot spots to be encountered and the sound head must be kept moving at a faster pace to prevent the high intensity location to be concentrated on one area.

Modes of Transmission

Ultrasound can be delivered in a continuous or a pulsed mode. Continuous ultrasound has an uninterrupted transmission of sound vibrations. This mode is generally associated with the thermal responses, although nonthermal responses occur as well. With pulsed ultrasound, however, the sound intensity is interrupted at specific intervals. When the energy is interrupted, some of the energy is dissipated, creating less of a thermal effect (146). The interruptions in the sound that create the pulsed mode of ultrasound are specified by a designated duty cycle. The duty cycle is the ratio of the amount of time the energy is on over a designated period of time (Table 6.10).

The typical duty cycles are 20% and 50%. Because the energy is delivered only a portion of the time, pulsed ultrasound provides a lower average intensity over a specified time, causing negligible thermal responses (44). For example, a 50% duty cycle with an intensity of 1.5 W/cm^2 would deliver only 0.75W/cm^2 (1.5 × 50%) or half of the temporal average intensity that continuous ultrasound at the same intensity would provide. The thermal responses that may occur are also dissipated during the off time of the pulsed mode.

Application

The patient receiving ultrasound treatment should be positioned for comfort with the target area exposed. The duration of treatment is generally 5 minutes for an area two to three times the ERA (19). Covering too large an area at one time or moving the sound head too fast minimizes the amount of energy exposed per unit area, causing decreased effects. Speed of the sound head is recommended to be 2 to 4 cm per second, depending on the BNR. Units with high BNRs should be moved faster to prevent the concentration of the high intensity in one specific area. Ultrasound can be applied using linear or circular motions of the sound head, with each stroke overlapping the previous one.

A conducting medium is required to allow adequate transmission of the sound waves to the treatment area (15). Acoustical energy travels poorly through gases, and the therapeutic value of the energy would otherwise be lost to the environment during the application of ultrasound. Even with direct contact to the skin surface, air present in the pores of the skin results in poor transmission and less absorption in the soft tissues. Therefore a liberal amount of a conducting agent should be applied to the treatment area. In addition, this inability of sound waves to be transmitted through air makes it essential that contact be maintained throughout the treatment so that the sound head does not become damaged. The sound waves can be reflected back onto the crystal and since there is no mechanism to dissipate the energy, the crystal can be damaged.

Commercial gels, lotions, mineral oil, and water can be used as conductive media with similar transmission qualities. However, when using combined electrical stimulation and ultrasound, mineral oil should not be used since it is not a good conductor of electrical current. Agents that are somewhat viscous such as gels are easy to work with since the coupling media stays at the treatment site and does not drip (18).

When treating irregular surfaces, such as the hands or feet, a submersion technique or indirect ultrasound can be used to maintain contact throughout the treatment. Ideally, degassed water is used for this technique as ultrasound travels poorly through gases. Water can be degassed by allowing tap water to sit for several hours before use. The clinician should wipe away bubbles that appear on the sound head or on the patient. Using ultrasound in a whirlpool just after agitation is not advised because of the aeration that has occurred. Cool water can negate the thermal effects with ultrasound, even with relatively higher dosages (39).

During the application of indirect ultrasound, the sound head and treatment area are submerged. The administration of ultrasound is the same except that the sound head should be kept 1 to 2 cm away from the surface to be treated. The intensity usually must be increased by 0.5 w/cm^2 to compensate for the absorption of ultrasound by the water and for increased distance from the sound head (41). When using this technique, electrical safety should be considered, making sure all cables to the machine are sealed.

During the treatment of ultrasound, the patient should not experience discomfort or excessive warming of the area. If an increase in surface temperature is sensed or if the conducting medium is becoming heated, one should question the effectiveness of the sound penetration. This situation may indicate that the energy is being absorbed at the surface of the skin, leaving less energy to be delivered to the deeper tissues (18). It has been found that the improvement in the quality of conducting media has minimized this concern. The sound head should be inspected for damage or the submersion technique should be considered if increased surface temperatures continue.

Treatment Parameters

As the instrumentation, regulation, and materials of ultrasound become more refined, treatments are becoming more specific. The classic factors to consider when determining the treatment parameters include frequency, duration, intensity, and mode of transmission—pulsed or continuous. One must also consider the type of injury, the stage of healing, the part being treated and the amount of surface area to be treated.

Intensity or strength of the ultrasound energy is referenced as watts per square centimeter (W/cm^2). This is the total power emitted over the crystal's radiating surface. The average output of an ultrasound treatment ranges from 0.5 to 3.0 W/cm^2. Newer units may have lower peak intensity outputs owing to the refinement of the equipment regulations that enhanced the efficiency and accuracy of the units.

The intensity of the ultrasound treatment depends on the desired results, the stage of the injury and the amount of soft tissue covering on the target area. When treating chronic conditions, it is generally desired to create a vigorous heating in the tissues with deep penetration. To achieve these results, higher intensities of ultrasound ranging from 1.5 to 2.0 W/cm^2 should be used. In more acute conditions when thermal effects should be minimized, lower intensities are recommended (0.5 to 1.0 W/cm^2) (44). When treating areas with a minimal soft tissue coverage of bony parts, lower intensities should be used to reduce the possibility of periosteal irritation if a higher frequency unit is not available. As discussed previously, the depth of penetration of energy depends on the frequency of the sound, which is often a preset variable of the ultrasound unit. Lower intensities are required to treat superficial areas because the depth of penetration is a function of the frequency and cannot be altered.

Suggestions for selecting treatment intensities have been made, but there is little to substantiate the consistency and accuracy of the suggested dosages for various tissue types in a clinical situation. One guideline for vigorous heating is to increase the intensity to elicit periosteal irritation (achiness) and then decrease intensity by 10% (80). This method relies on immediate feedback from the patient. However, there are times when periosteal irritation and burns do not elicit achiness and pain until several hours after the treatment. Attempts have been made to clearly define half-value thicknesses which is the depth in certain tissues in which half of the intensity of ultrasound has been absorbed (19). For example, in thick muscles such as the quadriceps, half of the intensity of 1-MHz ultrasound has been absorbed at approximately 3 cm. If the lesion is expected to be deeper, a higher intensity may be required to achieve a therapeutic dosage at the target depth. However, if the lesion is more superficial, a lower intensity may create desired therapeutic effects. Half-value thicknesses attempt to improve clinical decision-making, however, the values have primarily been determined using nonliving tissue, which may not be generalized to a normal biologic or pathologic tissue.

Higher frequencies such as the 3-MHz unit also can affect the ultimate energy delivered to a target area. Since the higher frequency does not penetrate as deeply, there is greater absorption in superficial tissues. Therefore the energy becomes more concentrated in these areas and a lower intensity can create similar thermal or nonthermal effects. Generally the intensity can be lowered by 0.25 to 0.5 W/cm^2 when using 3MHz (42).

Ultrasound should not cause pain, and the clinician should ask the patient about perceptions of discomfort and warmth during treatment. Pain during the application of ultrasound may indicate periosteal irritation in which case treatment parameters should be adjusted or the use of ultrasound discontinued.

Thermal Responses

The thermal responses that occur with ultrasound include increased collagen fiber extensibility, changes in nerve conduction, increased pain thresholds, increased enzymatic activity and changes in contractile tissue (21,52). The degree that the tissues are heated depends on several factors, including the absorptive capacity of the tissues to ultrasound, the dosage (intensity and duration) of ultrasound delivered to a given surface area, and the mode of transmission.

The ultrasound energy can be either absorbed or scattered by the tissues being treated. The better the absorp-

tive capacity of the tissue, the more ultrasound energy can be delivered to the tissues. If scattered, the energy is lost to the surrounding areas and is of minimal benefit. Absorption of ultrasound energy is greatest in tissues with a high collagen content (19). These tissues, namely, muscle, nerve, capsule, and bone are therefore selectively heated. The selective heating of these tissues occurs with a minimum of superficial tissue heating, which is one of the chief advantages ultrasound has over diathermies. Diathermy can be absorbed and therefore can heat superficial tissues such as adipose to dangerous levels before significant penetration occurs.

Ultrasound has excellent penetration through homogeneous tissues such as adipose, causing minimal absorption and subsequent heating in these superficial regions. However, at tissue interfaces, standing or shear waves develop, creating a concentration of energy that generates heat. The standing waves are found to be most significant at the bone-muscle interfaces. This concentrated heating is thought to be the cause of the periosteal pain and burning that can occur with ultrasound treatments. Tissues around these areas are heated by conduction. Therefore, ultrasound should be applied prudently.

Selective heating has been shown to increase collagen extensibility. The most effective method to achieve an increase in extensibility of the tissues is to combine ultrasound with stretching. The heating of the tissues increases the molecular bonding activity, therefore allowing plastic deformation to occur when that body part is placed under a stretch (82). This method can be used to help increase range of motion and flexibility.

Studies of the effects of ultrasound on blood flow have produced various results, largely due to the variations in treatment parameters used by the researchers (112). The thermal effects may not be responsible for the changes in blood flow that some have reported since the subcutaneous tissues in which ultrasound energy is concentrated do not have the same receptors and body-cooling mechanisms that the skin has. Muscle is under metabolic control and prearteriole sphincters dilate in response to the demand on the muscle and the need for more oxygen at these tissues. The potential for change in blood flow supports the moving technique of application of ultrasound versus the stationary technique. Stasis of blood flow, blood flow aggregation, and endothelial damage of blood vessels were found to occur at therapeutic dosages with the stationary technique (112).

The mechanism by which ultrasound decreases pain is uncertain. Ultrasound has been found to increase the pain threshold of peripheral nerve fibers (142). This effect was attributed to the generation of heat that transpires and to a nonthermal mechanism. Results of the effects of ultrasound on nerve conduction velocities are inconclusive (30,50). Some authors have reported that the dosage of the ultrasound treatment ultimately affects the nerve conduction. Dosages of 1 to 2 W/cm^2 caused a decrease in nerve conduction, whereas dosages below 0.5 and above 3.0 W/cm^2 caused an increase in nerve conduction (50). It is generally felt that increased temperature will increase nerve conduction velocity.

Nonthermal Effects

The nonthermal effects of ultrasound may be presented in conjunction with the thermal responses or may be present alone, as with the pulsed mode of ultrasound transmission. These nonthermal responses are cavitation and acoustic microstreaming (50,83). As sound is transmitted through the tissues, it causes regions of molecular compressions and expansion (condensation and rarefaction). The molecular oscillations affect small gas bubbles present in the blood or tissues. This vibrational effect on gas bubbles is cavitation. Cavitation may be stable, creating positive effects by increasing cellular activity or can be harmful (transient) if the gas bubbles become too large and collapse suddenly. The transient form of cavitation can be minimized by the atmospheric pressure and by maintaining contact on the treatment surface with the sound head.

Acoustical microstreaming is an event that produces velocity gradients and subsequent fluid movement along cell membranes. This movement results from the mechanical vibrations caused by the sound waves or from the stable cavitation's vibrating bubbles. Changes in chemical gradients result in ion migration through cell membranes and vessel walls. This stimulates protein synthesis, which is responsible for tissue regeneration. This effect, caused by an increase in fibroblast activity, was found with low-intensity ultrasound (less than 0.5 W/cm^2; pulsed at 20%) and is attributed to acoustic streaming (44).

Therapeutic Effects and Uses of Ultrasound

Ultrasound may be indicated for numerous problems encountered in a sports medicine environment. The therapeutic uses of ultrasound include pain relief, decreasing muscle spasm, promoting tissue healing, increasing range of motion, reducing inflammatory conditions, and phonophoresis. Therefore ultrasound can potentially benefit a multitude of entities.

Methods of pain relief and its effect on muscle spasms have been addressed previously. The treatment of inflamed soft tissues with pulsed ultrasound has not been studied extensively, but empirical findings substantiate its use with this type of problem. Caution should be used, however, when employing continuous ultrasound over an area of inflammation. A latent exacerbation of symptoms has been experienced by athletes even when moderate dosages (1.0 W/cm^2 for 5 minutes) of continuous ultrasound. Using the pulsed mode of ultrasound, with its less

---

TABLE 6.11. *Contraindications of ultrasound*

Ischemic areas—areas of poor circulation should not be treated with ultrasound since the body may be unable to dissipate heat and burning may occur.

Areas of decreased sensation—ultrasound must be administered within pain-free limits to avoid burning of tissues or irritating the periosteum. In anesthetized regions, the patient cannot perceive these potential side effects.

Over the eyes—the danger to eyes includes retinal damage and lens opacities as a result of the selective heating of these tissues.

During pregnancy—temperature elevation in fetuses has caused numerous adverse effects that range from central nervous system to orthopaedic abnormalities. It is not advised to treat females in the low back or abdominal region if there is any chance of pregnancy.

Cancer—because of the threat of metastases if neoplasms are present, ultrasound is contraindicated in these situations. This similar concern is present with infections because ultrasound may cause them to spread.

Active infections

Over fracture sites—application of continuous ultrasound over healing fractures is not advised because a demineralization process can occur, affecting the callous formation. Also a disrupted periosteum can easily be agitated with ultrasound, causing pain. Ultrasound can therefore be an effective tool when attempting to diagnose stress fractures. Low-intensity ultrasound with a low duty cycle is being investigated for osteogenesis.

Caution over the spinal cord—transient cavitation, which may damage cells, is especially a concern with the central nervous system tissues because of the inability to regenerate. Caution should be exercised when sonating over the spinal cord, especially after laminectomies. It is generally believed, however, that with the bony protection the spinal cord is afforded, minimal sound reaches the neural tissues.

Over open epiphyses—caution should be exercised when sonating in regions of open epiphyses. Selective heating of the cells at the bone interface can cause abnormal growth patterns. Although therapeutic dosages are believed to be safe, adverse effects can occur.

Over cervical and stellate ganglia

Around pacemakers—sonating directly over or around a pacemaker is contraindicated because of the chance of electrical interference. With a pacemaker, ultrasound to other parts of the body is not a problem as it would be with the diathermies. Ultrasound directly over the heart has found EKG changes in canine studies and should also be avoided.

Metallic implants, polyethylene, and methyl methacrylate associated with joint prostheses have not produced adverse reactions to ultrasound treatments and are not contraindicated.

From refs. 146 and 147.

thermal effect, may be more advantageous even when superficial heat is well tolerated by the patient. Rather than an antiinflammatory effect, ultrasound is felt to be "proinflammatory." The inflammatory process is accelerated, especially with the degranulation of mast cells. This allows a more rapid progression to healing (44).

When treating scar tissue, dosages that elicit a thermal response are most effective in increasing range of motion. As discussed previously, flexibility exercises should be used to optimize the effects of ultrasound on connective tissue extensibility and range of motion.

The effect of ultrasound on mineral deposition in soft tissues is inconclusive. Although significant pain reduction often occurs with conditions suspicious of having calcific deposits present (calcific tendinitis, bursitis, or heel exostosis), no radiologic confirmation has shown a reduction in calcium deposits (10).

A condition very controversial with regard to ultrasound is application to a large hematoma. A complication that can result from this type of injury, especially to the quadriceps or anterior arm, is myositis ossificans. Theoretically, ultrasound would be effective in helping to resolve a large organized clot because of its penetrative ability. Clinicians have seen progress in range of motion when ultrasound was used in the treatment of a resolving severe contusion. It is proposed that ultrasound may cause deionization of calcium ions such that fewer calcium ions are deposited in the forming fibrin matrix needed for clotting (54). However, if the injury caused periosteal disruption and osteoblast proliferation within the hematoma, ultrasound may only exacerbate the condition from the mechanical agitation. Further stimulation of osteoblasts is why ultrasound is contraindicated in a condition when myositis ossificans is suspected until the condition is radiologically diagnosed as mature.

The time after the injury is a important factor to consider when using ultrasound to promote tissue healing. Tendon repair in animals was inhibited when ultrasound was administered immediately after surgery. However, dosages and duty cycles vary greatly when comparing studies (109). Low-intensity ultrasound in the pulsed mode of transmission is found to be most effective in tissue healing. Nonthermal effects are responsible for the healing since optimal intensities are very low (0.25 to 0.8 W/cm^2 at a 20% duty cycle) (43). Higher intensities may result in tissue edema. Early application of ultrasound at low intensities has been found to be most effective in promoting tissue healing (44,104).

The contraindications of ultrasound use are included in Table 6.11.

Phonophoresis

Phonophoresis is a technique in which chemicals, usually antiinflammatory or analgesic medications, are driven into tissues by means of ultrasound. The thermal response and acoustic streaming are thought to be the reasons the ions are driven through cell and organelle membranes (54). Clinical studies report that therapeutic responses with phonophoresis, especially pain relief and improved range of motion, were superior to those with placebo treatments or ultrasound alone (74,128). Treatments using 10% hydrocortisone ointments were found to be more effective than 1% ointments (12). To minimize the possibility of trapped air bubbles that impede transmission, the ointment is massaged into the treatment surface. The medication is ideally left in place for several minutes prior to ultrasound treatment to saturate the outer layer of skin (127). Conventional treatment parameters are used with phonophoresis, depending on whether thermal or nonthermal effects are desired. Research has not substantiated an optimal frequency, intensity, or duty cycle to enhance topical drug delivery.

Electric Stimulation and Ultrasound

Ultrasound is often combined with some form of electric stimulation. The sound head becomes the active electrode while administering ultrasound. This technique provides a mechanical massage in conjunction with the thermal response of ultrasound (61). The combination of modalities is believed to enhance circulation, help relieve muscle spasm, and loosen fibrotic tissues, although these results have not been found in controlled studies.

CONCLUSION

Therapeutic modalities are an important adjunct to help the injured and rehabilitating athlete. They are tools that may facilitate the recovery process by reducing symptoms and enhancing the healing environment of the damaged tissues. The health-care practitioner should remain knowledgeable of the tools that are available, but one should remember that physical agents can be used ineffectively or indiscriminantly. The ultimate modality is exercise and the other modalities are available to facilitate the use of exercise. These adjunct tools are frequently overused and often delay the progress back to activity. Be knowledgeable and discriminant in the use of physical agents.

REFERENCES

1. Airaksinen O, Kolari PJ, Miettinen H. Elastic bandages and intermittent pneumatic compression for treatment of acute ankle sprains. *Arch Phys Med Rehab* 1990;71:380–383.
2. Alon G. *High voltage—a monograph.* Chattanooga, TN: Chattanooga Corp, 1984.
3. Alon G, DeDomenico G. *High voltage stimulation: an integrated approach to clinical electrotherapy.* Chattanooga, TN: Chattanooga Corp, 1987.
4. Alon G. Principles of electrical stimulation. In: Nelson DP, Currier

RM, eds. *Clinical electrotherapy.* Norwalk, CT: Appleton & Lange, 1991:1–10.

5. American Physical Therapy Association. *Electrotherapeutic terminology in physical therapy.* Alexandria, VA: APTA Publications, 1990.

6. Barnes WS, Larson MA. Effects of localized hyper- and hypothermia on maximal isometric grip strength. *Am J Phys Med* 1983; 64(6):305–314.

7. Basbaum AI, Fields HL. Endogenous pain control mechanisms: review and hypothesis. *Ann Neurol* 1978;4(5):451–462.

8. Behnke RS. Cold therapy. *J Ath Training* 1974;9:178–179.

9. Belitsky RB, Odam SJ, Hubley-Kozey C. Evaluation of the effectiveness of wet ice, dry ice and cryogen packs in reducing skin temperature. *Phys Ther* 1987;67:1080–1084.

10. Bender LF, Janes JM, Herrick JR. Histologic studies following exposure of bone to ultrasound. *Arch Phys Med Rehab* 1954;35: 555–559.

11. Beninson J. Six years of pressure-gradient therapy. *Angiology* 1961;12:38–45.

12. Benson HAE, McElnay JC, Harland R. Phonophoresis of lignocaine and prilocaine from Emla cream. *Int J Pharm* 1988;44:65–69.

13. Borrell RM, Parker R, Henley EJ, Masley D, Repinecz M. Comparison of in vivo temperatures produced by hydrotherapy, paraffin wax treatment and fluidotherapy . *Phys Ther* 1980;60:1273–1276.

14. Bowman BR, McNeal DR. Response of single alpha motoneurons to high frequency pulse trains-firing behavior and conduction block phenomenon. *Appl Neurophysiol* 1986;49:121.

15. Brueton RN, Campbell B. The use of Geliperm as a sterile coupling agent for therapeutic ultrasound. *Physiotherapy* 1987;73:653–654.

16. Bugaj R. The cooling, analgesic, and rewarming effects of ice massage on localized skin. *Phys Ther* 1975;55:11–19.

17. Byl NN. The use of ultrasound as an enhancer for transcutaneous drug delivery: phonophoresis. *Phys Ther* 1995;75:539–553.

18. Cameron MH, Monroe LG. Relative transmission of ultrasound by media customarily used for phonophoresis. *Phys Ther* 1992; 72:142–148.

19. Castel C, Draper DO, Castel D. Rate of temperature increase during ultrasound treatments: are traditional treatment times long enough? *J Athletic Training* 1994;29:156.

20. Castel JC. *Pain management, acupuncture and transcutaneous electrical nerve stimulation techniques.* Topeka: PhysioTechnology, 1972.

21. Castel JC. Therapeutic ultrasound. *Rehab Therapy Prod Rev* 1993; 1:22–31.

22. Cheng N, Van Hoof H, Bockx E, et al. The effects of electric current on ATP generation, protein synthesis, amd membrane transport in rat skin. *Clin Orthop Rel Res* 1982;22:264–272.

23. Cheng RSS, Pomeranz B. Electroacupuncture analgesia could be mediated by at least two pain relieving mechanisms: endorphin and non-endorphin systems. *Life Sciences* 1979;25:1957–1962.

24. Chisar M. Utilizing electrical muscle stimulation for the retardation of atrophy. *J Ath Training* 1989;24:238–241.

25. Cohn BT, Draeger RI, Jackson DW. The effects of cold therapy in the postoperative management of pain in patients undergoing anterior cruciate ligament reconstructions. *Am J Sp Med* 1989;17: 344–348.

26. Coleridge Smith PD, Sarin S, Wilson LA, Scurr JH. *Improved venous ulcer healing using intermittent pneumatic compression,* 3rd ed. Nice, France: Colloque Franco-Britannique De Phlebologie, 1988.

27. Cosgrove KA, Alon G, Fischer SF, et al. The effect of two commonly used clinical stimulators on traumatic edema in rats. *Phys Ther* 1992;72:227–233.

28. Covington DB, Bassett FH. When cryotherapy injures. *Phys Sports Med* 1993;21:78–93.

29. Cummings J. Iontophoresis. In: Nelson DP, Currier RM, eds. *Clinical electrotherapy.* Norwalk, CT: Appleton & Lange, 1991:317–330.

30. Currier D, Greathouse D, Swift T. Sensory nerve conduction: effect of ultrasound. *Arch Phys Med Rehab* 1978;59:181–185.

31. Currier DP, Mann R. Muscular strength development by electrical stimulation in healthy individuals. *Phys Ther* 1983;63:915–921.

32. Currier D, Ray JM, Nyland J, Rooney JG, Noteboom JT, Kellogg

33. DeDomenico G. *Interferential current-a monograph.* Chattanooga, TN: Chattanooga Corp, 1988.

34. Delitto A, Rose SJ, McKowen JM, Lehman RC, Thomas JA, Shively RA. Electrical stimulation versus voluntary exercise in strengthening thigh musculature after anterior cruciate ligament surgery. *Phys Ther* 1988;68:660–663.

35. Denegar CR, Huff CB. High and low frequency TENS in the treatment of induced musculoskeletal pain: a comparison study. *J Ath Training* 1988;23:235–237.

36. Denegar CR, Perrin DH, Rogol AD, Rutt R. Influence of transcutaneous electrical nerve stimulation on pain, range of motion and serum cortisol concentration in females experiencing delayed onset muscle soreness. *JOSPT* 1989;11:100–103.

37. Denegar CR, Perrin DH. Effect of transcutaneous electrical nerve stimulation, cold, and a combination treatment on pain, decreased range of motion, and strength loss associated with delayed onset muscle soreness. *J Ath Training* 1992;27:200–206.

38. Denegar CR, Perrin DH. Effects of transcutaneous electrical nerve stimulation, cold, and a combination treatment on pain, decreased range of motion, and strength loss associated with delayed onset muscle soreness. *J Ath Training* 1992;27:200–206.

39. Draper DO. A comparison of temperature rise in human calf muscle following applications of underwater and topical gel ultrasound. *JOSPT* 1993;17:247–251.

40. Draper V, Ballard L. Electrical stimulation versus electromyographic biofeedback in the recovery of quadriceps femoris muscle function following anterior cruciate ligament surgery. *Phys Ther* 1991;71:455–464.

41. Draper DO, Hatheway C, Fowler D. Methods of applying underwater ultrasound: science versus folklore. *J Athletic Training* Summer 1991.

42. Draper DO, Sunderland S. Examination of the law of Grotthus-Draper: does ultrasound penetrate subcutaneous fat in humans. *J Ath Training* 1993;28(3):246–250.

43. Dyson M, Pond JB. The effect of pulsed ultrasound on tissue regeneration. *Physiotherapy* 1970;56(4):136–142.

44. Dyson M, Sucking J. Stimulation of tissue repair by ultrasound: a survey of the mechanisms involved. *Physiotherapy* 1978;64: 105–108.

45. Edmeads J. The physiology of pain: a review. *Prog Neuropsychopharmacol Biol Psychiatry* 1983;7:413–419.

46. Engles, M. Tissue response. In: Donatelli R, Wooden MJ, eds. *Orthopedic physical therapy.* New York: Churchill Livingstone, 1989:1–30.

47. Enwemeka CS. Inflammation, cellularity and fibrillogenesis in regenerating tendon: implications for tendon rehabilitation. *Phys Ther* 1989;69:816–825.

48. Enwemeka CS. Connective tissue plasticity: ultrastructural, biomechanical, and morphometric effects of physical factors on intact and regenerating tendons. *JOSPT* 1991;14:198–212.

49. Ersek RA. Relief of acute musculoskeletal pain using transcutaneous electrical neurostimulation. *JACEP* 1977;6:300–303.

50. Farmer WC. Effect of intensity of ultrasound on conduction of motor axons. *Phys Ther* 1968;42:1233–1237.

51. Frank C, Amiel D, and Akeson, WH. Healing of the medial collateral ligament of the knee. A morphological and biochemical assessment in rabbits. *Acto Orthop Scand* 1983;54:1917.

52. Gieck JH, Saliba EN. Application of modalities in overuse syndromes. *Clin Sports Med* 1987;6:427–466.

53. Green GA, Zachazewski JE, Jordan SE. Peroneal nerve palsy induced by cryotherapy. *Phys Sports Med* 1989;17:63–70.

54. Griffin JE, Echternach JL, Price RE, Touchstone JC. Patients treated with ultrasonic driven hydrocortisone and ultrasound alone. *Phys Ther* 1967;47:594–601.

55. Griffin JE, Karselis TC. *Physical agents for physical therapists.* Springfield, IL: Charles C. Thomas, 1982.

56. Griffin JW, Newsome LS, Stralka SW, Wright PE. Reduction of chronic post-traumatic hand edema: a comparison of high voltage pulsed current, intermittent pneumatic compression, and placebo treatments. *Phys Ther* 1990;70:279–285.

57. Guyton AC. *Medical Physiology.* Philadelphia: WB Saunders, 1981:41–54.

58. Hale JR, Jessen C, Fawcett AA, King RB. Arteriovenous anastomosis and capillary dilation and constriction induced by local heating. *Pflufer Archives* 1985;404(3):203–207.

59. Halvorson G. Therapeutic heat and cold for athletic injuries. *Phys and Sports Med* 1990;18:87–92.

60. Hanjurgens A, May HU. Differences between dynamic interference current analgesia and TENS analgesia. *Nemectron Medical* 1980.

61. Hayes KB. *Manual for Physical Agents*, 4th ed. Norwalk, CT: Appleton & Lange, 1993.

62. Healy WL, Siedman J, Pfeifer MD, Brown DG. Cold compressive dressing after total knee arthroplasty. *Clin Orth Rel Res* 1994;299:143–146.

63. Hill AV. Excitation and accommodation in nerves. *Proc Royal Soc* 1936;119–129.

64. Ho SSW, Illgen RL, Meyer RW, Torok PJ, Cooper MD, Reider B. Comparison of various icing times in decreasing bone metabolism and blood flow in the knee. *Am J Sports Med* 1995;23:74–76.

65. Hobler CK. Reduction of chronic post-traumatic knee edema using interferential stimulation. *J Ath Training* 1991;26:364–367.

66. Hocutt J, Jaffe R, Rylander R, Beebe K. Cyrotherapy in ankle sprains. *Am J Sports Med* 1982;10:315–319.

67. Hong CZ, Chen YC, Pon CH, Yu J. Immediate effects of various physical medicine modalities on pain threshold of an active myofascial trigger point. *J Musculoskeletal Pain* 1993;1:37–53.

68. Hooker DN. Electrical stimulating currents. In: *Therapeutic modalities in sports medicine*. St. Louis: Mosby, 1994:73–106.

69. Houglum, PA. Soft tissue healing and its impact on rehabilitation. *J Sport Rehab* 1992;1:19–39.

70. Hughes GS, Lichstein PR, Whitlock D, Harker C. Response of plasma beta-endorphins to transcutaneous electrical nerve stimulation in healthy subjects. *Phys Ther* 1984;64:1062–1066.

71. Kaempffe FA. Skin surface temperature reduction after cryotherapy to a casted extremity. *JOSPT* 1989;10:448–450.

72. Kahn J. *Low volt technique*. Syosset, NY: Churchill Livingstone, 1983.

73. Kahn J. *Principles and Practice of Electrotherapy*. New York: Churchill Livingstone, 1987:156.

74. Kleinkort JA, Wood F. Phonophoresis with 1% versus 10% hydrocotisone. *Phys Ther* 1975;55:1320–1325.

75. Kloth L. Electrotherapeutic alternatives for the treatment of pain. In: Gersh, MR, ed. *Electrotherapy in rehabilitation*. Philadelphia: FA Davis Co, 1992.

76. Kloth LC, Miller KH. The inflammatory response to wounding. In: Kloth, LC, McCulloch, JM, Feedar JA, eds. *Wound healing: alternatives in management*. Philadelphia: FA Davis Co, 1990:1–13.

77. Knight K. The effects of hypothermia on inflammation and swelling. *J Ath Train* 1976;8:7–10.

78. Knight KL. *Cryotherapy: theory, technique and physiology*. Chattanooga, TN: Chattanooga Corp, 1985.

79. Kots YM. Improvement of muscular strength with electrical stimulation. *Theory and Practice of Physical Culture* 1971;3:64–67 (Translated from Russian and French).

80. Kukulka CG. Principles of neuromuscular excitation. In: Gersh, MR, ed. *Electrotherapy in rehabilitation*. Philadelphia: FA Davis Co, 1992.

81. Lehmann JF, DeLateur BJ, Silverman DR. Heating effects of ultrasound in human beings. *Arch Phys Med Rehab* 1966;4:331–339.

82. Lentell G, Hetherington T, Eagan J, Morgan M. The use of thermal agents to influence the effectiveness of a low-load prolonged stretch. *JOSPT* 1992;16:200–207.

83. Lota MJ, Darling RC. Change in permeability of the red blood cell membrane in a homogeneous ultrasonic field. *Arch Phys Med Rehab* 1955;36:282–286.

84. Loy TT. Treatment of cervical spondylosis: electro-acupuncture versus physiotherapy. *Med J Aust* 1983;2:32–34.

85. Malone TR, Englehardt DL, Kirkpatrick JS, Bassett FH. Nerve injury in athletes caused by cryotherapy. *J Athl Training* 1992;27:235–237.

86. Mannheimer JS, Lampe GN. *Clinical transcutaneous electrical nerve stimulation*. Philadelphia: FA Davis, 1984.

87. McGraw WT. The effect of tension on collagen remodeling by fibroblasts: a stereological ultrastructural study. *Connect Tissue Res* 1986;14:229.

88. Melzack R, Wall PD. Pain mechanisms: a new theory. *Science* 1965;150:971–979.

89. Melzack R. Myofascial trigger points: relation to acupuncture and mechanisms of pain. *Arch Phys Med Rehab* 1981;162 114–117.

90. Mendel FC, Wylegala JA, Fish DR. Influence of high voltage pulsed current on edema formation following impact injury in rats. *Phys Ther* 1992;72:668–673.

91. Mendel FC, Fish DR. New perspectives in edema control via electrical stimulation. *J Ath Training* 1993;28:63–74.

92. Merrick MA, Knight KL, Ingersoll CD, Potteiger JA. The effects of ice and compression wraps on intramuscular temperatures at various depths. *J Ath Training* 1993;28:236–245.

93. Michlovitz S, Firuta H. Peripheral edema: pathophysiology, evaluation and management. *Post Graduate Adv Phys Ther*. Fairfax, VA: APTA, 1987.

94. Michlovitz S, Smith W, Watkins M. Ice and high voltage pulsed stimulation in the treatment of acute lateral ankle sprains. *JOSPT* 1988;9:301–304.

95. Morrissey MC, Brewster CE, Shields CL, Brown M. The effects of electrical stimulation on the quadriceps during post-operative knee immobilization. *Am J Sports Med* 1985;13:40–45.

96. Myer JW, Draper DO, Durrant E. Contrast therapy and intramuscular temperature in the human leg. *J Ath Training* 1994;29:316–322.

97. Nanneman D. Thermal modalities: heat and cold. *AAOHN* 1991;39:70–74.

98. Newton RA. *Electrotherapeutic treatment: selecting appropriate waveform characteristics*. Clifton, NJ: JA Preston Corp, 1984.

99. Newton R. High-voltage pulsed current: theoretical bases and clinical applications. In: Nelson DP, Currier RM, eds. *Clinical electrotherapy*. Norwalk, CT: Appleton & Lange, 1991:1–10.

100. Nolan MF. Conductive differences in electrodes used with transcutaneous electrical nerve stimulation devices. *Phys Ther* 1991;71:746–750.

101. Noonan TJ, Best TM, Anthony Seaber AV, Garrett WE Thermal effects on skeletal muscle tensile behavior. *Am J Sp Med* 1993;21:517–522.

102. Olson JE, Stravino VD. A review of cryotherapy. *Phys Ther* 1972;52:840–853.

103. Paris DL, Bayes F, Gucker B. Effects of the neuroprobe in the treatment of second-degree ankle inversion sprains. *Phys Ther* 1983;63:35–40.

104. Patrick MK. Applications of therapeutic pulsed ultrasound. *Physiotherapy* 1978;64:103–105.

105. Picker RI. Low volt pulsed microamp stimulation. *Clinical Management* 1990;9(2):10–33.

106. Poumerat G, Squire P, Lawani M. Effect of electrical stimulation superimposed with isokinetic contractions. *J Sports Med Phys Fitness* 1992;32:227–232.

107. Quillen WS. Neuromuscular electrical stimulation (NMES): ultilization in the rehabilitative treatment of muscular inhibition and atrophy. *Post Graduate Adv Phys Ther*. Fairfax, VA: APTA.

108. Reed B, Zarro V. Inflammation and repair and the use of thermal agents. In: Michlovitz SL, ed. *Thermal Agents in Rehabilitation*. Philadelphia: FA Davis Co, 1990:1–16.

109. Roberts M, Rutherford JH, Harris D. The effect of ultrasound on flexor tendon repairs in the rabbit. *Hand* 1982;14:18–22.

110. Robinson AJ. Basic concepts and terminology in electricity. In: Snyder-Mackler L, Robinson AJ. eds. *Clinical electrophysiology*. Baltimore: Williams & Wilkins, 1989:1–20.

111. Robinson AJ. Physiology of muscle and nerve. In: Snyder-Mackler L, Robinson AJ, eds. *Clinical electrophysiology*. Baltimore: Williams & Wilkins, 1989:59–94.

112. Robinson SE, Buono MJ. Effect of continuous-wave ultrasound on blood flow in skeletal muscle. *Phys Ther* 1995;75:145–150.

113. Rucinski TJ, Hooker DN, Prentice WE. The effects of intermittent compression on edema in postacute ankle sprains. *JOSPT* 1991;14:65–69.

114. Roesser WM, Meedks LW, Venis R, Strickland G. The use of transcutaneous nerve stimulation for pain control in athletic medicine. A preliminary report. *Am J Sports Med* 1976;4:210–213.

115. Selkowitz DM. Improvement in isometric strength of the quadri-

ceps femoris muscle after training with electrical stimulation. *Phys Ther* 1985;65:186–196.

116. Shealy CN. Management of acute pain in trauma. *Comprehensive Ther* 1979;5:15–18.

117. Sinacore DR, Delitto A, King DS, Rose SJ. Type II fiber activation with electrical stimulation: a preliminary report. *Phys Ther* 1990; 70:416–421.

118. Singer RN, Johnson PJ. Strategies to cope with pain associated with sport related injuries. *J Athl Training* 1987;22(2):12–15.

119. Sloan JP, Giddings P, Hain R. Effects of cold and compression on edema. *Phys and Sports Med* 1988;16:117–120.

120. Smith LE. Restoration of volitional limb movement of hemiplegics following patterned functional electrical stimulation. *Perceptual and Motor Skills* 1990;71:851–861.

121. Snyder-Mackler L. Electrical stimulation for tissue repair. In: Snyder-Mackler L, Robinson AJ, eds. *Clinical electrophysiology.* Baltimore: Williams & Wilkins, 1989:229–244.

122. Snyder-Mackler L, Garrett M, Roberts M. A comparison of torque generating capabilities of three different electrical stimulating currents. *JOSPT* 1989;10(8):297–301.

123. Snyder SH. Opiate receptors and internal opiates. *Scientific American* 1977;236(3):44–56.

124. Spielholz NI. Electrical stimulation of denervated muscle. In: Nelson DP, Currier RM, eds. *Clinical electrotherapy.* Norwalk, CT: Appleton & Lange, 1991:121–142.

125. Stanish WD, Valiant GA, Bonin A, Belcastro AN. The effects of immobilization and electrical stimulation on muscle glycogen and myofibrillar ATPase. *Can J Appl Sports Sci* 1984;7:267–271.

126. Starkey C. *Therapeutic modalities for athletic trainers.* Philadelphia: FA Davis Co, 1993:1–22.

127. Stewart HF, Abjug JL. Contraindications in ultrasound therapy and equipment performance. *Phys Ther* 1980;60:424–428.

128. Stratford PW, Levy DR, Gauldie S, Miseferi D, Levy K. The evaluation of phonophoresis and friction massage as treatments for extensor carpi radialis tendinitis: a ramdomized controlled trial. *Physiotherapy Canada* 1989;41:93–99.

129. Stratton SA, Smith MM. Effect of transcutaneous electrical nerve stimulation on forced vital capacity. *Phys Ther* 1980;60:45–47.

130. Strickler T, Malone T, Garrett W. The effects of passive warming on muscle injury. *Am J Sports Med* 1990;18:141–145.

131. Taylor K, Fish DR, Mendel FC, Burton HW. Effect of a single 30 minute treatment of high voltage pulsed current on edema formation in frog hind limbs. *Phys Ther* 1992;72:63–68.

132. Tomaszewski D, Dandorph MJ, Manning J. A comparison of skin interface temperature response between the ProHeat Instant Reusable Hot Pack and the standard hydrocollator steam pack. *J Athl Training.* 1992;27:355–359.

133. Underwood FB, Dremser MA, Finstuen D, Greathouse DG. Increasing involuntary torque production using TENS. *JOSPT* 1990; 12:101–104.

134. Urbscheit NL. Review of physiology. In: Nelson DP, Currier RM, eds. *Clinical electrotherapy.* Norwalk, CT: Appleton & Lange, 1991:1–10.

135. Vasudevan SV, Melvin JL. Upper extremity edema control: rationale of the techniques. *Am J Occ Ther* 1979;33:520–523.

136. Weston M, Taber C, Casagranda L, Cornwall M. Changes in local blood volume during cold gel pack application to traumatized ankles. *JOSPT* 1994;19(4):197–199.

137. Wigerstad-Lossing I, Grimby G, Johsson T, Morelli B, Peterson L, Renstrom P. Effects of electrical muscle stimulation combined with voluntary contractions after knee ligament surgery. *Med Sci Sports Exercise* 1988;20:93–98.

138. Wilkerson GB. External compression for controlling traumatic edema. *Phys and Sports Med* 1985;13:96–106.

139. Wilkerson GB. Inflammation in connective tissue: Etiology and Management. *J Ath Training* 1985;20:298.

140. Wilkerson GB. Treatment of the inversion ankle sprains through synchronous application of focal compression and cold. *J Ath Training* 1991;26:220–234.

141. Williams AR. *Ultrasound: biological effects and potential hazards.* London: Academic Press, 1983.

142. Williams AR, McHale J, Bowditch M, et al. Effects of ultrasound on electrical pain threshold perception in humans. *Ultrasound Med Biol* 1987;13:249–251.

143. Windsor RE, Lester JP, Herring SA. Electrical stimulation in clinical practice. *Phys and Sports Med* 1993;21:85–93.

144. Yackzan L, Adams C, Francis K. The effects of ice massage on delayed muscle soreness. *Am J Sp Med* 1984;12:159–165.

145. Zarins B. Soft tissue injury and repair: biomechanical aspects. *Int J Sports Med* 1982;3:9.

146. Ziskin MC, McDiarmid T, Michlovitz SL. Therapeutic ultrasound. In: Michlovitz SL, ed. *Thermal agents in rehabilitation.* Philadelphia: FA Davis Co, 1990:134–169.

The Injured Athlete, Third Edition,
edited by D. H. Perrin.
Lippincott–Raven Publishers, Philadelphia © 1999.

CHAPTER **7**

The Psychology of Injury and Rehabilitation

Robert J. Rotella, Elizabeth G. Hedgpeth, and Morris M. Pickens

After an injury, athletes may experience many different reactions. Athletes who sustain injuries not only have to deal with the physical consequences of not being able to participate in an activity they love, but must also deal with the roller-coaster effects of mood swings, increased levels of stress, and the loss of social support that once was met through being part of a team. Once athletes recover from the initial shock of being injured, they realize that their daily schedules are disrupted as they no longer spend hours on the practice field but instead spend hours in the training room going through rehabilitation. New surgical techniques, more elaborate exercise equipment, and intricate braces used for protecting an injury allows for the body to be physically ready far before the mind is prepared for a healthy, safe, and effective return to competition. This reality has created new concerns and considerations, which necessitates that careful attention is paid to the psychological aspects of injury and rehabilitation. Sophisticated sports medicine rehabilitation teams include team physicians, athletic trainers, and specialists in sport psychology.

This chapter will examine: (a) athletes' perceptions and reactions to injury, (b) the role of the sport psychologist in rehabilitation, (c) strategies for coping with injury, and (d) rehabilitation compliance and return to competition.

ATHLETES' PERCEPTIONS OF AND REACTIONS TO INJURY

Athletes may perceive similar injuries in vastly different ways. One may see the injury as a terrible disappointment, another may perceive it as an opportunity to show courage, and yet another may find it a welcome relief from the embarrassment of poor performance, lack of playing time, or a losing season. For even seriously injured athletes, some may view their situation as an opportunity to display their toughness, discipline, and dedication and get excited and motivated by the challenge, whereas others may become depressed and discouraged with a significant loss of energy, enthusiasm, and motivation.

Athletes who respond in counterproductive and self-defeating ways will need help. The sport psychologist must be alert as the athlete may experience emotional and irrational thinking. Some injured athletes may become lost in the work of worry, focus on discouraging thoughts, and become overwhelmed by anxiety. These self-defeating thought patterns may interfere with rehabilitation and recovery. When athletes are thinking irrationally, they may exaggerate the meaning of an event, disregard important aspects of a situation, oversimplify events as good or bad, right or wrong, generalize from a single event, or draw unwarranted conclusions, even though evidence is lacking or contradictory. For example, they may decide that the athletic trainer is giving preferential treatment to revenue-producing athletes over nonrevenue-producing athletes. They may exaggerate the meaning of an event, thinking their athletic career has certainly been ended by the injury and their future is out of their control. They may disregard important aspects of a situation and become terribly discouraged after 10 days of therapy, even though they were told it would take at least 2 or 3 weeks to complete. Some injured athletes may also oversimplify events or generalize from a single event. They may, for instance, know of another athlete who had a similar injury and, despite intensive rehabilitation, failed to recover. Because of this, they may believe that their personal efforts are nonproductive or worthless. Other athletes while in a discouraged state may decide they are injury prone. This thought may cause anxiety, and as a result may lead to more frequent injury. Andersen and

R. J. Rotella and M. M. Pickens: Memorial Gymnasium, University of Virginia, Charlottesville, Virginia 22903

E. G. Hedgpeth: Mindset–Attitude, 2429 Perkins Road, Durham, North Carolina 27706

Williams (2) suggest that athletes who perceive a situation as stressful exhibit greater muscle tension and attention disruption, which in turn places athletes at greater risk for injury.

All sports medicine teams recognize that there are certain athletes who are particularly difficult. A brief description of seven of the most typically difficult athletes is presented below. Some practical ideas for communicating with these athletes are suggested. Understanding and empathy are crucial components in working with this population.

Injury-Prone Athletes

Some athletes seem to be more prone to injury than are others, perhaps the athlete may not be warming up correctly or is not fully in shape. Their poor endurance leads to fatigue, a slower reaction time, and reduced coordination. Mentally, these athletes may be tense, depressed, or preoccupied with problems in school, social problems, or problems at home. The mental changes may be subtle, but the team physician, athletic trainer, or sport psychologist can often tell that something is wrong. These athletes may uncharacteristically jump the gun, start fights, miss shots, or otherwise not be concentrating on the task at hand. They may have trouble sleeping, show a change in behavior or mood pattern. Talking with these athletes will sometimes uncover the source of the problem, and the difficulty can start to be resolved.

False Image of Invulnerability

Athletes have been systematically taught that mental toughness and giving 100% effort all of the time are necessary for success in sport. Athletes can be taught that "trying your hardest" is not the same as "doing your best" and that giving 100% all of the time will simply guarantee mental weakness rather than mental toughness. The reality is that it is impossible to give 100% all of the time. A full acceptance of the false attitudes or an extreme reaction to these attitudes may increase the likelihood of injury and failure.

Many highly motivated athletes can learn to "play through" almost any kind of pain. Developing such an ability may make for often-injured athletes who seldom, if ever, perform in an optimally healthy state. Such athletes will commonly have short-lived athletic careers and lives filled with pain and suffering from masked injuries that they were tough enough to "play through."

Unfortunately, in sports and especially in contact sports, an abundance of rewards is provided to athletes who accept these attitudes. Such rewards often lead to an extreme psychological reaction by athletes wishing to win the admiration and respect of coaches, athletic trainers, teammates, and fans. As the rewards for displaying these attitudes are enjoyed, athletes become increasingly willing to do whatever is necessary to earn them.

Gradually, the well-intentioned appearance of mental toughness and dedication evolves into the projection of a false image of invulnerability. As athletes strive to live up to this impossible image, problems begin to appear. Gradually it is accepted as fact that "tough" athletes never need a rest, never miss a play, never go to the training room, and never let a "minor" injury keep them from playing. Failure to live up to this image of invulnerability is judged a sign of weakness. Unfortunately, for athletes with this belief system their pride is attached to never missing a practice or game. Their bodies are therefore left extremely vulnerable to injury. Their minds are left unprepared for the incapacitating injury or life-long pain that may follow.

A major change in attitude is required to ensure a healthy adaptation to injury, rehabilitation, and life in general. Without such change athletes who hold such views will not accept the reality that they are vulnerable, that they are human and can get hurt physically and scarred psychologically. This change of attitude is crucial if athletes are to accept injuries as a natural occurrence in sport and be capable of responding positively to them. Such acceptance will enable athletes to come closer to developing to their fullest ability and allow coaches, athletic trainers, sport psychologists, and physicians to effectively fulfill their respective roles. The hazards of these past mistaken attitudes must be realized before the specific psychological strategies presented can be utilized.

Dependent Attention-Loving Athletes

Athletes who need attention and who enjoy being dependent upon others frequently make constant and extreme demands on the sports medicine team. Their behavior reflects dependency in that these athletes want to make others feel responsible for them and their health. The normal services provided to other athletes on a day-to-day basis are never good enough. These athletes always want more attention, more time, and more help.

In general, athletes of this type have refused to accept the responsibility of taking care of themselves. They want to be taken care of by others and, often as a result of their athletic abilities, have always been able to find others quite willing to do so. These athletes have developed innocent and devious behaviors for attaching themselves to the nurturing type caregivers in the helping professions. The sports medicine team must take a firm stand by creating boundaries, and reasonable time limits must be set when working with the dependent attention-loving athletes. If not, the sports medicine team will give until worn out and unable to help others. Some athletes will respond to these boundaries with frustration, hostility, and hurt feelings. In the past these responses have commonly helped them get the attention they desire.

Resistant Athletes

Athletes who resist treatment make the sports medicine team's job more difficult. Whereas it is common for the dependent athletes to make the sports medicine team feel needed and respected, the resistant athletes are perceived as showing no respect or appreciation for the athletic trainers' rehabilitation skills. Although there are various reasons for the resistant behavior of such athletes, it is usually best to avoid psychological interpretations.

For most athletes of this type, the sports medicine team must not take personal offense at the athletes' attitudes. Many athletes will change their attitudes and behaviors when the sports medicine team's responses are combined with humor. After trying these strategies without satisfactory results, the sports medicine team can employ a more straightforward approach. It is best simply to tell these athletes that it is their decision, they can live with their injuries, suffer through an extremely slow recovery, or follow the recommended rehabilitation regimen. Make it clear that the sports medicine team can live with the athletes' injury and the lack of treatment if the athletes are able to do so. Letting the athletes decide often leads them to make a commitment to rehabilitation. Too often the sports medicine team is hesitant to leave such decisions in the hands of athletes who might choose to continue to refuse treatment. This response will not encourage the development of responsibility that is necessary to effectively complete the rehabilitation process.

Childlike Athletes

It is not uncommon for even the toughest and most mature athletes to regress to a more childlike state when they are injured. This reality makes sense, particularly for athletes with disabling injuries that require a prolonged rehabilitation period, when it is understood that, as with young children, many everyday activities require help from another adult.

Depending on the athletes' personality, a variety of behavior patterns will occur. Some athletes will like being waited on, some will withdraw and become quiet and shy, some will lose their tempers, and others will whine and get lost in self-pity. It is then appropriate to give the athletes some control and responsibility over their rehabilitation to foster more adult-like behavior.

Angry Athletes

Obviously no sports medicine team member enjoys being verbally attacked or ridiculed by athletes receiving treatment. Although athletes' angry response to injury is understandable, displays of prolonged or persistent anger, particularly when directed at the sports medicine team, should not be tolerated. Anger is best responded to immediately and directly. Rather than attempting to explain the anger, it is best to show empathy and firmness while asking questions of the athletes. Questions are intended to facilitate an understanding of the anger.

The major goal in working with angry athletes is to establish a workable relationship between the parties involved. To do so the sports medicine team members involved must stay calm while establishing the necessary boundaries. Sports medicine team members who respond to such athletes by attacking back and acting irrationally will only ensure that there will be no resolution. Likewise, allowing oneself to display bitterness toward the angry athletes will further hinder the desired relationship. In any case the sooner a calm and objective relationship is established, the better it will be to achieve rehabilitation goals.

Unmotivated Athletes

Athletes display a lack of motivation for many reasons. Some athletes arrive in the training room for treatment with an extremely negative attitude, which hinders progress. Others who are injured for the first time may know of friends who, despite efforts to rehabilitate themselves, did not make a healthy return to competition. As a result these athletes assume that there is no reason to be motivated. Still others are despondent about their injury and have developed a counterproductive habit of complaining and questioning everything they are asked to do.

In each case the underlying problem must be addressed. Athletes cannot be forced to have a great attitude; they can, however, be helped to develop a positive outlook toward their treatment. The athletes must also perceive that their attitude and behavior will play an important role in treatment efficacy and effectiveness. Athletes can be given numerous examples of other athletes with similar injuries who, as a result of a positively motivated attitude have successfully recovered. A variety of strategies are useful, including motivational tapes, anecdotes, or videos that help inspire athletes to think about how good they will feel upon their return to competition. The sports medicine team members must accept the fact that although they may be able to inspire athletes for a short time they cannot make athletes want something that they do not want.

ROLE OF THE SPORT PSYCHOLOGIST IN SPORTS MEDICINE

A great deal of literature has been written concerning the psychology of athletic injury (5,17,22,34,57), but literature regarding the direct application of sport psychology in sports medicine is limited (6,54). In working within the field of athletic rehabilitation the relationship between the sport psychologists and the athletic trainers is vital.

The sport psychologist should discuss the philosophy of sport psychology with the athletic trainers and offer a protocol to integrate sport psychology into the existing rehabilitation program. Sport psychology is a positive, growth-oriented, educational process that stresses mental discipline and personal responsibility that can facilitate rehabilitation performance. Although athletes are ultimately responsible for their recovery, physicians, athletic trainers, and sport psychologists are part of the team that helps athletes through rehabilitation and return to their sport. Ultimately, athletes must be aware that their personal role in the rehabilitation process is paramount.

The strategies used by the sport psychologist should be unobtrusive yet thoroughly integrated within the rehabilitation program. The sport psychologist engages in an interactive process with the athlete as well as with other members of the sports medicine team. Having a thorough understanding of the psychological issues of the rehabilitation process is necessary in order to be accepted and respected by the athletic trainers and athletes (24). Spending time in the training room, taking basic courses and reading the rehabilitation literature can facilitate an understanding of the rehabilitation process.

The initial meeting between an injured athlete and the sport psychologist is the appropriate time to assess if an athlete needs psychological rehabilitation. This initial meeting should take place as close in time to the occurrence of the injury. Although many athletes, especially those more seriously injured, may require psychological intervention, sport psychologists must remember that many athletes can effectively cope with injury by themselves (56), and thus do not need psychological intervention. As a member of the sports medicine team, two primary roles a sport psychologist fulfills are that of social supporter and educator (26,45). The sport psychologist attempts to provide athletes with emotional support and at the same time, offer effective strategies and techniques for handling the rehabilitation process. If the sport psychologist is successful in providing effective strategies for handling rehabilitation, and athletes are successful in implementing these strategies, athletes are likely to be mentally and emotionally prepared to return to competition once their bodies are physically healed.

STRATEGIES FOR COPING WITH INJURY

Athletes have a variety of choices in terms of how they view their injury and rehabilitation. The sport psychologist works with injured athletes to address their perceptions of injury. This educational process involves helping athletes identify the challenges they face, formulate a plan of action to cope with those challenges, and develop a thinking and feeling action plan to get through the rehabilitation process (24).

When injury occurs, athletes can be encouraged to view it in a rational, self-enhancing way rather than from a self-defeating perspective. Athletes may understand that when they perceive that their injury blocks the attainment of important goals, perceptions are likely to be distorted. Athletes may know that it is reasonable and appropriate to think that the injury is unfortunate, untimely, and inconvenient, and to feel irritated, frustrated, and sad. It is unproductive, however, for athletes to be convinced that the situation is hopeless, that the injury should be hidden from coaches or athletic trainers, that the season or their career has ended, or that they will never again be able to perform effectively. Athletes are encouraged to express their feelings, to establish rapport with the sports medicine team, and to balance accepting help from others while retaining independence. Giving athletes some control over rehabilitation has been shown to reduce the stress some athletes feel concerning their injury (29). Athletes must be taught that they have control over the way they perceive an event—it is a choice they make.

There are a variety of psychological interventions sport psychologists may utilize to supplement the physical rehabilitation process (29,46,55). These include, but are not limited to, support systems, relaxation, imagery, goal-setting, positive self-talk, pain management, the use of mastery and coping tapes, video modeling, and systematic rationalization.

Support Systems

The sport psychologist can enhance athletes' recovery by conducting educational seminars for sports medicine physicians, athletic trainers, parents, or teammates that cover topics related to the role of effective thinking in the rehabilitation process. Letting the athletes know that their recovery is truly a collaborative effort and that the sports medicine team is striving toward the same goal also increases the chance for full recovery. The sport psychologist can provide informational and inspirational literature and videos pertinent to rehabilitation. These can range from brochures covering what surgery will entail to a video of elite-level athletes performing at peak levels following recovery from an injury. When using videos, the sport psychologist should consider several principles that increase the effectiveness of a modeling program. Observers are more likely to attend to a model if the model is similar to the observer (35). In the rehabilitation setting, athletes are more likely to attend to models who play similar positions, are at the same competitive level, have a similar style of play, and have suffered a similar injury (15). Through the use of video modeling, injured athletes can gain knowledge about the rehabilitation process, learn strategies for coping with setbacks, and develop confidence that they, like the video model, can successfully return to competition.

Social Support Groups

One of the easiest, yet most beneficial ways to help athletes cope with injury is simply to provide them with support. Social support has been shown to decrease stress and increase feelings of well-being (23,41,42,47). Within the training room Gieck (16) has shown that athletes receiving support from peers, coaches, and athletic trainers show a greater effort to fit rehabilitation into their schedule. One way to effectively provide social support is through the use of injury support groups. Crucial to the success of such groups is the sport psychologist's ability to invite thoughts, emotions, and feelings without demanding them, and the ability to help athletes learn how to use strategies and techniques pertinent to recovery. It is important that athletes perceive the group meetings as useful and not as a requirement they must meet (56). Thus, changing the format of the meetings from round-table discussion to how-to seminars (led by athletes who have successfully recovered from injury) and to watching inspirational videos may be beneficial. These sessions can be videotaped and given to the athletes for personal use to reinforce the positive interactions.

Similar-Injury or Mentor Support

Another program that can help athletes cope with rehabilitation is a similar-injury mentor program (23,53,55). This program allows athletes to express feelings and thoughts about experiences and at the same time learn from others facing similar situations. In the similar-injury mentor program, an athlete who is currently injured is paired with an athlete who suffered a similar injury in the past and has returned to competition (53). It is crucial that the mentor models effective thoughts and behaviors for the injured athlete and that the mentor is someone the injured athlete respects and trusts (15). The same principles that make a video model effective are likely to make a mentor model effective. It is important for the sport psychologist to make athletes aware that this program is for their benefit and is not a way of checking compliance to rehabilitation.

Coaches' Support

Coaches can be supportive by making a videotape at the first of the year and express what expectations they have for athletes who are injured. This video can include guidelines for attending practices, attending away games and providing an update to appropriate coaches. If the position coaches or assistant coaches add their input into the video it may personalize the tape for athletes at particular positions. The position coach can mention a particular athlete that played a particular position and discuss how that athlete stayed involved with the team when going through the rehabilitation process. This reinforces the similar-injury groups and the similar-injury mentor programs. This video can include guidelines for attending practices, attending away games, and providing athletes with specific coaches' expectations.

Relaxation

Injured athletes may use relaxation training to help manage stress and anxiety and to control pain. Progressive relaxation techniques may not be equally effective for all athletes. Those who tend to be anxious about an injury or who have insomnia, tension headaches, or general tightness benefit most. Many other athletes have learned on their own how to cope with stress and have been coping well for years. They should not be forced to spend extra time on relaxation training.

Jacobson's (31) basic premise of progressive relaxation states that it is impossible to be nervous or tense in any part of the body when the muscles are relaxed. In addition the tenseness of the involuntary muscles and organs can be reduced if the associated skeletal muscles are relaxed. This process takes practice of about 1 hour a day for 4 weeks or more but the payoff for the athletes down the road is the ability to evoke the relaxation response in a matter of seconds. It is important to present this time frame to the athletes and equate it to weight training which also doesn't produce instant results but pays off in time.

The relaxation method involves the tensing and relaxing of muscles in a predetermined order. The athletes lie on the floor, in a quiet room with arms and legs uncrossed to reduce additional stimulation. Discourage the use of music because the athletes need to attend to listening to their body. The muscles are tensed and relaxed in order for the athletes to become familiar with the feeling of the muscle in a relaxed state. The order, according to Jacobson (30), of muscle groups is as follows: left arm to right arm, left leg to right leg, abdomen, back, chest, shoulder muscles, and neck and face muscles last. The arm-hand sequence is done first because it is easier to experience the difference between tense and relaxed in these muscle groups.

The use of relaxation with imagery makes the process more effective (1). The procedure is talked through by the sport psychologist for the first few sessions using a slow, quiet tone of voice with inflection on tensing and relaxing. It is effective to have the athletes make a tape of their own voice to use until it becomes second nature. The athletes then equate their own voice with the relaxation, the assumption being that in time, the tape would be running in their head rather than from a recorder. The cycles will be approximately 10 to 15 seconds for the tension segment and 15 to 20 seconds for the relaxation segment. It is suggested to use about three repetitions for each muscle group (40). After the relaxation training is underway and has been assessed and found to be effective, imagery can be introduced.

Imagery

Imagery has been defined as the use of visualization to imagine situations (3). Imagery has also been defined as the use of one's senses to create or recreate an experience in the mind (52). The use of imagery during the rehabilitation process is advocated by many (21,25,46).

Ievleva and Orlick (29) found athletes to use three types of imagery in the rehabilitation process. The three types are (a) healing imagery (attempting to see and/or feel the body part healing), (b) imagery during physiotherapy (imagining ultrasound increasing blood flow and thus promoting recovery), and (c) total recovery imagery (returning to sport and performing well again). Just as Ievleva and Orlick suggest incorporating different types of imagery in a rehabilitation program, Green (21) suggests incorporating imagery at different times during the rehabilitation process. Imagery can be used immediately after an injury as a means of projecting a positive outcome. Imagery can also be used throughout the rehabilitation process as a means of coping with obstacles inherent during rehabilitation (21).

Vealey (52) provides the following suggestions when helping athletes use imagery. First, relaxation should usually precede imagery practice because imagery is more effective when it is combined with relaxation than when it is used alone. Second, athletes should practice imagery from an internal perspective, seeing the image from behind their own eyes, as opposed to an external perspective, seeing the image from outside one's body as if with a video camera. Third, athletes should practice imagery with realistic expectations. Fourth, athletes should practice imagery in a quiet setting. In all cases it must be emphasized that imagery is only as useful as the amount of energy and focus that is put into it. It is of little utility if athletes just go through the motions. The quality of imagery is essential in order to create a déjà vu.

Goal Setting

Goal setting (Table 7.1) is a process where one specifies a standard to achieve, usually within a specified time period (33). It is well established in the psychological literature that goal setting is an effective means of attaining some standard of performance (20). In the rehabilitation setting, results from Ievleva and Orlick (29) indicate that athletes who were involved in goal setting on a consistent basis healed faster than athletes who did not utilize goal setting. Ievleva and Orlick (29) also suggest that goal setting is most effective when athletes list the specific steps required to reach their goals.

According to Gould (20), goal setting is most likely to be effective when goals are specific as opposed to general, difficult but realistic, short-term as well as long-term, performance-oriented instead of outcome-oriented, stated positively instead of negatively, and included for both practice and competition. Gould (20) also suggests that goal setting can be effective for all competitive levels.

Positive Self-Talk

Self-talk (Table 7.2) can be thought of as the things one says to one's self (7). These things are not necessarily spoken out loud, although they may be, and often an individual is not even aware that they are engaging in self-talk (7). Research in sport shows that positive self-talk can have desirable effects on performance (36), and that negative self-talk can have undesirable effects on performance (43).

Likewise, Ievleva and Orlick (29) report that for athletes undergoing rehabilitation, those whose self-talk was positive, self-encouraging, and determined healed quicker than those whose self-talk was negative, self-pitying, and unforgiving. When athletes are noted to be engaging in negative self-talk, sport psychologists can help athletes learn how to stop the negative thoughts and replace them with positive ones. One strategy for doing this is to have the athletes generate a list of negative thoughts experienced during rehabilitation. These negative thoughts are then coupled with positive thoughts that can be substituted for the negative thoughts (7). Changing negative self-talk to positive self-talk requires both an awareness of one's thoughts and the ability to respond with a countering thought (7).

Pain Management

Pain management involves the use of self-regulation skills to cope with the pain often experienced during rehabilitation (Table 7.3). Turk, Meichenbaum, and Genest (50) have identified the following six categories of pain-management strategies.

External focus of attention involves directing one's attention away from the pain being experienced and toward environmental events (the sunset). Pleasant imagining entails athletes utilizing an internal focus of attention on pleasant images (relaxing on the beach). Neutral imagining is the same as pleasant imagining except the focus is

TABLE 7.1. *Goal setting*

Goals set by athlete	Target date
Listen to mastery tapes	Daily
Get to training room on time	Daily
Relaxation	Nightly
Review progress with athletic trainer	Weekly

TABLE 7.2. *Self-talk*

Negative thought	Coupled with	Positive thought
Why did I have to get injured? It's so unfair.	>	Injury is a part of sport. Other athletes have been injured and recovered and so will I.
These stupid exercises aren't helping. I don't know why I even do them.	>	These exercises seem awkward but the athletic trainers must want me to do them for a reason. I'm sure they'll help in the long run.
The pain is so bad I can't continue. I'm not getting better anyway.	>	Pain is often a sign of progress. It means I'm getting better, even if only a little each day.

on obscure images (walking down stairs). In rhythmic cognitive activity, athletes engage in a repetitive mental task (counting backwards). Pain acknowledging involves a reinterpretation of the pain or a shift away from an ordinary style of attention (attempting to detach oneself from the pain). In dramatized coping, the client may imagine pain as if it is the result of a heroic effort (saving a child from a burning building).

Heil (25) notes that of the six strategies, four (external focus of attention, pleasant imagining, neutral imagining, and rhythmic cognitive activity) are dissociative, the focus being away from pain, whereas two (pain acknowledging and dramatized coping) are associative, the focus being toward pain. Dissociative strategies are used more often than associative strategies because of their diversity and because they can be easily learned. Of the four dissociative strategies, pleasant imagining is usually the most effective but every effort must be made to fit the strategy to the individual.

A note of caution regarding pain. Pain is a subjective experience and needs to be taken at face value: pain is whatever the individual says it is. ''The athlete must learn to differentiate performance pain from injury during performance and benign pain (that occurring routinely) from harmful pain during rehabilitation'' (25) (p. 141). Athletes must be careful not to block out pain signals that could otherwise warn of danger. There is no easy answer to how this is done, but it appears to be a subtle distinction based on previously healthy performances and prior injuries experienced by athletes. Athletes tend to have a very acute awareness of their bodies and are usually able to intuitively perceive the difference between a muscle ache

TABLE 7.3. *Pain management*

Strategy	Example
External focus of attention	Focus on sunset
Pleasant imagining	Imagine relaxing on beach
Neutral imagining	Imagine walking down stairs
Rhythmic cognitive activity	Counting backwards
Pain acknowledging	Imagining pain is connected to another object (i.e., chair)
Dramatized coping	Pain is result of saving child from burning building

that is from over training and muscle pain that signals damage.

Mastery and Coping Tapes

Previously it was suggested that athletes' positive self-talk could enhance rehabilitation. Mastery and coping tapes are a way of utilizing positive self-talk through an auditory medium (44). In the rehabilitation setting, mastery tapes can describe the ideal rehabilitation process, whereas coping tapes might describe how to positively cope with a less-than-perfect situation.

By listening to the tape over and over, athletes will likely gain a sense of control that can help them effectively handle the rehabilitation process (Box 1). According to Rotella and Heyman (45), coping rehearsal is the more realistic of the two strategies, especially when dealing with recovery from injury. In order for athletes to have effective mastery and coping tapes, it is recommended that the sport psychologist help athletes design the tapes (7). Mastery and coping tapes are usually audiotapes as opposed to videotapes because of the cost and the ability to be used in many settings.

Systematic Rationalization

In order to assist athletes in reducing stress related to rehabilitation, Hedgpeth, Sowa, and Striegel (24) suggest that athletes conceptualize concerns, set goals, and then take action. Systematic rationalization (49) is a framework that can be used by the sport psychologist in the training room to understand athletes' perception of stressful events related to rehabilitation. Systematic rationalization classifies stressful life events based on athletes' personal beliefs of control and their perception of the importance of the events. Three steps are utilized in this strategy: (1) identification of stressors by athletes, (2) classification of stressors by athletes, and (3) review of the stressors by athletes and the sport psychologist. Athletes are asked to list all the stressors in their environment that may impact on their reaction to injury and rehabilitation. This step allows for early referral if the stressors listed are outside of the expertise of the sport psychologist (e.g., alcohol, drug abuse).

BOX 1
Coping Rehearsal for Knee Surgery

I'm not looking forward to surgery—I'm anxious. I'm likely to become even more anxious as the day of surgery approaches. When I realize that my mind is running wild I'll say "STOP" to myself and replace these thoughts with positive thoughts such as "let go" and relax.

Rehabilitation will be long and demanding, challenging my self-discipline and willpower. But I can't let the injury beat me. I must have confidence in my ability to overcome this challenge.

What must I do? I'll make a plan that will prepare me for successful rehabilitation. I must keep my cool and not lose it. If I get uptight, I'll relax and become aware of my self-talk. If I'm thinking negative thoughts, I'll "STOP" and repeat positive thoughts to myself. If I become discouraged, I'll think of athletes who have overcome far worse injuries than mine. Successful athletes realize that successful rehab is part of being a successful athlete.

There will be many excuses for not going to therapy: "I can't find time," "I'm too busy," "I have a test tomorrow," "The training room hours are ridiculous." I will make sure that I'm ready for these excuses and realize that they will only work against me. I will always find a way to get to the training room.

There will be days when I'll see little or no progress. I may experience pain that is likely to make me tense, irritable, and frustrated. When these occur, I must remember to stay calm, to think positively, and to keep my sense of humor. Then the athletic trainers will enjoy helping me more, and I'll feel better about myself. Think how good I'll feel when my rehab is successful.

Stressors are defined as events associated with the injury that produce negative symptoms such as excessive tension, arousal, fear, or anger. The second step is to classify the stressors from the athletes' list into the four quadrants: controllable or uncontrollable and important or unimportant. Stressors are examined one by one as a particular athlete classifies each stressor as controllable or uncontrollable based on the athlete's personal ability to manage or act on the stressors and important or unimportant based on personal priorities for each outcome. For example, the stressor of rehabilitation is classified as important and controllable if the athlete perceives the rehabilitation as a priority and within the athlete's personal control. However, the stressor would be classified as uncontrollable and important if the rehabilitation is seen as outside the athlete's ability to control and yet is a priority in the athlete's life.

The third step is to determine what action is appropriate based on a review of classifications. The stressors listed as unimportant and controllable or unimportant and uncontrollable are dealt with first. In general these stressors are seen as hassles and the athlete is encouraged to let go of hassles in order to put time and energy into addressing stressors they perceive as important. If they are not able to let go of hassles then the hassles need to be reclassified as important and become issues of personal priority.

Stress reduction for stressors classified as controllable and important is accomplished by traditional performance enhancement and stress-management techniques (e.g., goal setting, positive self-talk, relaxation). The fact that the athlete classified these stressors as controllable indicates that the athlete already has some idea as to how to reduce the stress associated with the event. The intervention then is to motivate the athlete to turn their ideas into behavior.

The final stressors that are classified as important and uncontrollable are the most difficult to resolve. The sport psychologist must work with the athlete to change the perception of the event as well as the response to the event. The interventions used may be positive self-talk, cognitive restructuring or any coping skills that encourage the athlete to change the perception of the event. When the shift from important to unimportant takes place the athlete is then able to let go of the stress associated with the event. Another alternative is for the athlete to change the perception of the stressor from uncontrollable to controllable. It is a positive step to reinforce the fact that the athlete's reaction to an event is always controllable. The challenge is to cut through the emotion associated with the event in order to arrive at a rational solution.

For example, Derrick is a 23-year-old senior basketball player at a Division I school. He dreams of playing in the National Basketball Association (NBA) after graduation from college. In the second game of the season he hurt his back and is now trying to rehabilitate his back while he continues to play. The stressors Derrick lists are fear of reinjury, not being able to play professional basketball, concern that his teammates think he is not really hurt, and the difficulty of getting to the training room between classes and practice. Derrick classified his stressors and placed them in the systematic rationalization quadrants as seen in Table 7.1.

The unimportant stressors (both controllable and uncontrollable) were discussed first. The sport psychologist encouraged Derrick to express his feelings about his teammates' perception of his injury. Derrick was able to understand that he was not able to control how his teammates felt and that their feelings did not make a difference in the way he reacted to his injury. The stressors that are important and controllable were dealt with next as it is most likely that Derrick has some idea about how to handle these stressors. Derrick is encouraged to make a plan to act on these stressors such as the use of time-management skills to find time to come to the training room as well as discussing with the athletic trainer additional hours the athletic trainer would be available in the training room. The athletic trainer may also have exercises that Derrick could do on his own that do not require training room facilities. The final quadrant is the most difficult to work with as Derrick must change his perception of the stressor. This involves discussing with Derrick the fact that not playing professional basketball may be out of his control but getting back into the best shape he can is within his control. Reinjury is also not under Derrick's direct control but by working with the athletic trainer he can develop precautions to protect his back while playing and while engaged with activities of daily living. Derrick can be encouraged to understand that effective rehabilitation is his best insurance against reinjury, but there are no guarantees. The one guarantee is that with practice Derrick can control his perceptions and can adjust his attitude at will. Systematic rationalization is an ongoing process and Derrick can add stressors as they occur during the rehabilitation process. The entire process can be repeated as often as necessary.

Rehabilitation Compliance

A major concern in the rehabilitation setting is compliance, getting athletes to come to the training room, put forth effort, and to do the exercises necessary to successfully return to the playing field. Athletic trainers have the techniques to effectively retrain muscles damaged during an injury, but if athletes do not comply with the prescribed treatment, the rehabilitation process will not be effective.

There are no published statistics per se concerning compliance in the training room setting but in the field of exercise the drop-out rate in the first three months of beginning a program is somewhere between 30% to 70% (40). In the field of medicine the overall compliance rate is 50% (39). Self-improvement programs fare no better with the drop-out rate for smoking cessation, obesity control, and stress-management programs estimated to be between 20% and 80% (51). It is important for those involved in athletic rehabilitation to determine not only the compliance rate for athlete rehabilitation but what affects the compliance of athletes to rehabilitation. It is no longer enough for athletes to just show up and sign in to a rehabilitation center. Intensity, effort, patience, persistence, and proper form are necessary to fully recover from an injury as rapidly as possible.

Psychosocial factors that impact compliance according to both injured athletes and athletic trainers are social support, goal setting, and the rapport between athletic trainer and athletes (12,13,14). According to Caplan (9) social support is the interpersonal relationship that provides emotional support, assistance, and resources in time of need as well as supplying feedback: it is the relationship with others who share similar values and standards. Social support has been shown to be related to compliance and can come from sport psychologists, athletic trainers, family, coaches, and teammates (8,11,12). As discussed earlier, injury support groups and similar-injury programs are effective in helping athletes to be more compliant to the rehabilitation process. Goal setting is an effective motivator and attainment of goals can increase rehabilitation compliance (16,28,58). Goals need to be specific to each athlete as well as challenging yet attainable. Athletes must be able to see that meeting short-term goals will enhance the long-term aim of returning to sport participation. It is also important for athletes to trust the sports medicine team and believe that the treatment will produce the desired result (18,19). A true partnership between the athletes and the sports medicine team is most effective when athletes take responsibility for the rehabilitation process and the sports medicine team supports and guides the athletes through the process.

Return to Competition

Readiness to return to play is a major decision and should be made by a team consisting of sports medicine physicians, athletic trainers, the athletes, and the sport psychologists. While the physician and the athletic trainer decide if athletes are physically ready to return to play, the sport psychologist and the athlete need to be confident about the athlete's mental readiness to return to competition. Bill Bradley in *Life on the Run* (4) makes the point that only the athlete knows when he/she is ready to return to competition. ''Sometimes I have been told I could play when I knew I couldn't and sometimes I have been told I couldn't play when I knew I could'' (p. 133). The goal of the sport psychologist is to help the athlete return to competition fully prepared psychologically. If an athlete is not confident about returning or fears reinjury, the athlete is more likely to be reinjured (46). It is also recommended that the sport psychologist obtain input concerning the athlete's frame of mind from other members of the sport medicine team as well as just asking the athlete if he is ready to return. Again, the decision of when an athlete is ready to return to competition is best determined by the athlete, physician, athletic trainer, and sport psychologist as members of a team making a decision that first and foremost looks out for the best interest of the athletes.

From Injury to Return to Competition: ACL Reconstruction

The following is an example of a psychological rehabilitation program designed for an injured college football player. This program incorporates many of the strategies presented earlier and progresses from injury to return to competition.

During a mid-season Saturday afternoon game, Jim, a linebacker, tackles an opponent and as he does, he hears a "pop" and feels extreme pain in his left leg. As the athletic trainer gets to the player, he/she speaks in a calm voice and assures the player that everything will be O.K. Initial prognosis indicates a third-degree tear of the anterior cruciate ligament (ACL).

At the Sunday morning meeting, Jim, the sports medicine physician, and the athletic trainer decide to brace Jim's knee for the remainder of the season and have it surgically repaired after the bowl game. This allows him to stay involved with the team and also become mentally prepared for both the surgery and postoperative rehabilitation. During the preoperative phase of injury-recovery, Jim has 2 to 3 months to learn effective strategies for rehabilitation.

During this Sunday morning meeting, Jim is introduced to the sport psychologist by the athletic trainer. The focus of this meeting is for the sport psychologist to understand the athlete through active listening and assessing his need for psychological rehabilitation through general conversation. Strictly teaching from the outset will most likely not help establish a caring, trusting relationship crucial to the care of the athlete. There will be plenty of time for teaching in the months ahead. At the conclusion of this initial meeting, the sport psychologist and Jim set up a tentative schedule for meetings (assuming psychological rehabilitation is deemed appropriate).

At the first scheduled meeting, the sport psychologist outlines the months ahead and answers any questions about the upcoming surgery. This is also an appropriate time to ask what type of interaction (mentor groups, educational seminars) Jim prefers, and if not done previously, provide him with any literature or videos pertinent to his recovery. After this meeting, the sport psychologist should tell the athletic trainer what strategies will likely be used over the course of the rehabilitation program.

During the second meeting, the sport psychologist may instruct Jim how to use imagery and pain management for his upcoming rehabilitation exercises. This is also time for Jim, along with the help of the sport psychologist, to set appropriate goals for the upcoming months. These might include going through a quality workout each day, maintaining a positive attitude toward rehabilitation, and listening to his coping tape on a nightly basis. It is important to make sure the ability to reach these goals is under Jim's control.

Subsequent sessions could include other activities such as systematic rationalization and including Jim in an injury support group if possible. The sport psychologist continues to supply Jim with motivational messages and encourages others to keep supporting Jim.

Approximately a week prior to surgery, the focus of the meetings is switched from handling preoperative rehabilitation to surgery itself and postoperative rehabilitation. This is a good time for both the sport psychologist and Jim to evaluate what works and what does not work and adjust strategies accordingly. Again literature and video may be helpful in dispelling any fear Jim may have concerning surgery. Before surgery, the sport psychologist and Jim set up a meeting time as soon after surgery as possible. This first postoperative meeting includes new goals for upcoming postoperative rehabilitation.

Postoperative rehabilitation strategies will be the same or similar to preoperative strategies depending on the evaluation. Again the sport psychologist encourages Jim to stay involved in a mentor program or injury support group if possible. If not done previously, coping and mastery tapes may be made so that Jim can utilize these for the remainder of the program. Throughout the rest of the program the sport psychologist and athletic trainer remain in touch to effectively care for Jim until his return to competition.

Once Jim is physically ready to return to competition, the sport psychologist needs to be assured that Jim is also mentally ready to return. Active listening concerning Jim's return can provide an indication of his readiness. There is no easy way to do this; the point is that the athlete is not assumed to be mentally ready, but has been assessed and judged to be mentally ready.

Career-ending Injuries

In many cases, one of the major differences between athletes who will return to competition and those who have suffered a career-ending injury is their perception of their future life (27,37,38). Athletes who plan to return to competition often have hope of returning stronger, faster, or better than they were before, whereas athletes who will not return may feel hopeless, helpless, and in extreme cases, suicidal (27,48). Although both types of athletes may have been the topic of newspaper articles or television news stories at first, the media quickly forgets the athlete whose career is over. Meanwhile, the returning athletes are likely to have their rehabilitation progress covered by the media, and therefore may continue to receive "star" treatment. The sport psychologist must be aware of the different situations likely to occur and recognize the unique needs of athletes in either situation.

Athletes who have suffered a career-ending injury are faced with at least two obstacles different from athletes planning to return to competition. First, they must learn to function effectively on a daily basis given their disability. Second, they must reintegrate into society as a nonathlete or different-sport-athlete, such as a wheelchair basketball player (27,37,38). Therefore this situation requires the sport psychologist and the athlete to focus not only on overcoming roadblocks and regaining confidence, but also on helping the athlete accept a new way of life, which up to this point may have been unappreciated and devalued by the athlete (27).

There are at least three specific ways, in addition to those utilized for an athlete returning to competition, that a sport psychologist can counsel an athlete whose career has been ended by injury. The first is to understand that an athlete is likely to go through a sequence of emotions following such an injury. These emotions, according to Rotella and Heyman (46), based on the work of Kübler-Ross (32) are 1) denial, 2) anger, 3) grief and bargaining, 4) depression, and 5) acceptance. Although Ogilvie (37) describes the range and sequence of the emotions experienced somewhat differently, ([1] denial, [2] projection, [3]) resentment, anger, and hostility, and [4] depression) there is a general consensus among researchers that athletes who suffer a career-ending injury will experience a fairly predictable pattern of emotional reactions (27). By understanding as much as possible about what the athlete is going through, the sport psychologist can provide appropriate and effective counseling dependent upon which emotion the athlete is experiencing. It is important to note that not all athletes go through the pattern of emotions offered by either Rotella and Heyman (46) or Ogilvie (38) and that one athlete's reaction to injury may differ markedly from another athlete's reaction (27).

The second way a sport psychologist can counsel an athlete who will not return to competition is by educating the family and close friends of the athlete on how everyone's life will change. This education includes making them aware of the emotions previously described, teaching them the best ways to cope with their reaction to the athlete's injury, and providing outlets for their concerns. It is essential that family members and friends realize that the athlete's adjustment to, and perception of, a new lifestyle is in large part dependent upon the family's attitude toward the new lifestyle (27).

A third way in which a sport psychologist can help is by introducing the athlete to new careers and sports. For example, players who have lost the use of their legs might enjoy wheelchair sports such as tennis, golf, basketball or competitive fishing. Again, the perception of the athlete toward new endeavors may in large part be influenced by the values of others, and thus care should be taken to present every opportunity with an optimistic attitude (27).

The main difference between working with athletes who will return to competition and those who have suffered a career-ending injury is recognizing the experiences and emotions each is likely to encounter and devising a plan to meet their needs. This plan often entails viewing different injuries from different perspectives depending on the severity of the injury. The overall goal of rehabilitation and the process that will be followed during rehabilitation is different for a returning athlete than an athlete forced to retire, but the care with which the sport psychologist handles the athlete and the commitment of the sport psychologist to helping either athlete should not be different. In each scenario the sport psychologist is encouraged to treat the whole person, not just the injury.

CONCLUSION

When athletes are injured, they may perceive and react to the injury in a negative way. They often experience a setback not only physically but also mentally to their confidence and self-esteem. Today it is no longer appropriate to suggest that athletes who are not psychologically hardy are malingerers or lacking in toughness or are not willing to give 100%. Contemporary athletes are well educated in what it takes for optimal performance, which includes a sound mind as well as a fit body. Thus, it is important for sports medicine team members to be aware of what the athlete is likely to experience and be prepared to respond in effective ways. This entails addressing both the mental, physical, and emotional aspects of rehabilitation. The sports medicine team needs to address the psychological aspects of rehabilitation with the same vigor given to the physical aspects. The addition of a sport psychologist on the rehabilitation team can assist athletes as well as athletic trainers to better handle the long and sometimes arduous task of recovering from injury.

REFERENCES

1. Achterberg J. *Imagery in healing: Shamanism and modern medicine.* New York: Random House, 1985.
2. Andersen MB, Williams JM. A model of stress and athletic injury: prediction and prevention. *J Sport Exercise Psychol* 1988;10:294.
3. Block N. *Imagery.* Cambridge, MA: MIT Press, 1981.
4. Bradley B. *Life on the Run.* New York: Vintage, 1995.
5. Brewer BW, Jeffers KE, Petitpas AJ, Van Raalte JL. Perceptions of psychological interventions in the context of sport injury rehabilitation. *The Sport Psychologist* 1994;8:176.
6. Brewer BW, Van Raalte JL, Linder DE. Role of the sport psychologist in treating injured athletes: a survey of sports medicine providers. *J Appl Sport Psychol* 1991;3:183.
7. Bunker LK, Williams JM. Cognitive techniques for improving performance and building confidence. In: Williams JM, ed. *Applied sport psychology: personal growth to peak performance.* Mountain View, CA: Mayfield, 1986:235.
8. Byerly PN, Worrell T, Gahimer J, Domholdt E. Rehabilitation compliance in an athletic training environment. *J Athletic Training* 1994; 29(4):352.
9. Caplan G. Social support systems. In: Pines A, Aronson E, eds. *Career burnout: causes and cures.* New York: Macmillan, 1988.
10. Dishman RK. *Exercise adherence: its impact on public health.* Champaign, IL: Human Kinetics, 1988.
11. Duda JL, Smart AE, Tappe MK. Predicators of adherence in the rehabilitation of athletic injuries: an application of personal investment theory. *J Sport Exercise Psychol* 1989;11:367.
12. Fisher AC, Domm MA, Wuest DA. Adherence to sports-injury rehabilitation programs. *Phys Sportsmed* 1988;16(7):47.
13. Fisher AC, Hoisington LL. Injured athletes' attitudes and judgments toward rehabilitation adherence. *J Athletic Training* 1993;28:48.
14. Fisher AC, Mullins SA, Frye PA. Athletic trainers' attitudes and judgments of injured athletes' rehabilitation adherence. *J Athletic Training* 1993;28(1):43.
15. Flint FA. Seeing helps believing: modeling in injury rehabilitation.

In: Pargman D, ed. *Psychological bases of sport injuries.* Morganton, WV: Fitness Information Technology, 1993:183.

16. Gieck J. Psychological considerations of rehabilitation. In: Prentice WE, ed. *Rehabilitation techniques in sports medicine.* Boston: Mosby, 1990:107.

17. Gordon S. Sport psychology and the injured athlete: a cognitive-behavioral approach to injury response and injury rehabilitation. *J Canadian Athletic Therapist Assoc,* Fall 1988;4.

18. Gordon S, Milios D, Grove JR. Psychological adjustment to sport injuries: implications for athletes, coaches and family members. *Sports Coaches* 1991;14(2):40.

19. Gordon S, Milios D, Grove JR. Psychological aspects of the recovery process from sport injury, The perspective of sport physiotherapists. *Aust J Sci Med Sport* 1991;23(2):53.

20. Gould D. Goal setting for peak performance. In: Williams JM, ed. *Applied sport psychology: personal growth to peak performance.* Mountain View, CA: Mayfield, 1986.

21. Green LB. The use of imagery in the rehabilitation of injured athletes. *The Sport Psychologist* 1992;6:416.

22. Grove JR, Gordon AMD. The psychological aspects of injury in sport. In: Bloomfield J, Fricker PA, Fitch KD, eds. *Textbook of science and medicine in sport.* Champaign, IL: Human Kinetics, 1992.

23. Hardy CJ, Crace RK. The dimensions of social support when dealing with sport injuries. In: Pargman D, ed. *Psychological bases of sport injuries.* Morgantown, WV: Fitness Information Technology, 1993:121.

24. Hedgpeth EG, Sowa CJ. Addressing the stress of athletic injury rehabilitation in the training room. *The Sport Psychologist* 1996; (in press).

25. Heil J. *Psychology of sport injury.* Champaign, IL: Human Kinetics, 1993.

26. Heil J, Bowman JJ, Bean B. Patient management and the sports medicine team. In: Heil J, ed. *Psychology of sport injury.* Champaign, IL: Human Kinetics, 1993.

27. Henschen KP, Shelley GA. Counseling athletes with permanent disabilities. In: Pargman D, ed. *Psychological bases of sport injuries.* Morgantown, WV: Fitness Information Technology, 1993:251.

28. Ice R. Long-term compliance. *Physical Therapy* 1985;65(12):1832.

29. Ievleva L, Orlick T. Mental links to enhanced healing: an exploratory study. *The Sport Psychologist* 1991;5:25.

30. Jacobson E. Variation of specific muscle contracting during imagination. *Am J Physiol* 1931;96:101.

31. Jacobson E. *Progressive relaxation: a physiological and clinical investigation of muscular states and their significance in psychology and medical practice.* Chicago: University of Chicago Press, 1938.

32. Kübler-Ross E. *On death and dying.* New York: Macmillan, 1969.

33. Lock EA, Shaw KN, Saari LM, Lathram AP. Goal setting and task performance. *Psychol Bull* 1981;90:125.

34. May JR, Sieb GE. Athletic injuries: Psychosocial factors in the onset, sequelae, rehabilitation and prevention. In: May JR, Asken MJ, eds. *Sport psychology: the psychological health of the athlete.* New York: PMA, 1987:157.

35. McCullagh P, Weiss MR, Ross D. Modeling considerations in motor skill acquisition and performance: an intergrated approach. In: Pandolf KB, ed. *Exercise and sport sciences reviews.* Baltimore: Williams & Wilkins, 1989:475.

36. Meichenbaum D. Toward a cognitive theory of self-control. In: Schwartz G, Shapiro D, eds. *Consciousness and self-regulation: advances in research.* New York: Plenum, 1976.

37. Ogilvie BC. Counseling for sports career termination. In: May JR,

Asken MJ, eds. *Sport psychology: the psychological health of the athlete.* New York: PMA, 1987:213.

38. Ogilvie BC, Howe M. The trauma of termination from athletics. In: Williams JM, ed. *Applied sport psychology: personal growth to peak performance.* Mountain View, CA: Mayfield, 1986:365.

39. Podell RN, Gary LR. Compliance: a problem in medical management. *Am Family Phys* 1976;13:74.

40. Rice PL. *Stress and Health.* Pacific Grove, CA: Brooks/Cole, 1992.

41. Richman JM, Hardy CJ, Rosenfeld LB, Callanan RAE. Strategies for enhancing social support networks in sport: a brainstorming experience. *J Appl Sport Psychol* 1989;1:150.

42. Rosenfeld LB, Richman JM, Hardy CJ. Examining social support networks among athletes: description and relationship to stress. *The Sport Psychologist* 1989;3:23.

43. Rotella RJ, Gansneder B, Ojala D, Billings J. Cognitions and coping strategies of elite skiers: an exploratory study of young developing athletes. *J Sport Psychol* 1980;2:350.

44. Rotella RJ, Malone C, Ojala D. Facilitating athletic performance through the use of mastery and coping tapes. In: Bunker LK, Rotella RJ, Reilly AS, eds. *Sport psychology: psychological considerations in maximizing sport performance.* Ithaca, NY: Movement Publications, 1985:197.

45. Rotella RJ, Heyman SR. Stress, injury, and the psychological rehabilitation of athletes. In: Williams JM, ed. *Applied sport psychology: personal growth to peak performance.* Mountain View, CA: Mayfield Publishing, 1986.

46. Rotella RJ, Heyman SR. Stress, injury, and the psychological rehabilitation of athletes. In: Williams JM, ed. *Applied sport psychology: personal growth to peak performance.* Mountain View, CA: Mayfield, 1993:338.

47. Shumaker SA, Brownell A. Toward a theory of social support. *J Social Support* 1984;40(4):11.

48. Smith AM, Milliner ER. Injured athletes and the risk of suicide. *J Athletic Training* 1994;29(4):337.

49. Sowa CJ. Understanding clients' perceptions of stress. *J Counseling Develop* 1992;71:179.

50. Turk DC, Meichenbaum D, Genest M. *Pain and behavioral medicine: a cognitive-behavioral perspective.* New York: Guilford Press, 1983.

51. Turk DC, Salovey P, Litt MD. Adherence: A cognitive behavioral perspective. In: Gerber KE, Nehemkis AM, eds. *Compliance: the dilemma of the chronically ill.* New York: Springer, 1985.

52. Vealey R. Imagery training for performance enhancement. In: Williams JM, ed. *Applied sport psychology: personal growth to peak performance.* Mountain View, CA: Mayfield, 1986:209.

53. Weiss MR, Troxel RK. Psychology of the injured athlete. *Athletic Training* 1986;21(2):104.

54. Wiese DM, Weiss MR, Yukelson DP. Sport psychology in the training room: a survey of athletic trainers. *The Sport Psychologist* 1991;5:15.

55. Wiese DM, Weiss MR. Psychological rehabilitation and physical injury: implications for the sportsmedicine team. *The Sport Psychologist* 1987;1:318.

56. Wiese-Bjornstal DM, Smith AM. Counseling strategies for enhanced recovery of injured athletes within a team approach. In: Pargman D, ed. *Psychological bases of sport injuries.* Morganton, WV: Fitness Information Technology, 1993:149.

57. Williams JM, Roepke N. Psychology of injury and injury rehabilitation. In: Singer RN, Murphy M, Tennant LK, eds. *Handbook of research on sport psychology.* New York: Macmillan, 1993:815.

58. Worrell TW. The use of behavioral and cognitive techniques to facilitate achievement of rehabilitation goals. *J Sport Rehab* 1992; 1:69.

The Injured Athlete, Third Edition,
edited by D. H. Perrin.
Lippincott–Raven Publishers, Philadelphia © 1999.

CHAPTER 8

Research Methods and Injury Surveillance in Sports Medicine

Bruce M. Gansneder

The study of athletic injuries has come to be known as "injury surveillance." According to Webster, surveillance means to keep "close watch on a person or thing." So, injury surveillance means to keep close watch on or to track the occurrence of injuries. Since injuries are not planned or intentional, the study of them presents problems not found in experimental research. Injury surveillance has multiple purposes including documenting the incidence of various injuries, trying to understand why they occur, attempting to identify preventative measures, and even understanding how they are treated or could be treated in the natural setting. This chapter deals with the study of athletic injuries in natural settings. It explores the purposes of such studies, the major issues to be dealt with in the conduct of such studies (1,3,5), and presents a strategy for the conduct of such studies in sports medicine facilities.

THE PURPOSES OF INJURY STUDIES

Injuries occur on a day-to-day basis in all sports. Sports medicine personnel observe, diagnose, and treat injuries and try to do the best they can to help prevent them. Although they routinely record these injuries, it is unlikely that they study either the incidence of these injuries or the reasons why they happened. Consequently, their knowledge of injuries tends to be anecdotal and selective. Systematic injury studies can ultimately identify measures to prevent injuries, reduce their frequency, or reduce their severity. Injury studies attempt to understand how often various injuries occur and the factors that contribute to or cause the injuries.

B. M. Gansneder: Curry School of Education, University of Virginia, Charlottesville, Virginia 22903

The remainder of this chapter explores the following issues:

1. Choice of injury to study
2. Definition or classification of injuries
3. Injury recordings
4. Determination of incidence rates
5. Selected models for studying injuries
6. Study designs
7. Surveillance instruments
8. Developing a surveillance system for your facility

CHOICE OF INJURY TO STUDY

There are a myriad of athletic injuries in any sport or season. A comprehensive surveillance study would monitor all injuries that occur and try to explain why they happened. The time and costs associated with such a study are usually prohibitive. Accordingly we need criteria for choosing one injury over another. As can be seen in Table 8.1, injuries are chosen for study for practical and theoretical reasons, because the injury occurs a lot or because of its consequences, because it is easy to study, or because its occurrence and treatment needs to be documented.

INJURY CLASSIFICATION AND DEFINITION

At first glance, it would seem that the detection and classification of injuries would be simple. Someone would report an injury and describe the conditions under which it occurred, while noting the type of the injury and its severity. But because it is multi-faceted, classifying injuries can be done in terms of the nature of the injury, medical diagnosis, how long and in what manner the

TABLE 8.1. *Criteria for selection of injuries to study*

Time of occurrence
Sport or physical activity in which the injury occurred
Frequency of occurrence
Severity of injury
Cost of injury to the athlete or facility
Ease or difficulty of injury recording
Potential for quantification of injury
Importance of injury to outside agencies, e.g., insurance
     companies
Visibility or importance of the sport
Likelihood of lost playing time from the injury
Length of hospitalization or disability from injury
Potential of injury recurrence

injury is treated, financial costs associated with the injury, how the injury feels to the athlete, the effect of the injury on the athlete's performance or sport, time lost, or time lost to other activities such as work (6,9,11,13).

Insurance Classification

We could look at only injuries for which insurance claims are filed. These injuries are likely to be more severe. Filing an insurance claim necessitates effort on the part of the athlete and the person treating the injury. The athlete may avoid treatment and the person treating the injury may only file cases for which there is a high probability of reimbursement. The result would be that only the most serious injuries would be studied and other injuries would be ignored. We would then miss other injuries that occur and we would underestimate sports injuries.

Since only more serious injuries would be studied, relying on insurance claims would reduce the variance in the injury measure. This, in turn, would minimize the statistical relationship between "severity of injury" and other variables. As a consequence, we might underestimate how injuries (or severity of injuries) are related to gender, exposure time, experience.

Assessment by Medical Personnel

Studying injuries that have been treated by medical personnel might result in accurate and valid diagnoses of injuries. Injury data on athletes who are taken to the hospital could be recorded by hospital personnel. However, it is most likely that athletes will be taken to the hospital only when there is suspicion that an injury is serious. Less serious injuries would tend to be ignored. An option would be to have a medical person present at practices or games or available to come to the training room. Many high schools do not even have full-time athletic trainers. They are even less likely to have a full-time physician. Consequently, few high schools would be able to collect appropriate data.

Length of Incapacitation

This is probably the most common way to classify injuries. Length of incapacitation is an indirect measure of severity of injury, since it has a psychological component. Athletes don't all respond to injuries in the same way. They differ in their desire to please coaches, their tolerance for pain, motivation to play, and so on. The same level of injury may result in longer incapacitation for some athletes, shorter incapacitation for others. Length of incapacitation may also differ by sport. An injury that will restrict play in one sport may not impact an athlete's performance in another sport. A softball pitcher with a broken finger on her throwing hand may not be able to pitch, but a runner with the same injury may still be able to run. The runner's injury might not even be recorded since the length of incapacitation was zero. If it were recorded, we might believe that the runner's broken finger was less of an injury than that suffered by the softball pitcher. This suggests the importance of recording the nature and location of the injury as well as the sport within which the injury occurred.

Anatomical Tissue Diagnosis

Diagnosis to determine whether there has been damage to bone, muscle, tendon, or nerve tissue could be done by a physician. Noyes et al. (9) recommends this as the most objective way to determine whether there has been an injury.

Reduction or Loss of Function

The injured athlete may be unable to practice or to play in a game, but changes in function could be assessed manually or by using a machine. These changes could be measured against some predetermined standard or relationship to measures taken at the beginning of the season. Manual- or machine-based analysis of range of motion or strength could be done by a physician, an athletic trainer, or other allied health person.

RECORDING INJURIES

The reporting of the injury could be done by trained observers, by the athlete, a coach, an athletic trainer, a physician, or an allied medical person. The choice of the data recorder may affect the timing of the data collection as well as the diagnosis and classification of injuries. For example, since athletic trainers cannot legally diagnose injuries, they cannot be used to collect that kind of data. But there are a number of injury assessments they can make. They also may be the most qualified to record information about the conditions under which injuries occur. Sometimes individuals will need special training in the use of specific instruments.

Trained Observers

Injuries could be studied by using trained observers. They could attend practices and games and record the injuries as they occur. After the game, or if a player leaves the game, the observer could supplement his report with additional information gathered from the physician or athletic trainer. In addition, game and practice films could be analyzed to identify injuries. Although the purpose of game films is not to study injuries, normal filming often captures athletic injuries as they happen. A third alternative would be to place observers in the sports medicine facility where they would record the injuries that are presented.

The use of observers, however, normally restricts the amount of data that can be collected. This process is also extremely time consuming. To increase objectivity, an observation schedule would have to be developed, and observers would have to be hired and trained. Periodically, the training would need to be repeated. Observers might spend a great deal of time waiting to collect what might result in a small amount of data. These disadvantages suggest that this approach may be too costly in time, expense, and personnel. The use of certified athletic trainers and student athletic trainers to do the observation could reduce the cost since they are present during practice and games, but this could interfere with their work as athletic trainers.

Players

Players could be asked to complete an injury report form whenever an injury occurs, or at regular intervals during the season. A coach or athletic trainer could be designated to ensure that players complete these forms. However, athletes may over- or under-report the data. Other research suggests that both the reliability and validity of self-reports are affected by the time elapsed since the reported event occurred, the personal significance of the event, and the specificity of the reporting instructions. The longer the time between the occurrence of an injury and the athlete's report, the less accurate will be the report. Since subjects report significant events more reliably, reports of severe injuries may be more reliably reported than less severe injuries. To control for the specificity of reporting instructions, specific criteria could be provided on the reporting form. Athletes can be asked about the nature of the injury, the body part affected, and the conditions under which the injury occurred. Two other difficulties associated with self-reports cause two major problems. First, individuals exhibit wide variations in

their responses to injury and pain. Second, it may be difficult for individuals to provide accurate self reports. The accuracy of these self-reports may be increased by collecting them as soon after the injury as possible and by providing the individual with specific criteria to use in their self-reports.

Physicians

As mentioned above, the physician can provide an accurate medical diagnosis. She or he can correctly identify the severity of the injury. Reliance on physician-collected data, however, requires either that the physician be at all practices and games to be studied, or that the injured athletes be taken immediately to a physician for diagnosis. Unlike a major college that can support the costs of a team physician who would attend games and practices, the same cannot be said for a small rural high school. On the other hand, if injured athletes must be taken to a physician probably only those with more serious injuries will be taken. Once again, these kinds of studies would tend to reflect only the most serious injuries.

Coaches

Coaches, of course, would be at practices and games, and would be in a position to witness most injuries that occur. Unfortunately, coaches are not trained in the diagnosis of injuries, nor can they legally diagnose. Their primary responsibility is to attend to coaching and not to injuries. In addition, coaches may have a tendency to underestimate the severity of injuries. Once again, each of these factors may operate to reduce the recording of less severe injuries.

Athletic Trainers

Athletic trainers are also likely to be at practices and games. Although many secondary schools do not have full-time athletic trainers, most have at least part-time athletic trainers or access to an athletic trainer. As with coaches, however, athletic trainers are not allowed to diagnose injuries. Unlike coaches, however, they are skilled in the assessment of injuries. They are trained in manual and machine assessments, and can do performance assessments.

DETERMINING INCIDENCE RATES

Some authors (2) distinguish between incidence and prevalence. Incidence is the occurrence of injuries to the subjects studied over the duration of the study. Incidence includes only new injuries, not those that occurred prior to the study. Prevalence refers to all injuries that have occurred to the study group past and present but counted only at a single point in time. Respondents would be asked to report on injuries that had occurred in the present or in the past.

One of the reasons for collecting data on sports injuries is to determine the risk of injury that an athlete faces. Consequently, we need information about how often an injury occurs. We could then estimate the probability of an injury occurring. Assuming that we can define an injury and we know from whom we should collect the data, it would seem to be a simple matter, to just count the number of injuries and report them.

We could report that there were seven anterior cruciate ligament injuries (ACLs), four concussions, and so on. But, the meaning of these numbers depends on the total number of possible incidents or amount of exposure. There might be a total of 50 football players or 7 volleyball players. Injuries may occur over a period of time, such as seven ACLs this week, or this season, or last year, or the last 4 years. Injuries could be reported as a function of participation time such as minutes, hours, days, or sporting events (e.g., per game). Since many injuries (e.g., sprains, concussions) can occur repeatedly to the same person, they could be reported per person. Five of the 50 football players on a team could each play in one game for 30 minutes and sustain two concussions each. These are very different numbers that might lead us to very different conclusions.

When data are only available at the aggregate level it may be difficult to interpret incidence rates, since little is known about the number of players or the amount of exposure. This often happens when data are collected retrospectively. Coaches, for example, might be asked to report the number of concussions during the 3-year period before and after a helmet change. An analysis might be done to see whether there has been a reduction in the incidence of concussions. These data may be very unreliable. In addition, factors other than the helmet change may account for a decrease or increase in the number of concussions. It is possible that the number of players, or the average amount of playing time, or the number of games has changed across this time period.

Injury incidence ought to be tracked separately for each sport. For example, football players may be more likely to sustain injuries than volleyball players. We could simply count the number of injuries for football players and the number of injuries for volleyball players. At a given school there might have been 100 football injuries and only 50 volleyball injuries. It would appear that football players at this school are twice as likely to suffer an injury than volleyball players.

Variations in exposure or amount of participation will also change a player's opportunity for being injured. Obviously a player who participates 6 days a week for 4 hours a day is at less risk than a player who participates 7 days a week for 6 hours a day. The first player has 24 hours of participation per week whereas the second player has 42.

So injury rates or injury incidences need to be calculated relative to time period, number of players, and/or amount of exposure. We need to calculate the number of injuries for a given time period, per some number of players (say 100, or 1,000), per amount of exposure.

If data are collected on a day-to-day basis and recorded at the player/incident level along with information about the player's participation time, incidence rates can probably be calculated per game, per person, per week, or per hour. These rates could then be converted to a 1,000 hour or 10,000 hour base if desired.

If it is not possible to determine participation rates for each player, then rates could be estimated for the team or for players who "usually" participate at different rates. Team rates would be based on the total number of hours per week that the team is either in practice or playing games. Each week a football team might practice for five 4-hour days and play a 1-hour game for a total of 21 hours. This may occur over a period of 12 weeks for a total of 252 hours. Forty (40) players times 252 hours is a total of 10,080 hours a season. If there were 200 injuries during the season, this would equal 19.8 injuries for every 100 hours of exposure, 19.8 injuries for every 1,000 hours, and 198 injuries for every 10,000. These rates could be compared to injury rates in other sports.

When exact playing times can not be determined, it is sometimes possible to arrive at indirect estimates. The National Athletic Injury/Illness Reporting System (NAIRS) injury surveillance system classifies players as "star," "regular," or "substitute." Different estimates of playing time could be made for each type of player leading to the creation of injury incidence on the basis of exposure time. Then, comparisons could be made between the incidence of injuries across these three types of players.

Fictitious data on members of five men's teams and four women's teams for one season are presented in Tables 8.2 and 8.3. These are fall and spring sports that

TABLE 8.2. *A fictitious example: Number of athletes and length of season for five men's sports and four women's sports*

Men's basketball:	13 athletes, 150 days
Men's lacrosse:	25 athletes, 127 days
Men's baseball:	30 athletes, 127 days
Men's football:	100 athletes, 127 days
Men's track:	50 athletes, 127 days
Women's basketball:	15 athletes, 150 days
Women's field hockey:	25 athletes, 90 days
Women's softball:	25 athletes, 112 days
Women's track:	50 athletes, 127 days

occur from September to June. Data on injuries are collected from mid-August to mid-May. As can be seen in Table 8.2, there is a total of 333 athletes who spend a total of 1137 days per season. The number of athletes per team ranges from 13 to 100 and the number of days per season ranges from 90 to 150. During this time period, the 333 athletes incurred a total of 2,403 injuries. This represents an average of over 7 (7.22) injuries per athlete for the season. Since the number of days and hours in the season varies in sport, it makes sense to calculate incidence by the number of days or hours of exposure. These calculations result in about 6 (5.79) injuries for every 100 days of exposure and about one injury for every 100 hours of exposure. Clearly different ways of calculating injury rates result in very different numerical values. But these are aggregate indices.

If we calculate alternative injury rates by team as shown in Table 8.3, we get an entirely different picture. The largest absolute numbers of injuries occur in football, men's track, and women's track. But this is primarily a result of these teams involving more athletes. The highest average number of injuries per player are in football, lacrosse, and men's basketball. These three sports also have the highest per 100 days and per 1,000 hours of exposure. The rates per 100 days and per 1,000 hours or multiplicands of them could be used to compare injury rates at the high school level or even the injury rates of recreational athletes.

CONCEPTUAL MODELS FOR STUDYING INJURIES

An injury study can be as simple as keeping track of a single type of injury. The concern over the higher incidence of anterior cruciate ligament injuries in females would lend itself to this type of injury study. You might be solely concerned with the incidence and potential causative factors of ACLs in female athletes. One approach would be to make a list of all of the possible causes of the injury and then study them all. That approach would not be very efficient, thoughtful, or practical. Like other research in sports medicine, injury surveillance should be guided by theoretical or conceptual models of the phenomenon to be studied. For example, you might identify several anatomical factors such as quadriceps angle, hyperpronation, tibial varum, to measure in female athletes who rupture their ACL.

A number of conceptual models have been proposed by van Mechelen (11) to study the incidence (and prevention) of injuries. These models suggest factors or conditions that might increase (or decrease) the incidence of injuries. You could use one or another of the models to help focus an injury study. A brief overview of three of these is provided here: the stress/capacity model, the sports behavior model, and the stress/strain/capacity model.

Stress/Capacity Model

The stress/capacity model suggests that there are two major sets of factors that contribute to or "cause" injuries: stress factors and capacity factors. The stress factors are factors external to the person, and the capacity factors are internal to the person (Table 8.4).

Capacity factors might be physiological or psychological. van Mechelen suggests that injuries occur when there is an imbalance between stress factors and capacity factors. When a person has the capacity to deal with the stressors there is less likelihood of an injury occurring. Therefore, when we notice injuries occurring we try to identify the source of the imbalance. It may be a function of the playing conditions (e.g., the field, the weather); the behavioral demands (e.g., turning, twisting, hitting); the equipment being used (e.g., knee braces, taping); position played (e.g., guard, running back). It may be that players do not have the capacity to deal with these factors. The imbalance could be a function of the capacity of the player. It could be a function of the player's strength or flexibility; of the player's skill in making or playing a particular position; of the player's willingness to work harder at the sport. If we were to use this model to design

TABLE 8.3. *Alternative injury rates by team*

Sport	No. of players	Total no. of injuries	Average per player	Average per 100 days	Average per 1000 hours
Football	100	950	9.5	7.5	12.4
Lacrosse	25	213	8.5	6.7	11.1
Basketball	13	110	8.5	5.7	9.5
Basketball (Women's)	15	113	7.5	5.0	8.3
Field Hockey	25	163	6.5	7.2	12.0
Track	50	325	6.5	5.2	8.6
Track (Women's)	50	275	5.5	4.4	7.3
Baseball	30	165	5.5	4.1	6.9
Softball	25	88	3.5	3.0	5.0
Total	333	2403	7.2	5.8	9.6

a surveillance study, we would articulate the stressors and the capacity factors and then plan to collect data on all or some of these. Then we would see whether the incidence (or type) of injuries differs for the various factors.

We might be most interested in those factors over which we have some control. We might reschedule games in bad weather, for instance, or improve the equipment, train players better, or redesign conditioning programs. Part of our task would be to see whether we need to adjust the stressors or the person. For example, teeth may not have the capacity to withstand blows to the mouth. If so, this would be an imbalance between the capacity and the stressor. We are probably not going to be able to strengthen the teeth, but the addition of a mouthguard may restore the balance.

Sports Behavior Model

A second model is the sports behavior model. The sports behavior model adds psycho-social factors. It suggests that injury risk "is primarily dependent on the interaction between athletes and their personal characteristics, either physical or psychological, and the sports environment." The presence of these interactions suggests a dynamic model. The model van Mechelen proposes includes risk factors within which specific sports behaviors occur. The behaviors themselves are driven by an athlete's attitudes, feelings of self-efficacy, and by social influences. Risk factors are identified with regard to the athlete (physical and psychological factors), load, personal equipment, and environmental (physical and human factors) variables. Attitudes that have to do with expected consequences of the behavior are also relevant. These might have to do with fear of injury, the rewards associated with succeeding, or the punishments associated with losing. Social influences are influences from teammates, friends, the coach, and the crowd. Feelings of self-efficacy have to do with the athlete's belief that he or she is able to perform the behavior.

If we used this model to plan injury studies, we would still study the kinds of internal and external factors suggested by the stress/capacity model, but we would include psychological and sociological variables. We would want to determine whether an increase in injuries is related to the following kinds of variables: a player's orientation to risk-taking, social pressure to perform, motivation to succeed, or fear of failure. We would want to see how these psycho-social factors adjust the relationship between internal and external factors. It may be, for example, that by providing mouthguards we would trigger certain psycho-social factors. If players wear mouthguards (or other protective equipment), for example, they might have a false sense of security that would make them overly confident and lead them to more aggressive and risky sports behavior.

Stress-Strain-Capacity Model

The stress-strain-capacity model adds a time dimension within which short-term or long-term injuries may occur. The model defines stress as including both external (environmental) and internal (personal) factors that, in the context of the capacities the individual brings to the sports behavior, influence both short-term effects (strain) and long-term, or permanent, effects. In this model we would view an individual athlete as coming to a situation with certain capabilities including the ability to control the amount of strain in the activity. These factors may influence short-term effects (acute injuries) that go away before the next activity. They may also produce long-term effects, such as temporary incapacitation or permanent damage.

If we use this model in injury studies we would add a time dimension. We would consider the duration of the sports activity and the duration of the injury. It may be that injuries are different in shorter vs. longer term activities. It may also be that a sports activity that occurs year after year will produce different kinds of injuries. We would also pay more attention to the issue of short- and long-term injuries and to the issue of the repetition of injuries (such as repeated concussions).

These models remind us that a complex set of factors may be related to the occurrence of sports injuries. Most injuries occur in natural environments like a playing field, a track, a ski slope, or a street. The physical characteristics of these environments are not controlled in the way that we can control the temperature, lighting, or social environment of an experimental laboratory. Injuries happen to individual players who differ in skill and desire. Players wear different kinds of equipment and perform different types of sports activities with different types of competitors. All of this happens in some time frame. One sports event may be longer or shorter than another. Sports activities may occur only for a moment, or for a week, or over a period of years. Any of these factors may influence the incidence, type, or severity of injuries. Identifying the specific cause or set of causes of sports injuries is a diffi-

TABLE 8.4. *Internal and external factors contributing to injury from van Mechelen (1992) stress/capacity model*

Stress factors: Factors external to the person
  Weather
  Field condition
  Equipment
  Degree of risk
  Involvement of other participants
Capacity Factors: Factors internal to the person
  Strength
  Flexibility
  Personality
  Motivation
  Attitude

cult proposition. But models like these can help us define the scope and focus of our specific study.

STUDY DESIGNS (10,14,15)

The ultimate purpose of injury surveillance is to identify the causes of injuries so they can be prevented. To identify causes we need to provide solid evidence that a presumed cause is indeed the cause. To do this we need to: demonstrate that the cause and the effect are related, that the cause precedes the effect, and that other plausible causes can be ruled out. The designs presented below differ in the degree to which they accomplish these goals. As shown in Table 8.5, these designs differ in the degree to which the experimenter can exercise control over the research situation.

Randomized Experiments

In a randomized experiment, subjects may be formed into research groups in two different ways. They may be randomly sampled from some population and then randomly assigned to research groups. Random sampling allows us to generalize back to the target population. A random assignment allows generalization to a theoretical population and assures that differences between research groups, prior to the introduction of the independent variable, are random.

When it is not possible in experimental studies to sample from a population, researchers might take available subjects and then randomly assign them to treatment groups. We might randomly assign football players to wear a new kind of faceguard, while the remaining players continue wearing the current type. Then we would study the occurrence of facial injuries. In this case, although generalization might be made to a theoretical population, the specific identity of the population that they represent would be unknown. We would not know if the results can be generalized to football players in other age groups, or leagues.

In experimental studies, we can control the introduction and nature of the independent variable. In injury studies, the independent variable is some potential factor that we believe will affect the incidence of injuries. In experiments, the independent variable can be controlled in three different ways: the time of occurrence, the duration, and its intensity or nature.

First, we may control the exact time at which it occurs. It will be given now and not later, for instance. It will be given today and not tomorrow. This is critical because a treatment can be considered a potential cause only if it occurs before some potential effect. It is possible that more assertive players would choose to wear faceguards.

This might allow them to be even more assertive which might then increase their likelihood of injury.

Second, we may control how long the independent variable lasts. In injury studies, it would be important to control both the length of time of the study (e.g., a season) and the exposure time. We probably cannot control who starts and who doesn't start. When we cannot control factors, we need to compare them as they occur. Starters have more exposure time than those on the second or third team. We may need to compare results with starters to those of other players. Specific positions may result in more playing time. Consequently, we may need to make comparisons across playing positions.

Third, experiments control for the intensity at which the independent variable is delivered. How much of the face is covered? Of what kind of material is the faceguard made? We will probably not be able to control for the amount of force that is applied in contacts with the face, but we might compare players at different positions. We might also classify the intensity of the contact.

Controlling the Context or Environment under which the Independent Variable Is Introduced

We may control the context within which the independent variable occurs. In a laboratory situation we can remove other variables in which we have no interest. We can be sure that there are no noises, that the subject is alone in the laboratory, and that the temperature is appropriate. However, in a game or in a practice session, a host of other factors are present. It may be raining or sunny. There may be a large or small crowd. The opponents may be weak or strong. The playing field may be groomed or messy. We could limit our initial testing of faceguards to certain games (e.g., more or less competitive), or to certain game conditions (e.g., temperature or amount of rainfall).

In most studies we can control the time at which dependent measures are taken. Dependent measures can be taken at a single point in time or at multiple points in time. We might keep track of injuries only after the introduction of the faceguards. If subjects had been randomized to research groups, prior differences would be random. Post differences could then be attributed to the independent variable.

Multiple (e.g., weekly) measures of facial injuries could

TABLE 8.5. *Factors which researchers may control*

Control the selection or assignment of subjects
Control the introduction and nature of the independent variable
Control the context or environment of the study
Control the timing of the measurement of the dependent variable

be taken for 6 weeks before the faceguards are worn and then for 6 weeks while they are being worn. This would allow comparisons of scores on the measure from before the introduction of the treatment and after its occurrence. Of course, any number of measures could be taken before or after the introduction of the treatment.

Although it is possible to conduct experimental studies on the treatment of injuries (e.g., controlled studies can be made of the treatment of injuries with alternative modalities), the study of the causes of injuries does not easily lend itself to experiments. A recent survey of epidemiologic studies found that only 7% could be classified as experimental. For ethical reasons, researchers are unlikely to try out different ways to manipulate or "cause" injuries. An exception to this would be the study of the delayed onset of muscle soreness. Muscle soreness is manipulated and then studies are done on reduction of function or mobility and pain. Studies could also be done on the effect of various modalities on return to function, increased mobility, pain reduction, and the rates of recovery.

In studies of the natural occurrence of injuries, athletes are not randomly assigned to various injury conditions. Neither are they randomly assigned to various sports, athletic functions, or positions. Each of these variables might increase the risk of injury. All of these things occur for "natural" reasons and in "natural" kinds of ways. As a result, it becomes more difficult to pinpoint "causes." There may be many alternative explanations for the occurrence of injuries.

Although we cannot usually control the occurrence, duration, or intensity of these causative factors, we can usually control the selection of persons and situations to study, the type of data to be collected, the timing and quality of data collection, the source of the data, and the nature of the data.

We can do this with prospective or retrospective designs. Prospective designs are those that define and select the population and/or sample to be studied in advance of the occurrence of injuries. In retrospective designs data are collected on players after the occurrence of injuries.

Prospective Data Collection

First, a population or selected samples within an identified population are selected. At some appropriate time, such as the beginning of a season, data would be collected on each athlete. These data would include descriptive characteristics as well as factors that we might hypothesize would cause injuries. These data would serve as baseline data and function as explanatory variables in later analyses. Data on injuries incurred by each athlete would be recorded as they happened. Information would be recorded describing the time of the injury, the conditions under which it occurred, the nature of the injury, and its severity. At some later appropriate time, such as the end of the year or the end of the season, analyses would be done to describe injured and uninjured athletes and to make comparisons between them relative to the hypothesized causative or associative factors.

Prospective studies are most feasible at a single or a few sites. At the beginning of the season, the researchers would collect all of the basic data on each player in the sport. This would include demographic data and might even include social-psychological data. Basic physical information such as height and weight would also be collected. We would record those things that might be affected by injuries such as specific skills, flexibility, range of motion, balance, and strength, as well as measures of significant body parts. The variables chosen for study ought to be those that we expect are related to the occurrence of injuries. They might be variables that would increase the likelihood of injury. If it was believed that the amount of contact varied by position in women's field hockey, then one would collect data on players' positions. We might also record variables that would be diminished by an injury, such as strength. Initially researchers should probably start by identifying the most likely variables. These might be identified from the research or clinical literature, the models described above, or from the expertise or experience of the athletic trainers. The decision probably also should reflect what is manageable, doable, and affordable. Revisions could then be made from year to year on the basis of what is learned. The fact that the data are collected prospectively means that the same data are collected on injured and noninjured athletes, so the two groups can be compared.

This kind of study has a number of advantages. First, data are systematically collected on every athlete. This reduces the possibility that athletes in the study would be identified for irrelevant reasons. For example, it reduces the possibility that we would study only those athletes who complain about their injuries. In retrospective studies these athletes would be more likely to be studied. But the longitudinal nature of the prospective study, as well as its comprehensiveness, requires a lot of resources in terms of time, money, and personnel. It is also very difficult to do this on a state, regional, or national scale. Because that calls for complex sampling procedures, appropriate sites could be sampled and then random sampling (or stratified random sampling) could be done within each site.

Collecting Data on Injuries as They Occur

In this approach data would be collected only on injured athletes. This would reduce the number of persons studied as well as the amount of time needed for data collection, thereby reducing the cost of the system. It would be possible to track the incidence and nature of injuries. Other comparisons could be drawn between the types and severity of injuries occurring in different sports, under different conditions, or any of a number of other current factors. Since preinjury data are not available, it would be impossible to look at individual changes. Injured athletes could be compared with a sample of uninjured athletes, but differences might be preexistent.

Retrospective Data Collection

Retrospective studies collect data only after injuries have occurred. No predata are collected. At a given point in time athletes who are injured could be compared with those who have not been. This approach is limited because none of the design controls described above are present, and so pinpointing causes becomes very difficult.

Cross-Sectional Studies

Cross-sectional studies are retrospective studies in which the sampling is more sophisticated. In these studies the researcher carefully identifies the target populations from which he then draws a sample or samples at a single point in time. Then comparisons might be made of subgroups in the population. The researcher might sample injured and noninjured athletes from the university population at some point in time. Then through surveys or interviews, athletes might be asked to report on injuries they have sustained over some period of time (e.g., the last year). They might be asked to indicate the nature of the injury and the conditions under which the injury occurred. Depending on the focus of the study, a wide variety of questions could be asked to determine the athlete's exposure time and variables that might be related to the injury. These studies allow the collection of a lot of information with a minimum of time and cost. Analyses would focus on the relationship between injuries and any of the factors studied. A researcher might ask football players about their injuries as well as the turf on which they played when the injury occurred (e.g., natural/artificial). Comparisons could be then made to see if the type or severity of the injury was different on the two types of turf. Causal claims in this kind of study are very weak. Many other factors might be associated with the type of turf that would explain the difference in injuries. It could be that artificial turf costs more and so teams that have it have bigger, stronger players who inflict more damage on their opponents. These designs also suffer from their dependence on the respondent's (e.g., player, coach) recall since questions are asked only at a single point in time.

SOME SURVEILLANCE INSTRUMENTS

Large-scale surveillance studies are expensive and relatively rare because it is difficult to agree on appropriate definition and measures of injuries, and because injury surveillance is not a controlled experimentation methodology. The systems have tended to be very complex and require substantial time commitment from athletic trainers or other allied personnel on site.

Nevertheless, a number of exemplary systems have been developed (4,8,12). Damron reviewed some of these. Meeunisse and Love (7) reviewed 16 systems. Eleven are currently in use, one is being developed and four are no longer in use. A brief review of four systems is provided here. The National Electronic Injury Surveillance System (NEISS) was developed by the U.S. Consumer Product Safety Commission to collect data on injuries related to consumer products. NEISS data are collected on emergency room patients who have sustained a product-related injury that either requires medical help or restricts the patient's activity for at least one day. This system was designed to be national and to allow for the continuous collection of data electronically. Data are collected on hundreds of products including types of sports products.

The NCAA Injury Surveillance system has specific forms for different sports (e.g., football, baseball, volleyball). Table 8.6 lists the criteria for a reportable injury as defined by the NCAA system.

The National Athletic Injury Reporting System (NAIRS) was developed in 1974. As reported by Clarke (3) the NAIRS was developed to "provide immediate access to meaningful information on a continuous basis." Although nonsport injuries can be identified with this system, it was primarily developed to track coach-supervised practice or game play. The designers wanted it to be uniform, versatile, and inexpensive, while providing continuous input and output. It had simple recording methods and allowed for periodic in-depth studies and confidentiality. It acknowledged variability in diagnoses from site to site, included estimates of the severity of injury, and was controlled by an interdisciplinary committee. This instrument is no longer in use. Its development was very thoughtful and thorough and very comprehen-

TABLE 8.6. *Criteria for a reportable injury according to the NCAA injury surveillance system*

An injury is to be reported if it:
Occurs as a result of participation in an organized intercollegiate practice or contest
Requires medical attention by a team athletics trainer or physician
Results in any restriction of the athlete's participation or performance for one or more days beyond the day of injury
Causes any dental injury regardless of the loss

sive. It may have, in fact, been too comprehensive and collapsed under its own weight. But a sports medicine facility could revise parts of the instrument for local use.

Data collection was expected to be done by National Athletic Trainers Association (NATA) certified athletic trainers. A fairly complicated system was set up that included a NAIRS coordinator, a district coordinator, cluster coordinators, recorders, and the athletic director. Four forms were developed: the institution abstract, the sports season close-out abstract, the participant abstract, and the case abstract. Basic data on the institution were to be collected at the beginning of the year through the institution abstract. The sports season close-out abstract was to be completed after the season had begun. This form used to collect data on the physician and the coach as well as on the equipment and facilities. The participant abstract gathered information on each athlete. Each athlete was assigned a four-digit code and asked to provide information on his/her sport, skill level, years of experience, height, weight, and sex. The case abstract was used to document specific injuries. This form called for information on the nature of the injury, the date of injury, the conditions under which the injury occurred, the immediate actions taken, and the consequent management of the injury. Date of return to performance was also recorded on this form. This made it possible to study the relationship between many of these factors and the time to return to function. Specific codes were provided for each piece of information. In addition, codes were available for selected sports. Damron presents an example of the codes for volleyball. Codes are presented for the player's position, type of activity, playing surface, and equipment.

A computerized system called T-Whiz was developed by Human Kinetics in 1994. It is a general system that makes it possible for a training facility to keep track of personal and insurance data as well as equipment and supplies. It was designed for college and high school training rooms but could probably be adapted for any sports medicine facility.

Three kinds of data can be collected on any athlete: basic, personal, and demographic data; data on any injury the athlete sustains; and data on any treatment the athlete receives. Initially, a record is set up for each athlete and then these three separate but interconnected data sets are built. A separate computer screen is provided for the entry of each type of data.

Basic data includes the athlete's name and address, sport played, and insurance information. Six different medical notes or alerts can be entered to remind the athletic trainer of specific medical considerations the athlete may have, including allergies or prescriptions currently used. There is also room for 12 additional pieces of information such as whether the athlete has had a physical, wears eyeglasses, and so on. Presumably other kinds of fitness data (e.g., preseason strength or flexible values) could be recorded there.

A separate record or screen is provided for injuries. It includes the date of the injury, the body part or structure involved (e.g., eye, foot), the type of injury (e.g., tear, abrasion), the status of the injury, how many days the athlete was injured, the sport played, the surface on which the injury occurred, whether the injury occurred in a game or practice and at home or away, and the number of games or practices missed. There is also a place for the athletic trainer or other medical person to provide other details about the injury such as the kinds of assessments that were made and plans for treatment of the injury. Finally, there is a place to record insurance data including the status of the claim, when it was paid, the charges, and the expected and actual insurance payments.

The third record includes data on any treatments the athlete receives. Treatment data includes the date and time, the body part (i.e., structure), whether it was related to a previous injury, the sport within which the injury occurred, and the treatment modality. This computer program would seem to provide a sports medicine facility with a fairly comprehensive system for keeping track of injuries and treatments as well as equipment and supplies.

DEVELOPING A SURVEILLANCE SYSTEM FOR YOUR FACILITY

Although many large-scale injury surveillance studies have been reported in the literature, it does not appear that injury studies are regularly conducted in athletic training rooms at either the high school or college level. Few athletic trainers have the time to conduct comprehensive studies in their training room. Some do not think they have the skills needed to do this kind of work. Others believe it would interrupt their work as athletic trainers. Still others believe they already know all they need to know about injuries or that data provided by these systems are not relevant.

Perceptions that athletic trainers have of both the occurrence and causes of injuries could be very accurate, but too often day-to-day perceptions are selective and unsystematic. For the practitioner, the regular collection of injury data can help overcome selective memory about injuries. It may be that he or she can develop a simple and straight forward surveillance method that can be used in the sports medicine facility to collect relevant injury data. This may help to understand injuries better and to anticipate them, thereby reducing the likelihood of their occurring in the first place. If the resources staff, money, and time permit a comprehensive injury study, one of the national surveillance systems, or the computer program described above, can be adopted, otherwise a more limited study may be desired.

Steps in the Conduct of an Injury Study

Some of the steps in the conduct of an injury study are provided in Table 8.7.

Step 1. Decide on the Injury to Be Studied

In any training room many different types and levels of injuries occur. While it is possible to keep track of all of them at a general level, it is very difficult to collect specific data on each of them. Accordingly, you may need to decide which injury or injuries are most important to be studied. You should be guided by the criteria presented in Tables 8.1 and 8.2.

Step 2. Determine How to Assess the Injury

You will want to record the location, type, and severity of each injury. Location would indicate the area of the body injured such as head, neck, trunk, shoulder, arms, hands, hips, thigh, knee, legs, ankles, or feet. Type of injury include whether the injury was a fracture, sprain, strain, laceration, abrasion, or contusion. As mentioned earlier there are a number of different indicators of severity including referral to hospital, need for surgery, degree of injury, or the length of time that the athlete misses participation in the sport.

Steps 3, 4, and 5. Identify the Causes and Conditions of the Injury

Identify the causes and conditions of the injury as well as personal characteristics associated with the occurrence of the injury.

Steps 3, 4, and 5 have to do with the factors that are associated with the injury. The models presented earlier can help you with these steps. Potential causes are innumerable but can include specific physical movements or the presence or absence of protective equipment or materials (e.g., faceguards, taping). Conditions under which the injury could occur include characteristics of the sport, practice vs. competition, and environmental conditions (e.g., sun, rain, wind, temperature). Personal characteristics with which injuries might be associated would include sex, height, weight, physical condition, strength, commitment to sport, time spent on sport, or personality.

Step 6. Develop Your Study Design

Choice of design will be affected by the need, desire, and ability to control for subject selection and characteristics and to control for the time at which data are collected. The simplest design is just to collect data on injuries as they occur. Because of the limitations of this kind of design, you may want to collect data on all of the athletes at the beginning of the season as well as when injuries occur. With some revision, the instrument presented in Table 8.8 could be used both pre- and post-injury.

Step 7. Develop Instruments for Data Recording

In Table 8.8 I have developed an example form that could be used to record injuries. It is not intended to be comprehensive but to show you that essential information can be collected with a simple one-page form. This form can obviously be modified to reflect your needs. You would probably want to remove some items, add others, and possibly expand the content of some of the items. This instrument is not fancy or sophisticated, but it includes the major elements for studying injuries: identification of the recorder and of the athlete, characteristics of the athlete, factors and conditions associated with the injury, nature of the injury, and severity of the injury.

Step 8. Decide on Data Analyses

Before you begin your study, you need to identify the analyses you want to do. As someone once said, if you decide this after you conduct the study, the only thing you may be able to do is to do an autopsy and see what the data died of. Making these decisions before the study gives you a check on your study objectives as well as a check on whether this is the right data to collect. The data collected by the instrument presented in Table 8.8 could be used to calculate general incidence rates as well as incidence rates for different types and levels of injuries. They could also be used to compare the incidence, type, and severity of injuries by sport, sex, field and weather conditions, and location of the injury.

Some Practical Advice

1. Limit the scope of your study to attempt to find answers to questions that you feel are vital to your sports medicine facility.

TABLE 8.7. *Steps in the conduct of an injury study*

Decide on the injury to be studied
Determine how to assess the injury
Identify potential causes of the injury
Identify conditions under which the injury may occur
Identify personal characteristics with which the injury may be associated
Develop a study design
Develop an instrument for data collection
Decide on data analysis

TABLE 8.8. *Example form: a record of injuries*

Directions: *Please complete this form for each injury.*

Date: _____   Name of school: _____

Recorder name: _____

  Role of recorder
    Medical doctor   ( )
    Certified athletic trainer ( )
    Student athletic trainer ( )

Athlete
Name/number: _____

Sport	Men		Women
Basketball	( )		( )
Track	( )		( )
Baseball/softball	( )		( )
Lacrosse	( )		( )
Football	( )		( )
Field hockey	( )		( )
Soccer	( )		( )
Wrestling	( )		

Athletic information:

Year in school: ( ) 1st   ( ) 2nd   ( ) 3rd   ( ) 4th

Age: _____   Sex: ( ) Male ( ) Female   Height in inches: _____ Weight: _____

The injury:

Date of injury: _____

Where it occurred: ( ) Indoors   ( ) Outdoors
    ( ) Practice   ( ) Scrimmage

    ( ) Game: ( ) Home   ( ) Away

Playing surface: ( ) Grass   ( ) Astroturf   ( ) Asphalt   ( ) Wood

Weather/field conditions: ( ) Dry   ( ) Rainy

Contact during injury: ( ) Contact   ( ) Non-contact

Nature and severity of injury:

Principal body part injured: ( ) Recurrent   ( ) New

  Upper: ( ) Head ( ) Neck ( ) Trunk ( ) Shoulder ( ) Arms ( ) Hands
  Lower: ( ) Hips ( ) Thigh ( ) Knee ( ) Legs (Ankles ( ) Feet

Primary type of injury: ( ) Fracture ( ) Sprain ( ) Strain
    ( ) Laceration ( ) Abrasion ( ) Contusion

Referred to hospital: ( ) Yes ( ) No

Assessment: ( ) 1st degree ( ) 2nd degree ( ) 3rd degree ( ) 4th degree

Require surgery: ( ) Yes ( ) No

Length of time not participating (in days) _____

Insurance report filed: ( ) Yes ( ) No

2. Build a network of studies with other athletic trainers.
3. Develop a data collection device that is simple and easy to complete.
4. Develop procedures for data collection that fit with the clinical procedures in your training room.
5. Input data to a computer on a daily or weekly basis.
6. Select the injury to study that you are most concerned about.
7. Smaller is better. Plan a small targeted thorough study rather than a study to answer all questions about injuries. Use that study to learn and prepare for your next study.
8. Don't wait to do the best study that can be done. Do the best study you can do, NOW. If you wait to the best study that can done, you will probably never do any study at all.

REFERENCES

1. Albright JP, Noyes FR. The sports medicine research: guidelines for the investigator. In: Noyes FR, Albright JP, eds. *Sports injury research. Am J Sports Med* 1988;16:S10–S15.
2. Caine CG, Caine DJ, Lindner KJ. The epidemiological approach to sports injuries. In: Caine DJ, Caine CG, Lindner KJ, eds. *The epidemiology of sports injuries*. Champaign, IL: Human Kinetics Publishers, 1996, 1–13
3. Clarke KL. Premises and pitfalls of athletic injury surveillance. *Sports Med.* November/December 1975:292–295.
4. Damron CF. Injury surveillance systems for sports. In: Vinger PF, Hoerner EF, eds. *Sports injuries: the unthwarted epidemic*. Boston: John Wright, 1982:2–25.
5. Finch CF. An overview of some definitional issues for sports injury surveillance. *Sports Med* 24(3):157–163.
6. Janda DH. Sports injury has everything to do with sports medicine. *Sports Med* 1997;24(3):169–172.
7. Meeunisse WH, Love EJ. Athletic injury reporting. Development of universal systems. *Sports Med* 1997;24(3):184–204
8. Mueller F, Blyth C. Epidemiology of sports injuries in children. Clinics in sports medicine 1982;1(3):343–352.
9. Noyes FR, Lindenfeld TN, Marshall MT. What determines an athletic injury (definition)? Who determines an injury occurrence? In: Noyes FR, Albright JP, eds. *Sports injury research. Am J Sports Med* 1988;16:S65–S68.
10. Rudicel SR. How to choose a study design. In: Noyes FR, Albright JP, eds. *Sports injury research. Am J Sports Med* 1988;16:S43–S47.
11. van Mechelen W, Hlobil H, Kemper CG. Incidence, severity, aetiology and prevention of sport injuries. A review of concepts. *Sports Med* 1992;14(2):82–89.
12. van Mechelen W. Sports injury surveillance systems. One size fits all? *Sports Med* 1997;24(3):164–168.
13. van Mechelen W. The severity of sports injuries. *Sports Med* 1997; 24(3):176–180.
14. Wade CE. What is the question? In: Noyes FR, Albright JP, eds. *Sports injury research. Am J Sports Med* 1988;16:S38–S42.
15. Walter SD, Sutton Jr. McIntosh JM, Connolly C. The aetiology of sports injuries: a review of methodologies. *Sports Med* 2(1):47–58.

The Injured Athlete, Third Edition,
edited by D. H. Perrin.
Lippincott–Raven Publishers, Philadelphia © 1999.

CHAPTER 9

Maxillofacial Injuries

Gaylord S. Williams

Athletic injuries to the facial soft tissues and their under-lying bony and dental support framework comprise approximately 15% of all maxillofacial trauma cases seen in the United States. Fortunately, athletic injuries tend to be of less severity and magnitude than those caused by motor vehicle accidents, which are consistently the number one producer of maxillofacial injuries (21). Even minor injuries to the face, however, may produce permanent deformities and functional impairments if they are not diagnosed and properly treated. Many contusions, abrasions, and minor lacerations can be handled in the training room, but it may be critically important to recognize and refer to a specialist those injuries that may require more expert management.

FACIAL LACERATIONS

Because of the excellent blood supply through the abundant capillaries in the skin of the blush areas of the neck and face, lacerations in these areas tend to heal more rapidly and exhibit a greater resistance to infection than lacerations elsewhere on the trunk or extremities. A clean laceration on the face may safely be closed, with antibiotic coverage, for up to 24 hours. Tetanus prophylaxis should always be addressed whenever there is a laceration of the skin. A toxoid booster is indicated for any deep or contaminated wound and in any case in which the last immunization was more than 10 years prior to the injury or unknown (12). If an athlete sustains a laceration to his face on a road trip out of town, there is really no reason why he and a busload of his teammates should spend half an evening in the emergency room of that town while he has his lacerations closed by someone who will probably

never see him again in follow-up. It is quite reasonable in such a case to cleanse the wound with peroxide and saline, cover it with a sterile dressing, return home, and have the wound properly cared for by a local surgeon or emergency practitioner who can then follow the healing of the wound and provide continuity of care.

There is nothing wrong with "putting in a few sutures" to close an open facial laceration in a training room so that an athlete can return to participation in a contest or game. Such temporary suturing may prevent further contamination and stop bleeding so the athlete could continue in the contest. Current worries about infection with HIV and hepatitis viruses make it necessary to prohibit athletes with actively bleeding wounds from participation in sports where they may contact other players. A few well-placed sutures may, therefore, be necessary to return an athlete to the field of play. After the contest, these temporary sutures can be removed, the wound thoroughly cleansed and debrided, and carefully and accurately reapproximated with a definitive closure.

Lacerations involving features such as eyebrows, eyelids, nostril rims, and lips should be carefully repaired by someone skilled in the techniques of plastic repair. Small malalignments in these areas may result in highly visible defects that may be difficult to correct secondarily.

Local anesthesia is usually adequate for repair of simple lacerations of the face. Lidocaine containing epinephrine is recommended as the epinephrine will prolong the effect of the local anesthetic and constrict blood vessels to help reduce bleeding and swelling. After washing and prepping the laceration to be sutured, lidocaine can be safely injected with less pain by injecting the lidocaine around the edges of the wound through the open laceration. This is less painful than puncturing the skin with the needle outside of the area of the laceration. The skin is more sensitive to the pain of the needle stick than is the subcutaneous tissue. Slow injection of the local anesthetic is

G. S. Williams: Department of Plastic Surgery, University of Virginia Health Sciences Center, Charlottesville, Virginia 22908

recommended as the rapid injection of the local anesthetic contributes to the pain by hydraulically distending and stretching the tissues as the injection is made. An additional technique to help reduce the pain of the injection of xylocaine containing epinephrine is to buffer it with sodium bicarbonate. Xylocaine containing epinephrine, as it comes in the bottle, has a pH of approximately 5.2. This acid pH contributes to the sting of the injection. Buffering with sodium bicarbonate in a ratio of approximately 1:10 will raise the pH of the injected xylocaine containing epinephrine to approximately 7.2. At this much more physiologic pH, there is much less sting associated with the injection. It is essential that the buffered xylocaine containing epinephrine be prepared fresh and used soon after it is prepared. If left standing for more than 30 minutes, a precipitate may form in the xylocaine containing epinephrine and sodium bicarbonate and then it should not be used. This solution is easily prepared by aspirating 9 cc. of xylocaine containing epinephrine into a 10-cc. syringe and then aspirating 1 cc. of sodium bicarbonate into the same syringe. The solution is then well mixed by tilting the syringe several times and then the injection is made. Buffered xylocaine containing epinephrine is much less painful on injection, and penetration into nerve sheaths is facilitated, making the onset of anesthesia more rapid.

Wound closure techniques for facial lacerations should emphasize thorough cleansing and debridement of the wound with physiologic solutions. The wound should be thoroughly washed with saline or Ringer's lactate and irrigated with copious amounts of these solutions to remove dirt, contaminants, clots, and devitalized tissue prior to closure. Thorough wound irrigation may be easily accomplished using a 30-cc syringe and a 19-gauge needle to produce a high pressure jet of irrigation solution, which can be sprayed with considerable force into the open wound to dislodge and wash out all foreign material.

The closure of facial lacerations should emphasize the judicious use of subcutaneous sutures, fine accurate approximation of the wound edges with fine sutures placed close to the wound margins and not tied too tightly. Closure should result in eversion of the skin edges, producing a slight "pouting" of the wound at the closure line. Normal wound contracture with healing will result in a flat scar. If the wound edges are closed flat with no eversion at the edges, the final scar will be depressed. If the edges are inverted or rolled inward at the closure, the scar will be more depressed, wider, and highly visible when it heals. Skin edge eversion is facilitated by fine absorbable dermal sutures placed in an inverted manner in the dermis to "bury the knot," and by placing external skin sutures so as to include more dermis than surface skin in the suture loop (Fig. 9.1). Ugly scars are produced when large or heavy su-

ture material is used with sutures taken widely back from the wound margins, tied too tightly, and left in too long. In general, facial lacerations should be closed with 5-0 or 6-0 nylon and all external sutures should be removed within 7 days to avoid stitch marks. If only temporary wound closure is being performed, then larger suture material may be used. If this larger suture material is removed within a day or so, there will be no adverse effects or suture marks unless, of course, the heavy suture material has been too tight and caused necrosis of skin. Tape or steri-strip closures should be used for only the most minimal lacerations as they are not reliable as the sole means of holding the laceration closed—particularly in an athlete.

Scarring from facial lacerations can never be predicted with absolute accuracy. In general, people with darker and thicker skin tend to produce more hypertrophic scars than those with lighter pigmented and thinner skin. Infection, shear forces, tension, buried suture material, and genetic predispositions all may influence the outcome of the final resultant scar from any laceration.

If highly visible, deforming, or otherwise unsatisfactory scars result from facial lacerations, subsequent scar revision may be performed to improve the final result. Scar revision can be performed at anytime after the wound has healed, but, in general, it is usually preferable to wait until the inflammatory phase of wound healing is finished and the scar is mature before attempting revision. Scars in different areas of the face present different problems, and these must be individualized in deciding on the timing, indications, and type of revision.

Some caveats should be remembered in dealing with facial lacerations:

1. Never put anything into a wound to irrigate it or wash it out that you would not put in your own eye.
2. Do not shave eyebrows, they take a very, very long time to grow back out.
3. Be very slow to trim and discard any tissue on the face, particularly if it involves the eyelids, nose, or lips.

Abrasions and scrapes should be treated acutely by thoroughly cleansing the raw and denuded or de-epithelialized skin. Dirt or road grit that may be ground into the open abrasion may heal over and result in a permanent traumatic tattoo. The best time to remove this dirt is as soon as possible after the injury. The abraded area should be thoroughly anesthetized by xylocaine infiltration and scrubbed with a scrub brush or a sterile toothbrush or wire brush (Fig. 9.2). The abraded area is then covered with antibiotic ointment and a nonadherent Vaseline-type gauze. Abraded areas should be protected from direct sun exposure by covering them with a strong sunscreen for up to 6 months to prevent hyperpigmentation. Sunscreen protection is important in dark-skinned

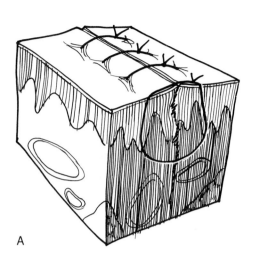

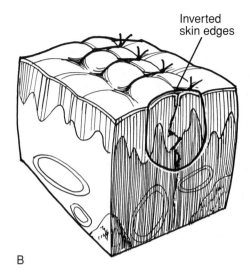

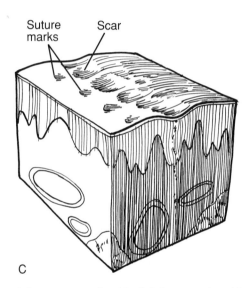

FIG. 9.1. A: Properly placed fine sutures should slightly evert the skin edges at the closure line. Heavy wide sutures with inverted or overlapped skin edges (**B**) will produce a wide, ugly, depressed scar (**C**).

people as well as fair-skinned people and severe hyperpigmentation can result if a sunscreen is not used on a dark-skinned person following an abrasion.

The boxer's face may be cut by friction from laces rubbed over it, by pinching of the skin between the boxing glove and the orbital bone, and by head butting. The cuts usually occur in the supraorbital region but may occur infraorbitally and in the lid. A supraorbital cut may trickle blood into the eye, interfering with the boxer's vision.

Cuts cannot be treated between rounds in the Olympic games, but a cut can be fixed in other amateur and professional bouts. The periorbital cut should be wiped clean and pushed shut and pressure applied: the cut should then be coated with an astringent. Pressure should not be used,

however, if there is a chance that the globe has ruptured. A layer of flexible collodion is next applied and Vaseline smeared around the cut so that further blows will slide off. After the fight, the cut should be minimally debrided and closed in layers to keep it from scarring down to bone. If not thus treated, the cut will open easily. Stitches should be placed about 2 mm apart, tied loosely, and a pressure dressing applied. To minimize scarring, the stitches may be left in only 3 to 5 days and the athlete should not box for 4 weeks.

The eyelid consists of two halves: the anterior half contains skin and orbicularis muscle; the posterior half contains the tarsus and conjunctiva. Vertical lid lacerations, and lacerations that include canthal tendons and

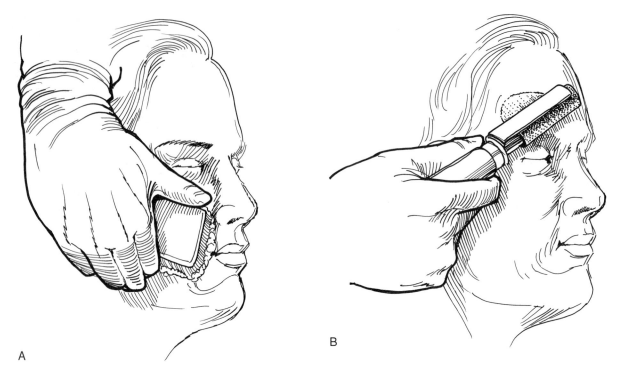

FIG. 9.2. "Road Rash" dirt, dust, or asphalt must be vigorously removed from the fresh wound by brush (**A**) or dermabrasion (**B**) to prevent traumatic tattooing.

lacrimal drainage system should be treated by a practitioner with experience in oculoplastic surgery. A thorough eye examination, including dilated fundus examination, should be done to exclude damage to the eyeball.

Boxers should wear headgear while sparring and during collegiate and service team bouts. The soft leather boxing headgear is padded with latex foam rubber or animal hair to protect the boxer's eyes, temples, and base of the skull; some models even protect the jaw.

FACIAL PROTECTION

Facemasks have helped significantly to reduce the number of facial injuries in tackle football, hockey, lacrosse, and motocross. In the 1950s, most tackle football injuries were to the face, such as bloody noses, cut lips, and dental injuries. In 1955, facemasks and mouthguards were recommended for high school football; by 1960 a facemask was required, and in 1962 the mouthguard was made mandatory. Players at first wore a single bar facemask, then a double bar. A vertical bar was added later, and more recently the birdcage facemask has become popular.

Quarterbacks, wide receivers, and running backs will often sacrifice protection for an unobstructed view. Faceguards do restrict the visual field slightly at knee level and below, making it harder to see a low opponent (31).

Special facemasks help to reduce injury; if a player must wear eyeglasses, for example, a specially designed facemask may be used. Mounting loops on a helmet allow the facemask to absorb blows.

The facemask must fit properly. If the bar style is fitted too low, it provides little protection for the facial area. If fitted too high, the bars obstruct vision and the mandible is exposed. By placing the facemask closer to the face, leverage is reduced if the facemask is grabbed by an opposing player. When a cage mask is fitted too close to the face, however, the angle of the mandible may be lacerated during the violent contact as the cage is driven back and bent. Facemasks should be checked each week for loosened screws and bolts. If no facemasks were worn, the large number of severe neck injuries probably would be reduced, because a player wearing only a helmet and mouthguard would be less likely to head-tackle, butt-block, or spear (30). Lost teeth or facial scarring would be a reasonable tradeoff for serious head and neck injuries. Without a facemask, however, the player might tend to close his eyes and drop his head, and even more injuries could result.

Before introduction of the facemask, eye injuries were common in ice hockey (26). Two-thirds of those injuries were caused by the stick and the rest by the puck, but blindness resulted equally from both objects. Full-face

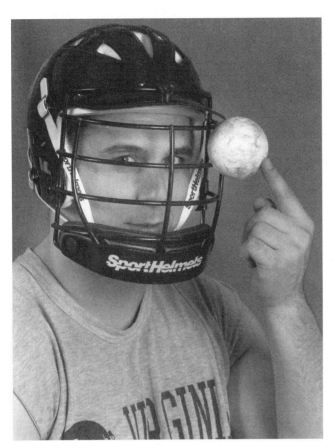

FIG. 9.3. The vertical bar greatly improves protection and has reduced the number of facial injuries.

wire mesh and polycarbonate hockey masks reduce facial injuries by preventing the stick or puck from penetrating. Although goaltenders often wear an expensive, molded fiberglass mask, the puck can still get through to cause a hyphema (blood in the anterior chamber) or worse injury. Plastic shield face protectors are satisfactory if kept in good condition but may fog up and scratch.

When lacrosse facemasks had only horizontal bars, the number of facial injuries was large because the stick and balls could squeeze through. The addition of a mandatory vertical bar has helped to reduce the number of facial injuries (Fig. 9.3).

Serious motor cross competitors wear a facemask, and such masks and helmets should be worn by all motorcyclists. The motorcyclist's mask keeps flying objects, stones, and bugs from injuring his eyes and helps a driver avoid losing control of his vehicle. A full-face helmet will give even better protection against severe facial injuries from motorcycle crashes.

EYE INJURIES IN ATHLETES

Because the opening to the eyeball is small, large objects, such as soccer balls and basketballs, may be de-

flected before their kinetic energy reaches the eye (3). Almost any kind of ball, however, may become deformed and seriously contuse the globe, despite protection provided by the skull's bony rims. Moreover, although the eyeball is surrounded by bony rims and is elastic and embedded in a resilient fat pad, minor trauma may cause eventual blindness, as when glaucoma develops after an injury.

Conjunctival Irritation

Dust and dirt from playing surfaces irritate an athlete's eyes, while sweat may be rubbed into the eyes by dirty fingers. If the conjunctiva becomes irritated, foreign bodies or corneal abrasions might be suspected. Antibiotic drops should be administered only by an ophthalmologist after a slit-lamp examination; they should never be given at the time of an initial corneal abrasion.

After a few hours in bright and reflected sun, a skier or yachtsman's cornea may suffer sunburn in which the eyes become irritated and the athlete is then unable to tolerate bright light. Dark glasses or goggles will prevent this type of sunburn.

Fingers in the Eye

In basketball, fingers are sometimes poked in the eye while players scramble for the ball, and a fingernail may scrape the eyeball. During cross-country skiing, a skier's cornea may be abraded by a tree limb. Such minor accidents may result in serious injury to the eye, including hyphema, dislocation of the lens, and a retinal detachment (Fig. 9.4). These conditions should never be overlooked on examination. All fingernails should be inspected and trimmed before games and practices and players required to remove rings and other jewelry that may endanger opponents or their teammates. Cross-country skiers are advised to wear eyeglasses or goggles while skiing in the woods.

To assess eye problems and to protect an injured eye, the physician should carry a local anesthetic, fluorescein strips, a concentrated light source, a small, near-vision card, eye patches, hard protective shields, and tape.

Fluorescein drops demonstrate superficial eye scrapes as bright green marks where the epithelium is absent. The marks are especially easy to see when a cobalt blue light is used for the examination. Scratched eyes should be patched. In this procedure, a pad is folded into the hollow of the orbit and then topped with a second pad. The athlete should be instructed to keep both eyes shut while wearing a patch, because blinking only further irritates the eye. Corneal injuries should be checked by an ophthalmologist because the abrasion may be a laceration. The eye patch should be worn for 24 hours, then the eye rechecked and

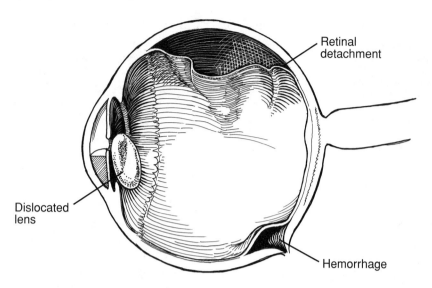

Retinal detachment

Dislocated lens

Hemorrhage

FIG. 9.4. Even slight or suspected injuries to the eye should be checked by an ophthalmologist to check for hyphema, retinal detachment, or lens dislocation.

patched for another 24 hours, which is usually sufficient time for healing to take place.

Foreign Body in the Eye

If a foreign body enters the athlete's eye, it may lodge in the upper or lower fornix or on the conjunctival or corneal surfaces, producing the sensation of being under the upper lid. Oblique illumination from a concentrated light source may be needed to determine its precise location. A foreign body at the lower lid is easily removed by pulling the lower lid down and gently wiping it away with a cotton bud.

When a foreign body is under the upper lid, an attempt should be made to move it to the lower lid. The athlete should first be asked to look down, and the upper lid should then be gently pulled over the lower lid to produce tears that may flush the object to the lower part of the eye. If the foreign body remains under the upper lid, the lid should be pulled out before folding it upwards over a cotton bud to expose the tarsal conjunctival surface. Another cotton bud may be used to wipe away the object.

Tennis Eye

Eye injuries may occur unexpectedly if an athlete is off guard, as in tennis when a player's eye is struck during a warm-up when more than one ball is in play. When volleying, players' eyes are vulnerable to hard-hit balls and to balls that skip off the net. Balls hit in anger or frustration after a player loses a point may strike an opponent who is not alert. Players with poor vision may have difficulty following the flight of the ball and be injured.

Squash balls and racketballs are especially dangerous

because they are small enough to fit into the orbit of the eye (8). The wild swings of inexperienced players send balls flying off at dangerous angles and velocities. In badminton, the 1.9-cm (0.75-in) diameter striking end of the shuttlecock similarly endangers the eyes.

In the excitement of a racket game, the player may underestimate the severity of a blow to his eye. The blow may cause temporary blurring with rapid recovery, but weeks or even years later the player may have serious vision loss from a detached retina that progressed from an asymptomatic peripheral break. For this reason, when a player's eye is struck by any small ball, an ophthalmologic checkup is desirable to rule out intraocular damage (33). An early funduscopic examination, with the pupil fully dilated, may reveal hemorrhage and edema in the peripheral retina, indicating a small tear. Proper observation and treatment will prevent extension of the tear. Any player with subjective disturbance of vision, altered visual acuity, loss of visual field or diplopia, excessive edema, and chemosis or hemorrhage into the anterior chamber should consult with an ophthalmologist.

A player looking around at a partner who is serving should have his racket up as a guard. Ordinary eyeglasses will not protect the eyes in tennis, since the lens may be pushed against the eye. To prevent this, tennis players should wear either an eyeguard or a sports frame with pop-out lenses and rotating earpieces. Closed eyeguards should be mandatory for squash and racquetball players, and novice badminton players are especially well advised to wear safety glasses because inexperienced players frequently suffer eye injuries.

"Black Eye"

Blows to a boxer's eye may rupture small blood vessels in the subcutaneous tissue of the eyelid. This skin is the thinnest in the body, and the subcutaneous supporting structures are equally tenuous. Hemorrhage here causes rapid and extensive swelling, shutting the lid. The eyeball should be checked for blood before it swells shut and the orbital bones palpated. A swollen eye should not be dismissed as a minor contusion because a blow may dislocate the lens or produce a hyphema, retinal edema, retinal hemorrhage, vitreous hemorrhage, retinal tear, or retinal detachment. The globe may have ruptured, causing intraocular hemorrhage and loss of vision. If the lids are swollen shut or if the eye is difficult to examine, it should not be forced open, and an ophthalmologist should be promptly consulted.

Swelling is usually self-limiting, and ice bags may be applied during the first 24 hours. Instant cold packs should not be placed over the eyes because they occasionally leak small amounts of chemicals through tiny holes. Some boxing handlers will cut a boxer's eyelid with a razor blade to evacuate blood, an unacceptable practice with little practical value, as the blood has spread diffusely through the tissues and is not localized. The blood supply to the lids will help resorb such interstitial blood within a few weeks. Bleeding into the periorbital tissues may dissect under the thin conjunctival covering of the globe and between it and the white sclera, producing a red patch. A thin hematoma here may remain red for weeks because the red blood cells remain oxygenated by absorption through the thin moist conjunctiva, but this will eventually clear completely.

Hyphema

A blow to the eye may damage small vessels of the ciliary body, which hemorrhage into the anterior chamber between the cornea and the iris. The athlete reports blurred vision, photophobia, and aching eye pain. The eye reddens and blood appears, producing a fluid level in the anterior chamber (see Fig. 9.4). Eyes with this condition should be shielded immediately and the athlete placed under the care of an ophthalmologist. Bed rest is obligatory since further hemorrhage occurs in the first few days and the second hemorrhage may be worse than the first. The hyphema may prevent a clear view of the retina for several days, but most hyphemas are absorbed within a week. After absorption takes place, the ophthalmologist can dilate the pupil to check for retinal damage, and the patient should be followed for life to avert the development of secondary glaucoma.

Retinal Detachment

A blow to the eye may be followed by detachment of the retina, especially in athletes with a predisposing familial history. Detachment is most likely to occur in persons with retinal degenerative lesions, such as myopia. Constant agitation of the vitreous body may be accompanied by retinal traction sufficient to cause breaks in the retina that is thin or diseased. For this reason, some ophthalmologists caution myopic people, especially those who have had previous retinal detachment, against jogging. A retinal detachment may occur weeks or months after an injury. Retinal breaks, with or without detachment, require the expertise of an ophthalmologist for full assessment and appropriate treatment.

BLOW-OUT FRACTURE OF THE ORBIT

If a fist, elbow, or ball strikes the orbit, blunt trauma may increase intraorbital hydrostatic pressure and break the inferomedial margin of the orbit (Fig. 9.5). Because this weak bone may fracture even without an associated orbital rim fracture, the athlete should be sent to an ophthalmologist with the eye shielded after any blunt trauma.

An athlete with a blow-out fracture of the orbit will develop periorbital edema and hemorrhage; when this subsides, he may have double vision. The infraorbital rim may feel abnormal, and the inferior rectus muscle may become tethered to the fracture, interfering with ocular movements. Such patients require evaluation and treatment by an ophthalmologist or maxillofacial surgeon.

Although conventional x-rays may demonstrate orbital floor blow-out fracture, computerized tomography is now the accepted standard for evaluation and accurate delineation of the extent of these fractures.

Contact Lenses

Many athletes wear contact lenses to avoid the disadvantages of spectacles, which may have heavy frames, fog up, and require cages, masks, and elastic straps (10). Spectacles can also be knocked off or a spectacle lens pushed into the orbit. Although hard contact lenses are particularly beneficial to athletes who have astigmatism, such lenses may slide off center, pop off, and be lost. Moreover, wind and dust particles may slide under them to cause serious eye abrasions. These sudden and often painful distractions may be dangerous in some sports, negating the advantages of such lenses. For the athlete who wears contact lenses, a cage or mask is still advisable because a broken contact lens may be more dangerous than a shatterproof spectacle lens.

Soft contact lenses are generally more comfortable than hard contact lenses (34). Vision is often not as crisp, however, and astigmatism not as well corrected with soft lenses. Swimmers usually can wear the soft lenses if goggles are used. These lenses require considerably more care than hard lenses and are more expensive. Proper care of soft lenses requires distilled water, saline solution,

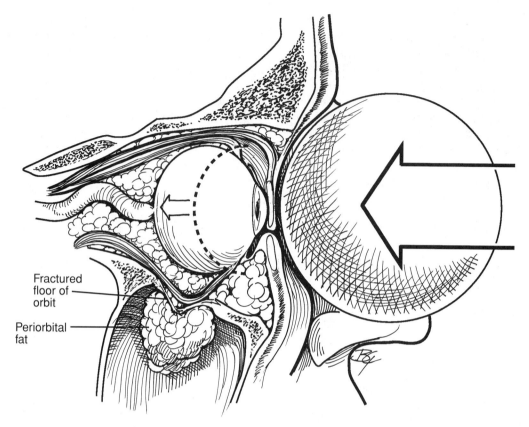

Fractured
floor of
orbit

Periorbital
fat

FIG. 9.5. A large blunt object striking the eye can fracture the thin orbital floor or medial wall without fracturing the surrounding orbital rims.

special lens cases, and a heating unit. The team physician and athletic trainer should know which athletes are wearing contact lenses, and if a wearer is knocked unconscious the lenses should be removed immediately.

Eyeguards

Because a badminton bird, squash ball, or racketball may cause eye injuries, some clubs require players to wear eye protectors. Such protection is important not only for myopic and novice players, but also for skilled players. The skilled player is less likely to give up control of center court, thus increasing the risk of eye injury from the racket or ball.

A myopic athlete's eyeglass lenses are concave, with the center section of the lens thinner than the outer edge, subjecting it to easy breakage. To give optimum protection, the lens center should be at least a 3-mm thick CR39 plastic or polycarbonate plastic (5). Plastic lenses have a higher resistance to breakage than do glass lenses and are lighter, give less surface reflection, and are less likely to fog (40).

Although plastic lenses do not easily break, they can be broken and may pop through an ordinary frame. Such lenses should be mounted in a sports frame made of nylon

with a steep posterior lip. When a lens in a sports frame is struck, it projects forward instead of being driven toward the eye. The athlete should wear a nylon frame with temples that rotate about 180 degrees. Currently popular metal frames should be avoided because they can cut the face or damage the eye easily.

All open eyeguards do not provide equal protection, and direct shots from a racquetball or squash ball can strike and damage the eye through the space between the upper and lower rims of the guards. Closed eye guards with either plain or prescription lenses will prevent such injuries. An open eye guard is, however, better than none because it will prevent slashes from rackets and damage from off-center hits (5,29). Sturdy goggles are recommended for skiers because cheap plastic goggles can shatter into tiny pieces.[a]

EAR INJURIES IN ATHLETICS

"Scrum Ear" and "Wrestler's Ear"

When an athlete's ear is repetitively rubbed or when it absorbs many blows or a single blow, blood may leak

---

[a] For a copy of eye protection recommendations or other information on eye safety in sports, contact the National Society to Prevent Blindness, 79 Madison Avenue, New York, New York 10016.

between the skin and the perichondrium. The ear then becomes throbbingly painful, tender, and swollen. After a few hours, a well-defined, smooth, rounded mass forms within the helix fossa. Blood and serum collect on both sides of the ear cartilage, isolating the cartilage from the soft tissue upon which its nutrition and vitality depend. The cartilage may then die and collapse. If the ear is not properly treated, the hematoma will organize and scar down within a few weeks, pulling the ear into a contorted, cauliflower-like configuration—the gnarled ear of a boxer, the scrum ear of a rugby player, or wrestler's ear.

Hot spots from friction during wrestling practice may be prevented by smearing Vaseline on the ears. The lubricant is, however, prohibited during matches. Wrestlers should wear ear guards, especially during wrestling practice, where the wrestler spends 95% of his time (Fig. 9.6). The headgear may rub and cause wrestler's ear.

If an ear has been rubbed and becomes hot, an ice pack should be applied promptly. Any hematoma should be aspirated sterilely because infection in this region may lead to chondritis, a long-lasting problem. After the hematoma has been aspirated, the region may be compressed with a collodion pack, plaster of Paris cast, mineral-oil-soaked cotton balls, or silicone mold. The collodion pack is a cast of cotton or strips of gauze soaked in flexible collodion (2). The collodion applicator should be kept well saturated to place collodion on the ear before the layers of gauze are started. After 24 to 48 hours, the pack may be removed and the ear checked for any reaccumulation before being repacked. The new pack should be left

in place as long as possible, and repeated if needed. Plaster of Paris may also serve as a packing, but a Q-tip should be placed in the ear canal while the plaster sets. Another technique uses a cotton "stent" moistened with mineral oil and placed into all of the convolutions of the auricular folds and also postauricularly. A mastoid dressing holds the stent in position for 10 days. As an alternative to aspirating the hematoma, it may be evacuated by making multiple incisions through the skin and perichondrium (7). Dental rolls are then sutured in place and a mastoid dressing applied.

These techniques are not without problems, as the collodion pack may easily dislodge and the collodion pack and plaster of Paris cast usually lack a vent. The problems may be avoided by fashioning a silicone mold pressure dressing around the end of an applicator stick, providing a tunnel through the mold that equalizes pressure between the external auditory canal and the outside atmosphere (11).

"Swimmer's Ear"

Swimmer's ear is an acute, diffuse external auditory canal infection usually caused by the bacterium *Pseudomonas aeruginosa* or, sometimes, by *Proteus*, *Escherichia coli*, or fungi (6,28). Humans lack the adaptations diving mammals have to prevent external ear problems. Porpoises, for example, have no external auditory canal opening, and a seal's ears are covered during dives by external skin flaps.

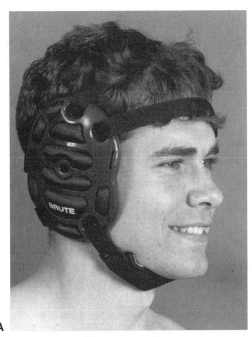
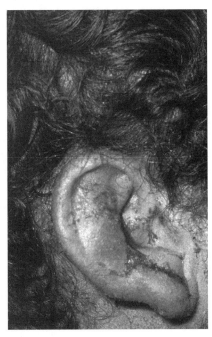

FIG. 9.6. Wrestlers and boxers wear ear protectors (**A**) to prevent against auricular hematoma (**B**).

Swimmer's ear may develop even if pool water is sparkling clean (36), because water washes away the ear's natural cerumen and the skin in the canal becomes irritated and itches. If the athlete then scratches in the ear, the continuity of the lining cells of the ear canal may be disrupted. These cells produce a protective acid mantle that retards bacterial growth, and individual variations in the mantle may explain why some athletes are more prone to develop swimmer's ear. An excessively curved, narrowed, or partly obstructed ear canal may trap water. Trapping also occurs when cysts, bone growths, ear wax, ear plugs, allergies, or dermatitis blocks the canal (20). In some cases, the infection moves inward to cause a middle-ear infection or to interfere with balance and hearing, or the infection may even advance to infect the brain.

Because the latency period for swimmer's ear is about 3 days, the association between swimming and swimmer's ear is sometimes overlooked. When the ear hurts and itches, the swimmer pulls the earlobe and rocks the jaw from side to side. On examination, the external ear canal is swollen and tender. Less often the infection is caused by a fungus; Candida produces yellow or white dots, and *Aspergillus nigra* forms a grayish-black membrane that coats the canal.

An infected ear canal should be reacidified with a solution of acetic or boric acid in alcohol (6). Antibiotic and cortisone drop combinations may also be used, and alcohol and glycol drops will decrease the moisture. A cotton wick that has been soaked in Burrow's solution (aluminum acetate) should be inserted to limit further swelling. The ear debris is then carefully removed, and acid-alcohol drops are instilled. The wick should be kept moist with drops of Burrow's solution applied to it every 2 hours to bring the solution to the full length of the ear canal and keep the canal open.

The swimmer can remove trapped water and prevent swimmer's ear by vigorously shaking the head and jumping with the head tilted to one side. The ears should then be fanned or blown dry with a hair dryer. Three drops of 3% boric acid in alcohol may be put into the ear canals before and after each swim to dry the canals. For good aural hygiene, three drops of glycerin may be placed in each ear canal after a shower and the canal covered with a cotton pledget that is removed after 1 hour.

Vinegar dropped into an ear may macerate the ear canal. If cotton buds are stuck into the canal or if the concha or tragal areas are vigorously rubbed with a hand or a towel, the delicate skin surface may break. Cotton buds may also push wax against the tympanic membrane or remove too much of the protective wax. Ear plugs should not be used because they are not watertight and may trap water and cause pressure necrosis.

Osteomas and Exostoses

Some swimmers and surfers develop small, bony masses in front of the tympanic membrane (4,6,9). Such growths are endemic in swimmers in cold California water but are not usually found in the ears of swimmers who swim in heated pools. Swimmers in cool ocean water should wear headgear to protect their ear canals.

A growth may be an attempt to protect against the cold water that bathes the tympanic membrane and may be an osteoma or an exostosis. An osteoma is a solitary unilateral bone growth attached to the tympanic squamous suture superficial or lateral to the canal isthmus. Exostoses are broad-based elevations of the bony canal that are usually multiple and bilaterally symmetrical. They lie deep or medial to the canal isthmus at the upper edge of the tympanic bone. These multilobed tumors of the external ear canal, unlike swimmer's ear, are painless but progressive. First, the inner bony part of the canal thickens with cobblestone-like swellings, and after further exposure to cold water the swellings become knuckle-like. Eventually, they completely block the ear canal to produce a conductive hearing loss.

Osteomas and exostoses may be excised. If a defect remains that rings more than one-third of the circumference of the ear canal, it may be closed with a skin graft (4).

Barotrauma

Divers may experience serious problems such as cerebral arterial air embolism, joint pains (the "bends"), or venous gas pulmonary embolism (the "chokes") (38). Divers who have chronic obstructive pulmonary disease, bronchial asthma, or lung blebs sometimes trap air when they ascend from deep water, causing a pneumothorax.

More common problems affect the air-filled cavities of the sinuses and the middle ear spaces of divers (36). These very susceptible, air-filled structures have rigid walls and small openings, and the air within them must be equilibrated, continuously, with the external air pressure. Proper equilibration demands that Eustachian tube and sinus ostia be patent (Fig. 9.7).

The barometric pressure outside and inside the body at sea level is 14.7 lb/in^2, and for every 33 feet of descent in sea water the pressure increases by this amount. Barotrauma may occur even in relatively shallow dives because the greatest volume changes within tissue cavities per foot of descent occur near the surface.

"Ear squeeze" may develop during the descent phase of diving as pressure differentials cause vascular tissues to dilate and the epithelium of the sinuses and middle ear to swell. This swelling is an autoregulatory mechanism that functions to lower the pressure differential. The engagement of the tissues decreases air volume in the cavity but may further occlude the ostia and prevent equalization of pressures. The pressure differential may then increase to produce transudation and, finally, blood vessel rupture, which reduces the pressure differential by adding blood

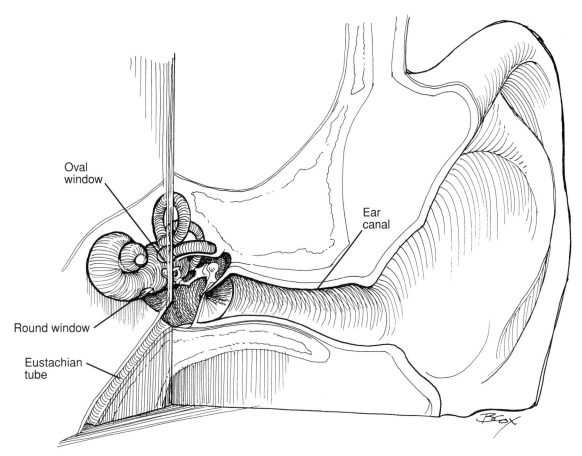

Oval
window

Ear
canal

Round window

Eustachian
tube

FIG. 9.7. Swimming and diving can damage the athlete's ear canal, the oval window, the round window, and the sinuses if excessive pressure differentials are encountered.

to the cavity. With ear squeeze, the diver notices ear pain, decreased hearing, ringing in the ears, inability to clear the ears, and sometimes blood-tinged sputum.

When the external canal is blocked by cerumen, an osteoma, the diving hood, or an earplug, an artificial air-filled cavity external to the tympanic membrane is created. The middle ear becomes overpressurized in relation to the closed cavity between the plug and tympanic membrane, and the tympanic membrane distends outward to produce a "reverse ear squeeze."

Inexperienced divers may not be able to equalize pressure (38). Infection, allergies, or vasomotor rhinitis may also swell the mucous membranes. Large adenoids, scarring from adenoidectomy, or congenital obstruction of the openings prevent pressure equalization.

The diver should keep the openings to the middle ear and sinuses clear by removing impacted cerumen. The ears should be checked for osteomas or exostoses, and pharyngeal masses that block air passages should be removed. Divers are advised to practice equalizing pressure and are cautioned not to dive when suffering from sinusitis or during a seasonal flare-up of allergic rhinitis. Per-

sons with disorders that might interfere with consciousness, such as seizure disorders or potential insulin reaction, should not dive.

A diver who takes a decongestant or antihistamine before diving should be aware that a "rebound" phenomenon may occur that produces swelling of the mucous membranes and barotrauma.

Tympanic Membrane Rupture

A blow to the ear in water polo, surfing, or water skiing may rupture the athlete's tympanic membrane. This injury used to be common in water polo, but players now wear caps with ear protectors, and thus the disorder is seen less often.

In competitive water skiing, the maximum boat speed is 58 km/h (36 miles/h), although the skier may go faster than the boat and a fall may rupture his tympanic membrane. The rupture occurs with a pop, and the athlete notices a decreased ability to hear. A ruptured membrane may admit cold water to produce a dangerous cold water caloric effect on the labyrinth, causing dizziness and nausea, which may panic the diver, water skier, or swimmer.

A ruptured tympanic membrane should be observed each day for signs of infection. If infection is present, antibiotic therapy should be administered; alternatively, antibiotic drops or systemic antibiotics may be given from the start to prevent infection. Steroid drops should be avoided because they retard healing. The membrane usually closes spontaneously within a week, although some otolaryngologists recommend early surgical closure of the rupture (25).

Caloric Labyrinthitis

Stimulation of the labyrinth of the ear by cold water produces caloric labyrinthitis with vertigo, loss of balance, and nausea.

Pipkin reported on caloric labyrinthitis in an otolaryngologist who dove from a dock into a lake (27). As cold water suddenly filled his external auditory canal, the doctor developed vertigo and lost his sense of balance. He understood, however, what was happening and, using his sense of touch, he crawled on the lake bottom to safety.

Ninety percent of all drowning victims drown within 9 m (10 yd) of shore; why so many strong swimmers drown is uncertain. Because caloric labyrinthitis may cause some of these drownings, no one should swim alone or in unfamiliar water, and all boaters should wear life preservers.

Round Window Rupture

The round window membrane may rupture in skin divers, free underwater divers, snorkelers, scuba divers, and weight lifters (6). The athlete's ear pops and a leakage of perilymph causes sudden deafness. This type of rupture demands prompt closure of the fistula, which may save some hearing. Unfortunately, the sudden hearing loss is often irreversible, making prevention essential.

Divers should be advised to avoid wearing earplugs and to forgo diving if they have an upper respiratory infection or allergic flare-up. Also, divers and weight lifters with already damaged ears should be advised that they risk more serious damage when they perform a Valsalva maneuver, which is increased pressure by forcible exhalation against a closed glottis.

Hearing Loss from Firearms

Repetitive impulse noise from the sudden explosive force of gunfire may produce hearing loss in marksmen and officials who must fire a starting gun at track meets. The "near ear" is subject to the greater acoustical trauma because it is closer and at a more direct angle to receive the assault (24). The left ear is the near ear of a right-handed rifleman, whereas the right ear is the near ear of a right-handed pistol shooter (22).

The noise from most guns is loud enough to cause hearing loss (23). The peak sound pressure level (PSPL) for the maximum endurable threshold of repeated impulses for ears of normal sensitivity is 150 dB. All shotguns and center-firing and rim-firing weapons have been found to exceed the damage risk level of 150 dB, except for the smaller 0.22 cartridges.

Less noise would preserve hearing and would allow marksmen to be more relaxed and to shoot more accurately (37). The amount of powder in the cartridge and its characteristics could be reduced to decrease the PSPL, but this would alter ballistic findings (23). Therefore, the most practical solution would be a modification of the gun barrel. In the absence of such a change, marksmen can help to reduce their hearing loss by firing on flat, open terrain and by wearing earmuffs that reduce noise by 20 to 45 dB (24).

NOSE INJURIES IN ATHLETICS

Nose Bleed

The athlete with nose bleed should sit or kneel in front of the physician and bend the head slightly forward. This position keeps him or her from swallowing blood, which may produce nausea and vomiting, and also lessens bleeding, since the head is above the heart. The physician places the thumb along the outside of the bleeding nostril and the index finger on the opposite side of the athlete's nose and applies steady pressure for several minutes.

When persistent bleeding occurs, the nose should be packed, but cotton ball packings are unsafe because the athlete may inhale a piece of cotton. A regular-sized tampon will serve as packing and may be referred to as a "nose plug"(1). The tampon must be cut to fit inside the nose. Once in the nose, the material expands and conforms to the nostril. The athlete may return to the game, since the tampon is too large to be inhaled, and the nose plug can be removed later. Several tampons, with strings removed, may be carried in the athletic trainer's kit.

Broken Nose

A nasal fracture may be determined by gently wiggling the athlete's nose at the cartilage line and above it on the bone to detect pain or grating. If displacement is noted, the nose should be splinted, and the fracture will need to be reduced (Fig. 9.8). When swelling prevents a proper evaluation of external nasal deformity, ice should be applied for up to 24 hours and the nose re-evaluated in 3 days. If

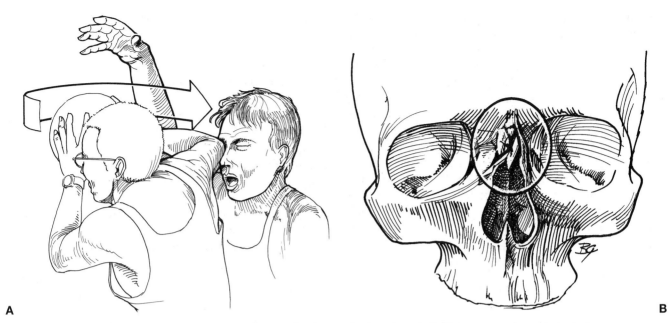

FIG. 9.8. Nasal fractures may vary from a simple nondisplaced crack (**left**) to a severely comminuted, displaced, deformation of the nose (**right**).

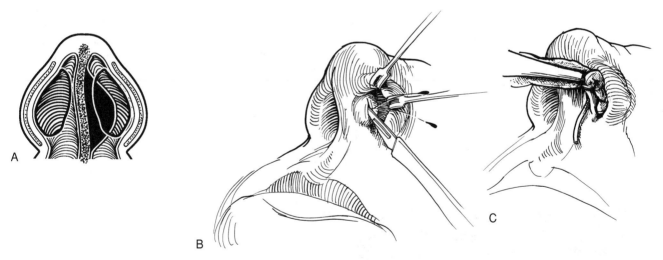

FIG. 9.9. A: A septal hematoma should be looked for in any nasal injury. When this occurs it should be drained (**B**) and packed (**C**) to avoid loss of the supporting septal cartilage.

the diagnosis of a nasal fracture is delayed for 2 weeks, the fracture may no longer be reducible by closed means. A corrective rhinoplasty may then be required to straighten the solidified displaced nasal bones and septum. Even though the nose contains very little bone, nasal defects may affect the Eustachian tube, making clearing of the ears by inflating the middle ear difficult or impossible.

A hematoma in the nasal septum is an emergency and must be incised or aspirated and the nose packed to pre-vent cartilage destruction, necrosis, and development of a saddle nose deformity. A bulge may also cause nasal obstruction (Fig. 9.9).

MOUTH INJURIES IN ATHLETICS

Mouthguards

Before facemasks were added to football helmets, 50% of football injuries were in or around the mouth; after the addition of facemasks, mouth injuries fell to 25% of the total. The facemask, however, offers little protection against blows under the chin from forearm blocking, from knees, and from kicks and does not block blows to the top of the head that snap the jaws shut.

Mouthguards were recommended for high school tackle football players in 1955 and made mandatory in 1962 but were not required to collegiate tackle football players until 1973 (16,18). Today's combination of facemask and mouthguard has made mouth injuries very rare. Mouthguards not only have reduced injuries to the mouth, such as split lips and broken teeth, but also have helped decrease concussions by absorbing the energy from blows, thus damping the transmission of forces to the brain (19,35).

Whether playing in recreational or competitive sport, every athlete should wear a mouthguard as a routine safety item (17), whether in practices or in an actual game.

The major types of mouthguards include custom-made, mouth-formed, and stock. Custom-made mouthguards are heavy-duty ones, made of dental vinyl or plastic pulled by vacuum over a plaster mold of the athlete's teeth. A mouth-formed, thermal-set, boiled, pliable, plastic mouthguard (Fig. 9.10) is satisfactory, but the stock rubber mouthguard is unacceptable because it may be a very poor fit. A well-fitted mouthguard is comfortable and offers very little interference with the athlete's speech and breathing. The volume of air intake in an athlete pushed to exhaustion decreases only by about 5% with a custom-made mouthguard (see Fig. 9.10) (13,32).

In tackle football, the mouthguard is often attached to the player's facemask or chin piece to keep him from misplacing it. A safety strap feature allows the strap to be pulled free of the mouthguard under unusual pressure to avoid stress injury to the player's teeth. Mouthguards must be checked for wear; many injuries occur when the guard has worn down.

Temporomandibular Joint

In addition to absorbing shocks, a mouthguard may also help to preserve an athlete's energy and to increase his strength by balancing the temporomandibular joints. When this joint is imbalanced, the nervous system picks up the fact of the malalignment when the athlete swallows and the teeth touch. As reflexes are activated, energy-sapping compensations for the malalignment occur in the athlete's back and limbs.

Some athletes have large mandibles with equally large mandibular condyles. If a large condyle is cradled in the base of an average-sized skull, there is less tolerance in the joint and a greater susceptibility to concussion. Athletes with deep overbite occlusion problems usually have small condyles and average-sized heads. These persons lack anterior muscle supports for their head and necks, resulting in an overuse of the posterior cervical muscles and more strained necks and pinched nerves (35).

An orthodontist can place a resilient bite plate between the occlusal surfaces of the upper and lower teeth to suspend the condyle away from the fossa, providing the temporomandibular joint with more tolerance. The plate also gives posterior occlusal support needed to balance the head.

Richard Kaufman, a sports orthodontist, fit the American luge team with mandibular orthopaedic repositioning appliance (MORA) mouthpieces to relax their tense head and neck muscles and reduce headaches and back pain (39). The MORA mouthpiece comprises two strips of

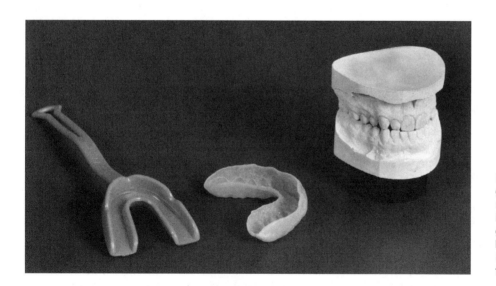

FIG. 9.10. A mouth-formed mouth guard (*left*) attaches to the face mask. A latex mouthguard (*center*) is custom made and even fills any gaps. Proper occlusion (*right*) can be obtained with an acrylic device (*not shown*) resting on the lower teeth.

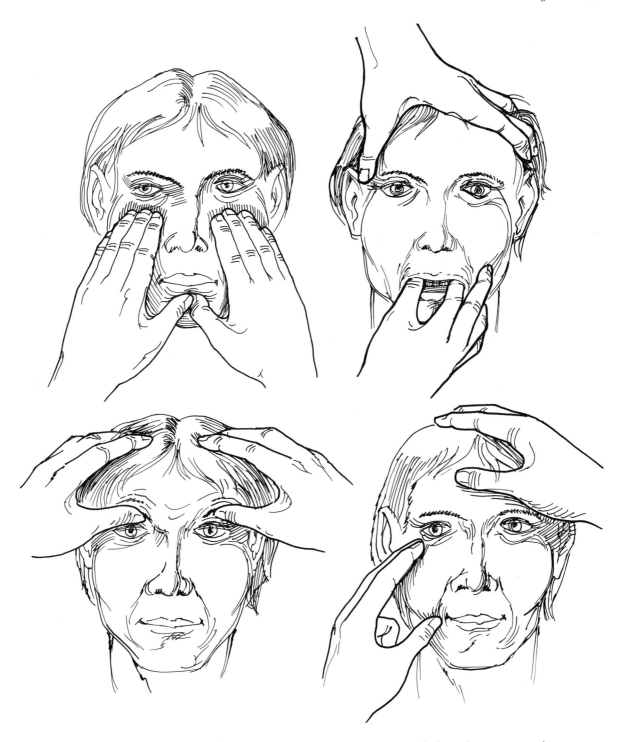

FIG. 9.11. Careful physical examination and bimanual palpation can disclose the presence of most facial fractures.

acrylic that fit precisely over the lower molars and bicuspids. The mouthpiece is held painlessly in place by two small stainless steel clasps that latch between the first and second bicuspids. The orthodontist adjusts the appliances, repositioning the condyles and balancing them from left to right as needed. With the MORA mouthpiece in place, the athlete can speak and breathe normally. The temporomandibular joint is thus balanced, reflex activity at the joint is reduced, and the athlete has added strength and endurance (39).

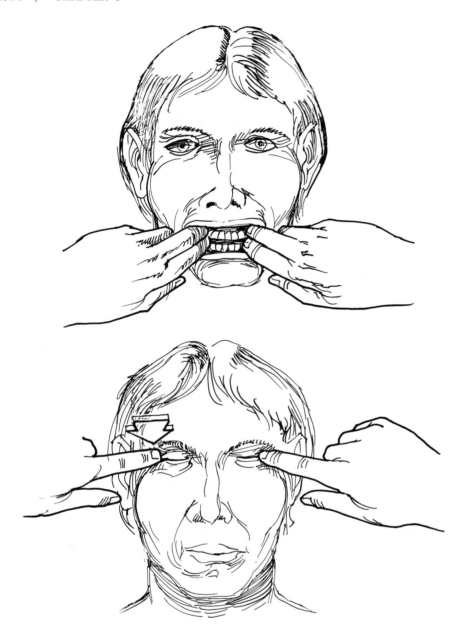

FIG. 9.11 *(Continued.)*

Tooth Problems

Tooth problems may be prevented by preseason check-ups and early dental care. Equipment for dental emergencies should include a kit containing forceps, sterile cotton, sterile saline, oil of clove (Eugenol), calcium hydroxide (Dycal), and temporary filling material (Cavit).

If an athlete loses a filling, forceps and sterile cotton may be used to clean the area and oil of clove and calcium hydroxide placed in the hole before a temporary filling is added. When a toothache accompanies the lost filling, the area should be cleaned with sterile cotton and a small cotton ball soaked in oil-of-clove placed into the cavity. The cotton is then covered with temporary filling material. The subject then bites down to compress the temporary filling. When a tooth is chipped and the nerve exposed, calcium hydroxide may be applied to the uncovered nerve area.

When knocked out, a tooth should be promptly washed with sterile saline but not rubbed. An ice pack may be applied to the face, with the athlete holding the tooth in its bed with the fingers or by keeping the mouth closed. He or she should then see a dentist, who may be able to align the tooth and keep it in place with arch bars or dental bands. If the periodontal membrane heals, the tooth will be reattached solidly.

A Panorex x-ray film should be taken to rule out alveolar or mandibular fracture after all moderate or severe injuries to the mouth.

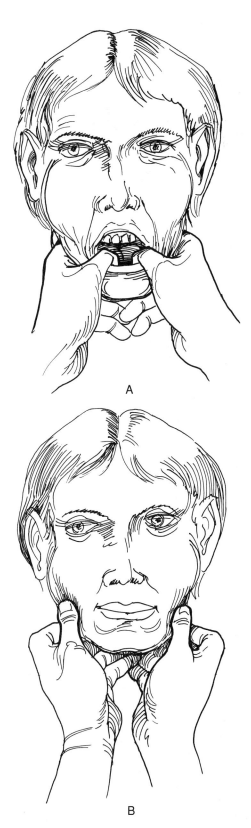

FIG. 9.12. The entire mandible can be examined bimanually except for the condyles.

Swallowed Bubble Gum or Chewing Tobacco

If an athlete chews gum or tobacco, the temporomandibular joint becomes overworked, and the chewing induces fatigue by sapping strength and endurance. The chewing athlete also risks aspirating the gum or tobacco and strangling.

The Heimlich or abdominal-thrust maneuver may save a choking athlete (14,15). Using this technique, the rescuer wraps both arms around the victim, and the victim's head and torso are allowed to slump forward. The rescuer then clasps the back of the wrist with the other hand so that the fist is pressed against the victim's diaphragm just below the ribs with a quick, hard squeeze. The squeeze is repeated as needed until the foreign body pops out like a cork. The victim should not be slapped on the back to dislodge the foreign body because such a slap may cause further inhaling of the foreign body.

If an athlete is knocked out and has gum or tobacco lodged in his throat, an oral screw may be used to force the mouth open to remove the foreign body. For an athlete who has an uncorrectable upper airway obstruction to breathing, a cricothyreotomy may be lifesaving.

Facial Bone Fractures

Virtually all fractures of the bones of the face can be suspected if not diagnosed by careful physical examination (Fig. 9.11). The smooth bones of the orbital rims can be palpated beneath the thin eyelid skin around the entire circumference of each orbit. Any areas of extreme tenderness or bony irregularity should raise the question of fracture. Tenderness and depression of the cheekbones and the areas of the zygomatic arch can readily be appreciated by the examining hand (Fig. 9.11). The entire mandible can be examined bimanually except for the region of the condyle (Fig. 9.12). Intraoral examination and palpation of the gums should disclose any fractures of the maxilla or mandible (Fig. 9.13). Aside from pain at the fracture site, the most common complaint with facial fractures is malocclusion of the teeth and pain on opening and closing the mouth. The treatment of facial fractures usually involves early open reduction and internal fixation and frequently necessitates mandibulomaxillary fixation to assure proper dental occlusion as the fractures heal. If a maxillary or mandibular fracture necessitates wiring the teeth into occlusion, an athlete may experience some real or imagined airway impairment and rather severe dietary modification while his jaws are wired together. This will usually result in some weight loss and loss of overall

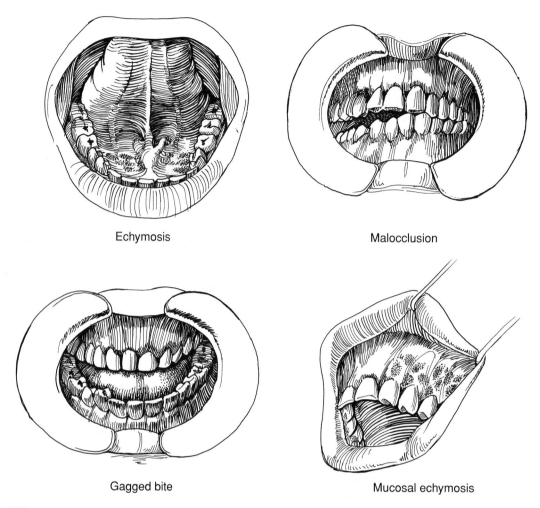

Echymosis

Malocclusion

Gagged bite

Mucosal echymosis

FIG. 9.13. Intraoral examination will reveal fractures by their accompanying hematomas, lacerations, and dental malocclusions.

strength and endurance that may extend beyond the period of having the teeth wired together.

Zygoma and Orbital Rim Fractures

The lateral and inferior orbital rims, the zygoma and its arch may be fractured from any severe blunt trauma delivered with a hard object to the cheek or side of the head. They are most commonly seen in contact sports in which the head is not protected with a helmet. Flailing elbows in basketball games and fist fights, which may break out in association with any athletic contest, are probably the most common causes of these fractures in athletes. Pain is noted immediately at the fracture sites and, if there is displacement, there may be a palpable bony irregularity or "step-off" in feeling around the orbital rim and noticeable depression of the bony prominence of the cheek. Since these fractures are usually due to a blow delivered from the side, the zygoma is

usually depressed downward and rotated medially. Since the lateral canthus of the eyelids is attached to the frontal process of the zygoma, downward displacement of this bone may produce an anti-mongoloid slant to the eyelids, drawing the outer canthus of the eye downward below the level of the medial canthus (Fig. 9.14). If the zygomatic arch is fractured, it may be depressed, producing a hollow of the lateral cheek in front of the ear. The depressed arch may impinge upon the temporalis causing pain and trismus when the injured athlete attempts to open the mouth. Virtually all fractures of these bones can be suspected on gross physical examination and x-rays should be taken in any case of suspected fracture. Treatment usually involves open reduction with internal plate or wire fixation of the fracture sites. These fractures develop fairly firm healing by ten to fourteen days and they should, therefore, undergo reduction and fixation within this time limit. Firm, solid, bone healing, however, requires 6 to 8 weeks. Most athletes could return to their sport after 8

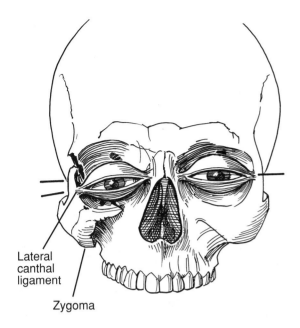

Lateral
canthal
ligament

Zygoma

FIG. 9.14. A depressed fracture of the zygoma may show a downward slanting of the eyelids and depression of the cheek.

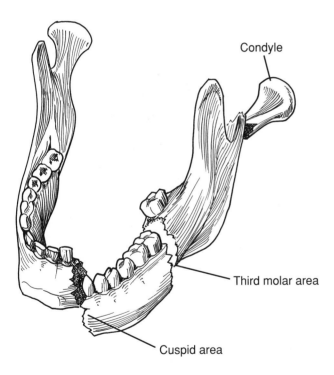

Condyle

Third molar area

Cuspid area

FIG. 9.15. Most mandibular fractures occur at these mandible weak spots.

weeks, but a boxer must wait 3 months before returning to the ring. A special molded plastic face mask may afford protection to an athlete after a fracture in this area and allow participation in sport earlier than these general guidelines.

Mandible Fractures

A blow to the angle of the jaw, the point of the chin, or the side of the chin may break an athlete's jaw. Since

the mandible is a U-shaped bone with the open ends of the U resting in a bony fossa at the base of the skull, the mandible usually fractures in two places when it is broken. Breaking the mandible in only one place is about as difficult as trying to break a lifesaver at only one point. The mandible is weakest at the canine teeth, the third molars, and the condylar necks (Fig. 9.15). Most mandibular fractures occur at these three anatomic locations. Fractures of the condylar neck are more difficult to diagnose on gross physical examination than are fractures of the body or ramus of the

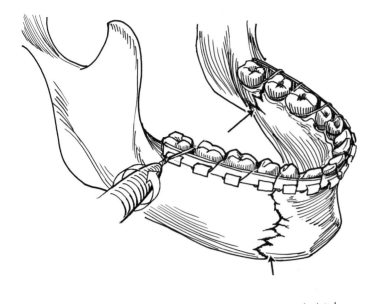

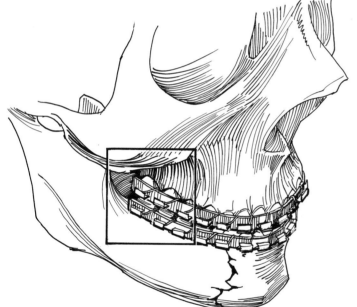

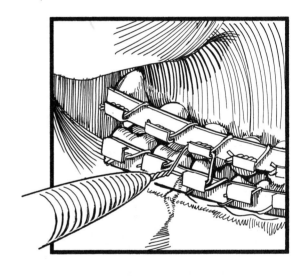

FIG. 9.16. Intermaxillary fixation is frequently required in the treatment of maxillary and mandibular fractures.

mandible. The latter areas can be examined bimanually. Condylar neck fractures can be suspected when there is pain in front of the ear on opening and closing the mouth and when the examining finger placed in the external auditory canal cannot feel movement of the condylar head as the injured athlete's mouth is opened and closed. Traction on the chin may also elicit condylar neck pain when it is fractured. Fractures of the mandible generally require placing the teeth in occlusion and wiring them together for some period of time to be certain that proper dental occlusion is restored as the fracture heals (Fig. 9.16). Careful and conscientious dental hygiene is essential while the teeth are wired in occlusion. A high caloric liquid or soft diet may minimize the weakening of an athlete while wired in dental occlusion.

Maxillary Fractures

Fractures of the maxilla are rarely seen in athletes, but may occur from freak accidents. Fitted mouthpieces, now worn in most contact sports, have helped to minimize the incidence of these fractures. Like the mandible, fractures of the alveolar portions of the maxilla may be heralded by malocclusion and lacerations or hematomas of the gums of the upper jaw. Crepitus or false motion elicited when one grasps with one hand the nose and with the other the upper incisor teeth is indicative of a maxillary fracture (Fig. 9.17). If the maxilla is fractured, this maneuver will be painful and will usually only be permitted once.

When fractures of the maxilla, mandible, zygoma, or other facial bones are suspected, facial CT studies

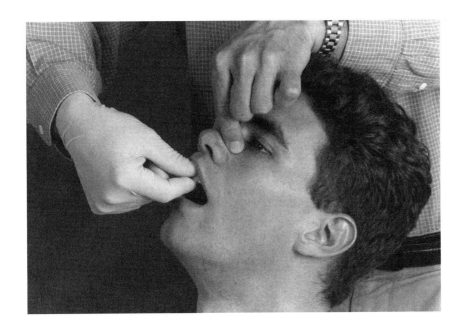

FIG. 9.17. Maxillary fractures can be detected by grasping the nose with one hand and the upper incisor teeth with the other. Crepitus or false motion and pain are indicative of maxillary fracture.

are now the accepted standard for accurately diagnosing, delineating, and evaluating the extent of these fractures and planning their surgical repair. Occasionally, an athlete may return to participation earlier wearing a special face mask to protect the healing fracture. In football, for example, an extra face bar may be added to the helmet to protect the player's injured jaw.

REFERENCES

1. Baker TE. A quick and easy method for controlling nosebleeds. *First Aider, Cramer* 1979;48(5):14.
2. Cooper DL, Fair J. Treating ''cauliflower ear.'' *Phys Sportsmed* 1976;4(7):103.
3. DeVoe AG. Injuries to the eye. *Am J Surg* 1959;98:384–389.
4. DiBartolomeo JR. Exostotic ear tumors—sea water sport peril. *Phys Sportsmed* 1976;4(7):60–63.
5. Easterbrook M. Eye protection for squash and racketball players. *Phys Sportsmed* 1981;9(2):79–82.
6. Eichel BS. Otologic hazards in water sports. *Phys Sports Med* 1974; 2(7):43–45.
7. Eichel BS, Bray DA. Management of hematoma of the wrestler's ear. *Phys Sportsmed* 1978;6(11):87–90.
8. Fowler BJ. Ocular injuries sustained playing squash. *Am J Sports Med* 1980;8:126–128.
9. Fowler EP Jr, Osmum PM. New bone growth due to cold water in the ears. *Arch Otolaryngol* 1942;36:455.
10. Garner AI. Athletes are endangered by unsafe eyewear. *First Aider, Cramer* 1977;47(3):3.
11. Gross CG. Treating ''cauliflower ear'' with silicone mold. *Am J Sports Med* 1978;6:4.
12. Handler SD. Diagnosis and management of maxillofacial injuries. In: Torg JS ed. *Athletic injuries to the head, neck, and face*, 2nd ed. St. Louis: Mosby Year Book, 1991.
13. Hayes D, Gregorasz TMJ, Maule JD. Effects of intraoral mouth guards in ventilation. *Phys Sportsmed* 1977;5(1):61–66.
14. Heimlich JH. The Heimlich Maneuver: where it stands today. *Emergency Med* 1978;10:89.
15. Heimlich JH, Uhley MJ. The Heimlich maneuver. *Clin Symp* 1979; 31(3):3–32.
16. Heintz WD. Mouth protectors: a progress report. *J Am Dent Assoc* 1068;77:632–636.
17. Heintz WD. The case for mandatory mouth protectors. *Sports Med* 1975;3:61–63.
18. Heintz WD. Mouth protection in sports. *Phys Sportsmed* 1979;7(2): 45,46.
19. Hickey JC, Morris AL, Carlson LD, Seward PE. The relation of mouth protectors to cranial pressure and deformation. *J Am Dent Assoc* 1967;74:735–740.
20. MacFie DD. ENT problems of diving. *Med Serv J Can* 1964;20: 845.
21. Manson PN. Facial injuries. In: McCarthy JG ed. *Plastic surgery,* vol 2. Philadelphia: WB Saunders, 1990.
22. Odess JS. The hearing hazards of firearms. *Phys Sportsmed* 1974; 2(10):65–68.
23. Odess JS. Acoustic trauma of sportsman hunter due to gun firing. *Laryngoscope* 1972;82:1971–1989.
24. Ogden FW. Effect of gunfire upon auditory acuity for pure tones and the efficacy of ear plugs as protectors. *Laryngoscope* 1950;60: 993–1012.
25. Oppenheimer P, Jules K, Wiley H, Kishin G. Repair of traumatic-myringorupture. *Arch Otolaryngol* 1961;73:328–333.
26. Pashby TJ. Eye injuries in Canadian amateur hockey. *Am J Sports Med* 1979;7:254–257.
27. Pipkin G. Caloric labyrinthitis: a cause of drowning. Case report of a swimmer who survived through self-rescue. *Am J Sports Med* 1979;7:260–261.
28. Roydhouse N. Earaches and adolescent swimmers. In: Eriksson B, Durberg B, eds. *Swimming medicine IV. International series on sports science*, vol 6, Baltimore: University Park Press, 1977:79–85.
29. Ryan, AJ (moderator). Roundtable discussion: eye protection for athletes. *Phys Sportsmed* 1978;6(9):43–67.
30. Schneider RC. *Head and neck injuries in football*. Baltimore: Williams & Wilkins, 1973.

31. Schneider RC, Antine BE. Visual fields impairment related to football headgear and face-guards. *JAMA* 1965;192:616–618.

32. Schwartz R, Novich MM. The athlete's mouthpiece. *Am J Sports Med* 1980;8:357–359.

33. Seelenfreund MH, Freilich DB. Rushing the net and retinal detachment. *JAMA* 1976;235:2723–2736.

34. Smith J. Contact lenses and athletes. Trainer's corner. *Phys Sportsmed* 1978;6(4):124.

35. Stenger JM, Lawson EA, Wright JM, Ricketts J. Mouthguards. *J Am Dent Assoc* 1964;69:273–281.

36. Strauss MB, Groner-Shrauss W, Cantrell RW. Swimmer's ear. *Phys Sportsmed* 1979;7(6):101–105.

37. Taylor GD, Williams E. Acoustic trauma in the sports hunter. *Laryngoscope* 1966;76:863–879.

38. Turcotte H. Scuba divers answer the challenge of the sea. *Phys Sportsmed* 1977;5(8):67–68.

39. Verschoth A. Weak? Sink your teeth into this. *Sports Illustrated* 1980;54:36–42.

40. Vinger PF. Sports-related eye injury. A preventable problem. *Surv Ophthalmol* 1980;25:47–51.

The Injured Athlete, Third Edition,
edited by D. H. Perrin.
Lippincott–Raven Publishers, Philadelphia © 1999.

CHAPTER 10

Athletic Injuries to the Head and Neck

Robert C. Cantu

The head and cervical spine are unique in that their contents are incapable of regeneration. The brain and spinal cord cannot regrow lost cells as can the other organs of the body, and thus injury to these structures takes on a singular importance. Every effort must be made to protect the athlete's brain and spinal cord because injury can lead to dementia, epilepsy, paralysis, and death (20,21,24).

Over the last 20 years there has been a dramatic decrease in the most serious head injuries, especially the incidence of subdural hematoma, due to multiple factors including rules changes such as outlawing spear tackling and butt blocking in football, equipment standards, better conditioning of the neck, and improved on-the-field medical care. The reduction of the most serious neck injury, quadriplegia, has been less impressive likely because there presently is no meaningful equipment to prevent this injury.

THE HEAD

Injury Recognition

Recognition of a head injury is easy if the athlete has a loss of consciousness. It is the far more frequent mild head injuries in which there is not a loss of consciousness but rather only a transient loss of alertness that is much more difficult to recognize. More than 90% of all cerebral concussions fall into this most mild category where there has not been a loss of consciousness but rather only a brief period of posttraumatic amnesia or loss of mental alertness. Because the dreaded second impact syndrome can occur after a grade I concussion, just as it can after more serious head injuries, it becomes very important to recognize all grades of concussion.

Mechanism of Injury

There are three distinct types of stresses that can be generated by an acceleration force to the head. The first is a compressive; the second is tensile, the opposite of compressive and sometimes called negative pressure; and the third is shearing, a force applied parallel to a surface. Uniform compressive and tensile forces are relatively well tolerated by neural tissue but shearing forces are extremely poorly tolerated.

The cerebral spinal fluid that surrounds the brain acts as a protective shock absorber converting focally applied external stress to compressive stress because the fluid follows the contours of the sulci and gyri of the brain and distributes the force in a uniform fashion. The cerebral spinal fluid, however, does not totally prevent shearing forces from being imparted to the brain, especially when rotational forces are applied to the head. These shearing forces are maximal where rotational gliding is hindered within the brain such as the dura mater—brain attachments, the rough, irregular surface contacts between the brain and the skull, which especially prominent in the floor of the frontal and middle fossa.

In understanding how acceleration forces are applied to the brain, it is important to keep in mind Newton's law: force equals mass × acceleration, or, stated another way, force divided by mass equals acceleration. Therefore, an athlete's head can sustain far greater forces without injury if the neck muscles are tensed such as when the athlete sees the collision coming. In this state, the mass of the head is essentially the mass of the body. In a relaxed state, however, the mass of the head is essentially only its own weight, and therefore the same degree of force can impart far greater acceleration.

Injury Assessment Techniques

In assessing a brain injury, if the athlete is unconscious, it must be assumed that she or he has suffered a neck

R. C. Cantu: Neurosurgery Service, Emerson Hospital, Concord, Massachusetts 01742

fracture and the neck must be immobilized. In assessing an athlete with a head injury who is conscious, the level of consciousness or alertness is the most sensitive criteria for both establishing the nature of the head injury and subsequently following the athlete. Orientation to person, place, and time should be ascertained. The presence or absence of posttraumatic amnesia, and the ability to retain new information such as the ability to repeat four objects 2 minutes after having been given them, or the ability to repeat one's assignments with certain plays of the contest should be determined. It is also important to ascertain the presence, absence, and severity of neurologic symptoms such as headache, lightheadedness, difficulty with balance, coordination, sensory or motor function. Whereas a complete but brief neurologic examination involving cranial nerve, motor, sensory, and reflex testing is appropriate, it is the mental exam and especially the level of consciousness that should be stressed.

Glasgow Coma Scale

When time permits the use of the Glasgow coma scale (Table 10.1) can be very useful in not only predicting the chances for recovery but also in assessing whether the injured athlete is improving or deteriorating from a given head injury. An initial score of greater than 11 is associated with more than a 90% chance for an essentially complete recovery, whereas an initial score of under 5 is associated with more than an 80% chance for death or a vegetative state.

Differential Diagnosis

The differential diagnosis with a head injury includes a cerebral concussion (see Table 10.2 for severity of con-

TABLE 10.1. *Glasgow coma scale =*
E + M + V

Eye Opening	**(E)**
Spontaneous	(4)
To Speech	(3)
To Pain	(2)
No Response	(1)
Motor Response	**(M)**
Obeys Commands	(6)
Localizes Pain	(5)
Withdraws From Pain	(4)
Decorticate Posturing	(3)
Decerebrate Posturing	(2)
No Response	(1)
Verbal Response	**(V)**
Orientated	(5)
Confused Conversation	(4)
Inappropriate Words	(3)
Incomprehensible Sounds	(2)
No Response	(1)

TABLE 10.2. *Severity of concussion*

Grade	Feature	Duration of feature
Grade I (Mild)	PTA	<30 Minutes
	LOC	None
Grade 2 (Moderate)	PTA	>30 Minutes, <24 Hours
	LOC	<5 Minutes
Grade 3 (Severe)	PTA	>24 Hours
	LOC	> 5 Minutes

PTA, Posttraumatic amnesia; LOC, Loss of consciousness.

cussion), the second impact or malignant brain edema syndrome, intracranial hemorrhage, and postconcussion syndrome.

Concussion

Concussion is derived from the Latin concussus, which means to shake violently. Initially it was thought to produce only a temporary disturbance of brain function due to neuronal, chemical, or neuroelectrical changes without gross structural damage (12). We now know structural damage with loss of brain cells does occur with some concussions.

In a grade I concussion, which is the most common type of cerebral concussion accounting for 90%, there is no loss of consciousness and the period of posttraumatic amnesia is brief. It is often difficult for the physician on the sideline to recognize that the player has sustained a concussion. The word ding is commonly applied to this injury. With a grade II or grade III concussion, there are periods of unconsciousness and the injury is obvious to medical personnel. Occasionally one sustains a grade II or grade III concussion because of extended periods of posttraumatic amnesia when the athlete has not actually been unconscious. By definition, periods of posttraumatic amnesia lasting greater than thirty minutes but less than twenty-four hours, even in the absence of unconsciousness, would equate with a grade II concussion whereas a period of posttraumatic amnesia greater than twenty-four hours would equate with a grade III concussion.

Second Impact Syndrome

Second impact syndrome (SIS), rapid brain swelling, and herniation following a second head injury are more common than previous reports in the medical literature have suggested. Between 1980 and 1993, the National Center for Catastrophic Sports Injury Research in Chapel Hill, North Carolina, identified 35 probable cases among football players alone. Autopsy or surgery and MR imaging findings confirmed 17 of these cases. An additional 18 cases, though not conclusively documented with autopsy findings, most probably are SIS. Careful scrutiny excluded this diagnosis in 22 of 57 cases originally suspected.

In addition, SIS is not confined to football players. Head injury reports of athletes in other sports almost certainly represent the syndrome but do not label it as such. Fekete, for example, described a 16-year-old high school hockey player who fell during a game, striking the back of his head on the ice (16). The boy lost consciousness and afterward complained of unsteadiness and headaches. While playing in the next game 4 days later, he was checked forcibly and again fell striking his left temple on the ice. His pupils rapidly became fixed and dilated, and he died within 2 hours while in transit to a neurosurgical facility.

The autopsy report revealed occipital contusions of several days' duration, an edematous brain with a thin layer of subdural and subarachnoid hemorrhage, and bilateral herniation of the cerebellar tonsils into the foramen magnum. Though Fekete did not use the label SIS, the clinical course and autopsy findings in this case are consistent with the syndrome.

Such cases indicate that the brain is vulnerable to accelerative forces in a variety of contact and collision sports. Therefore, physicians who cover athletic events, especially those in which head trauma is likely, must understand SIS and be prepared to initiate emergency treatment (25).

Recognizing the Syndrome

What Saunders and Harbaugh called the second impact syndrome of catastrophic head injury in 1984 (36) was first described by Schneider in 1973 (37). The syndrome occurs when an athlete who sustains a head injury—often a concussion or worse injury, such as cerebral contusion—sustains a second head injury before symptoms associated with the first have cleared.

Typically, the athlete suffers postconcussional symptoms after the first head injury. These may include visual, motor, or sensory changes and difficulty with thought and memory processes. Before these symptoms resolve—which may take days or weeks—the athlete returns to a competition and receives a second blow to the head (10,11).

The second blow may be remarkably minor, perhaps involving a blow to the chest, side, or back that merely snaps the athlete's head and indirectly imparts accelerative forces to the brain. The athlete may appear stunned but usually does not lose consciousness and often completes the play. The athlete usually remains on his feet for 15 seconds to a minute or so but seems dazed, similar to someone suffering from a grade I concussion without loss of consciousness. Often the athlete remains on the playing field or walks off under his or her own power.

What happens in the next 15 seconds to several minutes set this syndrome apart from a concussion or even a subdural hematoma. Usually within seconds to minutes of the second impact, the athlete, conscious yet stunned, quite precipitously collapses to the ground semicomatose with rapidly dilating pupils, loss of eye movement, and evidence of respiratory failure.

The pathophysiology of SIS is thought to involve loss of autoregulation of the brain's blood supply. This loss of autoregulation leads to vascular engorgement within the cranium, which in turn markedly increases intracranial pressure and leads to herniation either of the medial surface (uncus) of the temporal lobe or lobes below the tentorium or of the cerebellar tonsils through the foramen magnum. The usual time from second impact to brainstem failure is rapid, taking 2 to 5 minutes. Once brain herniation and brainstem compromise occur, coma, ocular involvement, and respiratory failure precipitously ensue. This demise occurs far more rapidly than that usually seen with an epidural hematoma.

Prevention Is Primary

For a catastrophic condition that has a mortality rate approaching 50% and a morbidity rate nearing 100%, prevention takes on the utmost importance. An athlete who is symptomatic from a head injury must not participate in contact or collision sports until all cerebral symptoms have subsided, and preferably not for at least 1 week after. Whether it takes days, weeks, or months to reach the asymptomatic state, the athlete must never be allowed to practice or compete while he or she has postconcussion symptoms (10,11,25).

Players and parents as well as the physician and medical team must understand this. Files of the National Center for Catastrophic Sport Injury Research include cases of young athletes who did not report their cerebral symptoms. Fearing they would not be allowed to compete and not knowing they were jeopardizing their lives, they played with postconcussional symptoms and tragically developed SIS.

Intracranial Hematoma

With an intracranial hematoma there is usually a loss of consciousness. With the epidural hematoma there may be a regaining of consciousness shortly thereafter. This lesion typically occurs with a temporal skull fracture from a blow received in the temporal area. There usually is no associated brain injury, and death usually results from the mass of the rapidly expanding blood causing brain herniation. Typically this athlete will have a headache and will then have deteriorating levels of consciousness fifteen to thirty minutes after the initial injury.

On the other hand the subdural hematoma, which is the most common cause of athletic head injury death, and continues to carry a 30% to 40% mortality rate even at the finest neurosurgery centers, is usually associated with a loss of consciousness and the athlete not regaining consciousness. It is the severe associated brain injury that causes death in a significant percentage of cases.

The intracerebral hematoma usually occurs deep within the brain and is associated with an extremely severe acceleration injury to the head. Typically consciousness is not regained unless this lesion is extremely small.

Subarachnoid hemorrhage may be seen from a ruptured congenital vascular lesion such as an aneurysm or arteriovenous malformation. This condition can also result from a severe contusion or bruise of the brain.

Diffuse Axonal Injury

This condition results when severe shearing forces are imparted to the brain and axonal connections are literally severed in the absence of intracranial hematoma. The patient is usually deeply comatose with a low Glasgow Coma Scale and a negative head CT. Immediate neurologic triage for treatment of increased intracranial pressure is indicated.

Immediate Treatment

With a head injury the ABCs of first aid must be followed. Before a neurologic exam is undertaken, the treating physician must determine the airway is adequate, and that circulation is being maintained. Thereafter the physician may direct their attention to the neurologic exam.

Definitive Treatment

Definitive treatment of Grade II and Grade III concussions as well as the second impact syndrome and intracranial hematoma should take place at a medical facility where neurosurgical and neuroradiologic capabilities are present. In the case of the intracranial hematoma, definitive surgical evacuation is indicated, and in cases of the closed head injuries and more severe degrees of concussion, observation is appropriate with careful neurologic monitoring.

What Tests to Order and When to Order

After a grade I concussion, observation alone may be all that is indicated. In instances of grade II and grade III concussion, however, a computerized tomography (CT) scan or magnetic resonance imaging (MRI) of the brain is recommended. It is recommended that these athletes be removed from the contest and sent to a definitive neurologic facility where such imaging can take place upon arrival of the patient. In the case of the second impact

syndrome and intracranial hemorrhage, emergent scanning with either a CT or MRI is also appropriate.

When to Refer

All head injuries other than a grade I concussion should be referred for neurologic or neurosurgical evaluation following removal of the athlete from the contest (26,32).

When to Operate

Closed head injuries such as concussions and diffuse axonal injury of the brain do not require surgery. However, significant intracranial blood accumulations whether epidural, subdural, or intracerebral may require prompt surgical evacuation. Congenital vascular anomalies such as an aneurysm or arterial venous malformation may require planned deliberate surgical intervention.

Appropriate Time Course for Resolution

Table 10.3 provides guidelines for return to competition after a cerebral concussion whether grade I, grade II, or grade III, and whether this was the first, second, or third concussion sustained in a given season (4–9). An athlete who has sustained a second impact syndrome and who is in the small minority that survives without significant morbidity would not be allowed to return to a contact or collision sport. So too an athlete who has undergone surgery for an intracranial hemorrhage would be ill advised to return to contact or collision sports. Both the surgery and the underlying hemorrhage causes an alteration of cerebral spinal fluid dynamics and impairs the ability of the cerebral spinal fluid to protect the brain from subsequent head injury.

Principles of Rehabilitation and Return to Play Criteria

Neural tissue itself is incapable of being rehabilitated per se. In the situation where there has been significant neurologic impairment, the athlete would not be allowed to return to competition. Only after complete neurologic recovery would the athlete be allowed to return to competition. While other guidelines exist (23,25), I prefer those in Table 10.3. Return is allowed only when and if his or her general physical condition and conditioning, especially of the neck muscles, had returned to preinjury status.

Other conditions that would preclude return to contact/collision sports include spontaneous subarachnoid hemorrhage, permanent neurologic sequellae from head injury, and a posttraumatic seizure disorder.

TABLE 10.3. *Guidelines for return after concussion*

	First concussion	Second concussion	Third concussion
Grade I (Mild)	May return to play if asymptomatic[a] for 1 week	Return to play in 2 weeks if asymptomatic at that time for 1 week	Terminate season; may return to play next season if asymptomatic
Grade II (Moderate)	Return to play after asymptomatic for 1 week	Minimum of 1 month; may return to play then if asymptomatic for 1 week; consider terminating season	Terminates season; may return to play next season if asymptomatic
Grade III (Severe)	Minimum of 1 month; may then return to play if asymptomatic for 1 week	Terminate season; may return to play next season if asymptomatic	

[a] Asymptomatic means no headache, dizziness, or impaired orientation, concentration, or memory during rest or exertion.

Knockout

The most common knockout blow is to the chin or "button." This twists and distorts the brain stem and overwhelms the reticular-activating mechanism (sleep-wake center), sending a sudden bombardment of impulses to the brain and rendering the boxer, for instance, unconscious. When a boxer is knocked down, striking the ring floor may cause more serious damage than the blow from his opponent. Ring floors are more safely constructed today than before, being made of canvas stretched over shock-absorbing Ensolite. The boxer may also be knocked out as his head strikes the cable ropes, or ring posts, or from a succession of hard blows. A blow to the eye or neck may produce severe pain, causing loss of consciousness, and a blow to the carotid sinus, heart, or solar plexus may block blood flow and cause the boxer to lose consciousness. Punches to the thin-walled temporal area may lead to loss of balance and dizziness.

Unfortunately, former fighters or steeple chase jockeys who have suffered many blows to the head may develop brain-stem hemorrhages that result in diffuse neuronal destruction and the clinical appearance of dementia pugilistica (punch drunk). Such persons become irritable and depressed, with slurred and monotonous speech. They move slowly with an unsteady gait, have tremors, and may endure dull headaches and seizures.

Stroke

In young athletes with little or no atherosclerosis, brain stem stroke may result from vertebral artery trauma after neck rotation and extension. In this condition, the rotation or extension of the spine compromises vertebral artery blood flow.

The vertebral arteries ascend in transverse foramina up to the level of the axis. They then abandon their vertical course and are susceptible as they pass upward and outward to reach the transverse foramina of the atlas, from which point they enter the skull to form the basilar artery.

Most of the movement during neck extension and rotation occurs at the atlantoaxial and atlanto-occipital joints, where the vertebral arteries lie unprotected. Excessive rotation may sublux the atlantoaxial joint, and the contralateral vertebral artery may be especially vulnerable to stretching and compression within the transverse foramen of the atlas, reducing blood flow to the brain. Two thirds of all persons have significant discrepancies in the size of their vertebral arteries, with the left usually being larger than the right. Ischemia is more likely when the smaller vessel is compressed. Hyperextension causes the atlas to slide forward and stretch and compress the vertebral arteries within the transverse foramen of the atlas.

In one case, a wrestler who hyperextended and rotated his neck while bridging had several half-Nelsons applied to him shortly thereafter. He then developed vertigo, ataxia, numbness of the left side of his face, and tingling in his body. Transient singultus prevented him from swallowing when he tried to drink water. Similar neck manipulations in yoga may also cause a stroke involving the brain stem.

Another cause of stroke with a neck injury involves the carotid arteries. By either extremes of lateral flexion or extension or a forceful blow by a relatively fixed, narrow object such as a stiffened forearm or a cross-country ski tip impaling one's neck in a forward fall, the inner layer (intima) of the carotid artery may be torn. This can lead to clot formation at the site of the injury, resulting in emboli to the brain or, more commonly, a complete occlusion of the artery causing a major stroke.

On the Field Evaluation of Head Injuries

If an athlete is lying on the field unconscious, a head and neck injury should be assumed until proven otherwise. The rescuer should grasp the athlete's jaw and pull it forward to protect from swallowing the tongue. This should be done gently because there may be a major neck injury. Ammonia ampules should not be placed under the athlete's nose because this may cause him or her to jerk the head away and damage his spinal cord.

The athlete is placed on a backboard with the head and neck immobilized between sandbags or held fixed with a four-way strap or traction device. The facemask should be removed; the helmet is not removed because improper removal may cause undue neck motion. Some masks are hinged, or the rubber facemask mounting loops may be cut to allow the mask to swing away. If the facemask must be cut, heavy-duty bolt cutters or a Trainers Angil will do the job sufficiently. Bolt cutters should always be at hand, taped to the headboard. If the player's helmet must be removed due to an inadequate airway after face-mask removal, at least two persons must do the job. One applies longitudinal traction whereas the second places one hand behind the player's neck and grasps the player's jaw with the other hand. Traction is maintained while the first rescuer spreads the helmet and removes it from the injured player's head.

Athletes who wear contact lenses should be identified so that the lenses may be removed if the athlete is knocked unconscious.

Footballer's Migraine

Blows to a player's head from a soccer ball, especially unexpected and accidental blows, may initiate migraine headaches by distorting the player's intracerebral vessels. At the beginning of a match, the soccer ball will weigh 400 g, but old leather balls become much heavier on a wet pitch. The balls may travel at 50 km/hour (30 miles/hour); thus they have a heavy impact. Migraine headaches have also been reported after blows to the side of the head in wrestling and other sports, a condition attributed to trauma-induced cerebral vasospasm. Tunnel vision, tingling in the hands, general headache, and vomiting may accompany a migraine headache. These cases demand a careful neurologic examination.

HELMETS

Tackle Football

Tackle football helmets have changed dramatically since the 1890s, when the first unpadded leather headgear was worn. In the late 1930s internal suspension systems were added, and in 1950 rigid outer shells with pneumatic and hydraulic inner suspension systems became available (Fig. 10.1).

Better energy-absorbing systems are being placed into helmets to protect against brain injury, and helmets have become so sophisticated and protective of the head that they now endanger the wearer's neck and his opponent's body. One study showed that helmets were responsible for 12% of the total injuries in high school football. Similarly,

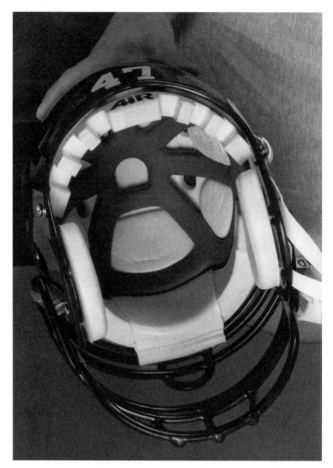

FIG. 10.1. The interior of this football helmet contains individual vinyl foam air cushions that conform to the shape of the player's head and absorb shock. Other helmets have inflatable air cells, liquid cells, and suspension systems.

almost 10% of professional tackle football injuries are produced by a blow from an opponent's helmet.

Minimum protective standards are now compiled by the National Operating Committee on Standards for Athletic Equipment (NOCSAE). Helmets are tested by dropping them from heights of 3, 4, and 5 feet to land on an Enso-lite-covered steel block. The helmet is positioned to land on its top, front, rear, right and left front, and right and left rear sections under varied environmental conditions. Football helmets must have rebound capabilities, unlike those used in motor sports racing that are designed to absorb a high impact only once. All National Collegiate Athletic Association institutions now require that helmets meet NOCSAE standards, and high schools must also meet these minimum standards.

A poorly fitted helmet is a dangerous piece of equipment, but when properly fitted it affords the athlete a remarkable degree of protection. Faulty technique is the real villain in the risk of neck injury. Most legal claims have been associated with such injuries, even though the helmet was not shown conclusively to be at fault. As a result of legal judgments against helmet manufacturers, about one half of the cost of a helmet is absorbed by liability premiums.

Baseball

Little league baseball rules require protective helmets for batters, catchers, baserunners, first and third base coaches, and on-deck hitters. These helmets have saved many lives, as a pitched ball may travel 112 km/hour (70 miles/hour) and a batted ball more than 160 km/hour (100 miles/hour). For further protection, the on-deck circle should be in a safe location and all dugouts fenced in. Major leaguers usually wear a modified batting helmet while at bat, but the helmet only protects one side of the head, and if the batter ducks the wrong way he can be struck in the bare temple.

A cricket cap may soften a blow from the 154 g (5.5 oz) leather cricket ball. The bowler stands only 6.6 m (22 ft) from the batter, and the ball may bounce unpredictably at the batter from the turf or may glance off his bat. Peaked caps, such as baseball and kayak caps, block the sun's rays from striking the athlete's forehead and help to prevent headaches. The kayak cap may also be dunked in water and put on as a refreshing headpiece.

Bicycle

Many bicyclists forgo helmets, even though they achieve high speeds on hard roads with potholes and traffic dangers. Among head protectors, "leather hairnets" can prevent scrapes but provides only minimal shock absorption. Vegetable bowl-shaped styrofoam helmets are better and can protect the cyclist's head in a fall from saddle height. They do not, however, cover the vital temporal region that can strike curbs. In addition to protecting the head, a white or fluorescent helmet helps to identify a cyclist.

Equestrian

Almost all serious head injuries in our equestrian study occurred to helmetless riders (17). Fewer than 20% of all horseback riders wear a helmet, and even if they do the helmet usually flies off when the rider falls because most riders fail to fasten the chin strap. Most helmets are little more than decorative shells anyway and afford little protection if they do stay on the rider's head.

Steeplechase jockeys who suffer many falls may, like boxers, become punch drunk with traumatic encephalopathy and epilepsy. The Jockeys Association in Great Britain and the British Standards Association have cooperated in the design of helmets for jockeys and for exercise boys and girls. These rigid shells contain energy-absorbing liners and floating cushions with temple protection and a secure cap retainer. Wearing this headgear has resulted in dramatically reduced numbers of severe and sometimes fatal head injuries.

Hockey, Lacrosse, and Jai Alai

A hockey helmet should have a shock-resistant lining and padding in the temporal regions. The helmet not only protects a player's head but also serves as an anchor for the facemask. A hockey helmet with a suspension system but without padding leaves the player's head susceptible to a depressed skull fracture from the hard puck. Lacrosse helmets, although only thin shells with a small visor, serve to anchor the facemask. Jai alai players also wear hard, plastic caps that are unfit to protect their heads from balls almost the size of baseballs and harder than golf balls that travel faster than 160 km/hour (100 miles/hour).

Motorcycle

Although motocross competitors are required to wear crash helmets, motorcyclists are not required to wear a helmet on the highways in most states. Motorcycle crash helmets are designed to absorb a high impact only once, and they have poor rebound capability. The helmet also serves as a place to attach the facemask that prevents stones and bugs from striking the driver's eyes. The best protection against facial injury is a full-face helmet.

Laws requiring the use of crash helmets by motorcyclists have been repealed in many states, and deaths have doubled where such laws have been repealed. Those who argue for repeal claim that a helmet decreases the driver's ability to hear, lowers peripheral vision, and increases neck injuries and that the requirement is a violation of a person's rights.

These arguments are countered by studies showing that hearing is not reduced because there is no change in the signal-to-noise ratio. Even wrap-around, full-face helmets allow 109 degrees of peripheral vision on each side of the nose, an amount that satisfies Department of Transportation safety standards. There is no evidence of increased neck injuries. With respect to the rights issue, taxpayers must often underwrite lifelong medical bills and maintenance costs for head-injured cyclists, who frequently do not have insurance.

THE NECK

Injury Recognition

The neck is subject to some of the most devastating injuries in athletics, and sports rank second only to automobile accidents as a leading cause of injury to this area. Two thirds of all catastrophic injuries in football and half of wrestling deaths involve a cervical spine fracture with spinal cord injury.

The same traumatic lesions that affect the brain may also occur to the cervical spinal cord, that is, concussion, contusion, and the various types of hemorrhage. Unlike the head where subdural hematoma is the most common and lethal hemorrhage, the subdural hematoma is uncommon in the spine. Since I have been associated with the National Center for Sports Injury Research (NCSIR), there have been no spinal subdural hematomas. Instead the intraspinal (within the cord) is the most common and the epidural is next most common type of hemorrhage. Also, all spinal hemorrhages have been in the cervical region and none have been seen in the thoracic or lumbar region.

Mechanism of Injury

The cervical spine is composed of seven vertebrae joined by multiple ligaments, intervening cartilages, and muscles. In the lateral view, it is curved convex forward (lordosis). The ligaments consisting of elastin and collagen provide the primary stabilizing component of the cervical spine. Elastin fibers arranged in a parallel manner longitudinally allow the ligaments to stretch up to twice their length and yet return to their original length. The main ligaments are the anterior and posterior longitudinal, intertransverse and capsular, interspinal and supraspinal, and ligamentum flavum.

The muscle groups posterior to the spine column are significantly greater than those anterior to the spine. This, coupled with the fact that the neck movement in flexion is limited by chin contact with the sternum whereas extension is possible until the head strikes the posterior chest wall, makes extension injuries potentially more serious for an equivalent amount of force. Thus, the spine is more resistant to flexion than extension.

The head weighs about 4.5 kg (10 lb) and is supported by the smallest, most delicate part of the spine. The first cervical vertebra, the atlas, comprises a ring with lateral masses and no central body. Its articulations are curved to provide flexion and extension between the overlying occiput and itself. The second cervical vertebra, the axis, has curved articulations that allow rotation between the atlas and the axis. Most of the rotation in the cervical spine occurs in this area.

The odontoid is the superior projection of the body of the axis. The transverse ligament holds the anterior tubercle of the atlas adjacent to the odontoid. Stability of the atlas and axis depends on the transverse ligament of the atlas and the odontoid process of the axis. The third through seventh vertebrae are similar to each other, providing some flexion, extension, tilt, and rotation. The vertebral arteries ascend in the vertebral foramen of each lateral mass from C-6 through C-1.

X-ray films of the cervical spine should include anteroposterior, lateral, and oblique views and an open-mouth view to show the odontoid and the lateral masses of the atlas. Sometimes the lower cervical spine is especially difficult to visualize after an injury because muscle spasms cause the shoulder shadow to obscure the region. In these instances, the athlete's head is stabilized and his arms are gently pulled down to allow this area to be seen. If this technique is unsuccessful, a swimmer's view is obtained in which one arm is abducted 180 degrees and the other arm is pulled down along the athlete's side. To obtain a clear view of the lower cervical spine, the beam is then directed at a 60-degree angle to the neck.

Prevertebral soft tissue swelling of 5 mm or more at the anterior-inferior border of C-3 provides indirect evidence of a cervical spine injury. Although an x-ray film may show normal alignment, momentary subluxation may have occurred at the time of injury, causing severe damage to the spinal cord. The mechanisms of cervical spine injury include neck compression, pure flexion, flexion and compression, flexion and rotation, hyperextension, and lateral flexion.

External forces can flex, extend, rotate, or compress the spine. In flexion injury (Fig. 10.2), the anterior elements are compressed, causing anterior wedge vertebral body fracture, chip fracture, and occasionally anterior dislocations. The posterior elements are injured, which results in rupture of the posterior longitudinal, interspinal, and supraspinal ligaments as well as the ligamentum flavum. Occasionally, rupture of the posterior half of the disk is seen.

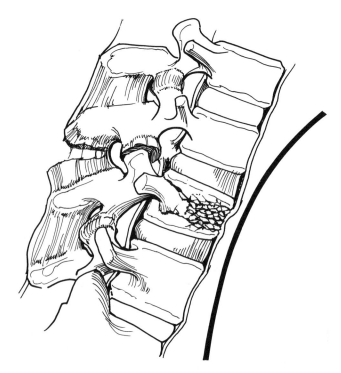

FIG. 10.2. Flexion injury to the spine.

Flexion Injuries

In a pure flexion injury, the athlete's chin sometimes strikes his sternum before his neck breaks. A facemask such as the birdcage facemask used in tackle football blocks further flexion. Flexion of the neck may produce a stable wedge fracture of a vertebral body. A pure flexion injury, as from a fall on the back of the head, may also rupture the transverse ligament. The odontoid then is no longer restrained, and an atlantoaxial dislocation results. After such an injury, as the athlete leans his head forward, the atlas slides forward, and he becomes dizzy, developing a headache from pressure on the greater occipital nerve and a tingling in his feet. As he leans backward, the dislocation reduces.

If the distance between the odontoid and the anterior arch of the atlas on a lateral x-ray film exceeds 5 mm, the supporting structures probably have failed. A distance of more than 10 mm implies the loss of all ligamentous stability. A lateral x-ray film with the neck flexed is most important, since overlooking this instability could result in an athlete's death (3). If he survives this dislocation, his neck is firmly immobilized, and an early occipitoaxial fusion or an atlantoaxial fusion with wire and an iliac bone graft is performed.

When an athlete falls on the back of the head, he or she may fracture the odontoid. Such fractures usually occur at the weakest part of the dens, its base. A slight tilt of the odontoid on the open-mouth view will serve as a clue to a fracture and is an indication for tomograms and flexion and extension films. When a fracture is suspected but no fracture line is seen, the lateral film should be checked for prevertebral soft tissue swelling as a clue to the presence of a fracture.

Flexion/Compression Fractures

A player's neck may buckle during head tackling (Fig. 10.3).

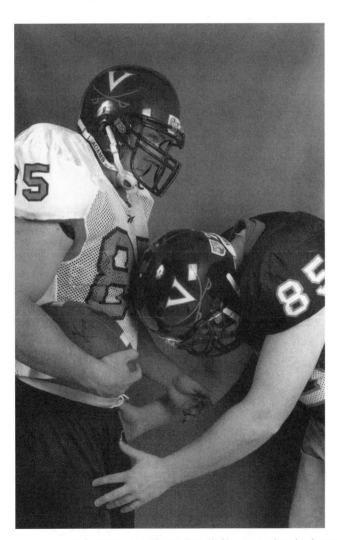
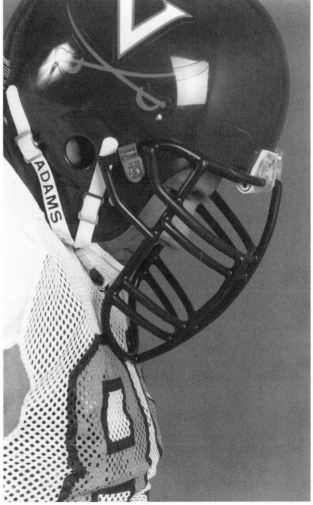

FIG. 10.3. Head tackling (*left*) can seriously damage the tackler's neck and even paralyze him. The bird-cage mask (*right*) can help to block full flexion.

This happens most commonly in high school defensive backs who wear single or double-bar facemasks, the kinds least likely to block flexion. Major stress occurs at the C-5–C-6 level, where the mobile part of the cervical spine joins the less mobile part. Flexion and compression forces produce a wedge-shaped or a teardrop fracture, which is a chip broken off the anterior lip of C-5. The injured athlete's neck will be unstable if the posterior soft tissue elements are completely torn, but otherwise the compression fracture may be stable. The entire vertebral body may crumble, with the posterior part split off and displaced.

Flexion and Rotation Injuries of the Cervical Spine

A combination of neck flexion and rotation may dislocate or fracture one or both facet joints. If a player is lying on the field and the head locked in one position, no attempt should be made to straighten it, since the facet joints may be locked. If the rotational component of the injury force is great, the pedicles may be fractured. With complete unilateral facet dislocation, x-ray films show the vertebral body to be subluxed about 25% anteriorly. When both facets are locked, the body is displaced anteriorly about 50%. Traction may unlock the facet joints, but sometimes operative unlocking is needed.

Lateral Flexion Injuries

Lateral flexion of an athlete's neck may cause a fracture through the lateral mass of a pedicle, a vertebral foramen, or a facet joint. Such an injury may produce a Brown-Sequard syndrome in which damage is limited to the lateral half of the athlete's spinal cord, producing an ipsilateral corticospinal muscle palsy and contralateral hypersthesia to pain and temperature. Lateral flexion may also produce a nerve pinch.

Extension Injuries

With an extension spine injury (whiplash, Fig. 10.4), the anterior elements are distributed and the posterior elements are compressed. This leads to rupture of the anterior longitudinal ligament and anterior disk, with posterior bony injury to the spinous processes, facets, and the neural arch.

Hyperextension Injuries

When a player's facemask is grabbed and levered backward or an athlete's face is struck by a knee, his occiput may actually contact his thoracic spine, causing neck injury (Fig. 10.5). The force needed to hyperextend the neck is not too great, since the anterior muscles of the neck are far weaker than the posterior muscles. Such

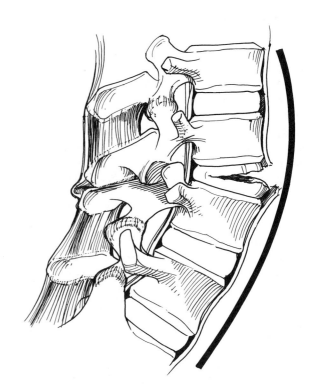

FIG. 10.4. Extension injury to the spine.

injuries may produce vertebral artery ischemia or thrombosis, with a momentary feeling of paralysis or tingling in the limbs. Compression and spasm of spinal arteries produce acute paralysis, numbness, and more tingling in the lower limbs, then in the upper limbs, but the athlete may recover even before being transported from the field.

Hyperextension is the most common mechanism of nerve root injury. Injury to the C-5 nerve root affects the shoulder and deltoid muscle; the C-6 nerve root controls the biceps and conveys sensation from the radial aspect of the arm and thumb; C-7 conducts sensation from the index and middle fingers; and C-8 controls the intrinsic muscles of the athlete's hand and innervates the ring and little fingers and the inner arm.

Hyperextension of an athlete's neck may fracture the laminas or pedicles of the axis, or a lamina may fracture along with an avulsion of an anterior-superior chip of a vertebral body. Tomograms and oblique x-ray films may be needed to diagnose such fractures. The athlete may have a complete spinal cord injury, but an x-ray film may show only a widened interspace anteriorly. Hyperextension may also produce an odontoid fracture; the only external sign of the injury may be a bruise on the athlete's forehead or face.

Hyperextension may produce a central cord syndrome, the most common incomplete cord syndrome. This occurs mostly in middle-aged persons who have osteoarthritic spines. The spinal canal is narrow, and the cord is crushed between the anterior osteophytes and an infolded ligamentum flavum posteriorly. Central spinal cord vessels

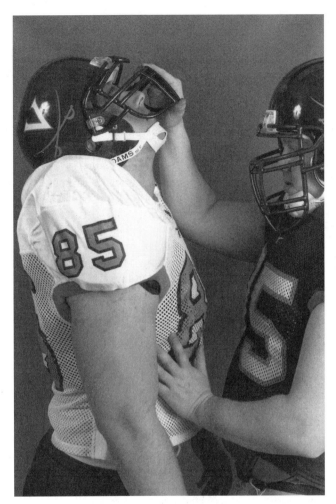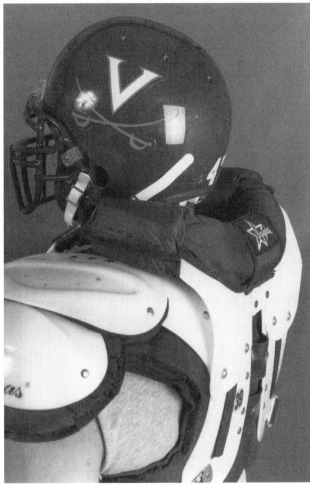

FIG. 10.5. A player's neck may be hyperextended by leverage on his face mask (*left*). A neck roll (*right*) can help to block hyperextension posterolaterally and the posterior-inferior margin fracture pushed into the spinal canal. The disk between C-5 and C-6 may also be expelled back into the spinal canal. These fractures frequently produce a transverse lesion of the cord and quadriplegia.

are injured, venous circulation is impaired, and there is progressive hemorrhage and thrombosis of vessels, with edema ensuing. Damage to the anterior horn cells in the central gray matter of the cord will produce a severe, flaccid lower motor neuron paralysis of the upper extremities, whereas damage to the central part of the corticospinal and spinothalamic long tracts in the white matter produces upper motor neuron spastic paralysis of the trunk and lower extremities. The medial parts of the lateral pyramidal tracts are affected, but there is sacral sparing. Motor and sensory functions often return to the athlete's lower extremities and trunk, but recovery of hand function is poor.

Cervical collars will limit extension of the neck, but defensive backs and wide receivers object to collars, arguing that a collar restricts their movements.

A compression or burst injury (Fig. 10.6) occurs with vertical loading of the spine, such as from a blow to the vertex with the neck flexed. This leads to vertebral endplate fractures before disk injury. At higher forces, the entire vertebrae and disk may explode into the spinal canal. Analysis has shown this to be the major mechanism of cervical fracture, dislocation, and quadriplegia not only in football (spearing, butt blocking), but in diving injuries as well as the recent increase in Canadian ice hockey neck injuries (38).

With the normal head-up posture the cervical spine has a gentle lordotic curve, and forces transmitted to the head are largely dissipated in the cervical muscles. When the neck is flexed, the cervical spine becomes straight with the vertebral bodies lined up under one another. The forces of impact to the vertex of the head are directly transmitted from one vertebra to the next. This allows for minimal dissipation of the impact forces to be absorbed by the neck muscles. If the impact force exceeds the strength of the bone, it compacts it at one or more levels resulting in a compression fracture. If the fractured vertebra malaligns and is driven back into the spinal cord, quadriplegia may result.

A combined flexion-rotation injury (Fig. 10.7) is most

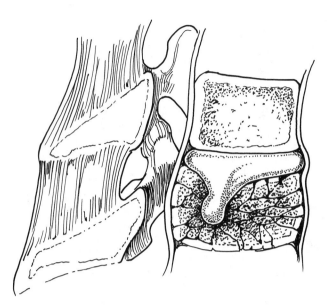

FIG. 10.6. Compression (burst) injury to the spine.

likely to result not only in a flexion injury alone, but also in anterior subluxation. Subluxation usually is found only in the presence of rotation and is more easily produced in flexion than in extension.

Most cervical spine flexion, extension, and rotation injuries occur with head trauma, but it is important to realize that such injuries can occur independently. Extension injury can occur with sudden acceleration forward, that is, a block or tackle from the rear. Flexion injury can occur with sudden deceleration, such as when the force is delivered from the front. Neck fractures without head trauma also may occur with sudden acceleration of the lower torso or buttocks cranially (as with a fall broken by landing on one's buttocks or by direct impact to the posterior cervical region by blunt trauma).

Injury Assessment Techniques

The major concern with a cervical spinal injury is the possibility of an unstable fracture that may produce quadriplegia. In the NCSIR registry, all cases of quadriplegia in the absence of spinal stenosis resulted from fracture dislocation of the cervical spine. At the time of injury, on the athletic field, there is no way to determine the presence of an unstable fracture. This requires appropriate radiographs to be taken. Also there is no way of differentiating between a fully recoverable and a permanent case of quadriplegia. If the patient is fully conscious, a cervical fracture or cervical cord injury is usually accompanied by rigid cervical muscle spasm and pain that immediately alerts the athlete and physician to the presence of such an injury. It is the unconscious athlete, unable to state that his or her neck hurts and that his or her neck muscles are not in protective spasm, who is susceptible to potential cord severance if caregivers are not aware of the possibility of an unstable cervical spine fracture. With an unconscious or obviously neck-injured athlete, it is imperative that no neck manipulation be carried out on the field. Definitive treatment must await appropriate radiographs at a medical facility. The athlete must be transported with the head and neck immobilized to the medical facility. There a detailed neurologic examination is carried out. If any motor, sensory, or reflex abnormalities are noted, the anal sphincter tone and sensation of the peripheral and sacral areas must be checked. If the neurologic examination is normal, the next step is a lateral cervical spine radiograph. If this is normal, a complete cervical spine series of anterior, posterior, lateral, oblique, and flexion-extension views must be obtained. As high as 20% of unstable cervical spine injuries may be missed when the cross-table lateral cervical spine radiograph is used alone (3). In the adolescent, displacement of the second cervical vertebra over that of the third occurs because of the hyper-

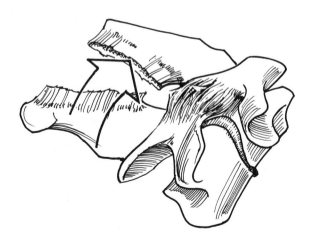

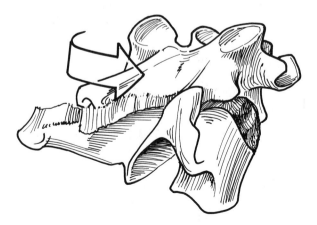

FIG. 10.7. Flexion-rotation injury to the spine.

mobility of those segments. Failure to recognize this normal of 1 to 2 mm of subluxation variation may lead to unnecessary treatment of this pseudosubluxation.

When there is spinal cord injury documented on the neurologic examination, a lateral cervical spine radiograph is taken on the still neck-immobilized patient. In this instance, oblique and flexion-extension views are not taken for fear of further injuring the spinal cord. Instead, one proceeds to a computed tomography of the cervical spine to define further the extent of the trauma and presence of spinal cord compression by bone, disk, or hematoma. A contrast positive cervical computed tomography often is more sensitive in showing spinal cord compression. In those tertiary institutions with a MR scanner this modality may be used to define especially intraspinal pathology further.

Immediate Treatment

As with a head injury so too with a neck injury, the ABCs of first aid must be followed. Before a neurological exam is undertaken, the treating physician must determine the airway is adequate, and that circulation is being maintained. Thereafter the physician may direct attention to the neurologic exam as discussed under injury assessment techniques.

Definitive Treatment

Definitive treatment of all cervical spine fractures or spinal cord injuries should take place at a medical facility where neurosurgical and neuroradiologic capabilities are present. All unstable or significantly malaligned spine fractures will require surgical realignment and stabilization. The surgical techniques are beyond the scope of this chapter.

What Tests to Order and When to Order

The tests to order and when to order them are fully covered in the Injury Assessment Techniques section of this chapter.

When to Refer

All neck injuries with neurologic symptoms or signs or evidence of fracture should be referred for neurologic or neurosurgical evaluation following removal of the athlete from the contest.

PRINCIPLES OF REHABILITATION AND RETURN-TO-PLAY CRITERIA

It is recommended that an athlete not return to competition after a neck injury until he or she is free of neck pain, has a full range of neck motion without discomfort or spasm, and has neck strength in flexion, extension, and on each side returned to preinjury levels. If a preinjury profile is unknown, strength should at least be symmetrical. Lateral neck radiographs should show return of lardotic curvature in the neutral view, and MR imaging should not reveal significant disk disease or functional spinal stenosis.

Because of their participation in the Special Olympics, it is important to realize that as high as 40% of children with Down syndrome may have abnormalities of the cervical spine (35). By far the most common abnormality is a subluxation at the atlantoaxial (C1-2) joint followed by atlanto-occipital subluxation (13). It is recommended that cervical spine stability be assessed in all patients with Down syndrome who wish to participate in athletic activities, especially those involving the head and neck, such as soccer.

BURNERS AND NERVE PINCH

The athlete may stretch his cervical plexus or his brachial plexus, damage a nerve root, or rupture a cervical disk that will press on a nerve root. These upper extremity nerve injuries are especially common in wrestling, hockey, and tackle football, as when a linebacker's neck is bent to the side when he tackles. Nerve injuries in motocross are quite severe and may include nerve root avulsions. Other athletes who may injure their upper extremity nerves are skiers whose poles catch on trees, diving soccer goalies, and mountaineers and hikers who carry heavy backpacks.

A burner, also called a stinger or a hotshot, is a stretching of the cervical plexus, the supraclavicular nerves, or the brachial plexus that occurs when the athlete's head is bent away from the side of the arm pain. Supraclavicular nerves convey sensation from the top and front of the athlete's shoulder, and injury to them produces a sensory loss but no motor loss. An athlete's brachial plexus may be contused (neurotmesis) beneath the clavicle on the surfaces of the first rib. If a nerve root is avulsed (axonotmesis), the axon degenerates distally. A nerve root may be pinched when an athlete's head is abruptly flexed laterally, and pain then radiates down the arm on the side to which the head is bent.

Knowledge of neuroanatomy is essential when examining the athlete's arm for nerve damage. The first and second cervical nerve roots contribute to the spinal accessory nerve. This is the motor nerve to the trapezius, but it lacks a sensory part. The contour of the trapezius should be examined and compared to its counterpart. Trapezius strength may be tested by having the athlete shrug the shoulders against manual resistance. The rhomboid muscles are innervated by the nerve to the rhomboids from the C-5 nerve root; the examiner should observe for wasting of this muscle. The serratus anterior receives its nerve supply by way of the long thoracic nerve; the athlete should perform a wall push-up as a check for his serratus anterior's ability to protract the scapula. The suprascapular nerve supplies motor impulses to the supraspinatus and infraspinatus muscles; atrophy of these muscles should be looked for. For evaluation of the muscles supplied by the brachial plexus, the examiner should ask the athlete to abduct the shoulder, flex and extend the elbow, and pronate and supinate the forearm against resistance. The examiner should note any numbness or tingling in the arm and do a pinprick sensory examination.

If the athlete's neck is extended and tilted toward the involved side during an examination after a nerve pinch or cervical disk rupture, the symptoms are aggravated. After a brachial plexus injury, pain will increase when the neck is tilted away from the symptomatic side. An electromyogram may help in differentiating between a cervical disk protrusion and an injury to the brachial plexus. With cervical disk protrusion, the electromyogram will show fibrillation in the athlete's paraspinal muscles. When the injury is to the brachial plexus, the paraspinal muscles are normal.

If an athlete suffers a burner or nerve pinch, his protective gear should be checked. His shoulder pads should be in good condition, fit correctly, be worn separately, and protect him from lateral flexion beyond safe limits. When he shows signs of clinical recovery, his neck shoulders and upper back should be restrengthened. He must recover full sensation and strength before being allowed to return to practice, and he may need protective straps or a neck roll. His blocking and tackling technique should also be reevaluated.

If an athlete feels well after a burner and the clinical examination findings are normal, he may return to the game. He should, however, be checked after the game, the next day, and several days later because there may be ischemia and delayed nerve damage. After neuropraxia, with damage only to the myelin sheath, the player may return to practice in 2 days to 2 weeks.

After the first injury, an athlete is more easily reinjured, possibly because of less space in the foramen owing to swelling and fibrosis. The nerve root remains trapped and vulnerable to movement that may stretch or compress it. An athlete may also have less range of lateral flexion toward the injured side and impaired facet joint function. Long after nerve pinches and burners, he may have neurologic changes and limited neck flexibility and note persistent weakness in his extensor—supinator or flexor—pronator groups of muscles, along with patches of radial or ulnar nerve numbness.

An athlete who suffers recurrent burners in a high-velocity collision sport may have an underlying cervical sagittal stenosis. The stenosis is usually asymptomatic until spondylolysis develops or a hyperextension injury or vertebral subluxation occurs, whereupon the subject may become transiently or permanently quadriplegic. If spinal stenosis is suspected, definitive diagnosis should include an MRI.

TRANSIENT QUADRIPLEGIA

Transient quadriplegia or bilateral neurologic symptoms after a player takes a hit in a contact sport raises the specter of spinal cord compromise (27,28). In some athletes, spinal stenosis may be a contributing factor. Though radiographic bone measurements can suggest that the problem may be present, physicians are cautioned against making the diagnosis of spinal stenosis with this technique alone. Instead, diagnostic technologies that view the spinal cord itself, especially MR imaging, contrast positive computed tomography, or myelography, should be employed (22). These imaging methods can determine if the spinal cord has a normal functional reserve: the space largely filled with a protective cushion of CSF between the cord and the spinal canal's interior walls lined by bone, disk, and ligament (Fig. 10.8). In addition, these techniques also determine whether the nerve tissue is deformed by an abnormality such as disk protrusion, bony osteophyte, or posterior buckling of the ligamentum flavum.

Controversy persists as to whether cervical stenosis increases the risk of spinal cord injury. The author believes very strongly that those who have had spinal cord symptoms from sports-related injuries and are shown to have true spinal stenosis on MR imaging should not be allowed to return to contact sports.

Though there are no hard data to back up that recommendation, there is a body of literature in the sports medicine, neurology, and radiology fields that indicates that spinal stenosis predisposes a patient to spinal cord injury (1,2,14,19,29,30,33,34,40).

Matsuura and his group (29), for example, compared the spinal dimensions of 100 controls with those of 42 patients who had spinal cord injuries. They found that the control group had significantly larger sagittal spinal canal diameters that did the patients who had spinal cord injuries. Furthermore, the National Center for Catastrophic Sports Injury Research has no instance of complete neurologic recovery in spinal stenotic athletes with fracture dislocation of the cervical spine, whereas there are a number of such complete recoveries in athletes with normal-size spinal canals. There are also several instances of permanent quadriplegia in athletes with tight spinal stenosis without fracture or demonstrated instability. Thus, we are adamant that following spinal cord symp-

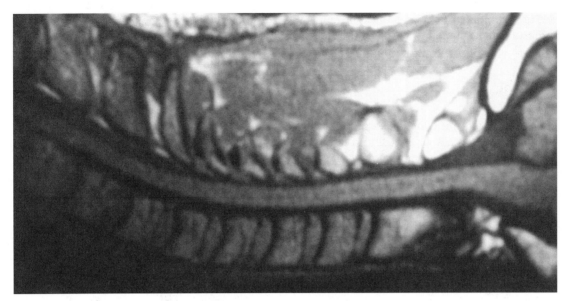

FIG. 10.8. Magnetic resonance imaging of the normal spine shows the cerebrospinal fluid-filled space between the spinal cord and the bony interior wall of the spinal canal.

toms, identification of functional spinal stenosis is a contraindication to further participation in contact collision sports.

TACKLE FOOTBALL

Deadly head injuries in tackle football have declined over the past two decades, but neck injuries have declined less. The helmet-facemask system effectively protects the player's head, but by doing so it allows the head to be used as a battering ram in tackling and blocking. Luckily, the helmet's slick outer plastic shell sometimes enables the head to glance off an opponent. At first, the proposal to place a soft outer lining on the football helmet may seem sound, but such a lining would produce an increased friction, and the tackler's head would stick to his opponent and absorb more force.

Football helmets are not designed to protect a player's neck; thus most fatal or paralyzing injuries occur when the player's neck is hyperflexed as he spears, head tackles, or butt-blocks (39). In head tackling and butt-blocking, the top of one's head is used as the contact point hitting the opponent in the numbers. Knee blows to the head or grabbing of the facemask tilts the facemask violently and hyperextends the neck. Tacklers sustain more than 70% of all neck injuries; specifically, defensive backs, who must tackle bigger running backs and ends, suffer the largest number of head and neck injuries.

Some assert that the grave risk of quadriplegia in tackle football has been concealed from players and parents. Others state that unless changes in technique are taught and rules are enforced, continued neck injuries and catastrophic paralysis will put football in severe jeopardy. If the number of neck injuries does not decrease appreciably, litigation against equipment manufacturers could conceivably remove helmets from the market, and football could end by default. Such criticism has resulted in a change in the definition of spearing, tightening of the rules, and a reappraisal of blocking, and tackling techniques. Spearing, for example, formerly referred to the impaling of a player who is out of the action with the use of one's helmet after a blown whistle. It is now redefined as an intentional use of the helmet to punish an opponent, and no player may now deliberately butt, ram, or strike an opponent with the top of his helmet. In the head tackling, the tackler drives in with his face to his opponent's numbers, propelling his helmet upward to the opponent's chin. Officials are now empowered to penalize players who use the head as a primary contact point. Instead of a 15-yard penalty for the use of the head, the player should be banished from the game. Officials who neglect to call penalties for spearing and butting should be replaced, and coaches who teach spearing should be fired.

Running backs should run with their heads up, avoiding the dangerous, flexed position. If the head nods slightly forward, the neck becomes a vulnerable straight column. In the correct bulled position, the player holds his head back some 10 degrees and tucks his chin so that shocks are absorbed by the neck muscles and upper back muscles. Proper tackling is done head to side with the tackler's head up, his eyes open, and initial contact made with the hands. The hand slides up along the opponent's side, and chest-to-chest contact is made. Strong leg drive is needed. Players should work on their tackling form in preseason practice. Shoulder blocking and tackling with the neck extended and tucked in a bulled position must be taught, and players must be trained to fall forward and backward, rolling on their shoulders and quickly getting up.

Diving

Immature, reckless young men with impaired judgment who lack training are the ones most likely to suffer a neck injury while diving, often ignoring warnings of shallow water. The water slows a diver's speed of fall, but only when a depth of 1.5 m (5 ft) has been reached. The force of the water spreads the unskilled diver's arms apart, and his head may strike the bottom. Many drownings may be due to quadriplegia when the diver strikes his head on the bottom, resulting in wedge or burst fractures of C-2.

Recreational divers rarely even lock their thumbs, but this precaution is insufficient to prevent their hands from pulling apart on entry. A stronger grasp may be achieved by holding the thumb with the opposite fist or by using the competitive diver's interlocking technique (18).

Safety efforts are best directed toward the prevention of diving accidents, with widely publicized warnings about the hazards of diving into shallow water, including the fact that the underwater rocks may not be clearly seen with changing light conditions later in the day.

Equestrian

A fall from a horse may result in a cervical spine fracture and quadriplegia. Such injuries are a significant problem for steeplechase riders, who often tumble from their mounts (17).

Equestrian athletes should practice dressage to bring the horse's hindquarters underneath the body and to achieve balance. As the horse's gymnastic skill increases, the horse should move more easily. Riders should stay on familiar terrain and check tack routinely. Learning how to fall and roll to protect the neck is advisable. A few steeplechase jockeys wear spinal protectors to prevent neck injury.

Young Tackle Football Players

Death rates do not accurately reflect the incidence of neck injuries in high school tackle football, and juniors and seniors have especially high rates of injury. Many injuries in this age group go unrecognized; thus when the symptoms of neck injury, such as radiation of pain into an arm or numbness and tingling in a limb, are explained to high school players, they frequently reveal a history of such injury.

Of 108 college freshman tackle football recruits in one study, 35 showed x-ray evidence of previous injury, such as old compression fractures, posterior element fractures,

disk narrowing, and ligamentous instability (1). Only about half of these athletes had been seen by a doctor and x-ray films had been taken only in 13 cases.

Youths who complain of neck pain should be examined (15). The examiner sometimes may find congenital instability in an immature neck. Lack of an odontoid, for example, puts the player at great risk for serious injury. Players should be informed about the symptoms of neck injury, and any player who misses a practice or game because of neck pain should have an x-ray taken. The player must have full, pain-free range of motion in his neck before returning to practice.

REFERENCES

1. Albright JP, Moses JM, Feldick HG, Dolan KD, Burmeister LF. Nonfatal cervical spine injuries in interscholastic football. *JAMA* 1976;236:1243–1245.
2. Alexander MD, Davis CH, Field CH. Hyperextension injuries of the cervical spine. *Arch Neurol Psychiat* 1958;79:146–150.
3. Blahd WH Jr, Iserson KV, Bjelland JC. Efficiency of the posttraumatic cross table lateral view of the cervical spine. *J Emerg Med* 1985;2:243–249.
4. Cantu RC. Guidelines for return to contact sports after a cerebral concussion. *Phys Sports Med* 1986;14:75–83.
5. Cantu RC. Head and neck injuries in the young athlete. In: Micheli LJ ed. *Sports injuries in the young athlete*. Philadelphia: WB Saunders, 1988.
6. Cantu RC. Head injury in sports. In: Grana WA, Lombardo JA, eds. *Advances in sports medicine and fitness*. Chicago: Year Book Medical Publishers, 1988.
7. Cantu RC. Criteria for return to competition after head or cervical spine injury. In: Cantu RC, Micheli LJ, ed. *American college of sports medicine: guidelines for the team physician*. Philadelphia: Lea & Febiger, 1991.
8. Cantu RC. Minor head injuries in sports. In: Dyment PG ed. *Adolescent medicine: state of the art reviews*, 2(1). Philadelphia: Hanley & Belfus, 1991.
9. Cantu RC. Criteria for return to competition following a closed head injury. In: Torg JS ed. *Athletic injuries to the head, neck, and face*, 2nd ed. Chicago: Year Book Medical Publishers, 1991.
10. Cantu RC. Second impact syndrome: immediate management. *Phys Sportsmed* 1992;20(9):55–66.
11. Cantu RC, Voy R. Second impact syndrome a risk in any contact sport. *Phys Sportsmed* 1995;23:27–34.
12. Committee on Head Injury Nomenclature of the Congress of Neurological Surgeons. Glossary of head injury including some definitions of injury to the cervical spine. *Clin Neurosurg* 1996;12:386.
13. Cope R, Olson S. Abnormalities of the cervical spine in Down's syndrome: diagnosis, risks, and review of the literature with particular reference to the Special Olympics. *South Med J* 1987;80:33–36.
14. Eismont FJ, Clifford S, Goldberg M, et al. Cervical sagittal spinal canal size in spine injury. *Spine* 1984;9(7):663–666.
15. Feldick HG, Albright JP. Football survey reveals missed neck injuries. *Phys Sportsmed* 1976;4:77–81.
16. Fekete JF. Severe brain injury and death following minor hockey accidents. *Can Med Assoc J* 1986;99:1234–1239.
17. Gierup J, Larsson M, Lennquist S. Incidence and nature of horse-riding injuries. *Acta Chir Scand* 1976;142:57–61.
18. Good FP, Nickel VL. Cervical spine injuries resulting from water sports. *Spine* 1980;5:502–506.
19. Grant TT, Puffer J. Cervical stenosis: a development anomaly with quadraparesis during football. *Am J Sports Med* 1976;4:219–221.
20. Gruber R, Bubl R, Fruttiger V. Anticonvulsant therapy after juvenile craniocerebral injuries: a retrospective evaluation. *Z Kinderchir* 1985;40:199–202.
21. Guthkelch AN. Posttraumatic amnesia, post-concussional symptoms and accident neurosis. *Eur Neurol* 1980;19:91–102.

22. Herzog RJ, Wiens JJ, Dillingham MF, et al. Normal cervical spine morphometry and cervical spinal stenosis in asymptomatic professional football players: plain film radiography, multiplanar computed tomography, and magnetic resonance imaging. *Spine* 1991; 16(6 suppl):S178–S186.
23. Hugenholtz H, Richard MT. Return to athletic competition following concussion. *Can Med Assoc J* 1982;127:827.
24. Jennet B. Late effects of head injuries. In: Critchley MO, Leary JL, Jennet B, eds. *Scientific foundations of neurology*. Philadelphia: FA Davis, 1971:441.
25. Kelly JP, Nichols JS, Filley CM, Lillehei KO, Rubenstein D, Kleinschmidt-DeMasters BK. Concussion in sports: guidelines for the prevention of catastrophic outcome. *JAMA* 1991;266(20):2867–2869.
26. Lindsay KW, McLatchie G, Jennet B. Serious head injury in sport. *Br Med J* 1980;281:789.
27. Maroon JC, et al. A system for preventing athletic neck injuries. *Phys Sportsmed* 1977;5(10):77–79.
28. Maroon JC, Steel PB, Berlin R. Football head and neck injuries: an update. *Clin Neurosurg* 1980;27:414.
29. Matsuura P, Waters RL, Atkins RH, Rothman S, Gurbani N, Sie I. Comparison of computerized tomography parameters of the cervical spine in normal control subjects and spinal cord-injured patients. *J Bone Joint Surg (Am)* 1989;71(2):183–188.
30. Mayfield FH. Neurosurgical aspects of cervical trauma. In: *Clinical neurosurgery*, vol 2. Baltimore: Williams & Wilkins, 1955.
31. Meggyesy D. *Out of their league*. Berkeley, CA: Ramparts, 1970: 125.
32. Murphey F, Simmons JC. Initial management of athletic injuries to the head and neck. *Am J Surg* 1959;98:379–383.
33. Nugent GR. Clinicopathologic correlations in cervical spondylosis. *Neurology* 1959;9:273–281.
34. Penning L. Some aspects of plain radiography of the cervical spine in chronic myelopathy. *Neurology (Minneapolis)* 1962;12:513–519.
35. Rosenbaum DM, Blumhagen JD, King HA. Atlantooccipital subluxation in Down's syndrome. *AJR* 1986;146:1269–1272.
36. Sanders RL, Harbaugh RE. The second impact in catastrophic contact sports head trauma. *JAMA* 1984;252(4):538–539.
37. Schneider RC. *Head and neck injuries in football: mechanisms, treatment and prevention*. Baltimore: Williams & Wilkins, 1973.
38. Tator CH, Edmonds JE. National survey of spinal injuries in hockey players. *Can Med Assoc* 1984;130:875.
39. Torg JS. Epidemiology, pathomechanics, and prevention of athletic injuries to the cervical spine. *Med Sci Sports Exerc* 1985;17:295.
40. Wolfe BS, Khilnani M, Malis L. The sagittal diameter of the bony cervical spinal canal and its significance in cervical spondylosis. *J Mt Sinai Hosp* 1956;23:283–292.
41. Yarnell PR, Lynch S. The "ding" amnestic states in football trauma. *Neurology* 1983;23:196.

The Injured Athlete, Third Edition,
edited by D. H. Perrin.
Lippincott–Raven Publishers, Philadelphia © 1999.

CHAPTER 11

The Shoulder

Kirk L. Jensen

ANATOMY AND BIOMECHANICS

The shoulder is composed of four joints: sternoclavicular (SC), acromioclavicular (AC), glenohumeral, and scapulothoracic (Fig. 11.1). The shoulder's remarkable range of motion, which is necessary for throwing and other upper extremity activities results from a dynamic balance between articular geometry, capsular, and musculotendinous structures. Any injury to these structures will result in abnormal function and diminish athletic performance.

The sternoclavicular joint is a diarthrodial joint and the only true articulation between the upper extremity and the axial skeleton. It is freely movable and functions like a ball-and-socket joint in that it has rotation in all planes. Its range of motion is determined by sternoclavicular joint incongruity, as less than 50% of the medial clavicle articulates with the sternum. Therefore the structural integrity of the mobile sternoclavicular joint depends on the strength of the surrounding ligaments; the capsular ligament, interclavicular ligament, and the costoclavicular ligament.

The AC joint, also a diarthrodial joint, has a fibrocartilaginous intraarticular disc, which is rarely functional past the fourth decade. The joint is surrounded by a thin capsule that is reinforced circumferentially by ligaments. The fibers of the deltoid and trapezius muscles blend with the superior acromioclavicular ligaments and provide horizontal stability to the AC joint.

The coracoid process of the scapula is closely related to the AC joint and extends forward and laterally like a crow's beak—hence the term *coracoid* from the Greek *korax* (the crow). The coracoid serves as the insertion for the pectoralis minor tendon and the attachment for both the coracoacromial and coracoclavicular ligaments. It functions as the origin of the coracobrachialis and the short head of the biceps. The movements of the clavicle and scapula, the so-called synchronous sternoclavicular rotation, are coordinated through the attachments of the coracoclavicular ligaments. These are the conoid and trapezoid ligaments, which are very strong ligaments, and whose fibers run from the lateral inferior surface of the clavicle to the base of the coracoid (Fig. 11.2). They are the primary ligaments connecting the distal clavicle to the scapula and vertically stabilize the AC joint.

The glenohumeral joint is well suited for mobility. The large spherical humeral head articulates with the small, shallow glenoid fossa of the scapula. The middle, and inferior glenohumeral ligaments, which are thickenings of the glenohumeral capsule, are important static stabilizers that resist anterior and inferior humeral head translation with abduction and external rotation (112) (Fig. 11.3). The superior glenohumeral and coracohumeral ligaments both resist inferior, and to some extent posterior translation of the humeral head (29). The glenoid labrum, the fibrocartilaginous origin of the joint capsule, functionally deepens the glenoid 2.5 mm (28) (Fig. 11.4). The humeral head is maintained within the glenoid through the action of the "rotator cuff" muscles (19,112). These consist of the two posterior external rotators; the teres minor and infraspinatus, the supraspinatus that centers the humeral head, and the subscapularis that is a strong internal rotator. Together, and in concert with the scapular rotators and the glenohumeral ligaments, the rotator cuff retains the humeral head in the glenoid and maintains the instant center of rotation on the glenoid within 2 to 3 mm throughout the shoulder's range of motion (76,89).

The supraspinatus muscle is active with any motion involving elevation; that is, abduction and forward flexion. Physiologically, the supraspinatus muscle accounts for less than 15% of the total cuff strength, and its insertion onto the humerus above the axis of rotation makes it a compressor and abductor of the humeral head, but not a head depressor (75). The magnitude of the force

K. L. Jensen: Division of Orthopedic Surgery, San Francisco General Hospital, San Francisco, California 94110

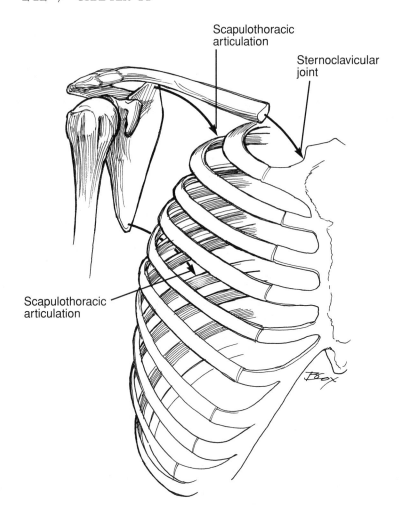

Scapulothoracic
articulation

Sternoclavicular
joint

Scapulothoracic
articulation

FIG. 11.1. The shoulder and upper extremity are attached to the thorax via the sternoclavicular and scapulothoracic articulations.

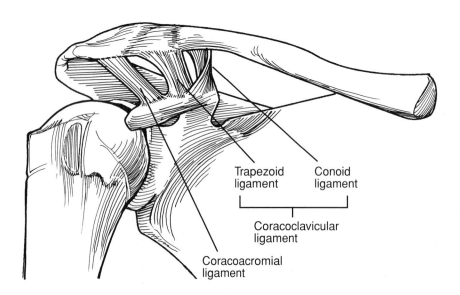

Trapezoid
ligament

Conoid
ligament

Coracoclavicular
ligament

Coracoacromial
ligament

FIG. 11.2. Anatomy of the acromioclavicular and coracoclavicular ligaments. The attachments of the conoid ligament and trapezoid ligament to the coracoid process are demonstrated. Also shown is the acromioclavicular ligament.

generated by the rotator cuff and biceps combined is equivalent to that of the deltoid muscle during forward elevation and scapular plane elevation, as revealed in studies using selective nerve blocks (110). Therefore the supraspinatus does not initiate abduction or forward flexion but functions together with the other short rotators to "fine tune" glenohumeral motion (50).

The three major portions of the deltoid are the largest and most important of the glenohumeral muscles. The anterior deltoid originates from the lateral clavicle, the middle part from the acromion, and the posterior deltoid from the spine of the scapula. They merge and insert together on the deltoid tubercle of the humerus. The multipennate middle portion, with its greater size and strength, takes part in all movements that elevate the humerus.

The tendon of the long head of the biceps originates at the supraglenoid tubercle with an attachment to the superior labrum (85). The tendon extends extrasynovially, but intracapsularly, through the shoulder joint. It then passes under the transverse humeral ligament into the bicipital groove that lies between the lateral greater tuberosity and the medial lesser tuberosity. The tendon of the long head of the biceps functions as a static humeral head depressor (116).

The coracoacromial arch is comprised of the coracoid, the acromion, and the coracoacromial ligament that connects these two bony processes. The underlying space contains the subacromial or subdeltoid bursae, the rotator cuff tendons, and the long head of the biceps (see Fig. 11.3). Processes such as inflammation, osteophytes, or developmental variations in acromion shape may decrease the space under the arch and lead to painful impingement of the soft tissues between the greater tuberosity below and the overlying coracoacromial arch.

When the athlete abducts the shoulder, the humerus is

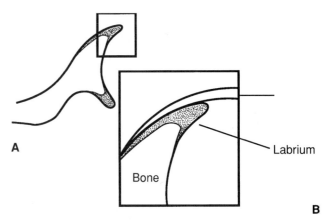

FIG. 11.4. A. Axial view of the glenoid and glenoid labrum. The glenoid labrum increases the surface area and depth of the glenoid fossa. **B.** Transverse section of the glenoid, the capsule attaches to the labrum, then continues with a periosteal attachment to the glenoid.

depressed by the rotator cuff muscles as they maintain the instantaneous center of rotation of the humeral head within the glenoid. This allows the greater tuberosity to pass posteriorly under the coracoacromial arch without impingement as the arm is externally rotated for complete overhead elevation. External rotation of the humerus also allows full elevation by loosening the inferior capsular ligaments that act as an inferior checkrein and places the shoulder in a more stable position (75). Experiments have shown that if the humerus is forcibly maintained in internal rotation, then forward elevation is limited to 115 degrees (4).

Complete overhead elevation requires smooth scapulothoracic motion that is coordinated with glenohumeral motion. The resting position of the scapula is in approximately 30 degrees of anterior rotation on the trunk. During the first 30 degrees of elevation, variably greater motion occurs at the glenohumeral joint. The last 60 degrees occurs with an equal contribution of the glenohumeral and scapulothoracic motion. The overall ratio throughout the entire arc of elevation is approximately two to one (65).

EXAMINING THE SHOULDER

Prior to the examination, a careful and thorough history should be obtained from the athlete; noting any traumatic events, the position of the shoulder and arm at the time of injury, duration of symptoms, provocative positions that reproduce the symptoms and any treatment given prior to being assessed by the examiner.

The athlete's shoulder should be examined systematically with the neck and both upper limbs easily viewed. Initial observation should assess skin color, muscle hypertrophy or atrophy, as well as deformities such as the prominence of an acromioclavicular joint separation.

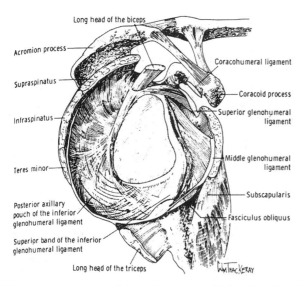

FIG. 11.3. Anatomy of the glenohumeral joint; the glenoid and surrounding capsule, ligaments, and tendons.

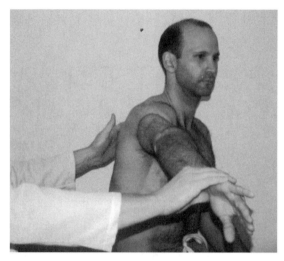

FIG. 11.5. Isolated testing of the supraspinatus tendon; resisted abduction (45 to 90 degrees) of the arm in the plane of scapula (30 degrees of forward flexion) and in internal rotation (thumb down).

Scapulothoracic rhythm is next assessed as the athlete abducts both shoulders simultaneously to an overhead position, then back to the side to determine if there is any asymmetry in a normally smooth synchronous motion. The stability of the scapula should also be observed during this movement, as scapular winging may be due to weakness or injury to one of the major scapular rotators; the serratus anterior, trapezius, or rhomboids.

The athlete's neck should always be examined during a shoulder evaluation, since a neck disorder may be the source of referred shoulder pain. As the athlete rotates the neck, with the chin turned to one side, the examiner presses on the vertex of the athlete's skull to reproduce radicular symptoms indicative of a disc problem. A thoracic outlet compression may be ruled out by the modified

Adson maneuver, which is performed by having the athlete turn the head away from the side being tested. The examiner then extends and raises the arm while palpating the radial pulse. If the pulse disappears, further investigation is warranted (66).

A systematic shoulder examination should begin in the front and then progress to the back. The sternoclavicular joint is first visually inspected for bruising or swelling, then palpated to elicit pain or detect instability. The examiner then palpates the entire length of the clavicle, assessing the insertion of the trapezius and clavicular origin of the pectoralis major. The coracoclavicular ligament region and acromioclavicular joint are next palpated. The integrity of the AC joint may be tested by applying gentle pressure to the top of acromion and observing for a stepoff at the AC joint. The coracoid process is then palpated; however, even a normal coracoid may be tender to deep pressure.

Glenohumeral joint motion assessment should document active and passive range and the quality of synchronous movement. Forward elevation, external rotation with the elbow at the side and at 90 degrees abduction, as well as internal rotation should be examined in an upright position. Some overhead athletes, such as baseball pitchers or tennis players, will have increased external rotation and decreased internal rotation when compared to the opposite side. Athletes who do heavy bench presses in the off season may have pectoralis major tightness, resulting in an internal rotation contracture.

Functional muscle strength testing should next be performed, as the majority of athletic injuries are musculotendinous in nature. Weakness associated with pain usually is associated with tendinous inflammation although weakness without pain usually reflects incompetence or disruption of the tendon. The infraspinatus and teres minor are tested by external rotation against resistance with

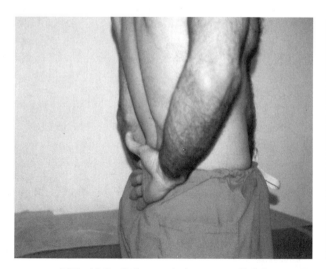
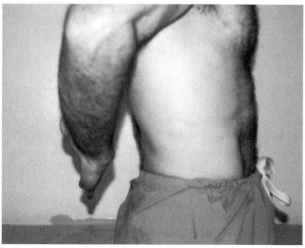

FIG. 11.6. Subscapularis test or "lift-off" test; the patient lifts the palm of the hand backwards, away from the small of the back. It is suggestive of a subscapularis tendon tear if the patient cannot lift off.

thc clbow at the side. The integrity of the supraspinatus is assessed by resisted abduction of the arm below 90 degrees, with the thumb pointing down, in the plane of the scapula (Fig. 11.5). The subscapularis is tested by the ''lift-off'' test; place the back of the hand on the middle of the back and lift the hand away from the back against resistance (Fig. 11.6).

Glenohumeral stability is difficult to assess in the muscular athlete, therefore performing maneuvers, both upright and supine, may help obtain an accurate clinical diagnosis. After the normal shoulder of the athlete is examined for stability, and the overall ligamentous laxity is assessed by testing for increased extension of the metacarpalphalangeal and elbow joints, the affected shoulder may be examined for instability. The acromion, the spine of the scapula, and the coracoid must be stabilized as the examiner applies directional stress to the humeral head to reproduce symptoms of subluxation. Usually the athlete allows only one reproduction of instability, then will involuntarily increase muscular tension to avoid a second painful subluxation. The apprehension test with the patient sitting or supine with the shoulder abducted to 90 degrees and a slow increase in external rotation should reproduce the feeling of impending anterior instability (Fig. 11.7). Pain alone, although often present, is not sufficient for a positive apprehension sign (54). Posterior instability is assessed by abducting the shoulder to 90 degrees, placing one hand on the other shoulder, and applying a posteriorly directed force through the elbow of the shoulder being tested (Fig. 11.8).

The bicipital groove, which contains the long head of the biceps tendon, can be palpated anteriorly as the shoulder is held in 10 degrees of internal rotation. Tenderness, which moves with rotation, should signify bicipital tendon pathology. A test for a dislocating biceps tendon, although a rare event, may be performed with the shoulder ab-

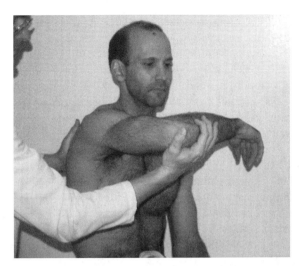

FIG. 11.8. Cross-body test for posterior glenohumeral instability. In a supine or standing position the athlete's arm is brought across the body, the scapula is stabilized, and a posteriorly directed force is applied at the elbow.

ducted to 90 degrees and the examiner rotating the arm from internal to external rotation. If a pop is heard or snap is felt, then the long head of the biceps may be dislocating from within the groove.

The examiner next abducts the shoulder to 70 degrees and palpates under the acromion from anterior to posterior for a tender supraspinatus tendon or subacromial bursa. At this level of abduction, the greater tuberosity just passes under the coracoacromial arch where impingement may occur. Crepitus may be felt or heard during rotation of the shoulder in this position indicating a thickened, inflamed bursa. The arm may be extended to palpate the anteriorly lying supraspinatus tendon and the posterior cuff tendons may be palpated when the athlete grasps the opposite shoulder. The examiner should also ask the athlete to simulate the shoulder motion that causes discomfort, and by offering resistance to this movement the examiner may be able to locate the trouble spot.

Finally the scapula is examined with the subject prone and the arm hanging over the examining table. The rhomboids and the large muscles that stabilize the scapula may then be palpated. The shoulder can be abducted to uncover the chest wall under the scapula, which then can be palpated.

SPECIFIC UPPER EXTREMITY INJURIES

Thoracic Outlet Syndrome

Thoracic outlet syndrome refers to compression of the brachial plexus or adjacent vessels by anatomic structures that narrow the space through which they course to the athlete's arm. These structures include the scalene and subclavius muscles, the first rib, anomalous cervical ribs,

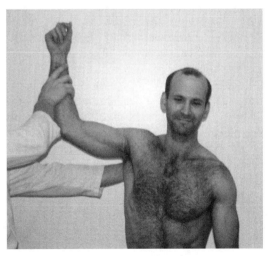

FIG. 11.7. Apprehension test (crank test). Abduction and external rotation of the patient's arm with the thumb applying anteriorly directed leverage.

excessive callous formation secondary to a clavicle fracture, the clavicle itself, or fibrous bands traversing the outlet. The symptoms most athletes present with are combinations of pain, paresthesias, and numbness in the ipsilateral upper limb and hand. Many of these patients have successful relief from surgical procedures, primarily resection of the first rib (104). It is less common for an athlete to have obvious ischemic vascular changes in the distal upper extremity with a Adson or modified Adson test. An even smaller group of athletes have a true neurogenic thoracic outlet syndrome, most of which have clearly recognizable anatomic anomalies and clearly recognizable objective clinical findings (66). If symptoms persist and clinical weakness or atrophy is evident, then further evaluation should consist of cervical radiographs and MR imaging, as well as electrodiagnostic studies. Very rarely, arterial occlusion of the second portion of the axillary artery occurs in an overhead athlete as extension, abduction, and extreme external rotation causes pectoralis minor compression (115).

Careful examination of the neck should also be performed to rule out a cervical disk problem. Magnetic resonance imaging (MRI) of the cervical spine should be considered in the clinical case of objective physical findings and supportive electromyography (EMG) results. Athletes with true neurogenic thoracic outlet syndrome typically have neuromuscular deficits and electrodiagnostic abnormalities that localize to the inferior cord of the brachial plexus. Initial treatment of compression problems include a sling, antiinflammatory medication, and exercises to maintain a full range of motion until a specific etiology is identified.

The vast majority of athletes who report paresthesias, pain, or fatigue in the arms and hands have a postural thoracic outlet syndrome. Typically these athletes are tennis players (91) or baseball players with "drooping" shoulders, as well as heavily muscled athletes such as weight lifters or rowers who perform strenuous, repetitive exercises. These individuals slump their shoulders forward and often have positive Adson maneuvers upon clinical exam. However, few have persistent vascular or neurologic deficits and rarely have abnormal electrodiagnostic studies. These symptoms usually respond to a rehabilitation program to improve posture and to strengthen the scapular rotators, rotator cuff muscles, and the three parts of the trapezius (20).

NEUROVASCULAR PROBLEMS

Quadrilateral Space Syndrome

The quadrilateral space is at the posterior aspect of the shoulder and is formed by the teres minor superiorly, teres major inferiorly, long head of the triceps medially, and the shaft of the humerus laterally. The axillary nerve and posterior humeral circumflex artery may be compressed by fibrous bands as they pass through this space (67). The athlete presents with posterior shoulder pain when the shoulder is abducted and externally rotated, as in the cocking phase of throwing. Physical examination usually is normal and EMG studies are not helpful. The diagnosis is confirmed by an arteriogram of the subclavian artery or MR angiography, which can assess the comparative patency of the posterohumeral circumflex artery in the adducted and abducted position (73). Rest and local corticosteroid injection may relieve the athlete's symptoms; however, surgical decompression of the teres minor tendon via a posterior approach is necessary if symptoms persist (8).

Suprascapular Nerve Entrapment

The suprascapular nerve can be injured at several different levels during its course to innervate the supraspinatus and infraspinatus. In the general population, entrapment most commonly occurs at the scapular notch and affects both muscles. The athlete may have entrapment distally as it passes around the base of the acromion to innervate the infraspinatus. This has been reported to occur in both volleyball (86) and tennis players (33), as well as pitchers (52). The athlete may present with various complaints of pain and examination will reveal atrophy of the infraspinatus muscle (13). The infraspinatus is not completely denervated and good results can be achieved with maximizing the remaining muscle function (90).

Brachial Plexus Injuries: Burner/Stinger

The terms *burner* and *stinger* refer to the acute onset of burning, stinging, paresthesias and pain throughout the upper limb, and occasionally associated with transient paralysis or weakness of the shoulder musculature. These injuries, seen in rugby and football players, typically occur following a downward force being applied to the shoulder or with lateral flexion of the head and neck to the opposite side. The pain may last from 15 seconds to 1 to 2 minutes; however, the numbness and paresis may last longer. This injury requires a careful, specific physical examination as it may be a precursor of a significant brachial plexus injury. The nerves most commonly involved are those of the upper trunk: the suprascapular, musculocutaneous, and axillary nerves. These may be assessed by testing the strength of the infra- and supraspinatus, the biceps, and the deltoid, as well as the sensation of the respective nerve distribution. Physical examination should reveal a normal, painless cervical range of motion, which distinguishes these lesions from other cervical spine injuries.

Clancy et al. (26) describes three grades of injury to the brachial plexus, which are not absolute and have mild, moderate, and severe categories of each grade. A grade I injury represents a neuropraxia of the nerves and the spectrum of injury includes weakness and parasthesia, which last minutes to hours. The athlete may return to play if the physical exam is normal and is withheld from returning to competition if an abnormal exam is present or persists. If clinical symptoms persist, cervical spine radiographs should be obtained immediately and electromyographical studies obtained at 18 to 21 days. A grade II injury exists when motor and sensory deficits persist longer than 2 weeks and represents axonotmesis. The EMG in this case will be abnormal and should be repeated to document reinnervation. Return to sports is allowed when full strength returns and the EMG reveals reinnervation (generally at 4 to 6 weeks). The grade III injury represents neurotmesis and clinical improvement is not appreciable at one year with abnormal physical and electromyographical exams. The athlete should reconsider involvement in contact sports in this situation.

Recurrent burners happen frequently, raising concern regarding cumulative injury. A preventative stretching and strengthening program for the cervical and shoulder muscles can prevent recurrence and various equipment combinations of shoulder pads and neck rolls are recommended for the football player.

STERNOCLAVICULAR JOINT INJURIES

The sternoclavicular joint is the only true articulation between the upper extremity and the axial skeleton. Therefore, many direct and indirect forces act through and may cause injury to the joint. Indirect forces such as landing on an outstretched hand or on the point of the shoulder are the most common mechanisms of injury to the SC joint. The ratio of anterior to posterior injuries is approximately 20 to 1 (82).

Radiographic examination is necessary and the serendipity view, a 40-degree cephalic tilt view of the manubrium, will provide information about displacement and direction. Tomograms may be helpful to distinguish between a dislocation and a medial clavicle fracture if computed tomography is not available. If a posterior dislocation is clinically evident, then all available x-ray techniques should be used to evaluate the SC joint, including, when necessary, combined aortagram-computerized tomography (CT) scan for potential vascular injuries (59). These radiographic studies should be performed prior to any attempt of closed reduction.

A mild sprain (intact rhomboid ligaments) occurs when the athlete complains of pain with movement of the upper extremity. The joint may be tender and swollen, but is stable. Treatment should consist of the application of ice for the first 24 to 48 hours and a sling should be worn for 3 to 4 days, followed by gradual use of the upper extremity.

A subluxation of the joint with partial ligament disruption will also have swelling and marked pain. Comparison to the normal side will reveal asymmetry due to the anterior or posterior displacement. Initial treatment should again consist of ice for 24 hours followed by the application of heat. Radiographic evaluation should precede reduction, and immobilization in a sling and swath is used to prevent movement of the upper extremity. The athlete should then be protected from further injury for 4 to 6 weeks.

A complete dislocation results in either anterior or posterior displacement of the medial clavicle. In either instance, a careful examination should pay attention to pulmonary and vascular symptoms. Anterior dislocations are reduced under local or general anesthesia by placing several towels between the shoulders, extending the arm, then applying gentle posterior pressure. Most dislocations can be reduced, but frequently these reductions are unstable. However, if the SC joint will remain reduced, the reduction can be maintained by a soft figure-eight dressing for 6 weeks. The athlete should be protected for 8 weeks from contact sports.

Posterior dislocations are potentially fatal as the great vessels and airway lie immediately posterior to the sternoclavicular joint and require reduction under general anesthesia. The athlete may complain of difficulty breathing or swallowing because of the posteriorly displaced medial clavicle compressing the airway or esophagus (59). Imaging of the sternoclavicular joint should be performed prior to any attempts at reduction. Reduction should be performed in the operating room, placing several towels between the shoulders, applying longitudinal traction to the abducted arm, and then extending the arm. The shoulders should be held for 8 weeks by a plaster of soft figure-eight splint to allow ligament healing.

Following the return to athletic activity from any of the above injuries, the athlete may develop pain, grinding, and popping of the SC joint, which may interfere with their performance. Arthritis of this joint may develop, requiring resection of the medial end of the clavicle or the intraarticular disc may need to be debrided (97). Generally anterior dislocations cannot be held in a reduced position and once the acute symptoms resolve the athlete may return to sport.

The medial clavicle epiphysis does not ossify until age 18 to 22 or fuse until age 25; therefore, most dislocations in this age group are displaced epiphyseal fractures. Tomograms or a CT scan should be obtained following reduction to ensure that the medial physis has been reduced.

THE CLAVICLE

The fractured clavicle accounts for approximately 10% of all fractures, with 85% occurring through the middle one third; 10% through the distal one third: and 5% through the proximal one third. The mechanism of injury is most commonly a directly applied force (e.g., tackling in a football game, hockey "board checking") (83). Again, careful physical examination at the time of injury should assess the neurovascular status of the upper extremity, as the brachial plexus and vessels pass under the mid-clavicle. Radiographic studies should include an anteroposterior (AP) view of the clavicle and a 20- to 45-degree cephalic tilt view.

Although anatomic reduction of the mid-clavicle fracture fragments is rarely obtained, full restoration of function with minimal cosmetic deformity is usually achieved. The figure-eight bandage is usually the form of treatment, held snugly to reduce fragment overriding and motion. It must be worn continuously until fracture callous is present on radiographic examination, then slow functional increase in use of the upper extremity while increasing range of motion and strength is encouraged. Collision sports and physically demanding sports should be avoided for an additional 6 weeks.

Distal clavicle fractures are generally divided into three groups (Fig. 11.9), depending upon the location of the fracture in respect to the coracoclavicular ligaments (79). In a type I, the fracture is distal to the intact coracoclavicular ligaments and is minimally displaced. The athlete may be treated with a sling for comfort, early isometric exercises, and discontinuation of immobilization as symptoms permit. In the type II fractures, the coracoclavicular ligaments are attached to the distal fragment allowing for superior displacement of the medial clavicle. These fractures are prone to nonunion and if weighted radiographs reveal displacement then surgical repair is indicated. The type III distal clavicle fracture extends into the AC joint and, depending on the size of the fragment, may be treated with a sling or if displaced, with open reduction and internal fixation. If posttraumatic symptomatic arthritis occurs, then resection of the distal clavicle must be considered.

Adolescent athletes with clavicle fractures should be treated nonoperatively unless an associated injury is present, because of the rapidity in fracture healing and potential for remodeling. All athletes with clavicle fractures should maintain their cardiovascular endurance through specific conditioning exercises such as stationary bike riding, aquatic running, and so forth.

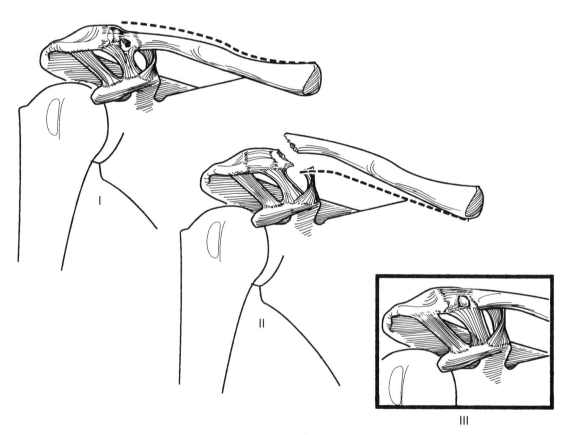

FIG. 11.9. Distal Clavicle Fracture Classification: Type I. Fracture distal to CC attachments, CC ligaments intact. Type IIa. Conoid and Trapezoid ligaments attached to distal segment. Type IIb. The conoid ligament is ruptured from displaced proximal fragment, while the trapezoid remains attached to the distal segment. Type III. Distal clavicle fracture involving the articular surface of the AC joint.

ACROMIOCLAVICULAR JOINT INJURIES

Weight Lifter's Shoulder

Atraumatic distal clavicle osteolysis is a poorly understood process affecting athletes with no history of trauma to the shoulder. The common precipitating factor appears to be repetitive loading of the AC joint; commonly seen in weight lifters (22,70). The athlete usually presents in the second to fourth decade of life with pain localized to the AC joint with overhead lifting activities. Aggravating maneuvers include the bench press, the clean-and-jerk, and body dips. Radiographs demonstrate distal clavicle osteolysis, cystic changes, and loss of subchondral bone. Initial treatment consists of avoidance of activities inciting pain (such as overhead lifting) and maintenance of shoulder range of motion. If patients do not respond following 6 months of conservative treatment or are unable or unwilling to modify their activities then open or arthroscopic distal clavicle excision is recommended with good reported results (1,24,41).

Shoulder Separations

The acromioclavicular joint is a true diarthrodial joint with articular surfaces and a fibrocartilaginous interarticular disk. The joint itself is surrounded by a thin capsule that is reinforced superiorly and inferiorly by the anterior and posterior acromioclavicular ligaments and by the superior and inferior acromioclavicular ligaments. More importantly the fibers of the trapezius and deltoid blend with the fibers of the superior acromioclavicular joint, providing strength and stability.

The most common mechanism for injury of the acromioclavicular joint is direct downward force applied to the point of the shoulder as may occur when falling while mountain biking or in-line skating. These injuries are also common in those involving high-impact collisions between participants such as football, hockey, rugby, and wrestling. The displacing force is transmitted to the acromioclavicular ligaments producing a mild or moderate sprain, depending upon the extent of ligament tearing. If the magnitude of the downward force is large, then the coracoclavicular ligaments are stressed, stretched or torn and the deltoid and trapezius fascial attachments to the distal clavicle may be ruptured.

If the athlete complains of shoulder pain after a fall or tackle, the shoulder should be examined with the shoulder pads off. The physical examination should note the presence of acromioclavicular joint deformity if the joint is tender and swollen. Manual depression of the distal end of the clavicle may determine if abnormal motion is present between the distal clavicle and the acromion. If swelling and tenderness of the acromioclavicular joint is noted, then ice and a sling are used for the first 72 hours. If the

player is sent back onto the field, a second blow may transform a type I injury into a more serious injury with a longer rehabilitative process.

Radiographic evaluation should be performed to assess the extent of the injury, determine if ligaments are disrupted, and therefore guide the appropriate treatment (Fig. 11.10). The acromioclavicular joint is best viewed when the tube is tilted up 15 degrees and the intensity is decreased. The integrity of the coracoclavicular ligaments should be tested by stress views of both shoulders, with 10 to 15 pounds suspended from the athlete's wrists. A comparison of the coracoclavicular distance between the injured and normal shoulder is then made.

Acromioclavicular injuries are graded I to VI (Fig. 11.11) (94), based upon the amount of damage to the acromioclavicular and coracoclavicular ligaments. A type I injury is a minor strain to the fibers of the acromioclavicular joint; the ligaments remain intact and the joint is stable. A type II injury consists of disruption of the acromioclavicular ligament and a sprain of the costoclavicular ligaments. The outer end of the clavicle may be slightly higher than the acromion and pain is present with palpation of the coracoclavicular interspace. Treatment of both type I and II injuries consists of ice, a sling for 72 hours and appropriate analgesic medication followed by cryotherapy and isodynamics or weight training within the athlete's pain tolerance (11). The athlete may return to competition when the shoulder is asymptomatic, and a painless range of motion of the shoulder when full strength is achieved (approximately 2 to 6 weeks). Protec-

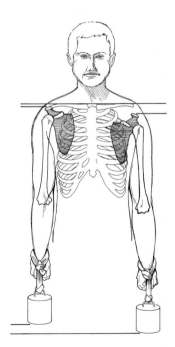

FIG. 11.10. Radiographic technique to differentiate type II and type III AC joint injuries. Measure the coracoclavicular distance on bilateral AP radiographs of the shoulder, with 10 to 15 pounds of weights hanging on both arms.

tive shoulder pads with a cut out doughnut configuration are available for use during competition.

The type III acromioclavicular joint separation is a complete tear of both the acromioclavicular and coracoclavicular ligaments, damage to the intraarticular meniscus, and disruption of the deltoid-trapezius sling of varying degree. Occasionally, the coracoclavicular ligaments remain intact, and this is associated with an avulsion fracture of part or all of the coracoid process. Moderate pain is present in the athlete's shoulder, and the arm is usually held close to the body and supported by the other arm to relieve the discomfort in the acromioclavicular joint. The lateral clavicle is quite unstable and appears to be floating free. It is important to realize that it is not the distal clavicle that is high-riding but the upper extremity that is drooping, due to the loss of attachment to the axial skeleton.

Treatment of the type III injury has been controversial in the past, as some orthopaedic surgeons advocate early operative repair and others advocate closed treatment. Individualization of treatment will result in the best outcome for athletes (30). The nonoperative treatment consists of symptomatic care initially with a sling and ice. Supine range of motion exercises are performed gently to maintain motion, and as pain resolves (usually within one to two weeks), active assistive range of motion and limited short-arc resistive exercises with cryrotherapy are instituted. A trapezius and deltoid-strengthening program with shrugs and resistive abduction can be initiated three to four weeks following injury. The athlete must be advised that the "bump" will persist and that some loss of strength will develop in the injured shoulder. Although special slings and taping methods have been advocated to reduce the distal clavicle, these are not recommended as they may cause skin pressure sores, prolong pain, and prevent early rehabilitation (94).

If the athlete is not involved in a contact sport and requires a strong stable shoulder or if pain and soreness with activity persists after six months of conservative therapy, then reconstruction of the coracoclavicular ligaments and repair of the torn trapezial-deltoid fascia is recommended (31). Although numerous surgeries have been devised and advocated over the years, several points have been well established. Primary distal clavicle excision without repair of the coracoclavicular ligaments will result in a shortened painful clavicle, which is still dislocated. Pins placed across the acromioclavicular joint may break and migrate (68).

The use of nonabsorbable suture in a figure-eight loop around the clavicle and the coracoid is commonly used. However, it may lead to a wear fracture and a return of the acromioclavicular dislocation (27). Excellent results have been reported using either a coracoclavicular lag screw or a PDS figure-eight loop (48) combined with repair of the torn coracoclavicular ligaments and trapezial-deltoid fascia (Fig. 11.12). The screw is re-

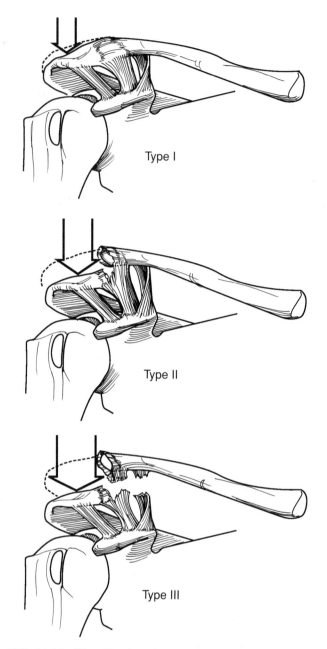

FIG. 11.11. Classification of acromioclavicular injuries. The differentiation between types I, II, III, and V is based upon the distance between the coracoid and clavicle on a standing AP radiograph. (*Continued.*)

moved at 6 to 8 weeks under local anesthesia. Gentle pendulum exercises are allowed during the time the screw is in place. Once the screw is removed, rehabilitation may begin and return to sport is possible once normal range of motion and strength necessary for participation is achieved.

If the injury is more than 4 weeks old the coracoclavicular ligaments are unable to be repaired and another source of tissue is necessary to reconstruct the ligaments and provide vertical stability to the upper extremity. In this situation, the coracoacromial ligament may be trans-

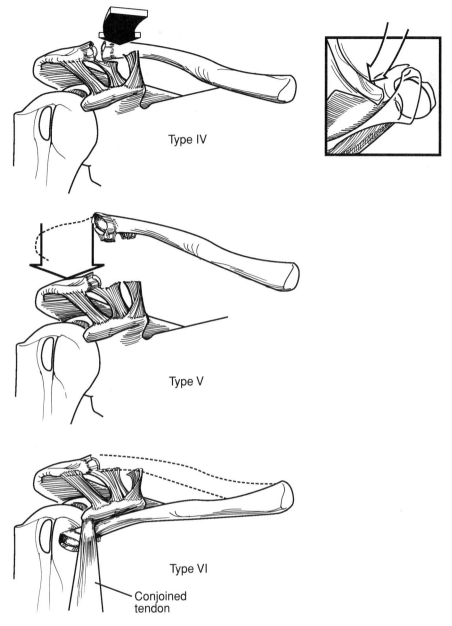

Type IV

Type V

Type VI
Conjoined tendon

FIG. 11.11. *Continued.*

ferred from the anterior acromion to the medullary canal of distal clavicle, as the distal 1.5 cm of the clavicle is resected. A coracoclavicular screw is placed for 10 to 12 weeks or a figure-eight loop of PDS suture is placed to relieve tension on the transferred ligament.

Type IV to VI acromioclavicular separations represent injuries that result from higher energy traumatic events and thus have a greater degree of anatomic disruption. In the type IV injury, the distal clavicle is dislocated posteriorly into the trapezius muscle and is best seen on the axillary lateral radiograph (Fig. 11.13).

The athlete will typically have much more pain, as the trapezius muscle is also injured. The type V injury is a severe type III in which the coracoclavicular distance is 1% to 300% displaced compared to the normal shoulder and the deltoid and trapezius muscles are detached from the distal clavicle. The type VI injury is rare and results from a traumatic abduction force to the extremity that displaces the distal clavicle under the coracoid. Operative repair of these injuries in the athlete is recommended, as the amount of muscle stripping from the distal clavicle results in a weakened shoulder. The

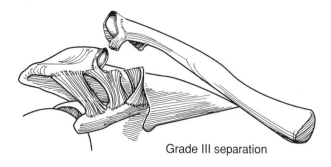

Grade III separation

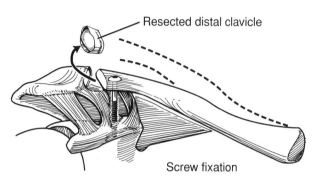

Resected distal clavicle

Screw fixation

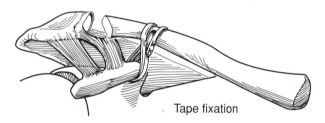

Tape fixation

FIG. 11.12. Surgical techniques for repair of acromioclavicular injuries. *Top:* Grade III separation. *Middle:* Coracoclavicular screw fixation. *Bottom:* Suture or mersilene figure-of-eight wrap.

rehabilitation process will be the same if repaired acutely.

Acromioclavicular Arthritis

The acromioclavicular joint may undergo degenerative changes similar to other articular joints as a result of repetitive microtrauma or traumatic injuries (70). Athletes who use across-the-body motions such as golfers, baseball players, or ice and field hockey players are susceptible to this entity. Football players who have had multiple acromioclavicular injuries will develop post traumatic arthritis. Radiographic osteoarthritic changes, such as joint narrowing and osteophyte formation, are best seen with the x-ray taken at a 10-degree cephalic tilt and reduced exposure. The patient will have pain localized to the AC joint with cross-body arm motion and overhead elevation. An intraarticular AC joint injection with 2 cc of 1% plain xylocaine should completely remove the athlete's pain if the AC joint is the source.

Initial treatment of acromioclavicular arthritis should include antiinflammatory medication, avoidance of overhead activity, and if unresponsive to these measures, an intraarticular AC joint steroid injection (31). If the athlete does not get relief, then a resectional arthroplasty of the acromioclavicular joint, either open or arthroscopic, should provide pain relief and return to athletic activity (1,41). Preoperative assessment should include weighted clavicle views to ensure costoclavicular ligament competence. The shoulder should be placed in a sling for one week with passive pendulum exercises starting immediately. Once tenderness has resolved, activities of daily living are performed with the shoulder, and active assistive exercises may be started after one week. Return to competition again depends on the sport; however, normal

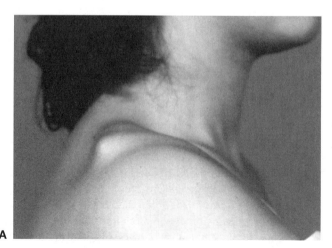

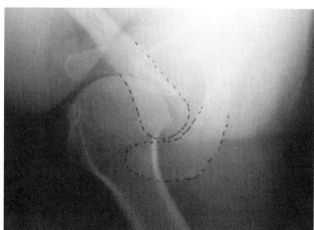

A

B

FIG. 11.13. Type IV acromioclavicular separation. **A.** The distal clavicle is displaced posteriorly into the trapezius muscle. **B.** This is best seen on an axillary lateral radiograph.

strength and motion should be present before considering contact sports (1,88).

THE SCAPULA

The athlete's scapula has an important role in overhead activities. Its position on the chest wall is controlled by muscles that arise on the iliac crest, ribs, and vertebral spinous processes, and then insert on the scapula. These muscles are the trapezius, rhomboids, and serratus anterior. They act in concert to place the scapula, and more importantly the glenoid in position for overhead activity. Because of the degree of movement on the chest wall, several bursae exist between the scapula and the chest wall.

Periscapular pain is frequent in shotputters, tennis players, and weight lifters. In putting the shot, the scapula muscles anchor the arm and must restrain the scapula during the follow-through. Pain in the rhomboids and scapulocostal bursitis are treated with massage, ultrasound, and, occasionally, steroid injections. During the backscratch position of the tennis serve, the inferior angle of the scapula may jam against the ribs to produce a bursitis, and the rhomboids may also be strained during the follow-through. Treatment is similar to that given for the shotputter's shoulder.

A weight lifter must strongly protract his shoulders. During this activity, the serratus anterior holds the scapula firmly to the lifter's chest wall. The muscle arises from his first eight ribs and inserts into the medial border of the scapula. In weight training, standing pull-overs may place traction on the long thoracic nerve, paralyzing the serratus anterior. This injury may be diagnosed by having the athlete do a wall push-up to elicit scapular winging. An electromyogram will show serratus anterior denervation. This injury may be prevented if pull-overs are done while the athlete is supine.

Snapping Scapula

A "snapping scapula" should not be considered a pathologic condition, as approximately 50% of the normal population have scapular sounds. However, painful scapular grating should be evaluated to assess the bony structure of the deep surface of the scapula and the chest wall. Scapular fractures, which are common in high-energy contact sports such as football, may become symptomatic due to exuberant fracture callous formation. An osteochondroma is the most common scapular tumor and may be present on the deep surface or a rib exostosis may develop. A chest CT is usually necessary to make these diagnoses as they are difficult to visualize on plain radiographs.

When an athlete has intractable periscapular pain, the examiner should evaluate the cervical spine for a radicular source. The athlete may report a recurrent stiff neck but usually without neurologic or electromyographic changes. Pain in the trapezius or other shoulder muscles or at the occipital-cervical junction may be due to nervous tension or afternoon fatigue or may follow prolonged flexion and extension of the neck. In these cases, the athlete should strengthen the neck muscles and try neck traction for relief of the shoulder pain.

Deltoid Strain and Shoulder Pointer

The deltoid muscle is the most exposed muscle of the shoulder girdle. A *shoulder pointer* is a contusion of the deltoid muscle as a result of a direct blow. In rugby the participants do not wear shoulder pads and deltoid strains are common. In football, protective wear theoretically decreases the risk of deltoid injury; however, this is offset by the increase in collision impact. The degree of injury to the deltoid or trapezial muscle fibers depends on the energy of the impact and may range from a mild bruise to actual deltoid avulsion. The recovery of shoulder function is related to the degree of irreversible muscle injury. Initial treatment consists of ice, rest, and appropriate analgesic medication followed by passive then active assistive range of motion. A hematoma should be treated aggressively with compression and heat to avoid formation of local ectopic bone. Local injections are not recommended as they may cause an infection and inhibit the healing response. Very rarely will there be avulsion of the origin of the deltoid. If a significant portion is involved then surgical repair should be performed before retraction and scarring of the deltoid occurs.

Pectoralis Major Tears

This injury generally results from extreme muscle tension, direct trauma, or a combination of both. The majority of cases occur in the 20 to 40 age group, are partial tears, and predominately avulse from the humerus (114). Diagnosis is based upon the clinical history and acute onset of shoulder dysfunction, pain, and significant swelling (12). A MRI may be obtained to provide information concerning the location of the tear, which affects treatment (72). Treatment of a complete tear in an active athlete requires early surgical intervention. A tendinous avulsion may be repaired anatomically to the humerus through drill holes; however, musculotendinous junction or intrasubstance tears offer poor material for direct repair, and imperfect results can be expected.

SUBACROMIAL SHOULDER PAIN

Subacromial pain generally exists in the overhead athlete as a result of several pathologic entities. The diagnosis and treatment of impingement, rotator cuff tendinopathies or tears, and calcific tendinitis will be discussed below. The specific treatment of subacromial pain in swimmers will also be addressed.

Repetitive overhead movements can lead to subacromial shoulder pain that has been given the term, "impingement"(78). Although this refers to a mechanical compression of the rotator cuff, biceps tendon and subacromial bursa, the same term may be applied to overuse tendinopathies of the rotator cuff (58). Impingement symptoms occur when the available space underlying the coracoacromial arch is decreased or when the contents are increased in size. Repetitive microtrauma from repeat overhead athletic activity may lead to subacromial bursae irritation with wall thickening, fluid accumulation, and adhesion formation. The rotator cuff tendons may become inflamed from overuse and develop altered tendon physiology that leads to thickening or tearing of the tendon. The overlying acromion may have an anterior hook as described by Bigliani (Fig. 11.14) (16), predisposing the athlete to develop subacromial symptoms. Another factor that may diminish available space is pathologic biomechanics of the shoulder joint secondary to occult anterior instability (54) or a tight posterior capsule (44).

The critical area of impingement as defined by Neer (77), consists principally of the area of the supraspinatus with variable extension to the anterior portion of the infraspinatus and long head of the biceps. This area corresponds to the region demonstrated to be hypovascular (69), which limits the tendon's ability to repair itself.

Classically, stage one impingement refers to reversible edema or hemorrhage of the tendon and bursitis in a young patient, typically less than 25 years old. Stage two impingement consists of chronic changes of fibrosis and tendinitis from repeated cuff microtrauma, which may be resistant to conservative treatment and occurs in the 25 to 40 age range. Stage three impingement occurs in the older athlete, rarely less than 40, and consists of anterior, inferior acromial osteophyte formation as well as partial or complete tears of the rotator cuff.

Pure impingement in the young athlete is a rare entity and more commonly is a result of underlying anterior instability or thoracoscapular weakness. Veteran athletes (over the age of 35) may develop primary impingement, as years of repetitive overhead activity may lead to the formation of anterior/inferior acromial spur formation or coracoacromial ligament ossification.

Calcific tendinitis generally occurs in the older athlete, between ages 35 to 45. Calcific deposits that occur within the rotator cuff, primarily the supraspinatus tendon, become symptomatic in 35% to 40% of patents. The etiology of this condition is subject to debate, as it is considered either a result of decreased vascular supply due to degenerative changes or a self-limited process. The major feature of an acute calcific tendinitis is unremitting pain at rest and with activity. A frozen shoulder may develop in about 10% and bicipital tendinitis may occur in 7% to 8% of patients with calcific tendinitis.

EXAMINING FOR SUBACROMIAL PROBLEMS

Careful examination of the subacromial space includes palpation of the bursa, as well as performing several provocative tests. These tests specifically determine the integrity of the rotator cuff, and the presence of impingement or instability. The examiner must also determine if generalized ligamentous laxity exists in the athlete by examining for hyperflexibility of the knees, elbows, and thumb metacarpolphalangeal joint.

Impingement

Subacromial pain caused by inflammation within the subacromial space may be reproduced by performing arm maneuvers that diminish the available space under the acromial arch and cause compression of the underlying structures. The classic impingement sign (Fig. 11.15A) is produced by forcible overhead elevation, which causes the supraspinatus tendon to impinge against the anterior-inferior acromion (78). If the tendon is inflamed this motion will produce pain. An alternative method is to forward flex the humerus to 90 degrees then forcibly internally rotate the shoulder, which brings the supraspinatus

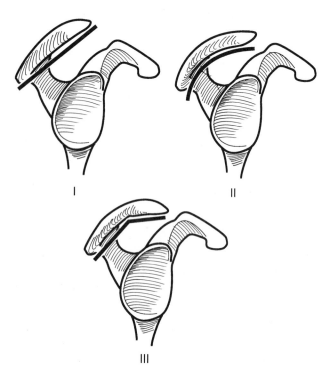

FIG. 11.14. Classification of acromial morphology based upon supraspinatus outlet view.

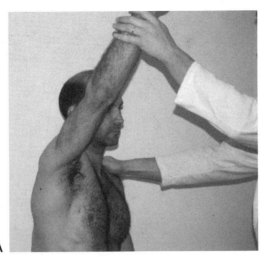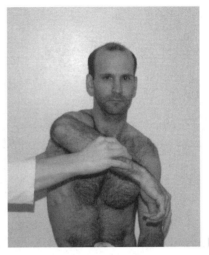

FIG. 11.15. Impingement tests: **A.** Neer impingement test, stressing at maximal forward elevation. **B.** Internal rotation impingement test, with the arm forward flexed 90 degrees, forcible internal rotation causes pain due to the supraspinatus impinging against the coracoacromial ligament.

tendon against the coracoclavicular ligament (see Fig. 11.15B) (45).

The *painful arc* refers to abduction in the coronal plane causing the athlete with impingement tendinitis and rotator cuff pathology to experience pain between 60 to 100 degrees of abduction. The athlete will sometimes unconsciously externally rotate the humerus at this position to clear the greater tuberosity posteriorly under the acromion and diminish the pain.

The *impingement test* localizes the athlete's pain to the subacromial space by documenting the response to an injection of lidocaine (10mL of 1% Xylocaine) into the subacromial bursa. Following the injection, the impingement test is repeated and a positive test is recorded if the athlete's previous pain is abolished.

The Rotator Cuff

If a tear of the external rotators or supraspinatus occurs, atrophy of the supra- and/or infraspinatus fossa should be apparent upon careful inspection and palpation. Generalized atrophy of the deltoid muscle from disuse may also be present and contribute to a patient's complaint of weakness. The painful grinding felt by the examiner by placing his hand over the painful shoulder and then raising the shoulder is typically related to a thickened bursa indicative of chronic bursitis.

Specific isolated testing of the rotator cuff muscles will elicit painful weakness indicative of tendinitis or a partial tear. Weakness without pain is suggestive of a complete tear. External rotation against resistance with the elbow at 0 and 90 degrees abduction is performed to assess the posterior cuff muscles, the infraspinatus, and teres minor. The supraspinatus muscle is tested against resistance with the arm abducted 90 degrees,

forward-flexed 30 degrees, and fully pronated. The subscapularis is isolated by performing the "lift off" maneuver; the back of the patient's hand is placed against his back, then is lifted off against resistance provided by the examiner. These maneuvers should be repeated following an injection of lidocaine into the subacromial space, therefore eliminating pain as a component of weakness. If the patient then has significant weakness without pain, then a complete tear of the rotator cuff tendon is most likely present.

Radiographic Evaluation: Plain Films, Arthrograms, and MRI

Several views of the shoulder are necessary to evaluate impingement. A shoulder AP in external rotation may reveal sclerosis or cysts at the area of insertion of the supraspinatus into the greater tuberosity of the humerus, or a calcium deposit in the supraspinatus tendon. However, a 30-degree caudal tilt view will best reveal the shape of the anterior acromion and the size of an anterior osteophyte (Fig. 11.16) (62). An axillary lateral radiograph will help rule out occult anterior instability by showing the shape of the anterior glenoid rim.

A shoulder arthrogram is the most accurate exam for revealing complete tears in an athlete's rotator cuff. However, the arthrogram will be normal in cases of tendinitis or in cases of an intratendinous tear and does not provide information regarding the size of the tear or the condition of the muscle. If the tear is a partial bursal tear the dye will indent the tendon, yet will not flow into the subacromial space. In a complete tear, the dye will leak through the torn tendon into the subacromial bursa (81).

Magnetic Resonance Imaging (MRI) is a modality that can provide noninvasive imaging of the shoulder. Its use

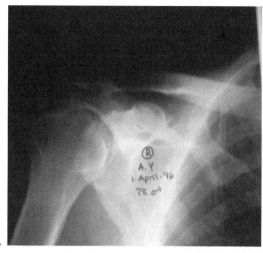
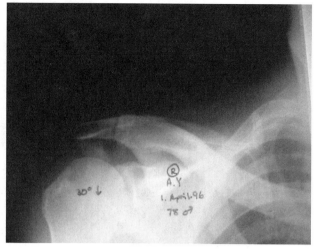

FIG. 11.16. A. Anteroposterior radiograph revealing no evidence of anterior acromial spurring. **B.** 30-degree caudal view revealing large anterior acromial spur.

in imaging the rotator cuff has increased in the past years with improvement in the images produced (51). Unfortunately, the main disadvantage of the MRI comes in its inability to differentiate tendinitis from partial or small complete tears unless combined with a contrast material. Saline or gadolinium MRI-arthrograms provide images that increase the accuracy in delineating the integrity of the rotator cuff tendons (Fig. 11.17) (107).

Treatment of Impingement

The treatment of subacromial impingement should be initiated early, when the athlete's symptoms do not affect performance. The preventative approach of daily stretching and strengthening will help avoid both secondary impingement in the younger athlete with occult instability and primary impingement in the older athlete.

Stretching consists of passive motion to an extreme

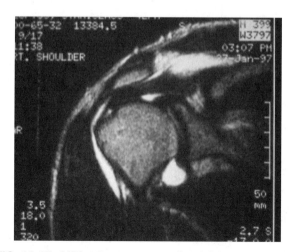

FIG. 11.17. MRI-arthrogram: revealing full thickness tearing of supraspinatus tendon.

within a specific plane of motion following a well-defined warm-up period. Capsule contractures are frequent in athletes and are dependent on the type of repetitive motion the athlete uses in his or her sport. Posterior capsule tightness is frequent in most overhead athletes and manifests itself as an internal rotation contracture. It can contribute to impingement by forcing the humeral head to migrate superiorly and anteriorly with overhead motion (44).

Strengthening of the shoulder girdle may seem trivial to the athlete who trains daily; however, the goal is not to achieve bulk strength, but to obtain the correct balance of strength. Weight lifters frequently concentrate on the trapezius and deltoid, neglecting the external rotators and subsequently develop an impingement syndrome. Reestablishing proper balance of the deltoid and rotator cuff by strengthening the cuff muscles will diminish the superior force on the humeral head and over time relieve the symptoms of subacromial pain. Patients with generalized laxity (i.e., swimmers and overhead athletes) may exhibit symptoms of impingement secondary to underlying multi-directional instability; these athletes respond to rehabilitation with an 85% success rate (21).

The approach to subacromial symptoms, once present, consists of abstinence from the offending athletic activity, antiinflammatory medication, daily stretching, and a careful strengthening program of the trapezius, rotator cuff, and scapular stabilizers (57,87,96). Occasionally subacromial corticosteroid injections can help break the cycle of inflammation. Surgery in the form of an open or arthroscopic subacromial decompression may be helpful in the older athlete (over 35) who has evidence of acromial pathology such as spurring. At the time of surgery the thickened subacromial bursa is excised, the prominent anterior, inferior acromion is removed, and the coracoacromial ligament is resected (57,96,105). It is very rare for a young athlete to require a subacromial decompression as the majority respond to conservative measures.

Treatment of Rotator Cuff Tears

There have been several different classifications devised to describe rotator cuff tears. Generally, none of these provide prognostic information, only different types or stages based upon the location (bursal or articular), size (1 to 5 cm), or completeness (partial or complete) of the tear.

Most rotator cuff tendon tears can be treated conservatively with a specific rehabilitation program to maintain a normal range of motion followed by a directed strengthening program of the rotator cuff, scapular stabilizers, deltoid, and trapezius (56). There are many professional athletes performing with tears of the rotator cuff. If a tear is traumatic in origin (for example, following a young athlete's fall onto his or her shoulder), then repair is indicated without acromioplasty or coracoacromial ligament resection. Nonabsorbable sutures are used to provide temporary fixation until the debrided tendon heals to a 3- to 5-mm bony trough (14,38,106). Arthroscopic repair of small complete tears is technically possible; however, no literature exists concerning the outcome in the athletic patient.

Partial (bursal or articular) tears are thought to be the result of repetitive eccentric microtrauma to the tendon that alters the normal tensile strength and subsequently breaks down. In the past these partial tears were often debrided arthroscopically in conjunction with an acromioplasty leaving behind a tendon that was thinner and temporarily relieving pain (37,39,101). This approach to the partial tear may allow 2 to 3 years of pain-free athletic activity, which can be important for the older athlete at the end of a career. However, the remaining tendon usually fails with time and requires rehabilitation or repair.

Rehabilitation Following Rotator Cuff Repair

After a rotator cuff has been repaired, rehabilitation is dependent upon the technique used and the type of athlete. If the surgeon had to detach the deltoid and then reattach it to the acromion, the athlete must not actively forward-flex the arm for 3 weeks. Passive range of motion may begin as early as the first postoperative day in the form of pendulum exercises and stretching of the external rotators. Rehabilitation proceeds from passive motion to active-assistive motion at 3 weeks and active motion may begin at 6 weeks. Resistive strengthening may begin at 12 weeks with Therabands. Light throwing may begin at 16 weeks, and return to limited noncontact practice for other athletes may be encouraged. Rehabilitation of the deltoid, trapezius, and scapular rotators must also be emphasized to ensure normal scapulohumeral rhythm. For the majority of athletes the return to competition occurs when a full range of motion with adequate strength is obtained. However, for a pitcher, more than a year of rehabilitation is often required before return to the previous competition can occur (Table 11.1).

Treatment of Calcific Tendinitis

Nonoperative treatment is successful in 90% of cases, as the deposits will resorb over time. Treatment of the *acute* calcific tendinitis should include a corticosteroid subacromial injection for pain relief and allow the athlete to maintain a normal range of motion through a daily program of stretching exercises. The shoulder should be iced prior to stretching in the acute case and heated in the chronic. If conservative treatment fails then excision of the calcific deposit with resection of the bursae and partial coracoacromial ligament resection should be performed. Open excision through a small deltoid splitting approach allows careful repair of the defect in the rotator tendon. Arthroscopic excision spares trauma to the deltoid; however, the deposit is simply decompressed and the remaining compromised tendon cannot be addressed (7). Postoperatively, a normal passive range of motion should be obtained by 2 weeks, active-assistive exercises started at 2 weeks, then resistive strengthening at 6 weeks.

Swimmer's Shoulder

As knowledge of shoulder pathophysiology has increased over the past decade, insight of "special" types of athletic injuries has allowed the care provider to be more specific. The term "swimmer's shoulder" (61) has become obsolete as it is too general and offers no information regarding specific shoulder pathology and subsequent treatment. However, it is true that swimmers, in general, tend to have shoulder pain due to pathology of a specific nature, such as impingement (60), anterior instability, or labral pathology (71), and subsequently require treatment that is appropriate for each entity.

The anterior shoulder pain, which is common in swim-

TABLE 11.1. *Rotator cuff repair rehabilitation goals*

Month 1	Decrease inflammation, increase motion. Passive forward flexion and external rotation.
Month 2	Full passive motion range of motion. Active-assistive exercises.
Month 3	Gain full active range of motion. Begin scapular stabilizer strengthening, rotator isometrics.
Month 4	May toss baseball 30 feet and increase the distance.
Month 5	Pitch 60 feet slowly.
Month 6	Increase to three-quarter speed.

mers, is usually an example of a stage 1 impingement lesion; the athlete is young, a repetitive overhead motion is the mechanism of injury, and the tendinopathy is usually reversible with conservative treatment.

The swimmer represents the extreme example of an overhead athlete. Undergoing a typical training regimen of 20 to 30 hours per week, an elite swimmer will perform 400,000 to 600,000 repetitive overhead motion cycles per year (93). The prevalence of a painful shoulder among swimmers has been reported to range from 3% (60) to 60% (36), clearly related to level of performance and training amount. The epidemiological surveys indicate that there are three main factors responsible for shoulder pain: swimming experience, training distance, and the use of hand paddles.

The butterfly, freestyle, and backstroke are all similar in technique, relying on internal rotation to generate power. Butterfly differs in that the amount of body roll is eliminated due to synchronous arm motion, this resulting in an increased amount of shoulder abduction during recovery. Shoulder pain in the breast stroker is no longer rare, as technique now requires shoulder abduction.

It has been estimated that approximately 80% of the swimmer's forward movement is due to the power generated by the upper extremities. During early pull-through the swimmer's arm is placed in front, the elbow is kept above the plane of the hand to improve the leverage of the internal rotators of the shoulder during pull-through. This position resembles an apprehension test as the shoulder is maximally flexed, abducted, and externally rotated. The backward thrust, generated during pull-through by internal rotation with the shoulder in an adducted, forward-flexed position, propels the swimmer forward and may "wring" the rotator cuff. The recovery phase also has the swimmer's shoulder in a internally rotated, extended, then forward, flexed position. The humeral head and the supraspinatus tendon can impinge upon the coracoacromial arch in this position if abnormal humeral head anterior translation occurs.

As stated previously, the rotator cuff tendons serve to maintain the humeral head centered in the glenoid. If fatigue of the rotator cuff musculature (specifically the supraspinatus) occurs, then abnormal superior humeral head translation may lead to symptoms of impingement. Relative muscle imbalance will develop, as the muscles that stabilize and elevate the scapula or externally rotate the shoulder are relatively weak (84).

Treatment

Treatment of a swimmer's shoulder pain should begin early, before the pain becomes continuous. The correct diagnosis needs to be made prior to embarking on a treatment/rehabilitation program as the different common pathologic entities have different prognosis and management.

If the cause of shoulder pain is determined to be an overuse tendinopathy then a specific program is initiated. Management of the elite swimmer may be difficult, as the concept of *rest* denotes a period of lost time in an endurance sport. Initially a concerted effort is made to identify specific changes in training or technique that have occurred prior to the development of shoulder pain. The use of paddles and weights should be discontinued and a stretching, strengthening program specifically aimed at reestablishing a normal balance of dynamic glenohumeral motion is begun. A nonsteroidal antiinflammatory medication should also be used for 2 to 3 weeks. Prior to training the shoulder should have moist heat applied for 20 minutes, then stretched. In addition, a change in emphasis to another stroke allows cardiovascular conditioning and avoids the aggravating movement. The swimmer should then ice the shoulder immediately after a workout.

If symptoms persist, then the swimmer should be switched to kicking drills without a kickboard and stroke modifications made to eliminate pain. Freestyle swimmers may need to increase the elbow height and body roll during recovery, as well as place their hand in less internal rotation during entry to decrease impingement. Occasionally a subacromial injection, followed by a period of rest from overhead activity while continuing the rehabilitation program, is necessary to break the cycle of chronic bursitis. Arthroscopic examination with coracoacromial ligament release and acromial smoothing has been inconsistent, due to difficulty of initial diagnosis.

If the swimmer complains of anterior shoulder pain with a clicking sensation, and examination reveals pain with rotation at 90 degrees abduction without apprehension or impingement signs then a labral tear should be considered. A complete stretching and strengthening program as described above should be initiated. If no improvement is seen after 2 to 3 months then a MRI-saline arthrogram should be obtained to assess labral pathology. An experienced skeletal radiologist should be consulted as variations in normal labral pathology can be misread. Arthroscopic labral resection may be recommended if a labral tear exists without underlying glenohumeral instability.

Instability as a cause of shoulder pain in the swimmer is a well-known etiology. Again, a specific rehabilitation program followed diligently will obviate the need for surgery in the majority of cases. Many swimmers (especially teenage females) demonstrate increased posterior and inferior humeral head translation indicative of multidirectional instability. Only if the athlete's symptoms are resistant to 12 months of continuous rehabilitation should surgical intervention be considered. An anterior capsular shift combined with repair of labral detachment if present will preserve external rotation and forward flexion

(74,80,95). Unfortunately, return of a swimmer with instability to the preinjury level is rare.

SHOULDER INJURIES IN THE THROWING ATHLETE

Throwing is an integral part of many sports; however, different throwing techniques are used, depending on the weight, size, and shape of the object propelled. An understanding of the simple biomechanics of throwing can help understand the underlying mechanics that can lead to shoulder injury. The main theme can be outlined as follows: the body weight and large muscles of the thrower are used to generate kinetic energy, which is then transferred through the shoulder in the direction of the thrown object. After release of the object, retained energy within the throwing arm is dissipated by reversing the process.

Beginning with a discussion of a baseball pitcher is useful as it is the most studied athletic activity and with minor modifications the same activity occurs in other athletic activities. The phases of pitching are windup, early cocking, late cocking, acceleration, and follow-through (Fig. 11.18A). In the windup phase, the pitcher picks up the contralateral limb, raising his center of gravity to the highest point possible. Early cocking begins with the ball leaving the glove and ends when the contralateral foot touches the ground. The most important event during early cocking occurs below the arm, as the pitcher falls toward the catcher to create an angular motion at an axis at the level of the foot. Late cocking occurs next, with the shoulder taken to maximum abduction and external rotation. Again, the important mechanical event is occurring below the arm, as the kinetic energy is transferred to the rotating torso. Acceleration begins with shoulder in maximal abduction and external rotation and ends with release of the ball from the fingers. Kinetic energy, which has been generated by the wind-up and cocking phases, is partially transferred to the thrown object; however, the majority remains in the throwing arm. Specific muscle groups are active during different phases (see Fig. 11.18B) and injury will interfere with normal smooth-throwing motion. Follow-through reverses the acceleration process with eccentric muscle contraction and internal rotation flexion of the humerus. The triceps decelerates the arm, and the thumb turns down as the forearm pronates. The overhead athlete will have hypertrophy of these muscles secondary to overuse that does not reflect a pathologic condition (Fig. 11.19).

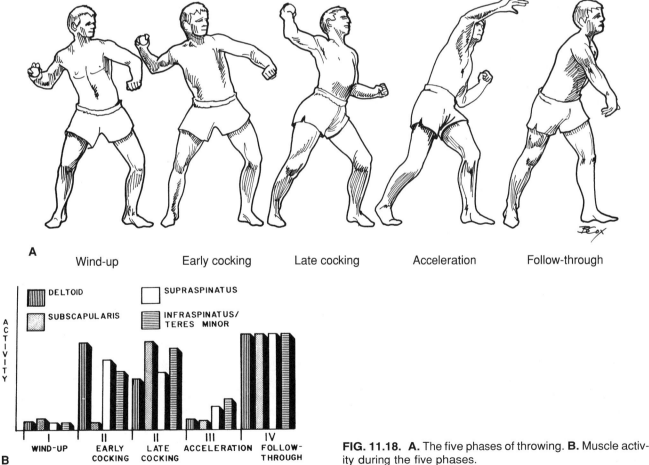

A. Wind-up   Early cocking   Late cocking   Acceleration   Follow-through

B. WIND-UP   EARLY COCKING   LATE COCKING   ACCELERATION   IV FOLLOW-THROUGH

DELTOID   SUPRASPINATUS
SUBSCAPULARIS   INFRASPINATUS/ TERES MINOR

ACTIVITY

FIG. 11.18. A. The five phases of throwing. **B.** Muscle activity during the five phases.

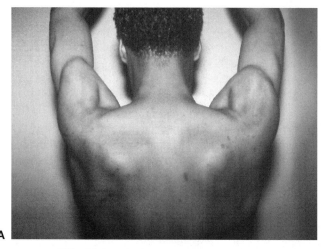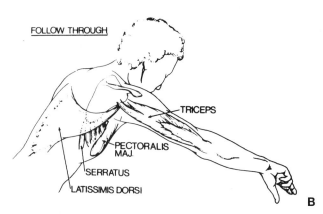

FIG. 11.19. A. Asymmetry of the pitcher's right arm due to hypertrophy of the posterior deltoid and triceps. **B.** Schematic drawing depicting the muscles responsible for deceleration.

The football pass is a pushing motion in which the cocking phase and follow-through are shorter than a baseball pitcher. Unlike a baseball pitcher, the football quarterback uses the same type of motion for each pass, with little variation.

Field event throws include the javelin, shot-put, discus, and hammer. Javelin throwers with good technique throw over the shoulder with elbow extension. *Round arm* throws are incorrect, and these throwers tend to develop shoulder and elbow problems similar to those of baseball pitchers. A shot-putter's fingers support the heavy shot, and the large, scapular-anchoring muscles must slow the arm down after the shot has been released. Discus and hammer throws are centrifugal motions that do not produce as many shoulder problems as do overhead events. Softball pitchers, hurlers, and ten-pin and duck-pin bowlers stress, and sometimes rupture, their biceps tendons during their underhand, flexion activities.

THE TENNIS SERVE

A brief comparison between the tennis player and baseball pitcher is useful for providing insight into the pathophysiology of shoulder injuries in the tennis player.

There are significant differences in serves per match versus pitches per game, pace versus speed, recovery time, amount of external rotation of the shoulder, and rotator cuff problems. A hard-fought three-set singles tennis match with scores of 6-4, 4-6, 6-4 requires that each player serve 15 games. Taking nine serves per game as an average, each player would hit 135 serves. In contrast, a major league baseball pitcher averages about 120 pitches in a game. The tennis player after serving 135 serves in a match may the same day play the next round of the tournament and serve the same number of serves or may play doubles and come right back the next day without shoulder trouble.

The tennis serving motion has been broken into 4 stages based upon a visual and electromyographical study: windup, cocking, acceleration, and follow-through. Although there are similarities in muscle activity the extent of external rotation and abduction appears to be less in the tennis player than in a pitcher.

While few young tennis players have major shoulder problems, impingement syndrome and glenohumeral instability are the most common etiologies of pain. The "drooped" shoulder common among highly trained tennis players is attributed to stretching of the shoulder-elevating muscles and to hypertrophy of the racket-holding extremity (45). This shoulder dependency causes a relative abduction of the extremity, which may result in impingement of the rotator cuff. Most rotator cuff problems occur in tennis players who are 30 to 50 years of age and have played for a long time (63).

Diagnosis and Treatment of Throwing Injuries

When diagnosing a throwing injury, the examiner should obtain a detailed history to determine which phase of the throwing motion is involved (56). In general there is a fine balance between scapulothoracic and glenohumeral motion; any injury to the muscles or tendons of the shoulder girdle can lead to weakness, abnormal motion, and diminishing athletic performance. In general the throwing shoulder will exhibit increased external rotation and limited internal rotation (Fig. 11.20). As mentioned previously, tight posterior capsules can lead to developing subacromial inflammation affecting the bursa or supraspinatus tendon. Therefore, a careful preventative program that consists of daily stretching to avoid contractures (see Fig. 11.20 B), strengthening of the entire shoulder girdle to avoid imbalance, and postperformance icing to avoid inflammation can help protect against injury (55).

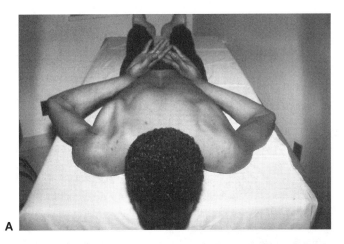

A

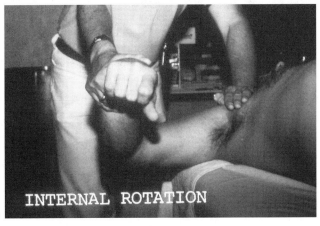

INTERNAL ROTATION

B

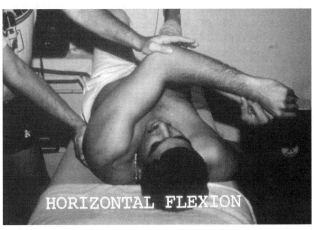

HORIZONTAL FLEXION

FIG. 11.20. A. Internal rotation contracture as evidenced by scapular winging. **B** (**left** and **right**). Daily stretching routine to avoid joint contracture.

When his arm is maximally abducted and externally rotated in the late cocking phase, the inferior glenohumeral complex of the capsule is the main static force resisting anterior movement of the humeral head. Repetitive microtrauma to the capsule can lead to capsule damage and the subsequent development of instability. As static stabilizers break down, the rotator cuff muscles and scapular rotators function beyond their usual limits, leading to fatigue (58). A pitcher will note an unstable feeling as his humeral head begins to slip forward in the glenoid, then moves back again. As this abnormal motion occurs the pitcher may notice a decrease in velocity or a sensation of having a "dead arm" (99,100). Examination of the shoulder should consist of several provocative maneuvers to reproduce the athlete's sensation of slipping. In the anterior drawer test, the examiner pushes the humeral head forward to determine if abnormal anterior laxity exists. The athlete may wince in apprehension of the feeling of instability when the arm is abducted to 90 degrees and externally rotated. Some pitchers normally subluxate their shoulders anteriorly and develop posterior shoulder pain from eccentric contraction injury of the posterior cuff muscles as they fire to prevent the humeral head from sliding forward.

At the late cocking phase the humeral head may also impinge on the posterior superior rim of the glenoid (kiss-ing lesion), causing a partial tearing of the posterior supraspinatus tendon or labrum (111). This phenomenon is usually associated with mild anterior laxity that may be missed due to the posterior shoulder pain.

At the start of acceleration, the pitcher's body is "opened up" and his arm is left behind. The strong internal rotators of the shoulder girdle then fire maximally as the arm catches up to the body. Apprehension may be felt by the pitcher at the beginning of the acceleration phase, and the anterior capsular pain may be reproduced when the examiner manually resists the acceleration motion.

Repetitive throwing too often may produce subacromial pain with subdeltoid and subacromial bursal adhesions (57). Frequently pitchers with these adhesions exhibit poor form, opening up too soon; that is, the pitcher leaves his arm behind his body after bringing his trunk around. As his arm drags behind, he tries to rush it forward to catch up by dropping his elbow, "short-arming" the ball.

Subacromial symptoms subside with rest, but once mature adhesions form the pain returns whenever throwing is resumed. At surgery, the subdeltoid and subacromial bursa are often obscured by a thick adhesion that involves the whole bursal complex. The bursae are thick and show myxoid degeneration. Unfortunately, all modes of treatment for fully developed subdeltoid bursitis seem to fail.

For this reason, a pitcher should not be asked to pitch through a painful shoulder and to risk irreparable damage from formation of dense adhesions.

A pitcher releases the baseball at ear level, and his arm then follows through toward the plate. The arm continues to rotate internally, soon catching up with the body. Now the arm must be decelerated by the long head of the triceps, which acts as a rein, putting traction on the area of origin of the triceps at the inferior lip of the glenoid. This traction may produce triceps origin microtrauma and produce pain with follow-through.

Ossification at the posteroinferior part of the glenoid "Bennett's lesion" is often associated with tears of the glenoid labrum and posterior capsule (40). The pitcher may complain of pain either in the late cocking or follow-through phases of throwing. The origin of this ossification has been the subject of controversy, as it is either a response to microtrauma to the posterior origin of the inferior glenohumeral ligament or direct impingement of the humeral head. More recently it has been associated with posterior subluxation of the humeral head due to capsular laxity. Stryker notch views are necessary to view the lesion and a CT-arthrogram may better delineate intraarticular pathology. If a pitcher develops posterior shoulder pain and x-ray films show bone at the posteroinferior glenoid the shoulder should be evaluated for instability. Arthroscopic labral debridement alone may resolve the athlete's symptoms as the ossific lesion is extraarticular and does not need to be surgically approached. If instability is not present when following arthroscopic debridement, the pitcher should continue general conditioning and limit throwing until the ossific lesion has matured and is nontender to palpation. If instability is present then an arthroscopic examination should be performed and then the instability should be addressed.

The concept of generalized conditioning in the baseball pitcher is important to maximize the efficiency of kinetic-energy transfer to the ball. If a pitcher is not fit, fatigue will occur in the torso muscles that position the scapula or in the legs and subsequently alter his pitching motion, exposing his glenohumeral joint to potential injury. Conditioning and training is a continuous process throughout the year. A postseason schedule should include flexibility exercises, muscle strengthening, aerobic conditioning, position-specific endurance training, and finally skill training.

Partial Avulsion of the Glenoid Labrum in Throwing Athletes

As a pitcher releases the ball, his biceps contract strongly (5). This contraction may avulse the *upper* portion of his glenoid labrum from the glenoid rim. In contrast, when a football player dislocates his shoulder while arm-tackling, the *lower* portion of his glenoid labrum is avulsed.

The pitcher's tear may extend to become a long, bowstring tear. It can catch in the shoulder joint just like a bucket handle tear of a knee meniscus. When a pitcher who has an avulsed labrum throws, his shoulder will catch and pop and feel unstable.

It may be difficult to clinically detect a glenoid labrum tear. Two maneuvers commonly used are the clunk test and the Obrien test. The clunk test is performed with the athlete supine and relaxed; the examiner supports the elbow with one hand and places his other hand behind the humeral head. He then raises the athlete's arm fully overhead and pushes the shoulder anteriorly while rotating the humerus. The test is positive if it produces a clunk or grinding, which may be associated with apprehension and pain as the humeral head strikes or snaps over the labral tear.

Arthroscopic examination will reveal the extent and nature of the labral damage. Superior labral anterior to posterior tears (SLAP lesions) have been classified into four types by Snyder (102) and surgical treatment, debridement or repair, depends on the type present (Fig. 11.21). Although the debridement does not stabilize the shoulder, it removes the offending labral tear that may be causing pain (3). Postoperatively, the athlete may begin passive range of motion the day after surgery and then strengthen his arm. By 3 weeks, he should be throwing easily, and by week 7 he should be ready to return to competition.

Competitive Season Shoulder Care

This includes monitoring and therapeutic interventions for the cumulative effects of pitching on the shoulder over the season. Postgame specialized care in the form of ice, massage, antiinflammatory medications, and electrical stimulation are used to maximize recovery and prepare the shoulder for the next game. A complete warm-up before pitching helps to prevent injury to a pitcher's throwing arm (4). The athletic trainer first applies moist heat to the pitcher's arm for about 20 minutes, followed by an ice rub or a cold, wet towel rub. The pitching shoulder may also be massaged with an analgesic rub. The athletic trainer then stretches the pitcher's arm. After the game, the arm should be iced down with a large ice pack held over the player's shoulder by an elastic wrap and the elbow soaked in cold water. The ice is analgesic, decreases swelling, and is antispasmodic. Cold reduces the metabolism of the tissues and lessens cellular damage and the inflammatory response. The ice should not, however, be left on for more than 15 to 20 minutes, or a strong reflex vasodilatation may occur.

Antiinflammatory medicines such as aspirin may be given 20 to 30 minutes before exercising. Some physicians give a decreasing dosage schedule of butazolidine, 200 mg four times daily for 2 days, then 200 mg three

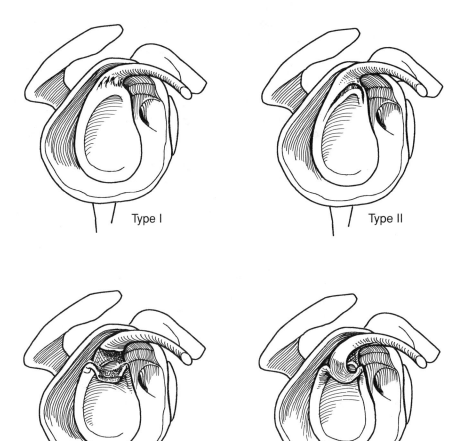

Type I

Type II

Type III

Type IV

FIG. 11.21. Superior labral anterior posterior (SLAP) lesion classification. **I.** Fraying with intact biceps anchor. **II.** Detachment of biceps anchor. **III.** Bucket-handle tear of superior labrum, biceps anchor intact. **IV.** Bucket-handle tear of superior labrum into biceps tendon anchor.

times daily for 2 days, and finally 100 mg three times daily for 3 days. Others use indomethacin (Indocin), ibuprofen (Motrin), tolmetin sodium (Tolectin), or naproxen (Naprosyn) for an antiinflammatory effect.

Despite the presentation of a simplified pitching motion, most pitchers vary in technique. Each pitcher has a different style and subsequently the number of innings or pitches, and even postgame care can vary greatly. Therefore, each pitcher should be involved in an intensive competitive season rehabilitation program designed to monitor subtle changes, such as postgame soreness or changes in range of motion, and to prepare the pitcher for the next game. Generally pitchers are divided into starting and relief pitchers.

Starting Pitchers

In general, starting pitchers know in advance of when they are pitching and can be involved in a day-to-day program during the season.

Although rotations can vary, typically, starting pitchers will pitch every 4 to 5 days (Table 11.2).

Relief Pitchers

To be available on a daily basis the relief pitcher must avoid postgame inflammation and soreness. Icing after an outing can accomplish this, although the number of pitches thrown and pitch velocity should be followed to avoid overuse. Relief pitchers typically warm up quickly and throw fewer pitches. They should follow a general conditioning program three times a week, consisting of running and leg strengthening.

BICIPITAL TENDINITIS

The tendon of the long head of the biceps arises at the supraglenoid tubercle and passes at an angle of 30 degrees into the bicipital groove, where it lies deep to the transverse humeral ligament. During shoulder motion, the ten-

TABLE 11.2. *Starting pitcher rotation*

Pitching day (Day 1)
  Pregame warm-up
    Stretching exercises
    Assisted stretching of dominant shoulder
    Massage
  Game warm-up
    Long ball toss for 5 minutes
    50–60 throws from mound
    Start of each inning: warm-up, 8 pitches
  Postgame care
    Ice to shoulder/elbow for 15–20 minutes
Day 2
  Conditioning, usually running
  Massage
  Assisted stretching program
  Shoulder strengthening at 100% resistance
  Light catch for 10–15 minutes
Day 3
  Conditioning, general aerobic and leg-assisted
    stretching program
  Light supervised pitching from mound
  Ice shoulder
Day 4
  Conditioning, general aerobic and leg-assisted
    stretching program
  Massage
  Light catch
Day 5
  Rest
  Assisted stretching exercises
  Limited shoulder exercises

don does not glide but remains fixed as the humerus slides along the tendon. During the follow-through in throwing, the humerus actually leaves the socket by as much as 2.5 cm to 3.75 cm (1 in to 1.5 in). Rubbing of the tendon by the groove and ligament is worsened by a tight groove, especially if the channel has a steep medial wall. In addition, many shoulders have a rough supratubercular area that irritates the tendon.

The biceps tendon itself is usually not palpable, therefore examination is largely by palpation of the bicipital groove. The groove points directly anterior when the arm is in 10 degrees of internal rotation and although one can roll the anterior edge of the deltoid beneath the fingers it should not be confused with the biceps tendon. While numerous tests have been reported, their reliability value in everyday practice is questionable.

The athlete with bicipital tendinitis usually reports a prodrome of shoulder pain. To localize the pathology to the biceps tendon, the tenderness should be over the bicipital groove and the area moves when the shoulder is shifted from internal to external rotation (35). The athlete's elbow is then flexed, with the arm at the side, and the shoulder is rotated. In bicipital tendinitis, the tenderness follows the movement of the bicipital groove. With the shoulder rotated internally, the tenderness is medial; at neutral position it

remains medial. When the shoulder is externally rotated, however, the groove lies in front or even lateral to the midline, and this becomes the tender area.

In examining for bicipital tendinitis, the athlete should be supine so that he or she is relaxed and his or her shoulder can be maneuvered easily. The examiner abducts the shoulder to 90 degrees and holds it in neutral rotation. The examiner supports the elbow and then rotates the shoulder internally about 15 degrees so that the bicipital groove points toward the ceiling. The examiner can now palpate the bicipital groove and the anterior deltoid easily. Further, by lowering the arm off the table, the biceps tendon bowstrings somewhat, becoming even more prominent. Next, the examiner rotates the humerus from external rotation to internal rotation and then back with the elbow flexed. If the tendon is subluxing, a snap or a pop may be heard or felt. If the athlete puts his hand on his head and then contracts his biceps, he may produce bicipital groove pain.

In Yergason's test for bicipital tendinitis, the athlete supinates the forearm against resistance. The examiner stands to the side and just behind the athlete. The athlete has the arm at the side and then flexes the elbow to 90 degrees with the thumb up. The examiner's hand is placed on the back of the athlete's hand and shadows the forearm; he asks the athlete to supinate against the examiner's resistance. In bicipital tendinitis, this movement will cause pain at the bicipital groove. To balance the athlete for this exercise, the examiner places his free hand on the athlete's opposite hip.

Speed's test is performed with the athlete standing and the arm at the side. The examiner stands on the affected side, putting one hand on the front of the athlete's forearm, providing resistance, and the other hand on the back of the athlete's hip for balance. The athlete is then asked to flex the shoulder, with the elbow straight, to approximately 60 degrees. A positive test elicits pain localized to the bicipital groove area and is considered the most useful in reproduction of bicipital pain.

The routine radiographic examination is frequently normal in biceps tendinitis. This has led to the development of special views to visualize the bicipital groove. The bicipital groove view, 30-degree caudal tilt view, and the outlet view are additional techniques that can reveal degenerative changes of the groove, a shallow groove, or extrinsic compression from anterior, inferior acromial osteophytes.

Biceps tendinitis usually occurs secondary to an impingement syndrome and rarely exists as an isolated entity. Therefore a careful history and physical examination should be performed. An injection of 1% Xylocaine into the subacromial space usually relieves all pain in an impingement syndrome. If the athlete has an associated bicipital tendinitis, pain may persist in the groove. Further injection anteriorly into the bicipital sheath with relief of pain will confirm the diagnosis of bicipital tendinitis.

Ice may be used in the early treatment of bicipital tendinitis and the athlete given a nonsteroidal, antiinflammatory medicine. Painful maneuvers should be avoided, and if the pain persists the arm should be rested. A local steroid deposit around the tendon often relieves the pain, but if it is injected into the tendinous substance it may provoke rupture. If the bicipital tendinitis is secondary to an impingement syndrome with acromial osteophytes then an open or arthroscopic subacromial decompression should be performed with careful examination of the intraarticular attachment. The surgical procedure for recurring bicipital tendinitis is identical to that for ruptures of the tendon of the long head of the biceps.

Dislocation of the Biceps Tendon

A checked swing in baseball, with a sudden forceful jerking back of the bat, or a direct blow to a quarterback's externally rotated passing arm, with the biceps tensed, may tear the transverse humeral ligament from its insertion on the lesser tuberosity. The main stabilizer of the biceps tendon is the subscapularis tendon and the coracohumeral ligament; therefore, dislocation of the tendon only occurs with injury to these structures and their integrity must be assessed with ultrasound, arthrography, or MRI.

The athlete with a dislocating biceps tendon has anterior shoulder pain with popping, cracking, and occasionally a locking sensation. The tendon slips and rolls over during throws, sometimes snapping back during internal rotation. Shoulder pain may occur when the shoulder is abducted to 90 degrees and then rotated externally and internally. The tendon dislocation can sometimes be brought out by manually resisting the throwing motion. Tenderness follows the movement of the bicipital groove. When the arm is internally rotated the tenderness is medial, and in neutral position the tenderness remains medial. When the arm is externally rotated, however, the groove lies in front of, or even lateral to the midline, and the tenderness shifts to this position.

For acute biceps tendon dislocation, the shoulder is iced and the arm rested in internal rotation. When dislocations recur, the operative repair must include repair of the rotator cuff and coracohumeral ligaments. In older athletes, the tendon substance may be severely worn with degenerative changes and tenodesis within the groove will provide good function.

Rupture of the Long Head of the Biceps Tendon

The biceps tendon becomes worn by persistent friction in a tight, steep-walled groove that has supratubercular rough spots. Further degeneration of the tendon occurs in swimmers as an avascular zone of the intracapsular part of the tendon is stretched over the humeral head. Rupture of the biceps tendon is not uncommon in the degenerated tendons of older athletes: It may follow an underhand delivery in fast-pitch softball or a snappy, underhand basketball pass. Even young athletes, especially gymnasts (34) and weight lifters, may rupture the tendon of the long head of their biceps. This type of rupture produces a bulging biceps in the arm.

The biceps spans two joints, and repairs usually restore only the part near the elbow. If the tendon is left unrepaired, the athlete will lose about 20% of elbow flexion power. Repair is usually not recommended for nonathletes, but repair may restore needed elbow flexion and supination to competitive athletes. In repairing this condition, the surgeon enters the shoulder joint through a small split in the rotator cuff or uses an arthroscope to preserve the integrity of the cuff. The intraarticular part of the tendon is then removed from the glenoid to prevent a buckling tendon remnant from interfering with shoulder action. Some surgeons roughen the floor of the bicipital groove and suture the tendon into the groove with mattress stitches. Others may choose a *trap door* technique in which the tendon is placed under an osteoperiosteal flap near the bicipital groove. After most of these operations, the shoulder must be rested. Because such long restriction of motion may freeze the shoulder, a keyhole technique that allows postoperative shoulder and elbow motion and rapid resumption of activities may be preferred (Fig. 11.22) (42).

ACUTE DISLOCATION OF THE SHOULDER

Acute dislocation of the shoulder is one of the oldest medical entities reported, as the earliest description was in the Edwin Smith Papyrus (3000 to 2500 BC). Perhaps the most important factor in determining the correct treatment of an acute shoulder dislocation is determining the direction of dislocation and amount of energy involved in the injury. Generally, shoulder dislocations are classified by their direction and by whether they are traumatic or atraumatic.

Acute Anterior Dislocation

In an anterior dislocation of the shoulder, the shoulder abducts and rotates externally, and the restraining forces of the subscapularis and anterior-inferior glenohumeral ligamentous complex fail with anterior or anterior-inferior displacement of the humeral head. The anterior capsule stretches, tears, and may be stripped from its attachment to the anterior glenoid rim. Occasionally the labrum strips from the glenoid with the capsule or is torn (9). The humeral head then slides below the coracoid and sometimes pops back into place but more frequently stays dislocated.

A player typically comes off the field supporting the

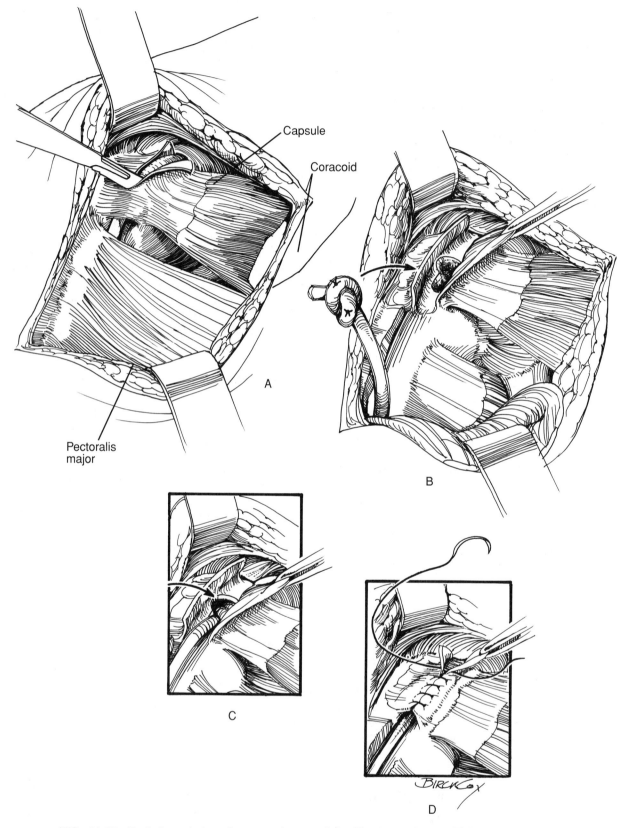

Capsule

Coracoid

Pectoralis
major

A

B

C

D

BIRCKCOX

FIG. 11.22. Keyhole technique for reattachment of the biceps tendon. **A.** The proximal end of the biceps tendon is mobilized, a burr creates the keyhole in the cortex of the proximal humerus. **B.** The tendon is tied in a figure of eight then placed into the keyhole (**C**). **D.** The transverse humeral ligament is repaired.

arm in slight abduction and external rotation. The acutely dislocated shoulder is very painful as muscles are in spasm attempting to stabilize the joint. The posterior shoulder is hollow beneath the acromion and the humeral head may be palpable. In a muscular athlete, this sign may be less apparent when the two shoulders are compared. However, an athlete with an anterior dislocation will usually not be able to touch the other shoulder, as he or she is incapable of full internal rotation. There is a frequent association with nerve injury, particularly the axillary nerve, and a careful assessment of neurologic status is necessary prior to reduction.

Although the shoulder will sometimes pop back after gentle traction on the field or sidelines, in most cases the athlete must be taken from the playing field for reduction of the dislocation. Early on, if muscle spasm is not profound, an ice pack anteriorly on the shoulder will provide analgesia and muscle relaxation. There are many different described reduction techniques and each individual involved in orthopaedic care has a favorite. The most atraumatic techniques are favored.

One method is to help the athlete to a prone position on the training table, with the arm hanging over the side. The physician gently pulls downward, with the athlete's elbow flexed to 90 degrees and his forearm supinated to relax the biceps. An assistant then rotates the inferior angle of the scapula toward the spine so that the glenoid faces the humerus. The combination of traction and scapular rotation allows the humeral head to slide easily back into the socket. A dislocation will sometimes even reduce spontaneously when the athlete lies prone on the examining table with a pillow under the chest and the arm hanging over the edge of the table.

The *countertraction technique* is an alternative method of reduction. While an assistant applies countertraction around the chest with a towel or sheet, the athlete's arm is pulled at about 30 degrees of abduction in line with the trunk (Fig. 11.23). The dislocated shoulder will usually reduce, but, in some muscular persons seen late and who have strong muscle spasm, a narcotic and an intravenous relaxant, or even general anesthesia, may be needed to facilitate reduction. If difficulty is encountered with reduction then a radiographic exam is necessary prior to a second reduction; an anteroposterior, an axillary lateral or a transthoracic lateral view x-ray film of the shoulder should be taken. Following reduction these films should be repeated to ensure reduction.

An athlete's first anterior dislocation should be immobilized for 3 to 4 weeks. Special immobilization devices or advanced exercise programs appear to have no effect on the recurrence rate of an anterior traumatic dislocation (49,98). The arm is usually placed in a sling, with abduction and forward flexion resistive exercises starting as soon as the early pain subsides. Otherwise, the anterior deltoid will atrophy rapidly. The athlete should also per-

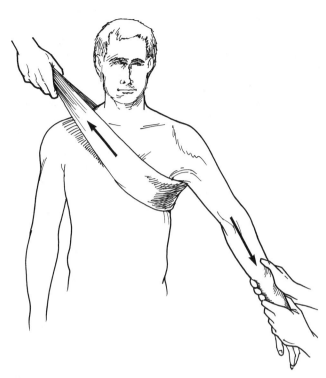

FIG. 11.23. Counter-traction technique for closed reduction of anterior-inferior glenohumeral dislocation.

form shrugs but should avoid external rotation early in retraining.

A fracture of the humerus or of the scapula sometimes accompanies a shoulder dislocation, and nerve damage may account for slow progress in regaining strength. In this situation, an arthrogram may be needed because a rotator cuff tear may also be present, causing shoulder pain and a poor return of strength.

Acute Posterior Dislocation

Recognition of a posterior dislocation may be difficult as there is not a striking deformity of the shoulder. A direct blow to the front of the shoulder may drive the humeral head out of the socket posteriorly, or, when a lineman comes up with shoulders abducted 90 degrees and flexed forward, his humeral head may slip out posteriorly. The athlete who has sustained a posterior dislocation will have the arm internally rotated and adducted at the side. The coracoid is prominent, the anterior part of the shoulder flat, and there is a posterior prominence compared with the normal side. He or she will have limited ability to abduct and to rotate the shoulder externally.

An anteroposterior x-ray film may look almost normal, but close inspection will show the medial margin of the humeral head to be overlapping the glenoid abnormally. Posterior dislocation should be suspected if there is a fracture of the lesser tuberosity. A lateral x-ray view along the spine of the scapula will reveal the humeral head to be dislocated posterior to the Y-axis of the scapula.

Patients with acute, traumatic posterior dislocation of the shoulder usually have more severe pain than an acute, traumatic anterior dislocation. The use of intravenous narcotics and muscle relaxants may be unsuccessful and general anesthesia may be required. Traction is applied in line with the internally rotated, adducted humerus to reduce a posterior dislocation. Sometimes the internal rotation may have to be increased to disengage the head. Pressure is then applied to the humeral head from behind to push it forward. Any external rotation during reduction should be avoided, as it may lead to fracture of the humeral head or shaft.

After the dislocation has been reduced, the humerus is most stable at neutral rotation and slight extension. Thus, the reduction is maintained for 3 weeks in a handshake cast in this position (25). This position allows healing of the injured posterior structures. External rotation and deltoid isometrics are performed during the period of immobilization. After removal of the cast the athlete should engage in a vigorous strengthening program of the external and internal rotators. Return to competition may occur when full range of motion is present, normal strength has been achieved, and at least 3 months have elapsed.

RECURRENT ANTERIOR DISLOCATIONS OF THE SHOULDER

Recurrence of anterior dislocations has been shown to be most closely associated with the age of the athlete at the time of the initial dislocation. The younger the athlete, the higher the incidence of recurrence. Some series have reported 90% or more recurrence rates for patients younger than 21 (6); however, these have a sampling bias and more closely controlled studies have recently reported 50% to 60% recurrence rates (49). The recurrence rates then decrease sharply as age increases; however, the incidence of rotator cuff tears increases in the older athletes.

Recurrence results from altered anterior glenohumeral anatomy secondary to the traumatic event. The anterior capsule may undergo plastic deformation in the form of lengthening up to 30% at the time of anterior dislocation and detach from the anterior cortex of the glenoid, with or without the labrum (15). As a result, the static restraining force of the anterior-inferior glenohumeral ligament complex is incompetent and unable to maintain humeral head reduction with abduction and external rotation of the shoulder. The labrum may also be detached from the glenoid rim; however, this by itself may have little effect upon recurrent anterior instability (103). Arthroscopic examination of the acute shoulder dislocation has revealed three different types of injury: a stable shoulder with capsular tears, an unstable shoulder with capsular

tears, and an unstable shoulder with capsular detachment (Fig. 11.24) (9).

Examination of the athlete will reveal posterior atrophy of the external rotators, apprehension when the shoulder is abducted and externally rotated, and occasionally increased anterior translation can be elicited with an anteriorly directed force. The athlete will be able to describe the positions that increase anxiety of recurrent dislocation, usually overhead activity with the shoulder externally rotated. With recurrence, the anterior-inferior glenoid rim may become worn or have loss of integrity due to repeated fractures. As the humeral head dislocates from the glenoid, it jams against the anterior glenoid rim. The firm cortical rim crushes the soft cancellous bone in the posterolateral part of the humeral head, producing a defect that appears on plain x-ray film as a posterolateral wedge of compressed bone (32).

Radiographic examination will reveal a posterior humeral defect on a west point axillary lateral and inferior glenoid wear and calcifications are visible on an apical oblique film. The torn labrum or detached capsule is not visible on a plain x-ray film, but an arthrogram or CT-arthrogram of the shoulder will more accurately define the presence of these lesions (53).

Some football players who have had an anterior dislocation of the shoulder may compete while wearing a shoulder strap that prevents redislocation. Gieck uses a 1.5-inch wide elastic belt (43), riveting the buckle to the shoulder pad on the side opposite the dislocation. The remaining part of the belt is then looped around the affected arm while the arm is held adducted and flexed slightly forward. The belt has several notches to allow the athlete to adjust the tension. Because it tends to stretch, the belt must be adjusted every week or two. The belt system is good for receivers, running backs, and defensive backs by allowing forward flexion of the shoulder for pass receiving and defending while limiting external rotation from a horizontal, extended, and abducted position. Recently, neoprene shoulder sleeves combined with a belt system have been worn by basketball players with recurrent dislocations in the midst of playoffs, as surgery is being postponed till after the competitive season. If recurrence interferes with athletic performance or activities of daily living, one of many surgical options may be recommended, including open reconstructive procedures (17,113), or arthroscopic repair (6).

The goals of surgical intervention have become more clearly defined; reestablishment of normal anatomical relationships and preserving normal motion (especially external rotation) is required for return to athletic activity. Therefore, many procedures used in the past have been discontinued and experience has revealed unacceptable high recurrence rates, high complication rates, or limitation of motion with subsequent arthritis. Recent reports have described the successful outcomes of capsular shift

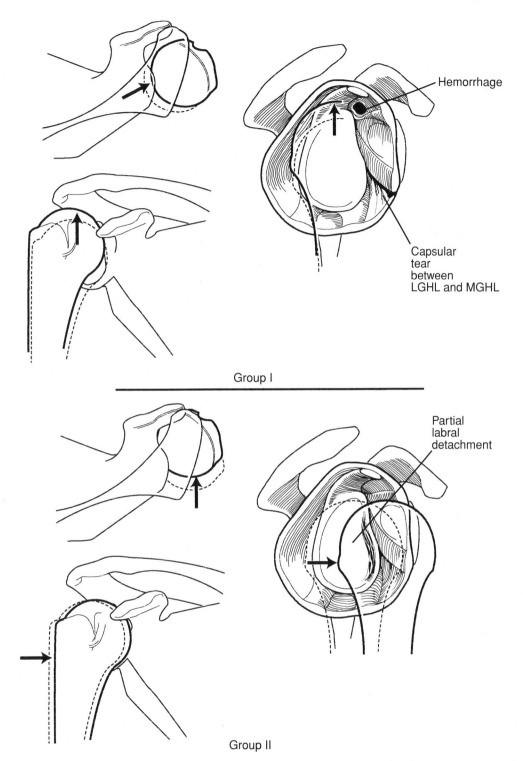

Group I

Group II

FIG. 11.24. Acute glenohumeral shoulder pathology classification. **Group I.** Capsular tearing without associated labral tear. **Group II.** Capsular and partial labral tears. **Group III.** Capsular and complete labral detachment (Bankart).

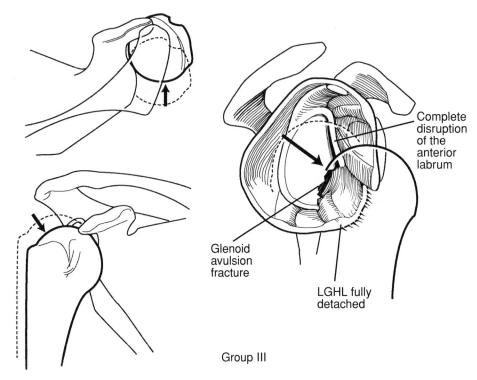

Complete
disruption
of the
anterior
labrum

Glenoid
avulsion
fracture

LGHL fully
detached

Group III

FIG. 11.24. *Continued.*

procedures combined with Bankart repairs in athletes (10,17,113). Arthroscopic repair has also become fashionable; however, recurrence rates have been reported to be 20% to 40%.

The Bristow operation (47) is a coracoid transfer that protects against dislocation while allowing better external rotation. In this procedure, the surgeon removes the tip of the coracoid process with the coracobrachialis and short head of the biceps still attached to it. He then roughens the bone at the junction of the middle third and lower third of the anterior glenoid rim and places the coracoid there. As the athlete abducts and rotates the shoulder externally after healing, the coracoid tip serves as a bone block, and the conjoined tendon of the coracobrachialis and short head of the biceps work as a dynamic sling that prevents the humeral head from dislocating. Some surgeons modify the coracoid transfer operation by using a screw to attach the coracoid tip to the glenoid, but the screw may loosen and even damage a blood vessel to produce an aneurysm. Although a coracoid transfer will sharply reduce dislocation (109), it limits external rotation to some extent, does not restore normal anatomy, has a high rate of arthritis (70% in some series), and is very difficult to revise. Because a throwing athlete needs full external rotation of the throwing arm shoulder, only rarely can return to the highest levels of performance and com-

petition if repair of a recurrently dislocating shoulder limits external rotation be achieved.

The best reported results in overhead athletes have been using an anterior capsulolabral reconstruction technique that also preserves the subscapularis tendon (74,100). Three techniques have been described, each with only a slight modification in the location of the capsular shift; glenoid-based T-shift (74), humeral-based T-shift (17,92), and the Rockwood shift (113). Each method preserves external rotation, preserves the subscapularis tendon, and restores normal anterior glenohumeral anatomy.

The rehabilitative process following anterior reconstructive procedures is as important as the procedure itself. Different surgeons offer different variations of the same theme, namely early range of motion within a safe zone, passive forward flexion, and external rotation without pain followed by active motion and resistive strengthening beginning at 6 to 8 weeks.

ANTERIOR SUBLUXATION

Anterior subluxation is a difficult entity to diagnose as physical examination may be unremarkable despite a clear description by the athlete. Subluxation may be traumatic or atraumatic and traumatic stability will be discussed in this section. Subluxation refers to abnormal anterior motion of the humeral head upon the glenoid without dislocation of the joint. The inferior glenohumeral ligament is usually stretched and incompetent due to repetitive microtrauma. This thickened area of the capsule is the prime anterior stabilizer of the shoulder and tightens as the arm is abducted and externally rotated. The athlete may also have this problem from an acute macrotraumatic event such as having wrenched the shoulder, for example, when sliding headfirst into a base or diving back to a base. Others report having had a direct blow to the shoulder or a history of heavy throwing or hard serving.

Subluxation may produce a ''dead arm'' syndrome in any overhead athlete, such as volleyball players, tennis players, pitchers, and water polo players. In the abducted externally rotated position of throwing, the humeral head moves into an abnormal anterior position on the glenoid and the rotator cuff muscles work to keep the head in position. Inefficient throwing results and the athlete complains of the arm *going out* or *going dead* as the velocity of the throw decreases. In short, he or she cannot use the arm forcefully in abduction and external rotation. In fact, the athlete may even drop the object he or she is throwing or holding. The quarterback will be unable to throw the ''long bomb,'' the volleyball player will be unable to spike, or a swimmer may have anterior shoulder pain. Occasionally, the athlete will complain of ulnar nerve symptoms, such as little- and ring-finger tingling.

Some athletes are clearly aware that the shoulder is slipping in the socket, others experience only sharp, paralyzing pain and are unaware that the shoulder is subluxing. A correct diagnosis is difficult to arrive at in the patient who is unaware that the shoulder is subluxing, and a careful history and symptoms must be elicited. Another group of people with shoulder subluxation are those who have had a previous shoulder operation. For example, young patients with a previous arthroscopic acromioplasty for relief of impingement with persistent pain may have instability as the primary pathologic condition.

Examination of the Subluxing Shoulder

In patients with glenohumeral subluxation, the anterior glenoid rim may be tender. However, the tenderness and pain are often posterior. For the shoulder to slide anteriorly, the tissues on the opposite end of the joint may be stressed, producing a posterior capsulitis or tendinitis. This explains the frequent posterior shoulder pain and tenderness in patients with anterior subluxation. Further, some posterior laxity may be found in patients with anterior subluxation because the posterior capsule has also been stretched.

The examination begins with the athlete sitting. Anterior instability is reproduced best when the shoulder is stressed in an anteroinferior direction. After examining

the normal shoulder, have the athlete sit in a relaxed position, hold the humeral head between the fingers and apply an anteriorly then posteriorly directed force, to determine the excursion. Next abduct the arm to 90 degrees in line with the scapula and externally rotate. Hold the arm with one hand at the elbow and press the humeral head forward, displacing it anteroinferiorly. At this time, the athlete may grimace and tighten the shoulder muscles because he or she feels pain or is apprehensive that the shoulder is about to dislocate (46).

Next, with the athlete supine on the examining table, externally rotate his shoulder. Excessive external rotation is common in anterior subluxation and in multidirectional shoulder instability. Sometimes, however, because the athlete is apprehensive, the affected shoulder may show decreased external rotation compared to the normal side or compared to an earlier baseline examination. As the shoulder is externally rotated, the pectoralis major may fasciculate. This sign is almost pathognomonic for anterior subluxation. With the patient still supine, and the shoulder abducted and externally rotated, place your hand posteriorly at the glenohumeral joint with your fingers on the humeral head and your thumb anteriorly with your other hand supporting the arm at the elbow and try to lever the humeral head anteriorly. Pain may be elicited with this maneuver and reversing the direction of force posteriorly, the relocation test, should abolish the pain if anterior subluxation is present (56).

Radiographic Exam

A complete radiographic series should be obtained along with a west point axillary lateral, which may reveal subtle Hill-Sachs lesions and an apical oblique view, which may show calcifications along the anteroinferior glenoid rim where periosteum may have been stripped from the anterior scapular neck. Arthrography may show dye extravasating into a large subscapular pouch that has resulted from avulsion of the glenohumeral ligaments from the glenoid. During this test, the athlete should abduct and rotate the shoulder inward. The subscapularis is tense in external rotation, and the underlying pouch might not be seen. Arthrography combined with CT (53) or MRI (107) provides the most sensitive exam to reveal labral tears and anterior capsular detachment; however, an experienced skeletal radiologist is necessary to interpret the scan.

Diagnostic Tests

If apprehension is the only positive instability finding when the arm is abducted and externally rotated, impingement must be excluded as the cause. Impingement and instability may both cause pain in this position, although with instability the pain is usually posterior. They may be differentiated, however, by injecting 10 mL of lidocaine (Xylocaine) into the subacromial space; impingement pain should be extinguished by the lidocaine.

Most people with anterior subluxation have been found to have a Bankart lesion. This is an avulsion of the labrum and capsule from the anterior glenoid rim. However, some have only laxity of the capsule and others have only a large opening between the tendons of the supraspinatus and subscapularis.

Treatment of Anterior Subluxation

After the first traumatic subluxation, the shoulder should be immobilized with a sling and swath for 2 weeks to decrease the possibility of a recurrence. Along with this rest, nonsteroidal antiinflammatory drugs lessen the inflammation. The athlete may then begin with regaining a full range of motion without stressing the anterior structures, then a rehabilitation program to strengthen the rotator cuff muscles, the deltoid, and the scapular rotators. Many will respond to a 2-month long exercise program with no further trouble.

If subluxations persist and interfere with athletic performance, surgical intervention may be necessary. The surgical procedure performed depends on the surgical findings. If the capsule is detached anteriorly then it will require reattachment. If capsular laxity is also present then a capsular shift should also be performed.

When there is no Bankart lesion but only a lax capsule, a modified capsulorrhaphy may be used to reef the capsule. In case of a interval lesion between the supraspinatus and the subscapularis tendons, the gap may be partly closed with interrupted sutures, care being taken not to limit the division of the two tendons around the coracoid. The capsular shift procedures described above, which maintain external rotation, are the favored surgical techniques and the Bristow, Putti-Platt, Magnusen Stack are no longer used in the athletic population. Arthroscopic surgical procedures were gaining popularity for treating anterior subluxations; unfortunately, the high failure has precluded its routine use.

POSTERIOR GLENOHUMERAL SUBLUXATION

Athletes will present with repeat episodes of posterior subluxation, which occurs in one of two ways: (1) from repetitive microtrauma or overuse, which stretches out the posterior capsule, or (2) from a single traumatic event that results in posterior subluxation with stretching of the posterior capsule, which then recurs. The athlete will feel shoulder pain during deceleration in the follow-through phase of throwing and pain when the shoulder is flexed, adducted, and internally rotated. The tenderness may be posterior or anterior. A history of a fall on the flexed arm or of a blow to the shoulder, driving the shoulder

posteriorly, is common. Athletes who perform heavy bench presses may also develop posterior subluxation. Some athletes are more uncomfortable when the humeral head leaves the glenoid, whereas others have discomfort when the head relocates. Pain results from the humeral head pressing against the posterior capsule and the cuff tendons of the infraspinatus and teres minor.

The examination for posterior subluxation begins with the athlete supine. This position calms the patient, relaxes the shoulder muscles, and eliminates the effects of gravity. The examiner first palpates the scapular neck and humeral head and controls the arm by supporting it at the elbow. The arm is flexed to 90 degrees and then horizontally abducted about 20 degrees. A posterior force applied to the arm may then sublux the shoulder (46). Often there will be a posterior bulge below the acromion. As the shoulder is horizontally abducted about 20 degrees more, the humeral head will reduce suddenly and the humeral head prominence will disappear. Remember that a shoulder may normally show considerable posterior laxity, one can normally get up to 50% posterior movement of the humeral head on the glenoid (44). Posterior subluxation may also be tested for by abducting the shoulder to 90 degrees, internally rotating it, and then horizontally adducting it. In posterior subluxation, the examiner will then feel the humeral head posteriorly. The athlete will usually say that this is the type of discomfort felt in his or her sport. As the arm is returned to neutral position at 90 degrees of abduction, the humeral head will reduce.

The athlete may be able to demonstrate the instability during the clinical examination; however, this does not mean that they are psychologically disturbed and they should be treated as if they could not voluntarily sublux their shoulder. The shoulder will sublux at a level of abduction that depends on the position of the arm at initial injury. Therefore, the probability of detecting a subluxation problem will increase if the amount of humeral rotation and the amount of abduction are changed and the examination repeated.

An axillary lateral x-ray film may show evidence of damage at the glenoid, such as a posterior capsular spur, bone chip, or calcification from throwing, or it may show a wearing away or erosion of the posterior glenoid with insufficiency of the posterior glenoid owing to repetitive heavy bench presses.

Treatment of Posterior Subluxation

The athlete should avoid bench presses and heavy pushing and pulling while the shoulder is symptomatic. Shoulder flexion should be avoided too, so that the humeral head will stay in the center of the glenoid away from the posterior aspect of the glenoid labrum and cuff. To strengthen the shoulder, the athlete does external rotations, starting the exercises at 45 degrees of external rotation with the arms at the side. If the athlete was to perform the exercises with less external rotation, the humeral head would shift posteriorly. The athlete should engage in a complete rehabilitation program to strengthen the rotator cuff muscles (specifically the external rotators), the posterior deltoid, and the scapular rotators. Approximately 70% will respond subjectively to a 6-month long exercise program and return to competition. In adolescents, strengthening will reduce the laxity as the posterior shoulder tightens and the shoulder matures. The older athlete with subluxation, however, is less likely to recover fully.

The surgical treatment of posterior instability has been controversial due to disappointing results in the past. A posterior capsulorrhaphy is now the recommended procedure with a capsular shift to obliterate posterior capsule redundancy (18). Postoperatively, the patient's arm and shoulder should be immobilized in 30 degrees abduction and neutral rotation for three weeks. If a preoperative CT scan reveals abnormal glenoid version, than an opening posterior glenoid osteotomy is combined with a capsular shift.

MULTIDIRECTIONAL INSTABILITY

The definition of multidirectional instability may be simply stated as instability of the shoulder in more than one direction. However, this condition is not that simple. Most athletes will experience instability in a primary direction which can be classified as anteroinferior or posteroinferior. The athlete may have multidirectional instability but only be symptomatic in one direction.

In patients with generalized ligamentous laxity, instability may develop in any direction with no or little trauma. In addition, significant inferior instability is the hallmark of generalized shoulder laxity with multidirectional instability. If the shoulder muscles become deconditioned then dynamic stability of the shoulder is lost and further instability develops, due to the lax integrity of the static stabilizers. Frequently, the athlete is an adolescent athlete who also has patellar subluxation problems, loose joints, and double-jointed thumbs.

On examination, athletes with multidirectional instability will commonly have signs of ligamentous laxity: hyperextension of the elbows, knees, and metacarpalphalangeal joints. The presence of a *sulcus sign*, inferior displacement of the humeral head when an inferior traction is applied to the grasped elbow indicates inferior instability. The gap between the humeral head and the undersurface of the acromion is usually less than 1 cm. This, when combined with excessive anterior or posterior humeral head translation, will support the diagnosis of multidirectional instability.

Treatment of Multidirectional Instability

Treatment of the athlete with ligamentous laxity and multidirectional instability has been controversial due to the poor surgical results of anterior procedures, posterior glenoid osteotomies, or posterior bone blocks. Fortunately, most athletes, 85% in some series, can be treated successfully with nonoperative rehabilitation (Fig. 11.25) (21).

The surgical findings of multidirectional instability are of capsular redundancy and superior rotator interval widening. Rarely is a capsular detachment or labral tear found. Therefore, surgical correction involves capsular shift procedures (Fig. 11.26) to decrease overall joint volume and closure of the superior interval lesion (2,80,113). Unidirectional anterior reconstructions such as the Bristow, Putti-Platt, or Magnusen-Stack may cause posterior displacement of the humeral head due to restricted external rotation and are not recommended.

THE HUMERUS

Hypertrophy of the humerus is a normal response to prolonged heavy arm exercise, and the cortical thickness of the humerus on the playing side of top-level male tennis players is thus 35% greater than on their nonplaying side. Top-level female players have a cortical thickness 28% greater on their playing side than on their control side (91).

One half of a large group of college gymnasts showed an asymptomatic cortical irregularity of the proximal humerus that simulates the cortical desmoid often found at the distal medial femoral condyle. This benign reactive process is located at the insertion of the broad, strong pectoralis major on the anteromedial cortical border of the humerus. Most athletes with this irregularity are all-around gymnasts who regularly perform strength moves, especially on the rings—hence the term *ringman's shoulder.*

Fractures of the humeral shaft have been reported in throwing athletes and wrist wrestlers. During the acceleration phase of throwing, the latissimus dorsi and the pectoralis major strongly rotate the athlete's shoulder internally, leaving the elbow behind. This torque may produce a spiral fracture of the humerus, especially in weak-armed but hard-throwing teenage pitchers with unrefined deliveries. When an outfielder throws from next to a fence or wall, he cannot use his body but must throw with his arm only. The torque may be so great as to fracture his humerus. Similarly, an arm wrestler may fracture the humerus during the losing phase of a contest. In the losing position, the elbow extends progressively, and there are changes in the direction of applied force during this eccentric muscle contraction. A spiral humerus fracture may occur at the lower third, with or without a butterfly fragment. These fractures are treated with a Sarmiento cast brace.

Little League Shoulder

Chronic stress syndrome in the proximal humeral epiphysis in the young baseball player is commonly re-

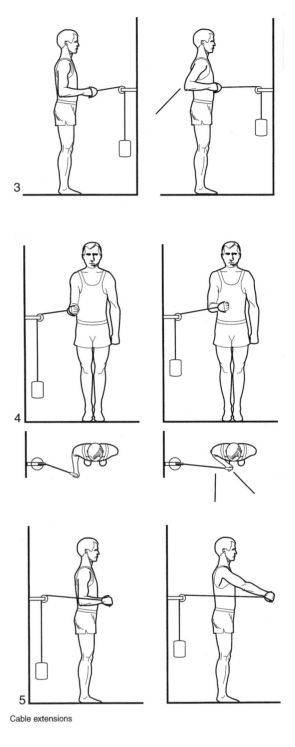

FIG. 11.25. A. Shoulder exercises to strengthen the rotator cuff muscles and the three parts of the deltoid. Initially the patient is given a set of three-inch rubber therabands, which progresses from one to five pounds of resistance. When proficient with these five exercises, the patient is progressed to a wall pulley with greater weight.

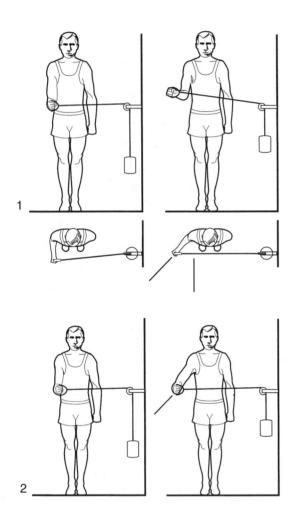

Cable extensions

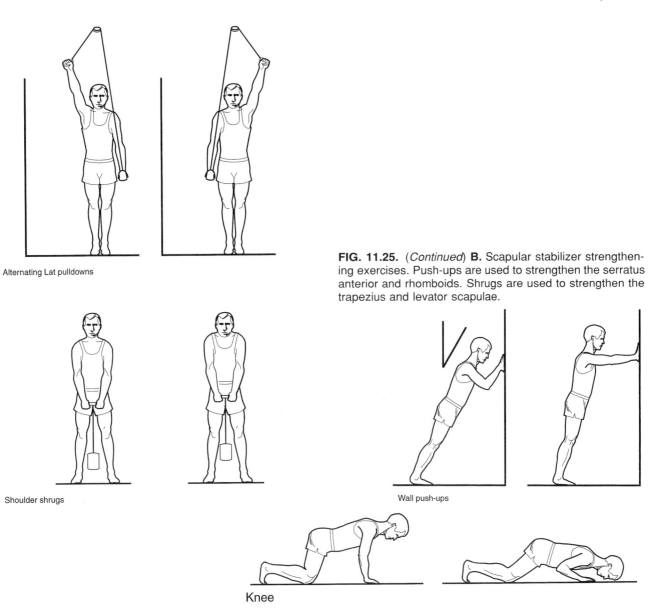

Alternating Lat pulldowns

Shoulder shrugs

FIG. 11.25. (*Continued*) **B.** Scapular stabilizer strengthening exercises. Push-ups are used to strengthen the serratus anterior and rhomboids. Shrugs are used to strengthen the trapezius and levator scapulae.

Wall push-ups

Knee

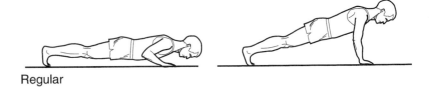

Regular

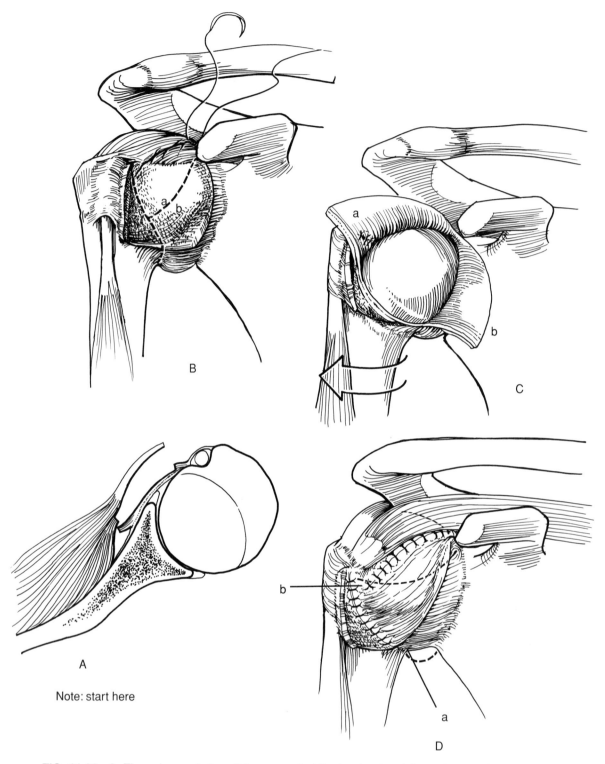

B

C

A

Note: start here

D

FIG. 11.26. A. The subscapularis split leaves part of the tendon to reinforce the anterior capsule. **B.** The split in the internal rotator is closed. **C.** Capsular flaps (*a* and *b*) are created. **D.** Flap *b* is brought superiorly and flap *a* inferiorly, eliminating capsular redundancy.

ferred to as "Little League shoulder" (108). The stress of rotary forces generated by the torque of the throwing motion create a reaction by the epiphysis of the proximal humerus (23). The shoulder may become tender and overhead activity painful. Palpation of the proximal humerus may become tender in extreme cases. The name "Little League shoulder" is a misnomer as this entity generally occurs in adolescents focusing on one repetitive overhead activity such as tennis, baseball, swimming, or gymnastics.

Radiographs will reveal widening of the humeral physis and a denser margin on the physeal side. Occasionally radiographic changes at the tip of the coracoid will also be seen. This condition responds well to rest and return to competition on a limited basis.

TENNIS SHOULDER

In the tennis serve, the racket is thrown up at the ball and decelerated over a very short distance from a speed of about 480 km/hour (300 miles/hour). The forces generated in this movement stretch the scapular-anchoring muscles, and the shoulder then droops, rotating forward from the pull of gravity on the increased mass of the arm.

The player with a drooped shoulder may develop anterior rotator cuff symptoms. A relative abduction of the shoulder is produced as the scapula tilts downward. There is less room for the rotator cuff, and it may be impacted, especially during serves and overhead returns. The player may also have pain on the backhand side when the arm ends high, especially with backhand volleys.

Signs and symptoms of compression at the thoracic outlet are thought by some to be associated with the drooped "tennis shoulder," causing neck and arm pain. However, a study over a period of 5 years of the players who competed in the United States Tennis Association National Clay Court Championships revealed that all players had drooped racket arm shoulders, but none have had symptoms of an outlet syndrome (63). The authors concluded that the tennis shoulder of a veteran player is a normal response to exercise and generally will not produce outlet difficulties. The younger and harder-hitting tennis professional may, however, develop outlet problems. If such a play is symptomatic, shrug exercises will help to elevate the shoulder, and if the symptoms persist a thorough workup should be conducted (64).

REFERENCES

1. Acus RW III, Bell RH, Fisher DL. Proximal clavicle excision; an analysis of results. *J Shoulder Elbow Surg* 1995;4:182–187.
2. Altchek DW, Warren RF, Skyhar HR, Ortiz G. T-plasty modifications of the Bankart procedure for multidirectional instability of the anterior and inferior types. *J Bone Joint Surg* 1991;73A:105–112.
3. Altchek DW, Warren RF, Wickiewicz TL, Ortiz G. Arthroscopic labral debridement: a 3-year follow-up study. *Am J Sports Med* 1992;20:702.
4. An KN, Browne AO, Korinek S, Tanaka S, Morrey BF. Three-dimensional kinematics of glenohumeral elevation. *J Orthop Res* 1991;9:143–149.
5. Andrews JR, Carson WG, MacLeod WD. Glenoid labrum tears related to the long head of the biceps. *Am J Sports Med* 1985;13:337–341.
6. Arciero RA, Wheeler JH, Ryan JB, McBride JT. Arthroscopic bankart repair versus nonoperative treatment for acute, initial anterior shoulder dislocations. *Am J Sports Med* 22:589–594.
7. Ark JW, Flock TJ, Flatow EL, Bigliani LU. Arthroscopic treatment of calcific tendinitis of the shoulder. *Arthroscopy* 1992;8:183–189.
8. Baker CL, Liu SH. Neurovascular injuries to the shoulder. *J Orthop Sports Phys Ther* 1993;18:360–364.
9. Baker CL, Uribe JW, Whitman C. Arthroscopic evaluation of acute initial anterior shoulder dislocations. *Am J Sports Med* 1990;18:25–28.
10. Bankart ASB. The pathology and treatment of recurrent dislocation of the shoulder joint. *Br J Surg* 1938;26:23–29.
11. Bergfeld JA, Andrish JT, Clancy WG. Evaluation of the acromioclavicular joint following first and second degree sprains. *Am J Sports Med* 1978;6:153–159.
12. Berson BC. Surgical repair of pectoralis major rupture in an athlete—case report of an unusual injury in a wrestler. *Am J Sports Med* 1979;7:348–351.
13. Biedert RM. Atrophy of the infraspinatus muscle caused by a suprascapular ganglion. *Clin J Sports Med* 1996;6:262–263.
14. Bigliani LU. Repair of rotator cuff tears in tennis players. *Am J Sports Med* 1992;20:112–117.
15. Bigliani LU, Pollock RG, Soslowsky LJ, et al. Tensile properties of the inferior glenohumeral ligament. *J Orthop Res* 1992;10:187–197.
16. Bigliani LU, Morrison DS, April EW. The morphology of the acromion and its relationship to rotator cuff tears. *Ortho Trans* 1986;10:216.
17. Bigliani LU, Kurzweil PR, Schwartzbach CC, Wolfe IN, Flatow EL. Inferior capsular shift procedure for anterior–inferior shoulder instability in athletes. *Am J Sports Med* 1994;22:578–584.
18. Bigliani LU, Pollock RG, McIlveen SJ, Endrizzi DP, Flatow EL. Shift of the posteriorinferior aspect of the capsule for recurrent posterior glenohumeral instability. *J Bone Joint Surg* 1995;77:1011–1020.
19. Blasier RB, Guldberg RE, Rothman ED. Anterior shoulder stability: contributions of rotator cuff forces and the capsular ligaments in a cadaver model. *J Shoulder Elbow Surg* 1992;1:140–150.
20. Britt LP. Non-operative treatment of the thoracic outlet syndrome symptoms. *Clin Orthop* 1967;51:45–48.
21. Burkhead WZ, Rockwood CA Jr. Treatment of instability of the shoulder with an exercise program. *J Bone Joint Surg* 1992;74A:890–896.
22. Cahill BR. Osteolysis of the distal part of the clavicle in male athletes. *J Bone Joint Surg (Am)* 1982;64:1053.
23. Cahill BR, Tullos HS, Fain RH. Little League shoulder. *Am J Sports Med* 1974;2:150–154.
24. Cahill BR. Atraumatic osteolysis of the distal clavicle. *Am J Sports Med* 1992;13:214–222.
25. Cautilli RA, Joyce MF, Mackell JV Jr. Posterior dislocations of the shoulder: a method of post-reduction management. *Am J Sports Med* 1978;6:397–399.
26. Clancy, WG Jr, Brand RL, Bergfield JA. Upper trunk brachial plexus injuries in contact sports. *Am J Sports Med* 1977;5:209–216.
27. Colosimo AJ, Hummer CD III, Heidt RS Jr. Aseptic foreign body reaction to Dacron graft material used for coracoclavicular ligament reconstruction after type III acromioclavicular dislocation. *Am J Sports Med* 1996;24:561–563.
28. Cooper DE, Arnoczsky SP, O'Brien SJ, et al. Anatomy, histology, and vascularity of the glenoid labrum. *J Bone Joint Surg* 1992;74A:46–52.
29. Cooper DE, O'Brien SJ, Arnoczsky SP, Warren RF. The structure and function of the coracohumeral ligament. *J Shoulder Elbow Surg* 1992;2:70–77.

30. Cox JS. The fate of the acromioclavicular joint in athletic injuries. *Am J Sports Med* 1981;9:50–53.

31. Cox JS. Current method of treatment of acromioclavicular joint dislocations. *Orthopaedics* 1992;15:1041.

32. Danzig LA, Greenway G, Resnick D. The Hill-Sachs lesion—an experimental study. *Am J Sports Med* 1980;8:328–332.

33. Daubinet G, et al. Paralysis of the suprascapular nerve and tennis. *Schweiz Z Sportmed* 1991;39:113–118.

34. Del Pizzo W, et al. Rupture of the biceps tendon in gymnastics: a case report. *Am J Sports Med* 1978;6:283–286.

35. Depalma AF, Callery GE. Bicipital tenosynovitis. *Clin Orthop* 1954:69.

36. Dominguez RH. Shoulder pain in age group swimmers. *Int Ser Sports Sci* 1978;6:105–109.

37. Ellman H. Arthroscopic subacromial decompression—analysis of 1- to 3-year results. *Arthroscopy-J Arthro Rel Surg* 1987;3(3): 173–181.

38. Ellman H, et al. Repair of the rotator cuff. *J Bone Joint Surg* 1986; 68A:1136–1144.

39. Ellman H, Kay SP, Wirth MA. Arthroscopic treatment of full-thickness rotator cuff tears: 2- to 7-year follow-up study. *J Arthro Rel Res* 1993;9:195–200.

40. Ferrari JD, Ferrari DA, Coumas J, Pappas AM. Posterior ossification of the shoulder the Bennett lesion. Diagnosis and treatment. *Am J Sports Med* 1994;22:171.

41. Flatow EL, Duralde XA, Nicholsen GP, Pollock RG, Bigliani LU. Arthroscopic resection of the distal clavicle with a superior approach. *J Shoulder Elbow Surg* 1995;4:41–50.

42. Froimson AI, Oh I. Keyhole tenodesis of biceps origin at the shoulder. *Clin Orthop* 1975;112:245–249.

43. Gieck JH. Shoulder strap to prevent anterior glenohumeral dislocations. *Athletic Training* 1976;11:18.

44. Harryman DT II, Sidles JA, Clark JM, et al. Translation of the humeral head on the glenoid with passive glenohumeral motion. *J Bone Joint Surg*, 1990;72A:1334–1343.

45. Hawkins RJ, Kennedy JC. Impingement syndrome in athletes. *Am J Sports Med* 1980;8:151–158.

46. Hawkins RJ, Mohtadi NGH. Clinical evaluation of shoulder instability. *Clin J Sports Med* 1991;1:59–64.

47. Helfet AJ. Coracoid transplantation for recurring dislocation of the shoulder. *J Bone Joint Surg* 1958;40B:198–202.

48. Hessmann M, Gotzen L, Gehling H. Acromioclavicular reconstruction augmented with polydioxanonsulphate bands. Surgical technique and results. *Am J Sports Med* 1995;23:552–556.

49. Hovelius L. Anterior dislocation of the shoulder in teenagers and young adults: five year prognosis. *J Bone Joint Surg* 1987;69A: 393–397.

50. Howell SM, Imobersteg AM, Seger DH, Marone PJ. Clarification of the role of the surpraspinatus muscle in shoulder function. *J Bone Joint Surg* 1986;68A:398.

51. Iannotti JP, Zlatkin MB, Esterhai JL, et al. Magnetic resonance imaging of the shoulder: sensitivity, specificity, and predictive value. *J Bone Joint Surg* 73A:17–29.

52. Jackson DL, Farrage J, Hynninen BC, Caborn DN. Suprascapular neuropathy in athletes: case reports. *Clin J Sport Med* 1995;5: 134–136.

53. Jahnke AH, Petersen SA, Neumann C, et al. A prospective comparison of computed arthrotomography and magnetic resonance imaging of the glenohumeral joint. *Am J Sports Med* 1992;20:695–701.

54. Jobe FW, Glousman RE. Rotator cuff dysfunction and associated glenohumeral instability in the throwing athlete. In: Tibone Paulos, ed. *Operative techniques in shoulder surgery*. Gaithersburg, MD: Aspen, 1991.

55. Jobe FW, Bradley JP. Rotator cuff injuries in baseball: prevention and rehabilitation. *Sports Med* 1988;6:378–387.

56. Jobe FW, Bradley JP. The diagnosis and nonoperative treatment of shoulder injuries in athletes. *Clin Sports Med* 1989;8:419–438.

57. Jobe FW, et al. Impingement syndrome in overhead athletes. *Surg Rounds Orthop* 1990;4:39–41.

58. Jobe FW, Kvitne RS. Shoulder pain in the overhand or throwing athlete. *Orthop Rev* 1989;18:963–975.

59. Kennedy JC. Retrosternal dislocation of the clavicle. *J Bone Joint Surg* 1949;31B:74.

60. Kennedy JC. Orthopedic manifestations of swimming. *Am J Sports Med* 1978;6:309–322.

61. Kennedy JC, Hawkins RJ. Swimmer's shoulder. *Phys Sports Med* 1974;2:35–38.

62. Kozo O, Rockwood CA Jr. Use of a thirty-degree caudal tilt radiograph in the shoulder impingement syndrome. *J Shoulder Elbow Surg* 1992;1:246–252.

63. Kulund DN, et al. The long-term effects of playing tennis. *Phys Sportsmed* 1979;7:87–94.

64. Kulund DN, McCue FC, Rockwell DA, Gieck JH. Tennis injuries: prevention and treatment. *Am J Sports Med* 1979;7:249–253.

65. Lauman U. Kinesiology of the shoulder joint. In: Kolbel R, ed. *Shoulder replacement*. Berlin: Springer-Verlag, 1987;125–173.

66. Leffert RD. Thoracic outlet and the shoulder. In: Jobe FW, ed. *Clinics in sports medicine. Symposium on injuries to the shoulder in the athlete*. Philadelphia: WB Saunders, 1983.

67. Linker, et al. Quadrilateral space syndrome: findings at MR imaging. *Radiology* 1993;188:675–676.

68. Lyons FA, Rockwood CA Jr. Migration of pins used in operations on the shoulder: current concepts review. *J Bone Joint Surg* 1992; 72A:1262–1267.

69. Macnab I, Rathbun JB. The microvascular pattern of the rotator cuff. *J Bone Joint Surg* 1970;52B:524.

70. Mathews LS, Simonson BG, Wolock BS. Osteolysis of the distal clavicle in a female body builder: a case report. *Am J Sports Med* 1993;21:150–152.

71. McMaster WC. Anterior glenoid labral damage: a painful lesion in swimmers. *Am J Sports Med* 1986;14:383–387.

72. Miller MD, et al. Rupture of the pectoralis major muscle in a collegiate football player. Use of magnetic resonance imaging in early diagnosis. *Am J Sports Med* 1993;21:475–477.

73. Mochizuki T, Isoda H, Masui T, et al. Occlusion of the posterior humeral circumflex artery: detection with MR angiography in healthy volunteers and in a patient with quadrilateral space syndrome. *AJR* 1994;163:625–627.

74. Montgomery WH III, Jobe FW. Functional outcomes in athletes after modified anterior capsulolabral reconstruction. *Am J Sports Med* 1994;22:352–358.

75. Morrey BF. Biomechanics of the shoulder. In: Rockwood CA Jr, Matsen FA III, ed. *The Shoulder*. Philadelphia: WB Saunders, 1990:208–245.

76. Morrey BF, Chao EYS. Recurrent anterior dislocations of the shoulder joint: clinical and anatomic considerations. In: Dumbleton Black JH, ed. *Clinical biomechanics: a case history approach*. New York: Churchill Livingstone, 1981:24–46.

77. Neer CS. Anterior acromioplasty for the chronic impingement syndrome in the shoulder. *J Bone Joint Surg* 1972;54-A:41–50.

78. Neer CS II. Impingement lesions. *Clin Orthop* 1983;173:70–77.

79. Neer CS II. *Shoulder reconstruction*. Philadelphia: WB Saunders, 1990:405–406.

80. Neer CS II, Foster CR. Inferior capsular shift for involuntary inferior and multidirectional instability of the shoulder. *J Bone Joint Surg* 1980;62A:897–907.

81. Nelson CL. The use of arthrography in athletic injuries of the shoulder. *Orthop Clin North Am* 1973;4:775–785.

82. Nettles JL, Linscheid RL. Sternoclavicular dislocations. *J Trauma* 1968;8:158–164.

83. Norfray JF, Tremaine MJ, Grove HC, Bachman DC. The clavicle in hockey. *Am J Sports Med* 1977;5:275–280.

84. Nuber GW, Jobe FW, Perry J, et al. Fine wire electromyography analysis of muscles of the shoulder during swimming. *Am J Sports Med* 1986;14:7–11.

85. Pal GP, et al. Relationship between the long head of biceps branchii and the glenoidal labrum in humans. *Anat Rec* 1991;229: 278–280.

86. Paladini D, Dellantonio R, Cinti A, Angeleri F. Axillary neuropathy in volleyball players: report of two cases and literature review. *J Neurol Neurosurg Psych* 1996;60:345–347.

87. Penny JN, Welsh RP. Shoulder impingement syndromes in athletes and their surgical management. *Am J Sports Med* 1981;9:11–15.

88. Petchall JF, Sonnabend DH, Hughes JS. Distal clavicular excision:

a detailed functional assessment. *Australian and New Zealand J Surg* 1995;65:262–266.

89. Poppen NM, et al. Normal and abnormal motion of the shoulder. *J Bone Joint Surg* 1976;58A:195.

90. Post M, et al. Suprascapular nerve entrapment: diagnosis and treatment. *J Shoulder Elbow Surg* 1993;2:190–197.

91. Priest JD, Nagel DA. Tennis shoulder. *Am J Sports Med* 1976;4:28–42.

92. Protzman RR. Anterior instability of the shoulder. *J Bone Joint Surg* 1980;909–918.

93. Richardson AB. The shoulder in competitive swimming. *Am J Sports Med* 1980;8;159–163.

94. Rockwood CA Jr, Young DC. Disorders of the acromioclavicular joint. In: Matsen FA III, Rockwood CA Jr, ed. *The shoulder.* Philadelphia: WB Saunders, 1990:423.

95. Rockwood CA Jr, Wirth MA, Blatter G. Specific capsular shift reconstruction for the management of patients with anterior shoulder instability. *Orthop Trans* 1994;17:972.

96. Rockwood CA Jr. Shoulder impingement syndrome: diagnosis, radiographic evaluation and treatment with a modified Neer acromioplasty. *J Bone and Joint Surg* 1993;75A:409–424.

97. Rockwood, CA Jr, Groh GI, Wirth MA, Grassi FA. Resection arthroplasty of the sternoclavicular joint. *J Bone Joint Surg* 1997;79A:387–393.

98. Rowe CR, Sakellarides HT. Factors related to recurrence of dislocations of the shoulder. *Clin Orthop* 1961;20:40–48.

99. Rowe CR, Zarins B. Recurrent transient subluxation of the shoulder. *J Bone Joint Surg* 1981;63A:863.

100. Rubenstein DL, et al. Anterior capsulolabral reconstruction of the shoulder in athletes. *J Shoulder Elbow Surg* 1992;1:229–237.

101. Snyder SJ, et al. Partial thickness rotator cuff tears: results of arthroscopic treatment. *Arthroscopy* 1991;7:1.

102. Snyder SJ, Karzal RP, DelPizzo W, et al. SLAP lesions of the shoulder. *Arthroscopy* 1990;6:274.

103. Speer KP, Deng X, Borreo S, et al. Biomechanical evaluation of a simulated Bankart lesion. *J Bone Joint Surg* 1994;76:1819–1826.

104. Strukel RJ, Garrick JG. Thoracic outlet compression in athletes: a report of four cases. *Am J Sports Med* 1978;6:35–39.

105. Tibone JE, et al. Shoulder impingement syndrome in athletes treated by anterior acromioplasty. *Clin Orthop* 1985;188:134.

106. Tibone JE, et al. Surgical treatment of tears of the rotator cuff in athletes. *J Bone Joint Surg* 1986;68A:887–891.

107. Tirman PF, Palmer WE, Feller JF. MR arthrography of the shoulder. *MRI Clin North Am* 1997;5:811–839.

108. Torg JS, Pollack H, Sweterlitsch P. The effect of competitive pitching on the shoulders and elbows of pre-adolescent baseball players. *Pediatrics* 1972;49:267–272.

109. Torg JS, Balduini FC, Bonci C, et al. A modified Bristow-Helfet-May procedure for recurrent dislocation and subluxation of the shoulder: report of two hundred and twelve cases. *J Bone Joint Surg* 1987;69A:904–913.

110. Van Linge B, Mulder JD. Function of the supraspinatus muscle and its relations to the supraspinatus syndrome: an experimental study in man. *J Bone Joint Surg* 1963;750–754.

111. Walch G, Boileau P, Noel E, Donnel ST. Impingement of the deep surface of the supraspinatus on the posteriosuperior glenoid rim: an arthroscopic study. *J Shoulder Elbow Surg* 1992;1:238.

112. Warner JJP, Caborn DNM, Berger R, et al. Dynamic capsuloligamentous anatomy of the glenohumeral joint. *J Shoulder Elbow Joint* 1993;2:115–133.

113. Wirth MA, Blatter G, Rockwood CA Jr. The capsular imbrication procedure for recurrent anterior instability of the shoulder. *J Bone Joint Surg* 1996;78-A:246–259.

114. Wolf SW. Ruptures of the pectoralis major muscle. An anatomic and clinical analysis. *Am J Sports Med* 1992;20:587–593.

115. Wright RS, Lipscomb AB. Acute occlusion of the subclavian vein in an athlete: diagnosis, etiology and surgical management. *Am J Sports Med* 1974;2:343–348.

116. Yamaguchi K, Riew KD, Galatz LM, Syme JA, Neviaser RJ. Biceps activity during shoulder motion. *Clin Orthop* 1997;336:122–129.

The Injured Athlete, Third Edition,
edited by D. H. Perrin.
Lippincott–Raven Publishers, Philadelphia © 1999.

CHAPTER 12

The Elbow, Wrist, and Hand

Frank C. McCue III, Thomas Sweeney, and Scott Urch

THE ELBOW

Anatomy

The elbow joint consists of three articulations: the humeral-ulnar, the capitellar-radial, and the radial-ulnar. The humeral-ulnar articulation determines the carrying angle of the elbow. When the elbow is flexed, the forearm is in line with the arm; as it extends, the trochlear course allows the forearm to move into valgus, producing the "carrying angle." Fractures at the elbow may alter this carrying angle. Pronation and supination take place around the capitellar-radial articulation, an area jammed during throwing. The radial-ulnar articulation is a small one that moves during pronation and supination.

The medial collateral ligament of the elbow is deep to the flexor mass. It has two parts: an anterior band and a posterior band. The thick anterior band is a major static stabilizer of the elbow, arising from the medial epicondyle to insert on the medial side of the coronoid process of the ulna. Some of its fibers are taut in all degrees of flexion and extension. The thinner and weaker posterior band functions only when the elbow is flexed to more than 90 degrees. The medial collateral ligament is stretched in baseball pitchers and round-arm-style javelin throwers, all of whom put extreme valgus stress on their elbows. Medial collateral ligament laxity may result from poorly reduced medial epicondyle fractures.

The flexor carpi radialis, palmaris longus, and parts of the flexor carpi ulnaris and flexor digitorum sublimis originate from the medial epicondyle. One head of the

pronator teres arises from the metaphyseal flare just proximal to the epicondyle. The flexor muscle mass exerts a strong pull on the epicondyle and may be partly avulsed in the young thrower. Because it is not yet fused to bone, the epicondyle sometimes is jerked from its bed and pulled into the elbow joint. Older tennis players, especially professionals who use spin serves, develop a large medial epicondyle as a response to heavy use.

The extensor muscles of the wrist and fingers arise from the lateral condyle of the humerus. The origin of the extensor carpi radialis brevis is often the site of damage in tennis elbow. It inserts at the base of the third metacarpal, the center of the hand. A fracture through the lateral condyle into the elbow joint sometimes heals slowly because the fracture site is bathed in synovial fluid containing fibrinolysin that prevents organization of the fracture hematoma.

The bony structures of the elbow joint are the capitellum, trochlea, and radial head. The capitellum lines up with the radial head on a lateral x-ray view of the elbow. If the radial head repeatedly jams against the capitellum, as in baseball pitching, capitellar avascular necrosis and osteochondritis dissecans may ensue. The trochlear sweep controls the carrying angle, and pieces from the medial edge of the trochlea may be chipped off during throwing.

Incongruity of the radial head after a fracture may result in osteoarthritis of the elbow with pain during pronation and supination. The orbicular or annular ligament arises from the humerus to surround the radial head. Adhesions between this ligament and the capsule of the elbow joint are responsible for some cases of tennis elbow.

When the elbow is fully extended, the olecranon fossa accepts the olecranon tip. The common supracondylar fracture in children extends through the very thin bone of this fossa and may lead to a bony build-up within the fossa that blocks full extension. Such a bony block affects throwing and also hinders a good follow-through in basketball shooting.

F. C. McCue III: Department of Orthopaedic Surgery, University of Virginia School of Medicine, Charlottesville, Virginia 22908

T. M. Sweeney: Department of Orthopaedic Surgery, Sarasota Memorial Hospital, Sarasota, Florida 34249

S. E. Urch: Methodist Sports Medicine Center, Thomas A. Brady Clinic, Indianapolis, Indiana 46202

A posterior fat pad resides in the olecranon fossa just external to the elbow joint (57). Intraarticular injury pushes this fat pad up so that it may be seen on a lateral x-ray film as evidence of intraarticular swelling. During throwing, the fat pad is normally pulled up by a slip of triceps, such as the articularis genu muscle of the knee, to prevent trapping and painful pinching of the fat pad between bone surfaces during rapid extension.

The biceps muscle is the main supinator of the forearm. Strong flexion of the elbow against resistance may avulse the biceps brachi from the bicipital tubercle of the radius. The brachialis muscle inserts into the coronoid process of the ulna. This muscle pulls chips from the coronoid in boxers, pitchers, and wrist wrestlers.

The major nerves near the elbow are the radial, median, and ulnar nerves. The deep and recurrent branches of the radial nerve may be trapped as they pass between the two parts of the supinator muscle. The median nerve may be impinged upon proximally in a tunnel under the ligament of Struthers, which sometimes runs from a supracondylar process of the humerus down to the medial condyle. Distally, the nerve may be trapped between the humeral and ulnar heads of the pronator teres as it seeks to lie on the substance of the flexor digitorum superficialis. The ulnar nerve courses behind the intermuscular septum and enters the forearm between the humeral and ulnar heads of the flexor carpi ulnaris. It may be trapped and irritated by fascial thickenings in the ulna groove behind the medial epicondyle; in such a case, the ulnar nerve may be decompressed or transplanted to the anterior compartment above the level of the medial epicondyle.

Fibers of the interosseous membrane descend medially from the radius to the ulna. If the athlete falls on his hand, the compression forces can be transmitted through this membrane from the strong lower radius to the strong upper ulna and humeral-ulnar joint. The triceps insertion fans out over the olecranon, and chips may be pulled off the olecranon tip in over-the-shoulder javelin throws or during missed jabs in boxing. The olecranon bursa lies at the elbow tip. It may become inflamed from repeated landings on the point of the elbow or after forceful elbow extensions. Sometimes loose bodies form within this bursa.

Fractures

Supracondylar

A fall from playground apparatus may fracture the thin bone in the supracondylar region of a child's humerus (Fig. 12.1). The fracture ends may then damage the intima of the brachial artery. Although the intima is torn, it may

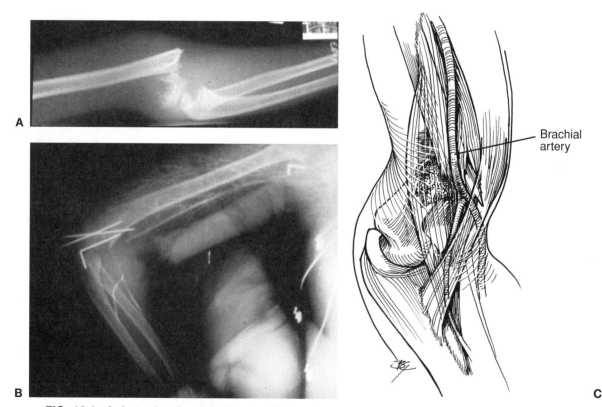

Brachial artery

FIG. 12.1. A. Lateral radiograph showing displaced type III supracondylar fracture. **B.** Lateral arteriogram image showing fracture after closed reduction and percutaneous pinning with disruption of brachial artery at the level of the fracture site. **C.** A supracondylar fracture of the humerus may damage the brachial artery and lead to a severe ischemic contracture of the forearm and hand.

take days for it to block the circulation completely. If the brachial artery is blocked, Volkmann's ischemic contractures of the forearm may occur, wherein the muscles die and the nerves fibrose, producing a useless limb. The vascular status and the nerve function of the limb should be evaluated both before and after reduction of the supracondylar fracture. The fracture is carefully reduced under axillary block or general anesthesia by applying traction and then flexing the elbow. The elbow should not be flexed initially without first applying traction, or else the brachial artery may be pinched.

A splint may be applied with the elbow in a flexed position for undisplaced or minimally displaced supracondylar fractures. If the elbow is flexed too much, however, the radial pulse may disappear. If this happens, it should be extended somewhat until the pulse returns. To treat a fully displaced fracture, a pin may be placed through the olecranon for overhead traction, and 10 days later a cast may be applied.

If there is no radial pulse and the youth has pain, pallor, paresthesia, and pain on passive extension of the fingers, overhead traction should be instituted. If pulse and feeling fail to return, then the brachial artery should be explored. Resection of a segment of the artery that contains the torn and folded intima may be needed to reduce the circulatory spasm. Prompt treatment of an elbow with danger signs may avoid the terrible complication of Volkmann's contracture.

Medial Epicondyle

The medial ligament of the elbow and flexor origin may be disrupted in a young thrower, gymnast, or wrestler who fractures the medial epicondyle (Fig. 12.2). Medial elbow stability depends on an intact medial collateral ligament and forearm flexors. Fibrous union of a displaced medial epicondyle fracture may cause chronic medial instability of the elbow and end a throwing career.

A routine elbow x-ray may not show much displacement of the medial epicondyle, compared to that which occurred at the time of injury. On x-ray film, the epicondyle may appear to be reduced, but in fact it may be rotated 90 degrees. This change in position of the medial epicondyle alters medial collateral ligament function and lessens the stability of the medial side of the elbow.

There are three types of medial epicondylar fractures (80). Type I occurs in youths who have open epiphyses. Here, the entire apophysis is avulsed, along with the forearm flexors and the medial collateral ligament. In type II fractures, the young athlete's epiphyses have closed. If the fragment is large enough to include the proximal attachment of the anterior band, the medial collateral ligament will be intact. Marked displacement, however, may tear the ligament. Type III fracture occurs in older children and adults. Here, a small chip is avulsed from the posterior aspect of the medial epicondyle with part of the

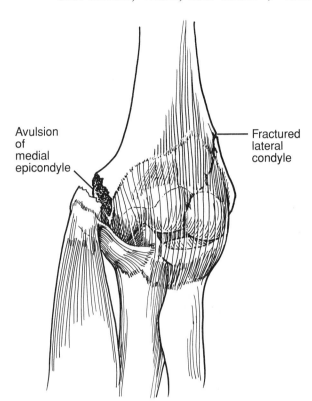

FIG. 12.2. A lateral condyle fracture allows synovial fluid to flow in and hinder healing. The medial epicondyle may be avulsed and even rotate from its normal position, obstructing the joint.

musculature, and the midportion of the medial collateral ligament tears.

A gentle test, the gravity stress test, is available for diagnosing acute medial instability of the elbow. With the athlete supine, the shoulder is rotated externally. Then his elbow is flexed 20 degrees to bring the olecranon clear of its fossa. The weight of the forearm and hand will usually exert enough valgus force to open the medial side. In larger, more muscular persons, a 0.45 kg or 0.9 kg (1 lb or 2 lb) weight may be strapped around the wrist. If the elbow is unstable, gravity stress test x-rays will show that the joint has opened and the medial epicondylar apophysis has become displaced distally.

Exploration of the medial side of the elbow is indicated if the medial epicondyle is displaced more than 1 cm or if it lies in the elbow joint. Moreover, a throwing athlete's elbow is usually explored if it is unstable on the gravity stress test. Exploration is also indicated with a posterior or posterolateral dislocation, since the epicondyle was probably very displaced and is now rotated.

Lateral Condyle

Fractures of the lateral condyle of the elbow are intraarticular ones that heal slowly and may become displaced (see Fig. 12.2). Synovial fluid seeps from the joint into the fracture site and contains fibrinolysin, which disrupts the fracture hematoma and may lead to a delayed union or to a nonunion.

A displaced fracture of the lateral condyle demands pin or screw fixation. Even if a lateral condylar fracture is undisplaced, however, the elbow should be x-rayed intermittently until it has healed, because an initially undisplaced fracture of the lateral condyle may become displaced. A malunited fracture alters the carrying angle of an athlete's elbow, and the range of elbow motion may also suffer.

Dislocation

Most elbow dislocations are posterior or posterolateral ones. Both of these types may have associated fractures of the medial epicondyle. Fortunately, even if the elbow is unstable medially, the forearm flexors are usually functionally intact and give satisfactory dynamic support for most elbow activities. In a thrower, however, a ligamentous repair is more likely to restore optimum function. Operative exploration is indicated in throwing athletes if the medial epicondyle has been fractured, since the epicondyle was probably very displaced and is now rotated.

The dislocation may be reduced on the field or in the locker room before muscle spasm sets in. It is best performed, however, with the athlete lying prone on an examining table with the elbow hanging off the side. First the lateral displacement is reduced and then straight traction applied. The elbow should not be directly flexed before reduction because this flexion maneuver could damage the brachial artery.

The athlete's elbow is rehabilitated with active range-of-motion exercises. Passive stretch should be avoided because it may cause elbow stiffness or myositis ossificans. When the athlete it ready to return to practice, the elbow should be taped in slight flexion, or a custom-made padded elbow strap may be wrapped around the arm and forearm and connected to allow full flexion but prevent hyperextension (Fig. 12.3) (33).

The Elbow in Throwing

During the acceleration phase of throwing, the thrower's arm is pulled forward dramatically. The forearm lags behind, and thus a valgus stress is placed on the elbow (Fig. 12.4). The forearm flexors then flex the wrist and fingers to propel the baseball, which is released in a flinging motion at about ear level. During follow-through, the forearm pronates and the olecranon jams into the olecranon fossa (2).

Types of Elbow Injuries

Little League Elbow

Young baseball players may develop elbow problems from a heavy pitching schedule (46). The Little Leaguer is allowed to pitch as many as six innings per week and averages 18 pitches per inning. A professional pitcher throws about 120 pitches in a nine-inning game, averaging 11 to 15 pitches per inning. Although a Little Leaguer throws fewer pitches than does a professional pitcher in a week of competition, he may throw hard on days between games. He may be a catcher for his team as well, and thus throw even more.

Adams studied the x-ray films of both elbows of 162 boys, aged 9 to 14 years, and compared pitchers to nonpitchers and to youngsters who were not playing organized baseball (1). He found that changes at the medial epicondyle, the radius, and the capitellum were in direct proportion to the amount of throwing and whether the youngster threw curve balls. All of the 80 pitchers that he checked had some degree of bony hypertrophy and separation and fragmentation of the medial epicondyle apophysis. Only a small number of the x-ray films of nonpitchers and control subjects showed these changes.

In the Houston study, 595 Little League pitchers were examined (31). Seventeen percent had elbow symptoms, and 12% had a limitation of elbow extension. Many radiologic anatomical variants were noted at the elbow. The medial epicondylar lesions were thought to be stress fractures, and if the youngster rested his arm these lesions were said to result in no functional deficits. The bony hypertrophy and enlarged medial epicondyles were considered to be normal anatomic variants.

In the Eugene study, 120 pitchers, aged 11 and 12 years, were examined (42). Twenty percent had elbow symptoms, and 23% had x-ray changes related to traction on the medial epicondyle. Ten percent of these pitchers had limitation of elbow extension. Five percent of these youths had more serious lateral compartment x-ray changes, but none of them had symptoms related to that area. The investigators concluded that the elbow symptoms of Little League pitchers did not correlate with the x-ray findings.

Studies that show negligible epiphyseal involvement in Little League baseball players may be misleading, since the youths present to physicians with symptoms when they are 13 or 14 years old and have already graduated from Little League baseball (10). The elbow trouble has an insidious onset, symptoms being early but subtle (4). These young athletes may fail to report elbow pain to the coach, and even if they do the coach may not have the soreness thoroughly investigated.

Most problems are at the medial side of the elbow, and Little League elbow has been defined as an avulsion of the ossification center of the medial epicondyle (8,23,72).

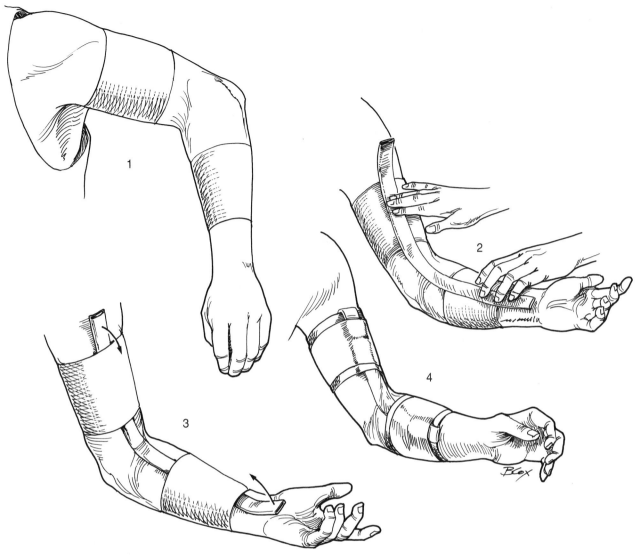

FIG. 12.3. Taping may prevent hyperextension of the elbow. Elastic tape serves as an anchor. Four strips of 3.8 cm (1.5 in) white tape are then stacked and folded longitudinally to form a strong band, which is held in place with more elastic tape. The ends of the band are folded over and secured with white tape.

The valgus stress of throwing may cause fragmentation, irregularity, mild separation, enlargement, or breaking of the medial epicondyle. The worst, chronic problems, however, are found on the lateral side of the elbow in which repeated jamming of the radial head against the capitellum may cause osteochondritis of the capitellum, avascular necrosis of the radial head, osteochondritic loose bodies, and osteoarthritis (74). Eight percent of young pitchers have lateral changes, and it is not uncommon to see loose bodies in the olecranon fossa of teenagers who began pitching at a young age.

The most serious of the elbow findings in young pitchers is osteochondritis dissecans of the capitellum. Valgus elbow stress during the acceleration phase stretches the medial collateral ligament of the elbow, and ultimately the radial head impinges against the capitellum. Osteo-chondritis dissecans occurs mostly in pitchers but does occur in some catchers. The average age of onset is 12.5 years, with the youths having played organized baseball for an average of 3.5 years (10).

X-ray films show ill-defined, patchy decalcification or cystic areas on the capitellum, radial head irregularity and hypertrophy, and early partial closure of the proximal radius growth plate. In contrast to normal closure, however, the fusion of the radial head growth plate begins on the lateral aspect and proceeds medially. These conditions are not benign but mark the end of hard, painless throwing for the teenage athlete. The prognosis is poor despite treatment, and these lateral side problems may reduce the athlete's ability to participate in throwing or racket sports later in life.

When elbow symptoms are marked and rest measures fail, the most consistent results follow curettage of the frag-

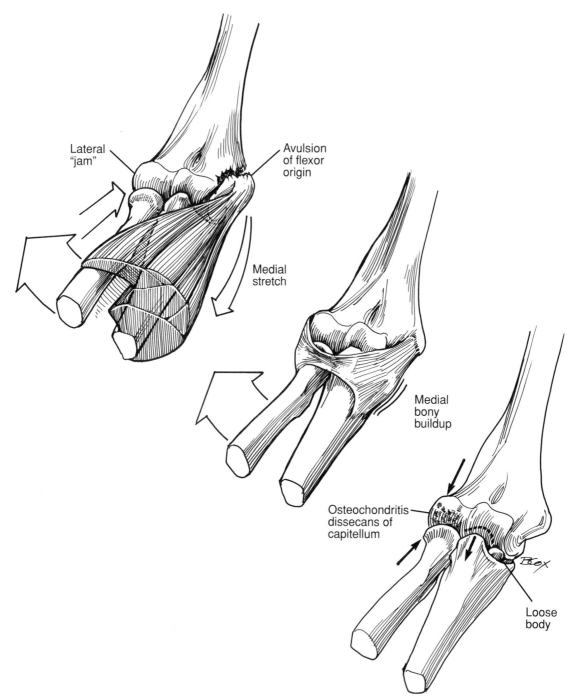

FIG. 12.4. Valgus stress to the elbow stretches the medial side and jams the lateral side, producing avulsions, bony buildups, osteochondritis and loose bodies.

mented capitellum down to bleeding bone and removal of all fragments that are either loose or attached to bone. In a study of young throwers with osteochondritis of the capitellum, 13 of 15 operated on had loose bodies (28). Surgery will not produce a normal elbow, but the pain does lessen and the youngster usually regains more elbow extension.

To prevent elbow problems in young pitchers, good throwing mechanics must be taught, and youngsters should especially avoid "just throwing with the arm." Proper pre-game warm-up is important, and the pitcher should ice his shoulder and elbow after the game. Young pitchers should be encouraged to report elbow soreness. In youth baseball, sore arms are often treated like the sore arms of professional players with ice, reducing the pitching, or missing a rotation. Soreness in youngsters, however, is more likely to be due to epiphysitis, and thus x-ray films are needed. If x-ray findings are abnormal, the youngster should refrain from pitching during that season.

Little League pitchers are at a disadvantage compared to their Big League counterparts. Foremost, the Little Leaguer's elbow is always immature. Professional pitchers have skilled pitching coaches who emphasize good body mechanics, using the large muscle groups, body turn, and proper push-off and follow-through. The professional pitcher has conditioning programs for muscle strength, endurance and flexibility, postgame icing, and expert medical care. The Little Leaguer usually lacks these advantages. Coaching is not expected to improve because there is no requirement that these well-meaning coaches be trained and certified to instruct their young players.

Baseball Elbow

When pitchers throw hard for years, their elbow joints wear out. Veteran pitchers develop an elbow flexion contracture, medial collateral ligament traction spurs or medial collateral ligament rupture, tardy ulnar nerve palsy, articular cartilage degeneration, posterior compartment lesions, and loose bodies.

The flexion contracture results from traction on the anterior capsule, biceps, and brachialis, microtears of the wrist and finger flexors, and pronator tears with resulting fibrosis (4,34,36). Bone may build up on the coronoid process and chip off to cause acute elbow pain (18).

Reactive bone spurs form in the distal part of the medial collateral ligament owing to valgus overload. Sometimes a spur breaks off to entrap and irritate the ulnar nerve. Spurs can be removed before they break off.

Medial Collateral Ligament Tears

A throwing athlete may rupture the medial collateral ligament of his elbow (79). He may report that he has had soreness medially for years. Suddenly, however, he feels a snap in the elbow; it gives way and he is unable to throw. Then when he makes a fist, he has pain in the flexor muscle mass or over the anterior oblique ligament. The examiner may find valgus instability, and x-ray films may show calcification or ossification medially. To check for stability, the examiner first flexes the elbow to about 50 degrees and then applies a valgus stress. Tears of the medial collateral range from complete ruptures, some of which are repairable and some of which are not, to chronic problems that result in attenuated ligaments.

If the ligament has been chronically stretched, the humeral portion may be moved up and forward on the humerus and fixed with a screw and washer. In tears that are unrepairable and in the case of ligaments that are stretched and markedly attenuated, the palmaris longus tendon may be transferred to the elbow and tied as a figure-eight.

In this tendon transfer operation, the surgeon incises the flexor muscle mass longitudinally to expose the liga-

ment and its pathology (34). He frees the ulnar nerve and holds it aside with care to preserve muscular branches of the nerve. He then harvests the palmaris longus tendon from the same side, drills holes in the humerus and ulna through which he passes the tendon, and then ties it. He then transfers the ulnar nerve anteriorly; otherwise the nerve may become encased in scar tissue.

After palmaris longus substitution for the medial collateral ligament, the athlete is not permitted to throw for about 5 months. He then throws for 15 minutes a day for about 2 months and then increases to three-quarter speed; by 12 months he may be back pitching. During rehabilitation, the tendon assumes ligamentous properties and becomes stronger.

Ulnar Nerve Entrapment

The throwing athlete with ulnar nerve entrapment may give a history of having fallen on his elbow or may report a twang at the elbow during pitching. He will have soreness near the ulnar groove (Fig. 12.5), and numbness of the little finger and the lateral side of his ring finger and may have some weakness of grip. An electromyography (EMG) test may be positive and x-ray films may show spurs.

If the ulnar nerve subluxes during pitching, it may produce a traumatic twang with tingling pain in the ring and little fingers with each pitch. If chronic neuritis develops, the nerve may be transferred anteriorly. With the nerve in this new anterior position, the pitcher can usually continue at a high level of throwing.

In transferring the ulnar nerve anteriorly, the surgeon should free the nerve all the way up to the arcade of Struthers and remove the intermuscular septum. He should also free the nerve all the way down through the fascial covering in zone III.

In a baseball pitcher, the transplanted ulnar nerve should be positioned under the muscle. If it is placed just on top of the muscle, it will probably twang when he throws. A little carpet of muscle should be left along the course of the nerve to prevent scar tissue from forming. When the nerve is transferred, the surgeon should also look for reactive bone spurs and posterior loose bodies.

Articular Cartilage Degeneration

Articular cartilage degeneration at the radiohumeral joint may disable a player. Moreover, in the acceleration phase, as valgus stress is applied to the elbow and it rapidly extends, an osteocartilaginous piece may be chipped from the trochlea, and the athlete will feel an acute, severe pain.

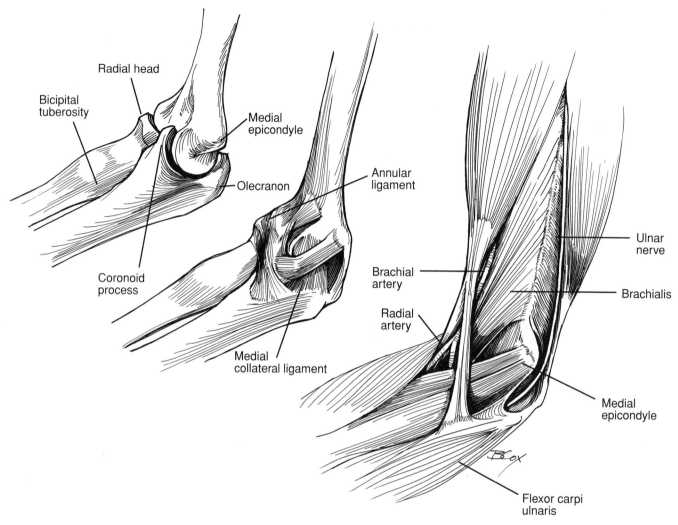

FIG. 12.5. At the medial side of the elbow, the ulnar nerve passes in a groove behind the medial epicondyle.

Olecranon Fossitis and Posteromedial Olecranon Bone Spurs

Posterior compartment lesions may be equally disabling. The olecranon process jams into the fossa, especially in pitchers with a poor follow-through who snap the elbow into extension. This jamming produces olecranon fossitis and new bone formation. The overgrowth of bone from the olecranon tip may fracture, causing severe elbow pain and leaving loose bodies at the tip of the olecranon. There is a toggle effect at the elbow during throwing as the olecranon bumps against the medial side of the olecranon fossa. This bumping may produce spurs at the olecranon tip and medial olecranon spurs. Further, the cartilage of the olecranon fossa may become soft. The spurs can be removed by resecting the tip of the olecranon and a portion of the medial side of the olecranon with an osteotome.

Surgery for Loose Bodies

Surgery on a pitcher's elbow usually comprises a combination of medial soft tissue surgery with removal of spurs and posterior intraarticular surgery. A posterolateral incision is generally chosen so that after the olecranon is observed and the loose bodies removed, the radial head and capitellar articular surfaces can be evaluated. The operation may well be effective if only one loose body is found and removed. The prognosis for a pitcher, however, is generally not good when many loose bodies are found because of coexisting traumatic arthritis. The surgeon's observations of the radiohumeral joint allow a prognosis as to when the pitcher may return to competition and a realistic appraisal of his future in baseball (34).

Javelin Thrower's Elbow

A javelin thrower may develop elbow trouble with either the correct arm action or an incorrect, round-arm method (55). The types of injuries suffered with each of these throwing styles, are, however, different.

The correct arm action for throwing a javelin is an over-the-shoulder throw with a bent-arm carry. The elbow is flexed and held well above and in front of the shoulder and close to the head. The elbow is then brought forward early and forcibly extended to launch the javelin. This violent extension may fracture the olecranon tip (76).

When the javelin is thrown with an incorrect round-arm method, the elbow comes around at the level of the shoulder, and internal rotation of the shoulder transmits force to the javelin. These throwers, like baseball pitchers, sprain the medial collateral ligament of the elbow and spurs form. The athlete may be able to develop the correct arm action by changing to a middle-finger hold, with the index finger extended under the javelin and the middle finger placed behind the binding. This change twists the hand inward to reduce the stress on the medial collateral ligament.

Tennis Elbow

Tennis elbow most often refers to pain at or near a player's lateral epicondyle (66) and is generally caused by faulty backhand stroke mechanics (32,64). The player with a faulty backhand often uses an Eastern forehand grip or a fistlike grip with the thumb extended behind the handle for more power. The stroke usually starts high with a hurried backswing. The body weight is on the back leg, and power is generated at the wrist and elbow. As the elbow extends, the wrist strongly hooks into ulnar deviation, which is a strong, commonly used motion for opening doors, chopping wood, and swinging a baseball bat. The beginner, however, may incorporate this motion, which comes so easily, into the stroke as a bad habit. The follow-through usually will be short and low and end with a jerk.

Combined elbow extension and ulnar hooking of the wrist cause the extensor mass, especially the deeply located extensor carpi radialis brevis, to rub and to roll over the lateral epicondyle and the radial head. Along with this irritation from rubbing over bony prominences are tugs on the extensor origin resulting in microtears. Rubbing, rolling, and microtears result in a painful elbow.

In an attempt to heal the damage, nerve-laden granulation tissue forms. This tissue is ill-suited to withstand constant use because it swells, stretches, and becomes painful. Adhesions also form between the annular ligament and the joint capsule. The pain worsens from the constant strain of the faulty backhand and the transmission of vibrations to the elbow from a too tightly strung racket with too small a handle or from heavy, wet balls and off-center hits.

Players with tennis elbow have pain in the region of the common extension origin, especially when they try to extend their middle finger against resistance with the elbow extended. The extensor carpi radialis brevis inserts into the base of the third metacarpal, and extension of the middle finger tightens the fascial origin of the muscle. The lateral epicondyle is tender, and the player notes pain when gripping the racket and extending the wrist.

For a quality backhand, either an Eastern backhand or a Continental grip is used. The arm and racket form an "L" (69). The racket is unhurriedly taken back low, and the stroke starts low. The player's other hand can help support the racket during the backswing. The player then shifts the body weight and swings from the shoulder to achieve pace. At impact, the player's weight has been transferred to the front foot. The wrist is firm and locked in a cocked position, a position that corrects the hooked wrist, which in turn cures the leading elbow. The ball is met in front, and the follow-through is long and high.

The player with a faulty backhand should be taught proper form and master the wrist-cocked L position. If this cannot be learned, then the player should work on a two-handed backhand, since tennis elbow only rarely affects players who use a two-handed backhand. A right-handed player hits a two-handed backhand like a one-handed left-handed forehand, with the right elbow slightly bent at contact. The player's left hand prevents the right wrist from hooking and also absorbs most of the impact and vibration. The player follows through by driving with the left arm.

A proper grip size prevents torque. A player determines grip size by measuring from the proximal palmar crease to the tip of the ring finger, along the radial side of the ring finger. More simply, the player can grip the racket and then place the free index finger between the ring finger and the base of the thumb. If the index finger just fits, then the grip size is usually correct.

A player with tennis elbow should avoid a rigid racket (30). A racket with a large sweet spot or a fiberglass or graphite racket helps to reduce vibration. Some metal rackets vibrate like a tuning fork. A racket should not be strung too tightly; usually between 50 and 55 pounds of tension is best.

Stretching and strengthening the wrist extensors are effective and major parts of the treatment for tennis elbow (5,40). Soreness is a guide for all stretching, isometric, and weight work. If the elbow becomes sore, the player has done too much exercise. The player's elbow is first immersed in a 40°C (104°F) whirlpool before beginning exercises. The player then performs isometric radial deviation-extension wrist cocking, holding each contraction for 6 seconds. When the player can do these at full force without pain, he or she advances to cocking a tennis racket. Next, a 0.67 kg (1.5 lb) weight is added to the neck of the racket. More weight is added slowly until the player is lifting 2.25 kg (5 lb). The player may have been lifting 6.75 to 9 kg (15 to 20 lb) before this episode of tennis elbow; thus it must be explained to him or her that exercise should start off with lighter weights.

The tennis player may also wind up a weight attached

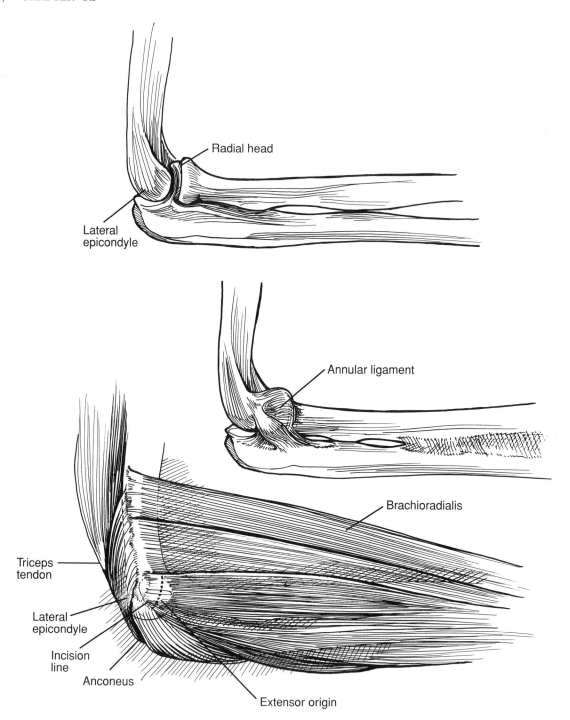

FIG. 12.6. Intractable pain at the lateral epicondyle may be relieved by percutaneous section (*dotted line*) of the extensor origin.

to a broomstick by a rope. Exercise starts with 20 repetitions of 0.56 kg (1.25 lb) and then gradually increases to 2.25 kg (5 lb). After the acute period, deep friction massage is an excellent way to break up adhesions at the elbow, to increase circulation, and to eliminate wastes.

After doing well in flexibility, isometrics, and weight programs, the player may hit against a wall for 5 minutes and then build up to 7.5 minutes, 10 minutes, and 15 minutes a day. It is important that the player use an Eastern backhand or Continental grip, hold the wrist cocked, and that the arm and racket form an L. Theoretically, however, hitting against a wall invokes a longer grip time than hitting with a partner, and therefore places a prolonged stress on the extensor origin. The grip pressure of better players is of short duration and peaks just before ball impact and then immediately relaxes. In average players the grip lasts longer. If there is no soreness after hitting against a wall for 15 minutes a day, the player may begin rallying. The elbow should be iced for 15 minutes after the stroke work.

Tennis players should keep their elbows warm, especially on cool or windy days. Some tennis players cut the toe section out of a wool sock, place the sock around their elbows, and secure it with a light strip of adhesive tape to prevent it from sliding down. Neoprene elbow sleeves perform the same function. While the player sleeps, he or she should wear a splint that cocks the wrist up, as he or she may otherwise be flexing the wrist at night and stressing the extensors.

The symptoms of tennis elbow may resolve with rest, but they are sure to recur unless the player starts a strengthening and flexibility program and hits with a cocked wrist. If the arm were put in a cast, the muscles would atrophy, the proprioception would decrease, and recovery would take longer.

The counterforce brace, a nonelastic, curved strap that the player fastens around the upper forearm (24), is supposed to remove stress from the extensor origin. Then his extensor muscles contract during the stroke; the brace essentially serves as a new origin for the muscles. It may reduce the sliding of the extensors over the lateral condyle. The brace also acts as a flag, reminding the player to concentrate on the backhand stroke mechanics.

A short, tapering course of phenylbutazone will usually alleviate the symptoms of acute tennis elbow. The chance that the drug may cause aplastic anemia or other serious problems is, however, too great for routine use. A white, chalky residue may accrue if a long-acting steroid is injected, and steroid injections may cause some of the tissue necrosis seen at operation for tennis elbow.

If tennis elbow does not resolve after the above changes have been made and the player has followed a complete flexibility and strengthening program and improved the mechanics of his stroke, an exploration of his lateral epicondyle region and an extensor slide operation may be proposed (40,67). The extensor origin is explored and the extensor carpi radialis brevis exposed. This muscle lies under the extensor carpi radialis longus. Damaged tissue is removed from its undersurface. The elbow joint is then entered and checked for adhesions and synovial pannus. Any adhesions that bind the capsule to the orbicular ligament are lysed, and a partial synovectomy is performed. The extensor origin is then allowed to slide distally and left in this position. After operation, the player resumes the same exercise program recommended for the treatment of acute tennis elbow. Less successful operations include removal of the radiohumeral meniscus—a pannus of synovium growing between the radial head and the capitulum—which may be pinched, excision of the orbicular ligament to relieve tension in the elbow joint, and a procedure to elongate the extensor carpi radialis brevis. However, if the soreness is only at the lateral epicondyle, a percutaneous sectioning of the extensor origin may relieve the pain completely (see Fig. 12.6, *dotted line*).

A medial tennis elbow most commonly affects veteran tennis players and professionals who hit hard with good stroke mechanics (60). Their strong wrist flexion in the tennis service and forehand ground strokes leads to medial epicondylar hypertrophy, avulsion of chips of bone from the medial epicondyle, and tears at the flexor origin. In the acute phase, rest and antiinflammatory drug therapy may be beneficial. A player's warm-up procedures should be checked, especially the shoulder warm-up. The elbow must be iced after practice and after matches. Massage to the sore area rids it of waste products and breaks up scar tissue.

Boxer's Elbow

When a boxer misses a jab, pieces of bone may chip from the tip of his olecranon process as it jams into his olecranon fossa (29). These chips may then become loose bodies in his elbow joint. Direct impacts of the olecranon against the trochlea may shear off pieces of the trochlea, and traction on the coronoid process may avulse bone. Elbow pain is usually not related to one specific blow and is most painful when a jab is missed.

These elbows are operated on arthroscopically if the loose bodies cause locking or catching. The joint is irrigated, loose bodies are removed, and any pieces of articular cartilage that are partly attached but appear ready to break free are removed.

Olecranon Bursitis

Direct blows to the point of an athlete's elbow, or repetitive rubbing there, may irritate the olecranon bursa to produce synovial fluid that swells the bursa (22). Olecranon bursitis is common in football receivers who land on hard artificial turf and also has been noted in recreational dart throwers trying to throw the darts *through* the board (43). If the bursa is often irritated, the bursal wall will thicken. Fibrinous or cartilaginous loose bodies may form within the bursa and feel like bone chips.

An acutely swollen olecranon bursa should have an ice pack. The bursa is then sterilely aspirated of fluid and an elastic wrap snugly applied over a cotton roll for 24 to 48 hours. If the wall of the bursa has been thickened from recurrent bursitis or if it contains cartilage chips, the bursa may have to be removed. The incision should not be placed over the point of the elbow because such placement may produce an adherent, painful, and easily bumped scar. Olecranon bursitis may be prevented by wearing well-fitting elbow pads (63).

THE WRIST AND THE HAND

Injuries of the hand are common in athletics, probably because the hand is characteristically in front of the athlete in most sports and frequently absorbs the initial contact (53). Further, the hand is used in almost every sport in one way or another. There is a tendency to minimize the severity and importance of these injuries because the hand does not bear weight and injuries to the hand usually do not totally disable the athlete. This is particularly true of young, poorly supervised athletes who may return to vigorous activity and unprotected use of the extremity long before adequate healing.

The key to proper care of hand injuries is early, accurate diagnosis and precise and proper treatment, which must be followed by an appropriate rehabilitation program (12). Conservative treatment measures are preferable for most injuries of the hand, and most athletes can be rapidly returned to their normal activities (21). Primary surgical repair is indicated, however, in a small number of cases, and secondary reconstructive surgery may be needed in injuries that have been neglected or improperly treated.

The wrist is probably the most complex joint in the human body because of its multiple joints and their varied anatomic configurations. Reaching an accurate diagnosis necessary for proper treatment can be difficult in many cases. In many of the more significant problems, however, a specific treatment of choice has not yet been perfected; despite the growing realization about the functional importance of the wrist, there has been a dearth of optimal results of treatment of many of its disabilities. There is still need for further research and study in this area. As in all examinations, a careful history is important and should include the location, duration, and intensity of pain, whether repetitive activity or a single traumatic event has occurred, the mechanism of injury, the previous treatment program, what activity aggravates the problem, a medical history (including previous diseases, past surgeries, and injuries) and what specific activities are limited and to what degree.

A complete physical examination of the upper extremity should include examination of the appearance of the extremity, localization of the tenderness, measurement of strength of grip and pinch, and examination of all involved structures. The presence of instability and any "click," particularly if it is reproducible, is extremely helpful and important, particularly in light of recent awareness of the various instabilities that can occur in this intercalated joint. A knowledge of the kinematics and biomechanics of this complicated joint is also extremely important, and our knowledge of these components has significantly increased over the past several years.

A basic radiographic profile will include many views, depending on the individual problem. It is more efficient to have a basic series of wrist views supplemented by clinical findings. A basic profile may include a neutral PA view, and AP or PA (anterior posterior or posterior anterior) views in radial and ulnar deviation. A true lateral view in the neutral position is particularly important in potential instabilities involving the lunate. Occasionally, laterals in palmar flexion and dorsiflexion are also indicated. A carpal tunnel view is particularly important to visualize the tunnel itself and the hook of the hamate for possible fracture. A closed-fist view with the forearm in supination allows axial compression and also increases the instability at the scapholunate joint in rotatory instability of the scaphoid. Obtaining a carpal tunnel view after an acute injury may be difficult because of the pain, and an oblique view with the forearm in midsupination or in pronation with approximately 20 degrees of elevation from the flat surface and the wrist in some dorsiflexion may be helpful in visualizing the hook of the hamate. Other oblique and rotational views, as indicated by the specific problem, are often valuable.

Also often necessary are secondary diagnostic studies, including wrist arthrography that, under fluoroscopic control, often shows perforations in the various ligamentous structures. However, some communications are a normal variant, some are found in increasing numbers with age, and there is difficulty in correlating the findings as a potential source of the patient's disability. The perforations at the radiocarpal joint and the radioulnar joint increase with age, whereas those at the scapholunate and the triquetral-lunate joint almost always denote pathology. Because of the high percentage of false-positives, the information must be carefully correlated with other findings of the examination in order to be helpful.

Bone scan may be helpful, but the generalized findings are not specific, with two abnormal patterns commonly seen: the diffuse pattern of increased uptake with generalized metabolic diseases, osteoporosis, rheumatoid and synovitis-type involvement; and a localized pattern seen in specific degenerative arthritic changes, fractures, tumors, and other vascular problems of the bone, such as Kienbock's and Preiser's diseases.

The computed tomography (CT) scan has been particularly helpful in evaluating distal radioulnar stability and is the single most accurate study to determine incongruities at this joint. The plane lateral radiographs are accurate only in the perfectly neutral position, but the CT scan demonstrates dislocation or incongruity in all degrees of pronation and supination and also gives an accurate picture with a plaster cast on the extremity.

Cineradiography is very useful in localizing wrist instability, especially when the patient has a "snapping" wrist and the normal synchronous motion is broken by the instability. This study is particularly enhanced by combination with arthrography.

Tomograms, particularly trispiral tomograms, have been helpful in visualizing irregularities, such as seen in Kienbock's disease, fractures, displacements, angulation, cysts, and other similar problems.

Magnetic resonance imaging (MRI) availability and quality is improving. Better definition has been obtained with the use of wrist coils. Avascular necrosis and some ligamentous tears can be effectively evaluated (58,81). However, the utility of wrist MRI is heavily dependent on the technical expertise of the radiologist.

Wrist arthroscopy is indicated when the physical examination and radiographic imaging studies do not elucidate a diagnosis or when a specific intraarticular lesion is suspected that may be treated by arthroscopy. Observation, splinting and limitation of activity may not be an acceptable approach for the athlete who needs to return to competition at the earliest safe opportunity (77). In acute and chronic injuries, arthroscopy affords diagnosis and treatment options for loose bodies, intrinsic ligaments, extrinsic ligaments, fractures, and the triangular fibrocartilage complex (54,56,71).

Some areas of confusion show up on radiography, such as accessory ossification centers, congenital absences and traumatic fusions, variation in size and shape of the bones, periarticular calcific deposits, cystic deformities, and tumors.

Injuries to the Wrist

Most wrist problems in athletics are produced by acute falls on the outstretched hand or result from repetitive stress with the wrist in extension (45). These injuries are frequent in weight lifters during the catch in the clean-and-jerk, gymnasts during floor exercise, and wrestlers and push-up enthusiasts. When the wrist is extended to extremes, the dorsal articular surfaces impinge and are compressed. If the wrist is forced beyond this point, the compressed contact areas are sheared. This force may pinch the synovium or produce osteocartilaginous damage. These extension forces may produce scaphoid impaction, triquetral-hamate impaction, or synovial cysts. More serious injuries include fractures and instabilities.

Radial-Scaphoid Impaction

With extension and radial deviation, the dorsal rim of the radius and the dorsal scaphoid rim collide (Fig. 12.7),

resulting in pain, weakness, and tenderness at the dorso-radial aspect of the wrist aggravated by wrist extension.

The examiner tells the athlete to point to the site of discomfort with one finger and should then ascertain the point of maximum tenderness carefully. The wrist may be tender over the dorsal scaphoid rim with the wrist in moderate flexion and ulnar deviation. A radiographic film, taken with a "skin-pin" (a small piece of paper clip) over the tender point, may show a bone spur or a little, loose piece of bone over the dorsal aspect of the scaphoid. In this case, the athlete should rest the wrist. When the athlete returns to practice and competition, he or she may have to change the wrist position for the exercise and have the wrist taped. If the disability is protracted, a surgical exploration may be needed. The surgeon may find synovitis dorsally and an area of chondromalacia and early osteophyte formation on the dorsal rim of the scaphoid. The rim may be hypertrophied, and the contiguous area of the dorsal radial rim may show chondromalacia. Sometimes, impaction of the scaphoid against the radius may avulse the osteocartilaginous fragment.

If a hypertrophic ridge on the scaphoid blocks extension, a cheilectomy (spur removal) of the dorsal rim of the scaphoid, synovial debridement, and perhaps removal of the dorsal radial lip are indicated (Fig. 12.7). This operation is similar to the cheilectomies performed for impingement at the anterior aspect of an ankle or at the big toe metatarsal-phalangeal joint. Postoperatively the athlete wears a splint for 2 weeks and then begins gradual range-of-motion and strengthening exercises.

Triquetral-Lunate Impaction

Forceful extension with ulnar deviation may occur in pile-ups in contact sports, during landings in floor exercise, with moves on the sidehorse, or swings in racket sports. Impingement occurs between the dorsal aspects of the triquetrum and the hamate.

Treatment includes rest and pulsed ultrasound, antiinflammatory medicine, a change of wrist position, and taping of the wrist. Exploration is indicated if the symptoms are unremitting. The surgeon may find inflamed synovium and chondromalacia at the hamate or triquetral rim and may need to remove the synovial infoldings and perform a synovectomy.

Occult or Overt Synovial Cysts

After damage to the wrist joint capsule, synovium may herniate to form a synovial cyst, especially in young female gymnasts. Wrist soreness is usually maximum in extension, but occasionally there is discomfort in flexion. The wrist is usually tender over the scapholunate interval, and sometimes the examiner can feel a mass there. Radio-

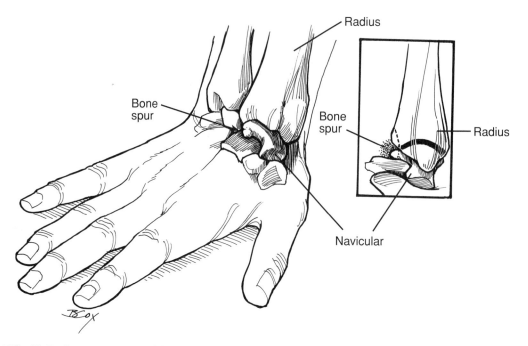

FIG. 12.7. Acute or repeated hyperextension of the wrist may result in a spur on the navicular and on the distal radius, producing a synovial cyst between. These spurs can be resected and the cyst removed.

graphic films are generally negative, and an arthrogram is usually not helpful.

Treatment includes rest in a splint, antiinflammatory medicine, a change of hand grip position, and taping. Aspiration rarely results in release of a jelly-like material and decompression of the cyst.

In recalcitrant cases, percutaneous needling may decompress the cyst and scar may form to prevent a recurrence. The cystic area is numbed and then stuck about 20 times with an 18-gauge needle. The athlete wears a splint for a few days and then resumes activities. If the needling does not work, an exploration may be necessary. The surgeon excises the cyst as it protrudes from the scapholunate ligament and sutures the ligament. The athlete should be informed that the cyst will sometimes, nonetheless, recur.

Radioulnar Joint

The distal radioulnar joint (DRUJ) allows forearm rotation of about 150 degrees in pronation and supination, with the radius and hand rotating around the ulna; some associated glide of the ulnar head in the radial sigmoid notch. The radius carries approximately 80% of the axial load of the forearm and the ulna; the associated connections with the triangular fibrocartilage complex carry 20%.

Understanding and knowledge of the ulnar aspect of the wrist have increased greatly in recent years, allowing greater awareness of proper diagnosis and thus more effective methods of treatment. A problem occurs in differ-

entiating the ulnar wrist pain arising from the radioulnar joint from the pain arising from the ulnocarpal complex. Painful pronation-supination of the forearm designates radoulnar involvement and, when painless, implies pain of ulnocarpal origin. Point tenderness, pain, subluxation with crepitus, and clicking, with or without stress, along with general hand and wrist examination, are important to localize the lesion.

Plain films, especially a direct lateral with the forearm in neutral position, are important, as are specific views to rule out other causes of pain. The CT scan is the most accurate method to evaluate the distal radioulnar joint, since it is easier to interpret and can be done with the cast in place. Arthrography may be helpful here as well.

Treatment of acute displacement of the distal ulna, in which accurate reduction can be obtained, consists of closed manipulation and reduction, held with a long arm cast for 4 to 6 weeks. The forearm should be positioned in full supination for dorsal displacement and in full pronation for volar displacement.

In chronic cases, many alternative methods of treatment are available, including ligamentous reconstructions, fusion of the DRUJ, proximal resection arthroplasty, ulnar shortening, and direct ulnar excision.

Triangular Fibrocartilage Complex (TFCC)

The mechanism is usually an ulnar blow to the hand, forcing the wrist into dorsiflexion and pronation. Local tenderness at the DRUJ, painful click or catch, or both, and occasionally radioulnar instability are diagnostic aids. Other causes of local pathology must be excluded, including subluxation of the extensor carpi ulnaris, lunato-triquetral instability, piso-triquetral degeneration, and general ligamentous laxity.

Partial ligamentous injuries may occur, and these should respond to protective casting until healing has occurred. If there has been a complete tear, however, repair with or without augmentation should be carried out in order to preserve the function of the TFCC in wrist stability, load resorption, axial compression, and motion of the wrist. Locking or intermittent catching may occur. Owing to injury and to the confined space, excision of the injured tissue may be indicated but should be carried out with caution and appreciation of its functional importance.

Carpal Instabilities

Stability of the wrist as an intercalated segment depends on the configuration of the joint surfaces in their articulation, plus the multiple ligaments connecting the bones. There are three longitudinal bony columns: thumb; radial force-bearing; and ulnar control. The force-bearing column, which transmits the force generated by the hand to the forearm, consists of the distal radial articulation, the lunate, the proximal two thirds of the scaphoid, the capitate, the trapezoid, and the bases of the second and third metacarpals. The control column on the ulnar side of the wrist consists of the distal ulna with its styloid and attached triangular fibrocartilage continuous to the distal radius, plus the triquetrum, the hamate, the capitate, and the bases of the fourth and fifth metacarpals. The thumb column comprises the distal third of the scaphoid, the trapezoid joint, and the base of the first metacarpal. Less force will be transmitted to the carpus with greater mobility at the carpometacarpal joint of the thumb.

The major ligaments of the wrist are intracapsular. They consist of the interosseous ligaments contained within the carpal row and the ligaments that cross the carpal row to guide the excursion of the proximal row upon the distal row. The volar ligaments are more substantial than the dorsal ligaments, with the prime stabilizer of the proximal pole of the scaphoid being the volar radioscaphoid ligament. Rotary subluxation of the scaphoid cannot occur unless this ligament is torn. The deep radiocarpal ligament is actually three ligaments: the radiocapitate, the radiolunate, and the radioscaphoid ligaments. The scapholunate interosseous ligament is a short, stout ligament standing dorsal to the palmar. These ligaments are difficult to repair individually, and repairs are carried out as complexes. The degree and the type of injury are determined by the position of the hand at the time of impact, the severity and velocity of the force involved, the type of loading of the joint surfaces, and the natural anatomic and biomechanical laxity of the individual involved. Most

commonly, a fall occurs with the wrist in extension and pronation, with the impact on the thenar side. The force carries the wrist into hyperextension, ulnar deviation, and intercarpal supination. The radiocapitate ligament is tightest in extension and ulnar deviation, whereas the radioscaphoid ligament is maximally taut in extension, with the proximal row stabilized to the forearm by five ligaments and the distal row by only the radiocapitate ligament. It has been shown that partial ligament failure can occur without complete disruption, and grossly intact ligaments can be associated with various carpal instability patterns. Also, in loose-jointed individuals, certain instability patterns can be seen, and it is often necessary to obtain stress views of the normal extremity as well.

Carpal Instability Patterns

The most frequent pattern is the dorsal intercalated segment instability (DISI) pattern in which the lunate is displaced volarward and flexed dorsally. In the volar intercalated segment instability (VISI) pattern, the lunate is displaced dorsally and flexed volarward. The DISI pattern can occur when the normal volar tilt of the distal articular surface of the radius is reversed, in addition to the ligamentous injuries. It is helpful to remember that, when a fracture of the radial styloid is present, the associated carpal instability pattern may be present as well. To determine these instabilities, a true lateral view of the wrist in neutral position is imperative.

The normal scapholunate angle averages 47 degrees (30 to 60 degrees), with greater than 70 degrees suggesting carpal instability and greater than 80 degrees, diagnostic. The capitolunate angle greater than 20 degrees is strongly suggestive of carpal instability. A scapholunate space of 1 to 2 mm is normal and greater than 3 mm abnormal, although occasionally this may be present bilaterally.

Diagnostically, the DISI shows a scapholunate angle of greater than 70 to 80 degrees and a capitolunate angle of greater than 15 to 20 degrees. The lunate is dorsiflexed, and there is increased overlap of the lunate and capitate on the AP view. The VISI shows findings of a palmar-flexed lunate, a capitolunate angle of greater than 30 degrees, dorsal subluxation of the lunate on the radius, overlap of the lunate and capitate on the AP view, and a scapholunate angle of less than 40 degrees.

The rotary subluxation pattern (Fig. 12.8) shows a scapholunate joint space of greater than 2 mm (see Fig. 12.8A), a shortening of the scaphoid due to vertical position with increased volar tilt, and a cortical ring sign, which is due to axial projection of the abnormally oriented scaphoid.

In the midcarpal instability pattern, the wrist assumes a VISI configuration until the final degrees of ulnar deviation, when the proximal row abruptly reaches dorsiflexion rather than making a smooth transition.

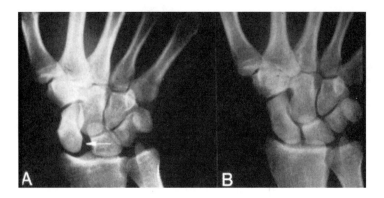

FIG. 12.8. **A.** The gap between the scaphoid and lunate (*arrow*) can be seen easily on this radiograph. **B.** The normal contralateral wrist.

Carpal Instability Treatment

Subluxation, in some cases, may be reduced and held in radial deviation and dorsiflexion, closing the scapholunate gap and restoring the alignment of the lunate and capitate. Usually, however, some type of fixation, open or closed, is necessary, since reduction may be difficult not only to obtain but especially to maintain in a satisfactory position. If the injury is fresh and normal alignment is obtained, it is generally better to use percutaneous K-wire fixation under the image intensifier after which a short arm cast is worn full-time for 6 to 8 weeks and then a removable splint for an additional 4 weeks. In the complete scapholunate instability, we approach the injury through both dorsal and volar incisions with repair of the anterior ligamentous complex and decompression of the median nerve and repair of the remnants of the dorsal interosseous ligaments, either directly or by roughening a bone and attaching through drill holes with a reefing of the dorsal capsule, using a flap of the dorsal carpal ligament routed beneath the extensor tendons. K-wire fixation is then carried out between the lunate and radius, between the scaphoid and radius, and between the scaphoid and capitate. The postoperative immobilization is essentially the same as for the closed reduction, with or without pinning. In deformity in which the normal volar tilt of the distal radial articular surface has been reversed, corrective osteotomy may be indicated.

In injuries seen after 2 months, before the appearance of degenerative changes, there are three main types of reconstruction. The first is repair of the ligament with grafting between the navicular and lunate, using a portion of a wrist extensor or flexor as a transfer. Most of these ligamentous structures do stretch out in time, but in most of our cases there was clinical improvement, especially in pain relief, and most of the individuals believe that they benefited functionally from the surgical procedure. Second, the tri-scaphe fusion between the distal scaphoid and trapezoid and trapezium, as described by Watson, did correct the increased gap on the neutral radiograph, but there tended to be a recurrence of the gap on ulnar deviation, as the lunate fails to rotate on the fixed navicular.

Also, a more rapid radioscaphoid arthrosis is seen in some cases. Third, a scapholunate fusion may be performed. This is logical but may be difficult to achieve; it certainly causes more stress on the adjoining articulations. Fourth, complete intercarpal fusion and, fifth, Silastic implant of the scapholunate may be used.

If degenerative changes are present, arthrodesis, proximal row carpectomy, or Silastic prosthesis may be the treatment of lunate triquetrum instability (VISI). In acute injuries, early treatment with casting for 6 to 8 weeks plus protective splinting until 3 months postinjury may be satisfactory. In chronic cases with dorsal subluxation and volar angulation of the lunate with compensatory dorsiflexion of the capitate, fusion of the triquetro-lunate joint is necessary. In most cases, ligamentous reconstruction eventually attenuates, although, again, symptomatic improvement may occur after these operations. When there is marked dorsal subluxation, soft tissue reinforcement is warranted postfusion.

Midcarpal Instability Treatment

All patients are started on a trial of conservative management, including immobilization, subjective symptomatic treatment, and antiinflammatory agents. In patients in whom these measures have failed, arthrodesis of the triquetro-hamate joint should be performed. Ligamentous structures have been used, but secondary attenuation tends to occur here as well.

Scaphoid Fracture with DISI

Most of these are fractures of the scaphoid waist, with the force causing dorsiflexion with collapse of the volar cortex. In acute cases, open reduction and internal fixation with a graft are carried out if volar collapse is present. In cases of scaphoid nonunion, treatment with electrical stimulation or bone graft can be carried out. It is important to correct this scaphoid angle with volar grafting if there is more than 30 degrees of angulation. The correction of this angulation will aid in the reduction of the lunate to a neutral position.

Lunate Dislocations

A lunate dislocation is seen more commonly than the perilunate dislocation; however, we believe that the lunate dislocation is secondary to a perilunate dislocation, which reduces spontaneously. With the reduction, the lunate is rotated and pushed volarly, where it may give symptoms of median nerve compression. The palmar radial lunate ligament remains intact, preserving the blood supply to the lunate. Diagnosis is easily made with lateral roentgenograms of the wrist.

The lunate is reduced with longitudinal traction, extension of the wrist, and pressure on the lunate from the palmar surface toward the dorsum. It is not unusual to have to recreate a perilunate dislocation to reduce the lunate, and then reduce the perilunate dislocation itself.

We protect wrist dislocations by holding them for 4 weeks in a cast with the wrist in slight flexion. At that time, we allow asymptomatic athletes to resume competition if they are protected for 4 more weeks in a silicone cast.

If an acute lunate dislocation is not diagnosed, open reduction is usually necessary. Median nerve palsies and flexor tendon constrictions are complications often seen and must be dealt with accordingly. The most common complication of this injury is late rotatory instability of the scaphoid.

Avascular Necrosis of the Lunate

Avascular necrosis of the lunate is also known as Kienbock's disease. The decreased blood supply to the lunate may be due to (1) primary circulatory problems; (2) traumatic interference with circulation, (3) ligament injury with subsequent degeneration collapse; or, more often, (4) single or multiple fractures with vascular impairment. This has not been found to be a common complication of lunate dislocation because blood supply is usually preserved. Repeated compression sprains or occasional single compressive episodes may be a cause.

The initial complaint is a weak wrist, with stiffness and pain with motion and on use, with the discomfort in the area of the lunate dorsally. There is weakness of grip, and early radiographs may be negative, except for an ulnar minus variant. It has been shown that, among randomly x-rayed wrists, about 51% have normal variance and 23% an ulnar minus variance. A relatively high percentage of individuals with Kienbock's disease show the ulnar minus variant of 2 mm or more. Over time, the typical x-ray findings of sclerosis, loss of lunate height, fragmentation, and proximal migration of the capitate may be seen, along with local and regional degenerative joint changes. The trispiral tomogram may be of diagnostic value to determine the degree of involvement and degenerative changes.

Treatment

The intraarticular effusion and reaction with unavoidable continuous stress on the carpal keystone interfere with attempts at healing. It has been postulated that, once the process of lunate collapse has begun, there is a progressive sequence of destruction in the face of anything other than operative treatment. However, we have seen a number of cases that have responded to splinting and conservative treatment over time without significant collapse or roughening of the articular surface. These, however, may be compression-type fractures, and thus conservative treatment is successful.

The search for an acceptable treatment plan continues, and many operative procedures have been described. One, a Silastic lunate implant, has been successful in our hands. The new Silastic is more resistant to wear. It is important to close the anterior structures, along with reinforcing the dorsal structures, to maintain the position, since the most common complication is subluxation of the implant. Even a subluxed implant, if not severely displaced, can be successful.

Intercarpal fusion is another treatment option. In cases in which there is less than 2 mm of collapse, there is fusion of the capitohamate joint only, and where there is a collapse greater than 2 mm, a capitohamate fusion with a Silastic lunate implant has been advocated. Also, fusion of the triquetrum and hamate has been described.

Ulnar lengthening and radial shortening to alleviate the stress of the ulnar minus variant allow revascularization of the bone. Various methods of wrist fusion and proximal row carpectomy are indicated as salvage procedures in cases in which there is degenerative arthritis of the wrist. Total wrist arthroplasty has also been used in cases of this type. The multitude of operative procedures reveals that an ideal method of treatment has not yet been yfound, but recent advances have shown a significant improvement in the knowledge and treatment of Kienbock's disease.

Tendinitis Near the Wrist

Overuse of the wrist and hand in athletics may result in tendinitis near the wrist. The athlete will complain of an aching pain and the involved tendon will be tender. The pain is accentuated by passive stretching of the affected tendon or by contraction of the associated muscle against resistance. X-ray films will usually have normal findings but may show a calcium deposit within the tendon sheath.

Oarsman's Wrist

Rowers, canoeists, and weight lifters who do curls may develop a traumatic tenosynovitis of the radial extensors of the wrist. This chronic and disabling overuse condition results in localized pain, tenderness, and a squeaky crepitus and swelling over the radial dorsal aspect of the forearm about 7 cm proximal to Lister's tubercle. The tenosynovitis results from hypertrophy of the abductor pollicis longus and the extensor pollicis brevis muscles that overlie the radial extensor tendons in the distal forearm and cross these underlying radial wrist extensor tendons obliquely (78). The extensor tendons and their enveloping paratenons are compressed against the deeper structures.

Treatment includes splinting, nonsteroidal antiinflammatory medicines, and, sometimes, a steroid shot. If pain persists, surgical decompression of the sheath of these muscles will relieve the pressure on the underlying paratenons of the radial wrist extensors. The release incision is made parallel to the muscle bellies of the abductor pollicis longus and extensor pollicis brevis obliquely over the dorsum of the distal forearm. This incision is dorsal and proximal to the site for decompression of these tendons for deQuervain's tenosynovitis. The APL and EPB are found to be hypertrophied where they cross the radial extensor tendons. The paratenons of the underlying extensor tendons are inflamed and adherent. The surgeon divides the sheath longitudinally from the musculotendinous junction to where the muscles disappear deep into the forearm. After a few days, the splint is removed and the athlete can exercise back to normal.

DeQuervain's Stenosing Tenosynovitis

Ulnar deviation of the wrist angles the tendons of the abductor pollicis longus and the extensor pollicis brevis under the retinaculum covering the first dorsal compartment of the wrist at the level of the radial styloid. Repetitive angulation produces tenosynovitis in this fibro-osseous tunnel. The area will be tender and Finkelstein's test positive. In this test, the wrist is ulnar deviated passively while the thumb is held adducted in the palm. This movement produces pain at the radial styloid. Treatment includes resting the wrist, putting the thumb in a splint and prescribing a nonsteroidal, anti-inflammatory medicine. In chronic cases, however, the roof is thick and pain persists. In such cases, decompression is indicated. While releasing the roof, the surgeon takes care to avoid the sensory branch of the radial nerve. He searches for a separate canal for the extensor pollicis brevis. Sometimes a synovial cyst is found in the compartment. The tendon may exhibit a fusiform enlargment just distal to the site of compression. After tendons are released, the wrist is splinted for a few days, then early motion begins.

Flexor Carpi Ulnaris Tendinitis

The flexor carpi ulnaris dominates wrist activity, and tendonitis of it is not uncommon after repetitive activity. The tendon of the flexor carpi ulnaris will be tender at the wrist, and wrist flexion or ulnar deviation against resistance will hurt. X-ray films usually have normal findings but may show a calcium deposit in the paratenon or tendon itself. Splinting, pulsed ultrasound, and nonsteroidal antiinflammatory medicines are usually effective.

The flexor carpi ulnaris inserts into the hook of the hamate and the bases of the fourth and fifth metacarpals. The pisiform bone is a sesamoid bone in the tendon. A synovitis may develop around the pisiform, or the pisiform-triquetral articulation may become arthritic (59). In such cases, the pisiform will be tender. With the wrist held flexed, pain is produced when the examiner pushes the pisiform laterally on its articulation with the triquetrum. A lateral x-ray film of the wrist may show a narrow joint space. In cases of arthritis of the pisiform, the surgeon may have to excise calcium deposits, lyse peritendinous adhesions, and excise the pisiform bone subperiosteally, leaving the insertion of the flexor carpi ulnaris intact. Postoperatively the wrist is splinted for a week, and then the athlete begins range-of-motion exercises and soon returns to his sport.

Flexor Carpi Radialis Tendinitis

Tendinitis is less common at the radial side of the wrist joint than at the ulnar side because motion is less frequent there. Wrist flexion against resistance will hurt, as will passive extension of the wrist. Resistant cases of stenosing tenosynovitis at the fibro-osseous tunnel of the flexor carpi radialis may be relieved by releasing the tunnel.

Scaphoid Fractures

The scaphoid spans the proximal and distal carpal rows. The proximal part of this bone is intracapsular, and the distal portion has many soft-tissue attachments. The vulnerable waist of the scaphoid is adjacent to the styloid tip of the radius, and most of the scaphoid fractures occur here. A fall on the outstretched hand or direct impact on the hand may fracture the scaphoid by forcing it against this styloid process. The athlete notes pain on power grip and is tender over the anatomic "snuffbox."

Scaphoid fractures often are diagnosed inaccurately as sprains, and inadequate treatment may result in nonunion. If an athlete has the above symptoms but x-ray findings are negative, a cast is applied, which incorporates the proximal phalanx of the thumb. Then, in about 2 weeks, the wrist is reexamined and another x-ray film taken. If a fracture is noted, another cast is applied that extends from three fourths up the forearm down to the interphalangeal joint of the thumb and is carefully molded about the base of the thumb.

Most scaphoid fractures are through the waist, some are through the proximal pole, and the least frequent are of the distal pole. Fractures of the distal pole heal fast because of good blood supply. Fractures at the waist or proximal pole may require prolonged immobilization, and nonunion, avascular necrosis, and collapse may occur.

Those scaphoid fractures that are unstable and displaced need primary open reduction and fixation and sometimes primary grafting. Delayed unions require prolonged casting; a decision should then be made as to whether the fracture should be grafted. If the decision is made to treat the fracture with a bone graft, we favor a volar approach and use the volar aspect of the distal radius as a donor site. Postoperatively, patients with these fractures are treated with the standard scaphoid cast, and postoperative healing still takes about 3 to 4 months. While the fracture is healing, the athlete may sometimes play his or her sport wearing a silicone rubber splint.

Protective Splint of Silicone Rubber

Under the rules of collegiate tackle football, sole leather or other hard or unyielding substances are prohibited on the hand, wrist, or forearm. Mindful of this rule, a protective silicone rubber splint or a cast with foam protection (Fig. 12.9) has been developed (3). The splint allows the safe return to competition of athletes who have had wrist sprains or fractures, such as a healing scaphoid fracture.

The silicone rubber protective splint can also be constructed with gauze impregnated with silicone rubber-RTV 11. The splint is easy to apply, conforms to the injured part, and is durable. First, a thin coat of lubricant cream is applied to the skin, and the gauze is wrapped smoothly on the body part. A catalyst is mixed with the silicone and a generous first coat of silicone applied. Usually three or four thicknesses of gauze are used, and the silicone is worked into each layer of the gauze with a spatula. The silicone takes about 3 hours to cure at room temperature. For removal, the splint is cut along the ulnar side. It can be secured again with adhesive tape. Because the silicone splint does not breathe, it is not used as a permanent cast but may be worn during practice and competition. A bivalved hard cast is worn at other times (3).

Hamate Hook Fractures

The hook of the hamate projects toward the palmar surface of the hand as a long, thin process of bone. The transverse carpal ligament and the pisohamate ligament both attach to the hook, and the flexor digiti minimi brevis and opponens digiti both arise from it. The tendon of the flexor digitorum profundus to the little finger lies on its radial side, and the motor branch of the medial nerve on its ulnar side.

The hook of the hamate may be fractured in a fall, but it breaks more commonly during a tennis, baseball, or golf swing (Fig. 12.10) (73). The butt of the handle may strike the hook and fracture it, or a violent contraction of the flexor carpi ulnaris can pull through the pisohamate ligament and jerk the hook.

An athlete with a hook of the hamate fracture will have wrist pain, a poor power grip, and a tender hook of the hamate. Routine x-ray films often do not show the fracture; thus a carpal tunnel view should be included with the wrist in maximum dorsiflexion. If the wrist is too painful for this view to be obtained, a maximum radial deviation view, with the wrist partly supinated, may show the fracture.

A short gauntlet cast, with an extension to the little finger, is applied for acute undisplaced fractures of the hook of the hamate. The nonunion rate for this fracture is high, owing to the intermittent pull of the muscular attachments. For a badly displaced fracture or a symptomatic nonunion, the displaced hook is removed.

The ulnar nerve or the flexor digitorum profundus to the little finger may become irritated at the fracture site and give symptoms of ulnar nerve neuritis or flexor tendinitis. To prevent a later tendon rupture, some surgeons remove the hook of the hamate even in painless nonunions. So that the ulnar nerve is not damaged during this procedure, it is exposed in the canal of Guyon and carefully followed.

Nerve Compression

An athlete's median nerve may be compressed in a tight carpal tunnel, or the ulnar nerve may be compressed

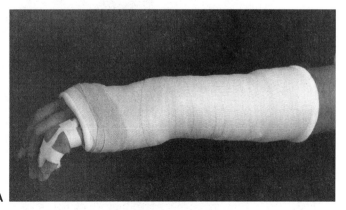
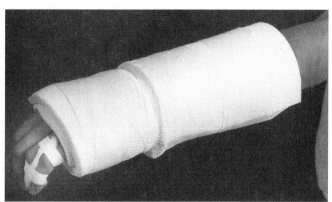

FIG. 12.9. Wrist and hand in cast (**A**) with foam protection (**B**) for particpation.

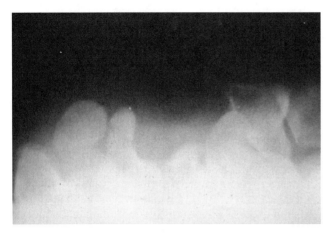

FIG. 12.10. The fracture of the hamate can be seen on a carpal tunnel view. The fracture sometimes fails to unite and irritates the nearby motor branch of the ulnar nerve; it may also cause a rupture of the flexor profundus to the little finger.

in the canal of Guyon. In the young, healthy athlete, rest and an antiinflammatory medication will usually relieve median nerve compression, but sometimes surgical decompression is needed.

Touring cyclists, especially on bumpy gravel roads, often develop numbness of the little finger and the ulnar half of the ring finger, with associated ulnar intrinsic muscle weakness (19,38). The numbness and weakness are caused by pressure from the handlebars on the ulnar nerve (Fig. 12.11) and may be relieved by wearing cycling gloves and thickly padding the handlebars. The ulnar nerve may also be compressed after a fracture of the pisiform or the hamate bone, and blunt trauma to the heel of the palm may also result in scarring within the canal of Guyon. This acute trauma may even produce a false aneurysm of the ulnar artery that may compress the ulnar nerve. Treatment consists of release of the ligament overlying the canal of Guyon and appropriate measures for the underlying lesion.

Bowler's Thumb

The hard edge of the thumbhole in a bowling ball may press against the base of a bowler's thumb during delivery and cause perineural fibrosis of the relatively subcutaneous ulnar digital nerve of the thumb (19,20,37,48,68). If fibrosis develops, the bowler will note pain, paresthesia when pressure is applied to this region, numbness of the ulnar-volar aspect of the thumb, and a fusiform mass.

If bowler's thumb is detected early, the bowler should modify his grip and use a larger, padded thumbhole. If the condition is noted later, after a mass has formed, the thumb is operated on. The thick, perineural sheath is incised and meticulously dissected free from the nerve fascicles. After neurolysis, the nerve may be transposed to a more dorsal-ulnar aspect of the thumb. Awareness of the

entity of bowler's thumb neuroma prevents unnecessary removal of the digital nerve. The symptoms may be relieved without excising the neuroma, and the critical sensation is maintained along the medial border of the thumb.

Thumb Metacarpal Fractures

Axial compression may injure a hockey player's thumb metacarpal when he takes off his gloves to throw a punch. The thumb may be driven down to shear off the base of the thumb metacarpal. A small medial fragment remains hooked to the strong volar ligament as the abductor pollicis longus pulls the main portion of the metacarpal proximally. This Bennett's fracture-dislocation may be treated by closed reduction and percutaneous pin fixation. In some cases, however, open reduction is needed to approximate the articular surfaces accurately. A Rolando's fracture is a proximal, intraarticular, T-shaped fracture of the first metacarpal. Here the flexor and extensor muscles pull the fracture fragments apart over the trapezium.

Although fractures of the metacarpal shaft are often angulated by muscle pull, a well-molded gauntlet cast can usually hold the reduction. Fractures of the proximal phalanx of the thumb may follow a twisting injury, such as when an equestrian's thumb becomes caught in a halter as the horse rears. These fractures are usually treated by a closed reduction and a gauntlet cast. Internal fixation may be required if the fracture slips.

Thumb Metacarpophalangeal Joint Dislocation

When the metacarpophalangeal joint of the thumb is forcefully hyperextended and dislocates, the membranous part of the volar plate may tear (Fig. 12.12). In a simple dislocation, the proximal phalanx lies dorsal to the metacarpal head and is standing straight up. Longitudinal traction should be avoided because the volar plate may slip

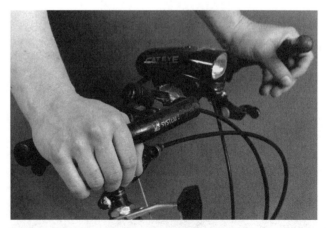

FIG. 12.11. A cyclist's ulnar nerve may be compressed at the wrist from pressure on the handlebars.

BOX 1:
Rehabilitation Progression for the Elbow, Forearm, and Wrist

OBJECTIVES

- *Strengthen:* Elbow flexors, extensors, pronators and supinators; wrist flexors and extensors; radial and ulnar deviators
  - *Flexibility:* Elbow flexors and extensors
    Wrist flexors and extensors
  - *Endurance:* Elbow flexors and extensors
    Wrist flexors and extensors

STAGES

- Initial
Cryokinetics (ice, pain-free active range of motion and resistive exercise)
- Intermediate
  Flexibility: Stretch the wrist into flexion for 15 seconds three times.
  Stretch the wrist into extension for 15 seconds three times.
  Strength: All of the following strength exercises begin with three sets of ten repetitions and progress to five sets of ten repetitions. When the athlete can handle five sets of ten, he or she then adds weight and begins again at three sets of ten repetitions.
- Holding a dumbbell, flex the elbow from the extended position. Then extend the elbow while forward flexing the shoulder and repeat.
- Use the T-bar to supinate and pronate. Choke up on the bar to flex the wrist and extend the wrist holding a dumbbell. Radially deviate and ulnar deviate with the T-bar.
- Advanced
  Progress to weight machines and other upper-extremity exercises with barbells.

between the metacarpal and the proximal phalanx, converting the simple dislocation into a complex one. Instead, the physician should push against the dorsal surface of the proximal phalanx and push the metacarpal dorsally.

When the volar plate is caught between the metacarpal and the proximal phalanx, the dislocation may be irreducible, x-ray films show a sesamoid bone within the widened joint space, and there is a dimple in the palmar skin. To reduce such a dislocation, the thumb metacarpal is first adducted and the thumb flexed to relax the intrinsics. Then the proximal phalanx is hyperextended, and the physician pushes against the dorsal surface of the proximal phalanx

and pushes the metacarpal up. If closed reduction fails, open reduction may be performed through a volar or dorsal approach.

After reduction, the thumb is immobilized in a plaster splint for about 2 weeks. The athlete often is allowed to resume competition while wearing a silicone splint. When the joint is completely stable and has a full range of motion, the immobilization may be discontinued.

Ulnar Collateral Ligament

Injury of the Thumb

Ulnar collateral ligament injuries of the thumb are often overlooked in young, poorly supervised athletes (51,52). There is a tendency to minimize the injury, but it may lead to a weakness of pinch and instability when the thumb is stressed in abduction. The injury occurs mostly in tackle football, from forced abduction of the thumb, but also in hockey players, who take off their gloves to fight, and in soccer goalkeepers, skiers, wrestlers, and baseball players (9,14,15,25,26,65). The skier's pole strap allows him or her to plant the pole harder by pulling down on the strap, and thus the pole need not be gripped as tightly. When the strap is wrapped around the wrist, discarding the pole is difficult, and the skier may land on it in trying to break the fall. A better method of holding the pole is with only the hand put through the loop.

The ulnar collateral ligament is usually torn from its attachment to the proximal phalanx. Sometimes a displaced rotated chip from the proximal phalanx may be seen on x-ray films (Fig. 12.13). Most of the tears are partial and can be treated by closed means, but acute, complete tears are treated with open repair and reconstruction. In more than half of these complete tears, the intrinsic aponeurosis is found to be lying between the ends of the ulnar collateral ligament and would block healing (51). The avulsed ulnar collateral ligament is reattached by a pull-out wire technique. If the ligament has been torn in its midportion, sutures are placed in it with the metacarpophalangeal joint flexed to 15 to 20 degrees, and the athlete must wear a splint or a thumb spica for 5 weeks.

Taping of the thumb allows an athlete to continue playing without jeopardizing a mild or moderate sprain and to play after surgery (Fig. 12.14). First the metacarpophalangeal joint is stabilized with the tape, and then the athlete's index finger is taped to his thumb, holding the thumb adducted and preventing abduction at the metacarpophalangeal joint. Alternatively, elastic tape may be used to hold the thumb adducted (Fig. 12.15).

An athlete with an old ulnar collateral ligament injury may have a long history of pinch weakness, pain, and instability at the metacarpophalangeal joint of the thumb. When the ulnar collateral ligament is thin or missing, it can be replaced by a slip of the abductor pollicis longus,

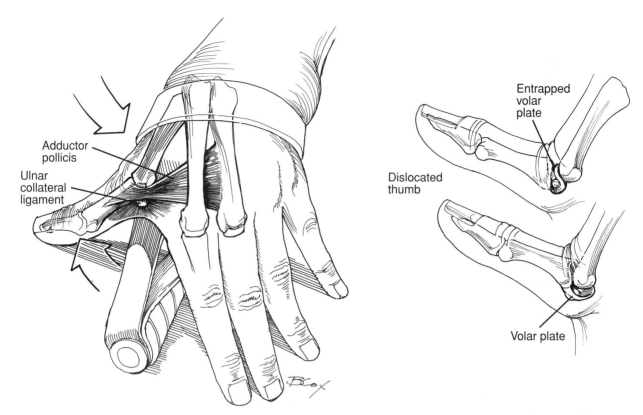

FIG. 12.12. Landing on a ski pole may dislocate the metacarpophalangeal joint of the thumb and the volar plate may become trapped in the joint. In other instances, the ulnar collateral ligament of the thumb may tear from its insertion into the proximal phalanx, and the tendon of the adductor pollicis may interpose to prevent healing.

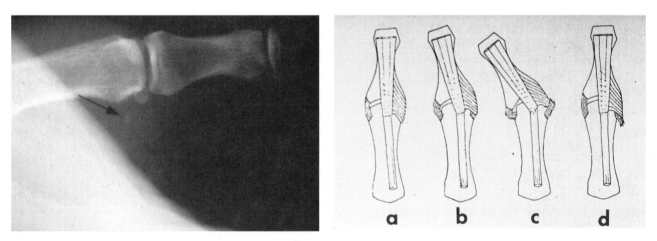

FIG. 12.13. Left: Radiograph showing displaced avulsion from proximal phalanx. **Right:** In complete tears of the ulna collateral ligament, the intact intrinsic aponeurosis may be found lying between the ends of the ulnar collateral ligament.

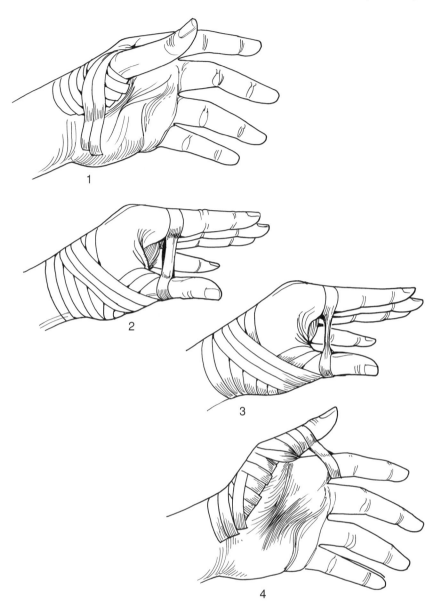

FIG. 12.14. A thumb taping with a "clincher strap" restricts thumb movement.

or a slip of the adductor pollicis may be advanced to the proximal phalanx as a dynamic repair.

Soft Tissue Injuries at the Metacarpophalangeal Joint of the Fingers

What may at first appear to be a dorsal dislocation of the proximal phalanx of a metacarpophalangeal joint is actually a volar dislocation of the metacarpal head. The head breaks through a buttonhole rent in the volar plate and is caught in this rent and between the lumbrical tendon and long flexors. This dislocation is usually referred to as an "irreducible dislocation" because closed reduction often fails. Although the index finger is most often affected, the little finger metacarpal or other metacarpals may also be dislocated. The affected finger is generally angled toward the ulnar, overlapping the adjacent finger, and a dimple appears in the skin at the midpalmar crease. Longitudinal traction actually prevents reduction, as the surrounding structures form a nooselike constriction around the metacarpal neck. An acute dislocation may sometimes be reduced by increasing the deformity and attempting to return the proximal phalanx through the tear in the volar plate. Once swelling has occurred, however, an open reduction is usually needed.

The dislocation may be reduced surgically through a volar approach. Great care must be taken to avoid damaging the very prominent palmar structures, especially the digital nerve and artery. Once reduced, the joint is surprisingly stable. The metacarpophalangeal joint is kept flexed about 30 degrees for 7 to 10 days, and then active flexion

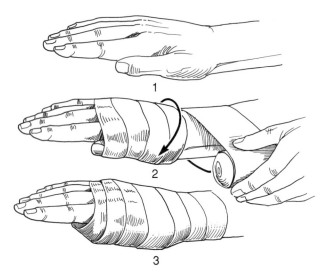

FIG. 12.15. A pancake thumb taping may protect a damaged ulnar collateral ligament of the thumb.

is begun from this position. An extension-block splint is worn, and extension and hyperextension are not permitted until 5 weeks after surgery. Nearly full flexion has usually been accomplished by the time the splint is removed.

A collateral ligament injury of a metacarpophalangeal joint is not nearly as common or as disabling as one involving a proximal interphalangeal joint. However, a piece of the proximal phalanx may be avulsed by the collateral ligament into the joint. Swelling, thickening, and the possible inclusion of the collateral ligament in the joint are the most disabling findings. Lateral instability is usually not a functional problem, since radial or ulnar control is maintained by the intrinsics.

Another soft tissue injury at the metacarpophalangeal joint is rupture of the extensor hood of the extensor digitorum communis. The extensor tendon can then slip into the valley between the metacarpal heads and produce a disabling snapping. A large mass of granulation tissue may form from hypertrophic synovium in the tear, preventing an athlete from gripping. The mass should be removed and the extensor hood repaired.

Hand Injuries in Karate

Karate means "empty hand" in Japanese. The fighting technique began in India more than 1500 years ago for self-defense against bandits, was later taught to Chinese monks, and developed further in Okinawa. In 1920, the martial art was exported to Japan and, after World War II, to the United States (16,27).

Karate enthusiasts scar their limbs, converting them into weapons to strike the sensitive areas of their opponents. This toughening may be achieved by striking a straw-covered, pliable post over a number of years, or the hands and feet may be driven into sacks of sand,

gravel, grain, or leather scraps (41). Scar tissue slowly increases, but, if rigid adherence to this program is replaced by a desire for quick results, the hands may be damaged (70).

Hypertrophic infiltrative tenosynovitis may develop around an extensor tendon that is greatly enlarged proximal to where it is trapped by a mass of scar tissue at the metacarpophalangeal joint (27). The scar tissue may be removed, but the incision should be placed so that it does not interfere with striking (27).

A correctly executed thrust and hand strike uses the index and middle finger metacarpal heads. Axial compression forces are transmitted from these metacarpals to the distal carpal row, which is dynamically splinted by the taut wrist extensors and flexors. These forces may produce intraarticular fractures (39). In contrast to correct technique, inaccurate thrusts, roundhouse blows, and the blocking of kicks will transmit angular torsional forces to produce oblique diaphyseal fractures of the metacarpals (35).

To lessen the chance of hand injury, a fist must be made properly (Fig. 12.16). A loose fist leaves the second and third metacarpals unsupported, and only their thick cortex and shaft may save them from breaking. To make a proper fist for karate, the interphalangeal joints are first maximally flexed. Then the metacarpophalangeal joints are flexed so that the thenar eminence gives support. The thumb is tucked out of the way. Striking is done only with the index and middle finger knuckles and with a maximally tightened fist. At impact the wrist is pronated, reminding the striker to maximally tighten the fist and also tearing an attacker's skin.

Metacarpal Fractures

Fractures of the finger metacarpals include proximal fracture-dislocations at the base of the fifth metacarpal that may be similar to a fracture-dislocation of the first metacarpal; metacarpal shaft fractures; fractures through a metacarpal neck, the "fighter's fracture"; and intraarticular fractures at the metacarpophalangeal joint.

A proximal fracture-dislocation of the fifth metacarpal may behave like an unstable Bennett's fracture-dislocation of the first metacarpal. Such a fracture is reduced and fixed with pins. Fracture-dislocations of the second, third, or fourth metacarpal are extremely rare, and the treatment must be individualized. Fractures of the proximal shaft of the metacarpals are controlled by metacarpal ligaments and are generally stable. They are protected in a short arm cast.

A fracture of a metacarpal shaft is usually only minimally displaced and may be controlled in a well-molded short-arm cast that is worn for 4 to 6 weeks. Occasionally percutaneous pins or an open reduction is necessary. Long, spiral fractures are more likely to require internal

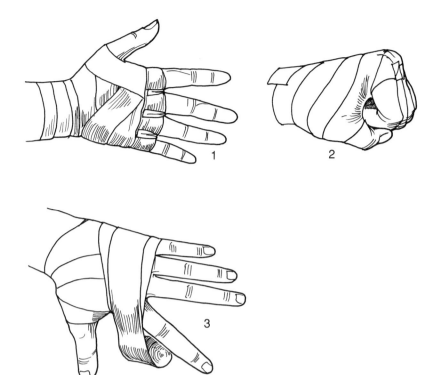

FIG. 12.16. In a properly made fist, the thumb supports the second and third metacarpals, but the lateral two metacarpals remain unsupported allowing a fracture to occur. The taping supports the boxer's metacarpals.

fixation to avoid compounding, rotatory deformity, and shortening of the metacarpal. When these fractures are treated closed, care must be taken to control the rotation of the digit, and it is often taped to an adjacent finger. Open reduction of a metacarpal shaft fracture may produce complications such as compromise of the bone's blood supply, fibrosis of the interosseous muscles, adherence of the extensor tendons, and local infection.

A fighter's fracture, or punch fracture, through the neck of the fifth metacarpal may follow a roundhouse punch. A boxer, with proper punching technique and taped hands, will more often fracture his second or third metacarpal than his fifth metacarpal. The boxer has the advantage of good technique, bandaged hands, and boxing gloves. His hands are bandaged with his fingers spread. When he flexes his fingers, the metacarpals are held strongly together. A boxing glove is really a mitten, with a firm leather band in the palm of the glove that supports all four finger metacarpals.

The fourth and fifth metacarpals are structurally weak, the fourth being the most slender, while the fifth is shorter and has a paper-thin cortex. The thenar eminence supports only the second and third metacarpals, leaving the lateral two metacarpals without support in a bareknuckled fist. The volar articular ridge of the metacarpal heads acts as a reinforcement and explains the obliquity of the fracture lines.

A fighter's fracture is common and often overtreated. Any rotation can usually be corrected by closed reduction with the metacarpophalangeal joint flexed so that the fragment is controlled by a tightening of the collateral ligament. Volar and dorsal felt pads are placed after the reduc-

tion. Then a molded plaster cast is applied, with an outrigger or with the little finger buddy-taped to the ring finger. Up to 40 degrees of angulation is acceptable in the more mobile fourth and fifth metacarpals. Holding the metacarpophalangeal and proximal interphalangeal joints in flexion with pressure over the dorsum of the proximal phalanx is unnecessary. Serious secondary stiffness and skin problems frequently follow such treatment. A fracture that is very unstable may require percutaneous pinning and, occasionally, open reduction with internal fixation.

If an appreciable part of the articular surface is involved in a fracture, the fracture must be anatomically reduced, usually by open reduction. An arthroplasty with a Silastic prosthesis may be needed in a joint that has been left grossly deformed by an old injury.

The complications of metacarpal fractures include rotatory deformity, localized Volkmann's ischemic contracture, limitation of flexion and extension at the metacarpophalangeal, proximal interphalangeal, or distal interphalangeal joints, and nonunion of the bone. In these cases reconstructive procedures may be needed to improve function.

Fractures of the Proximal Phalanx

The periosteum of the proximal phalanx is in contact with the extrinsic extensor and flexor tendons and the lateral bands. Because of this close association, these tendons readily adhere to fractures of the proximal phalanx, especially if they have been imperfectly reduced. Tethering of the tendons limits active and passive motion at the proximal interphalangeal and distal interphalangeal joints. Moreover, a fracture of the proximal phalanx may affect the metacarpophalangeal or the proximal interphalangeal joint. Restricted motion in either of these joints is disabling, but restriction of motion in both joints is disastrous.

The intrinsic and extrinsic muscles exert deforming forces on the fracture fragments. The proximal fragment is flexed by the intrinsics, and the distal fragment is controlled by the extrinsic flexors and extensors that span it. The collateral ligaments of the metacarpophalangeal joints aid closed reduction, controlling the metacarpophalangeal joint when it is flexed and maintaining control of the proximal fragment. A flexed position also lessens the deforming force of the intrinsic muscles, and flexion of the proximal interphalangeal joint relaxes the extrinsic flexors, reducing their deforming force.

An epiphyseal fracture of a young athlete's proximal phalanx may be angulated. Closed reduction is usually successful. The tough periosteum is often intact and aids in obtaining and maintaining the reduction. After reduction the finger is splinted, and when the reaction has resolved the injured finger is taped to an adjacent finger.

Inherently stable fractures of the shaft of the proximal phalanx and those that are stable after reduction may be controlled by splinting. After a thin felt pad is placed between the fingers, the injured finger is taped to an adjacent finger. For less stable fractures, a forearm splint is applied with an outrigger that holds the finger in the position of greatest stability. Remember that all the fingers should point toward the proximal tubercle of the scaphoid. Malrotation will occur if this relationship is not maintained. Early motion is particularly important after a fracture of the proximal phalanx to regain optimal finger motion.

Some proximal phalanx fractures present special problems. The spike of an oblique fracture may encroach upon the proximal interphalangeal joint just proximal to the articular surface and severely disrupt joint function. A spiral fracture can easily rotate and shorten to produce a deformity if it is not held well reduced. These are usually fixed percutaneously with pins, but when a closed reduction is not possible open reduction and pin fixation are done. A fracture involving the articular surface must be reduced anatomically and held with pins. When a proximal phalanx fracture is treated by open reduction and internal fixation, incisions must be placed properly and the tissue handled gently; otherwise, functional loss may be even greater than that after closed treatment. Prompt, appropriate treatment for proximal phalanx fractures is imperative. Secondary reconstructions for nonunions or for other bony or soft tissue abnormalities may not produce a fully functional finger.

Injuries to the Proximal Interphalangeal Joint

The anatomy of the proximal interphalangeal joint is complex for such a small articulation and must be understood for correct diagnosis and effective treatment of injuries to this joint. A hinged joint, it has a range of motion of from 0 to 120 degrees in the plane perpendicular to the palm. The lateral ligaments and volar plate are thick and strong. They are supplemented dorsally by the central slip of the extensor tendon and by the flexor tendons, less closely on the volar surface. The lateral bands and their extensions, the oblique and transverse retinacular ligaments, and Cleland's ligament radiating dorsal to the neurovascular bundle add some stability and must move and glide freely to allow proper motion. The volar cul-de-sac must be free of scar to allow full flexion of the finger, during which the base of the middle phalanx glides into the sac.

The proximal interphalangeal joint has limited lateral mobility and is particularly vulnerable because of its relatively long proximal and distal lever arms that transmit lateral stress and torque (50). Any fixed deformity of the proximal interphalangeal joint, either in flexion or extension, is extremely disabling. Because it is a small, non–weight-bearing joint, there is a tendency to minimize the severity of injuries to it. Poorly supervised athletes often return to unprotected use of the digit long before adequate healing has taken place.

Injuries to the proximal interphalangeal joint include articular fractures, fracture-dislocations, dislocations, collateral ligament injuries, buttonhole deformities, and volar plate injuries such as hyperextension and pseudo-buttonhole deformities.

Articular Fractures at the Proximal Interphalangeal Joint

Commonly seen articular fractures at the proximal interphalangeal joint include those that pass through one condyle of the head of the proximal phalanx, long and short oblique fractures, T fractures that split the condyles, fractures of the base of the middle phalanx, avulsion fractures of the articular surface, and comminuted fractures.

Stable fractures with little or no ligamentous instability, such as small chip fractures and avulsion fractures, should be splinted for 3 weeks with the proximal interphalangeal joint flexed to about 30 degrees. In most cases, the athlete may return to competition, wearing the splint for protection. Early protected flexion begins as soon as the acute reaction abates. Either a dorsal or volar splint should be worn during sports and other strenuous activities for an additional 4 to 6 weeks or until a full range of motion has been regained.

The indications for open reduction and internal fixation include displaced articular fractures that constitute more than one fourth of the articular surface, displaced volar lip fractures that invite subsequent dorsal subluxation, comminuted or displaced fractures, and dorsal avulsion fractures that include the insertion of the central slip of the extensor tendon into the base of the middle phalanx. Accurate restoration of the articular surface in this little, tight-fitting joint is important for a maximum return of function. Secondary reconstructive procedures, including Silastic implant arthroplasty, give less predictable results. Arthrodesis is a treatment of last resort and is rarely indicated.

Fracture-Dislocations of the Proximal Interphalangeal Joint

The most common fracture-dislocation of the proximal interphalangeal joint is one through the volar lip of the proximal phalanx (Fig. 12.17). Here the buttressing effect of the volar lip is lost, and, if untreated, the finger becomes stiff and painful and its function greatly impaired. The volar fragment may vary in size and communication. If the joint is stable, the digit may be splinted in flexion with a splint that blocks extension; if unstable, operative reduction and pinning are needed. Early flexion exercises should begin in 3 weeks, and the finger should be protected during sports activity for an additional 4 to 6 weeks.

An avulsion of the central slip of the extensor mechanism, with or without a bony fragment, and volar subluxation of the middle phalanx are rare injuries. They often demand an open reduction because the head of the proximal phalanx may be entrapped by the lateral bands to block a closed reduction.

Dislocations of the Proximal Interphalangeal Joint

If the proximal interphalangeal joint is hyperextended, the volar plate may rupture at its distal attachment, with or without an avulsion fracture from the base of the middle phalanx, and the middle phalanx will dislocate dorsal to the proximal phalanx (see Fig. 12.17). Reduction is usually easy and the joint generally stable because the collateral ligament system has usually remained intact. Once reduced, the joint is immobilized in 20 to 30 degrees of flexion for 3 weeks, whereupon the splint is removed and the athlete begins an active exercise program. The finger should be taped to an adjacent normal digit during sports activity for at least 2 more weeks until it is asymptomatic. With proper care and protection, full recovery should be expected, with an asymptomatic finger and a full range of motion.

For a lateral dislocation of the proximal interphalangeal

joint to occur, a collateral ligament and the volar plate must tear. The method of treatment for these dislocations depends on what instabilities exist after reduction. Some dislocations have a rotatory component, and the head of the proximal phalanx may become buttonholed between the central slip and the lateral band. These dislocations usually require open reduction. Open dislocations are meticulously cleaned, and then the torn tissues may be repaired. The athlete may begin active protected motion as soon as the skin heals.

"Buttonhole Deformity"

A disruption of the central slip of the extensor digitorum communis tendon over the proximal interphalangeal joint produces a classic buttonhole (boutonnière) deformity that consists of hyperextension at the distal interphalangeal joint (49). A central slip rupture is difficult to diagnose accurately. Unopposed pull of the flexor digitorum sublimis and pain and swelling at the proximal interphalangeal joint keep the joint flexed. The athlete's inability to extend the proximal interphalangeal joint is often attributed to the pain and swelling from the injury. The finger is splinted in the usual semiflexed position. When the extensor tendon is disrupted, however, this position favors a continued separation of the central slip and prevents healing. Later, as the athlete attempts to extend the finger, the tension on the lateral bands increases, causing them to drop volarly. These bands then become flexors, aggravate the deformity, and produce hyperextension at the distal interphalangeal joint.

To avoid developing a buttonhole deformity, a person with any injury associated with a lag of more than 30 degrees in proximal interphalangeal extension and tenderness dorsally directly over the base of the middle phalanx should be treated for an acute extensor rupture. The digit should be splinted with the proximal interphalangeal joint in full extension, and this splint should be worn for 6 to 8 weeks. Protective splinting should be continued during competition for another 6 to 8 weeks or until full flexion and maximum extension of the finger have returned. The metacarpophalangeal and distal interphalangeal joints may be left free to move. If there is residual restricted passive extension at the proximal interphalangeal joint, correction with a safety-pin splint is needed. In many of these cases, however, surgical reconstruction will be required. Many surgical procedures have been designed to correct chronic deformities, but owing to a variety of findings the results of these procedures are not predictable.

Volar Plate Injuries

The volar plate of the proximal interphalangeal joint has a proximal membranous portion attached to the proximal phalanx and a thick, cartilaginous distal portion

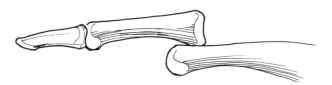

FIG. 12.17. A fracture of the volar lip of the middle phalanx may allow a dislocated proximal interphalangeal joint.

attached strongly to the base of the middle phalanx. An acute volar plate injury requires splinting for at least 5 weeks. The athlete may begin early protected motion at 3 weeks, wearing an extension-block splint to prevent extension of the digit.

An injury to the volar plate may result in either a hyperextension deformity or a flexion deformity at the proximal interphalangeal joint. Distal disruption of the plate may produce a "swan-neck" deformity. Surgical reconstruction is indicated only if the proximal interphalangeal joint locks in extension and interferes with normal function of the hand.

Damage to the proximal, membranous part of the plate may produce a "pseudoboutonnière deformity." This resembles the classic boutonnière deformity, but the central extensor slip is intact. With a pseudoboutonnière deformity, there is usually a history of a hyperextension or a twisting injury to the proximal interphalangeal joint. The signs of a pseudoboutonnière deformity include a flexion contracture of the proximal interphalangeal joint, which is more resistant to correction by passive extension than is the typical boutonnière, slight hyperextension of the distal interphalangeal joint, and radiologic evidence of calcification under the distal end of the proximal phalanx.

Static safety pin splinting is used in subacute, less-fixed pseudoboutonnière deformities. After correction, these fingers must still be followed closely because the deformity may recur. Chronic pseudoboutonnière deformities are much more resistant to extension with a safety-pin splint. If the deformity is disabling—usually past 40 degrees of flexion—or if it progresses or is a problem to the athlete, surgery is indicated.

Collateral Ligament Injuries

Collateral ligament injuries to the proximal interphalangeal joint are most common on the radial side of the digit. The proximal attachment of the collateral ligament is avulsed, and the volar plate may be partly or completely ruptured, depending on the magnitude of the injury force. If part of the collateral ligament is intact, as evidenced by some stability, the joint may be splinted in 30 degrees of flexion. The finger is splinted protectively for at least 3 weeks, but active motion exercises may begin at 10 to 14 days after injury. The splint is worn for another 4 to 6 weeks during athletic activity or until the joint becomes asymptomatic.

The treatment of choice for complete collateral ligament tears at the proximal interphalangeal joint is controversial. Some surgeons maintain that nonoperative treatment is satisfactory; however, the proximal end of the ligament frequently folds into the joint at the time of injury and remains stuck there. Thus, closed treatment often leaves the athlete with a swollen, tender, and unstable joint susceptible to further injury and prone to develop degenerative changes.

Surgery allows inspection of the joint and repair of the torn ligament. The surgeon must, of course, be well versed in surgery of the hand, or further damage may result from the operation. Reconstructive surgery may be needed in chronic cases, but the results are less satisfactory and less predictable than after a primary repair.

Fractures of the Middle Phalanx

Fractures of the middle phalanx are usually slow healing, oblique, or transverse through the hard cortical bone in the narrow waist of the shaft. The central slip of the extensor tendon inserts dorsally into the base of the middle phalanx, whereas the two slips of the flexor digitorum sublimis insert further distally into the volar surface of the shaft. This anatomy accounts for the characteristic deformities seen in the fractures.

The most common fracture site is distal to both insertions. In these, the stronger flexor sublimis tendon flexes the proximal fragment. Longitudinal traction and flexion of the distal fragment align the fracture, especially if there is an intact periosteal bridge. When a fracture occurs more proximally in the shaft, between the central slip of the extensor tendon and the insertion of the flexor digitorum sublimis, the proximal fragment will be extended and the distal fragment flexed. These fractures are reduced with longitudinal traction without flexion.

Fractures of the middle phalanx are held in a splint for about 3 weeks, whereupon exercises are begun. When the athlete is engaged in athletic competition, however, the splint must be worn for 6 to 8 more weeks or until the fracture is healed completely. Unstable fractures are fixed with percutaneous K wires and protected similarly. Occasionally, when satisfactory alignment cannot be obtained by closed means, open reduction and internal fixation are needed.

Avulsion of the Flexor Digitorum Profundus

Avulsion of the flexor digitorum profundus, "football finger," is more common than was earlier thought (7,13,44,91). The injury was misdiagnosed after or missed entirely, but increased suspicion and thorough examinations have led to an appreciation of its true incidence. The injury may occur in any digit but is most common in the ring finger. When a football player grabs an opponent's jersey, his little finger may slip, leaving only his ring finger holding on, the finger least able to be extended independently. The pull of the jersey forcibly extends the distal phalanx while the finger is being flexed actively. As a result, the flexor digitorum profundus is pulled from its insertion on the distal phalanx.

Even though the flexor digitorum is avulsed, it does not produce a diagnostic deformity. The examiner may decide wrongly that the athlete's inability to flex the tip of his finger is due to the marked soft tissue swelling and pain. The athlete's grip is weak and his proximal interphalangeal joint motion limited. The examiner should feel for a tender mass where the avulsed tendon has reacted into the proximal part of the finger or into the palm. X-ray films may show a small, avulsed fragment of bone.

The three common levels of retraction of the profundus tendon depend on the force of the avulsion. The least retraction occurs with an avulsion fracture of the volar lip of the distal phalanx as the volar plate remains attached to the fracture fragment. The plate tethers the flexor tendon near the distal interphalangeal joint to prevent further retraction. Greater force produces an avulsion of the tendon itself, which retracts to the level of the hiatus of the flexor digitorum sublimis and is held there by the vinculum longum. Intense force will completely avulse the tendon, and it will retract up into the palm.

The surgeon who treats these injuries must be familiar with the principles of hand surgery and well versed in the techniques of flexor tendon repair. Treatment must be individualized and adapted to each situation. In injuries that cause a large fracture through the volar lip of the distal phalanx with the volar plate attached, the fracture fragment is replaced. This reestablishes the continuity of the flexor digitorum profundus tendon. Postoperatively the finger is splinted in flexion for 3 weeks. The athlete then begins protected range-of-motion exercises, and the finger is splinted for another 2 weeks.

If the tendon has retracted to the hiatus, it still may be reattached for up to 3 weeks after the initial injury, and in some cases up to 6 weeks. If the injury is missed or neglected for a longer time, however, contractures will necessitate a secondary reconstructive procedure. When the tendon has retracted all the way into the palm, it may be reattached if the athlete is seen within 7 to 10 days after injury. However, the complete retraction of a sublimis tendon may disrupt its blood through the vinculum longum, and the tendon may die. By 10 days after these injuries, contractures develop, and a secondary repair is then indicated. The surgeon uses a free tendon graft because a primary repair at this time would result in a permanent flexion contracture of the digit. In reconstructing the tendon, any method that entails acute flexion of the finger must be avoided because this would produce a flexion contracture. For some surgeons, a fusion of the distal joint may be the treatment of choice. A solidly fused, pain-free distal interphalangeal joint at the end of a proximal interphalangeal joint that has a normal range of motion is far better than a stiff finger.

Distal Interphalangeal Joint Dislocation

In the usual dislocation of the distal interphalangeal joint, the phalanx dislocates dorsally. The injured athlete or a teammate usually reduces the dislocation by traction and manipulation before the athletic trainer or doctor sees it. After the reduction, the distal interphalangeal joint is generally stable; however, collateral ligament damage or interposition of the volar plate must be checked for carefully. After the dislocation has been reduced, a splint is worn during athletic activity for at least 3 more weeks or until tenderness is gone and a good range of motion regained.

Volar dislocations of the distal phalanx are much less common than dorsal ones. They are associated with damage to the extensor tendon mechanism or fracture of the dorsal lip of the distal phalanx. Open wounds are not uncommon with distal interphalangeal joint dislocations; they are cleaned and closed whenever possible and treated appropriately to prevent infection.

Injuries to the Extensor Mechanism of the Distal Interphalangeal Joint

Extensor mechanism injuries at the distal interphalangeal joint are common in athletics, expecially in football receivers, baseball catchers or fielders, and basketball players (Fig. 12.18). Compared to flexor tendon injuries, however, these extensor mechanism injuries are often inappropriately minimized. Two types of forces may cause extensor mechanism injuries: An extrinsic force can flex the distal interphalangeal joint against the active contraction of the extensor mechanism and rupture the extensor mechanism; and an extrinsic hyperextension can compress the athlete's distal phalanx against the middle phalanx. The middle phalanx then acts like an anvil to break off a large fragment of the articular surface, disrupting the extensor mechanism. In any type of drop finger deformity, the proximal interphalangeal joint must be examined clinically and roentgenographically. An injury to this joint frequently accompanies a drop finger injury and may result in serious residual disability if unrecognized and untreated.

The extensor tendon most commonly ruptures at the insertion of its conjoint tendon into the base of the distal phalanx to produce a "mallet" or drop finger deformity. The flexion deformity of the distal interphalangeal joint is, in many cases, associated with a hyperextension deformity of the proximal interphalangel joint (1). The proximal interphalangeal joint deformity develops after the central slip of the extensor mechanism has been disrupted distally. As the athlete repeatedly attempts to extend the distal interphalangeal joint, there is increased extension at the middle joint, with resultant dorsal subluxation of the lateral bands and a stretching of the volar plate. The intrinsic muscles thus gain a mechanical advantage, and the deformity increases. The flexor digitorum profundus, now lacking an antagonist at the distal joint, is placed under increased tension owing to the hyperextension of the middle joint. This gain in the mechanical advantage of the profundus produces an even greater flexion force across the distal joint.

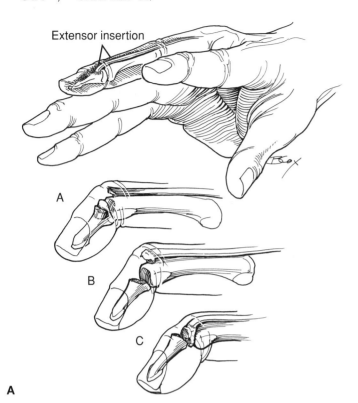

Extensor insertion

A

B

C

A

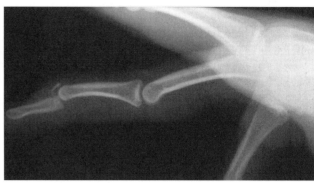

B

FIG. 12.18. A. The extensor mechanism may be disrupted at the distal phalanx by being stretched or torn. **B.** A bony fragment may be avulsed, or in the young, a fracture may occur at the growth plate.

There are several distinct anatomic types of distal interphalangeal joint extensor mechanism injuries, and the treatment needed depends on the type of injury. In some instances, the fibers of the extensor mechanism have been stretched and attenuated without being divided completely. In other cases, the tendon itself may rupture or may be avulsed from the base of the distal phalanx without any bony involvement. The tendon may also be avulsed with a small fragment of bone attached to it. This bony fragment appears on the x-ray film and may be used to localize the distal end of the retracted tendon.

A fracture may involve the articular surface of the distal phalanx. The fragment is usually large enough to affect the collateral ligaments of the distal interphalangeal joint and allow volar subluxation of the distal fragment in addition to the dropped finger deformity. Children may sustain a fracture-dislocation through the growth plate, which often involves the nail bed. The nail bed must be replaced to prevent later deformity and to facilitate healing.

A mallet finger, particularly in a young athlete, is usually treated by splinting alone if a large fragment of bone has not been avulsed. Stretching injuries often correct with time, but reinjury with complete rupture is a danger; thus they are treated like true ruptures. The distal joint is splinted in full extension or very slight hyperextension. If the distal joint were placed in extreme hyperextension, the blood supply to the skin might be impaired, resulting in a skin slough over the distal joint. Immobilization of the distal joint alone is satisfactory, allowing increased use of the hand and preventing proximal interphalangeal

joint problems that follow use of a longer splint. We have used this method successfully to treat mallet fingers that were first seen up to 12 weeks after the injury had taken place.

An athlete may continue to participate in sports with the finger splinted. We use either a custom-molded aluminum splint covered with moleskin or a thermoplastic orthoplast splint. The splint is worn continuously for 6 to 8 weeks and then for an additional 6 to 8 weeks only during athletics. The splint may be placed either volarly or dorsally. A dorsal splint allows more fingertip sensitivity, which is particularly important for football receivers and basketball players. The splint must be kept dry to prevent skin maceration and should be checked at regular intervals. When the splint is changed, however, the finger must not be allowed to drop down into any flexion.

When the articular surface of the distal joint is involved significantly, an open anatomic reduction with internal fixation is needed to correct the deformity, forestall volar subluxation, and prevent later traumatic arthritis. If there is any question about being able to maintain the splint properly, a thin wire is passed across the distal joint as an adjunct to the splint. The pin is removed after 4 weeks, but the finger must be splinted for an additional 3 to 4 weeks during athletic activity.

If an untreated drop finger is disabling to the athlete, a secondary surgical reconstruction may be indicated. Although these procedures are not technically difficult, the results are not entirely predictable. A good alternative for the symptomatic athlete is a fusion of the distal interphalangeal joint.

Fractures of the Distal Phalanx

Fractures of the distal phalanx mostly are direct crush injuries and usually are not displaced. If the fragments are displaced, the displacement is due to the initial traumatic force, since no deforming tendons span the fracture site. The distal phalanx is covered dorsally by the nail bed, which rests directly on the periosteum, and volarly by the fingertip pulp.

Undisplaced fractures of the distal phalanx are treated with a compressive dressing and splint. A painful subungual hematoma can be drained aseptically by piercing the nail with a heated paper clip. If the fracture of the distal phalanx is a displaced one, the nail and matrix may be disrupted. The matrix may lodge between the fracture fragments, block healing, and even cause a nonunion. A disrupted nail matrix must be replaced and repaired anatomically to allow proper healing and to prevent a nail deformity. The edges of the nail bed are approximated and repaired with fine absorbable sutures.

A nondisplaced nail may be used as a splint but should be removed unhesitatingly if the nail bed needs to be repaired. In addition, a nail may act as a foreign body or as a sequestrum. Although a nonunion is unusual in this area, it may occur, and reconstruction may be needed.

Hand Blisters and Calluses

Friction of the palm may cause blisters, which are collections of fluid between separated layers of epidermis, or produce calluses, which are protective build-ups of epidermis at friction areas.

During the season, calluses build up on a gymnast's hands (6). They should be kept trimmed or else will catch on the equipment and rip. They may be shaved down with a safety razor or reduced with sandpaper or a callus file. Ideally, calluses should be trimmed to the level of the surrounding skin. If they are completely removed, the underlying skin will be left tender and may tear.

Gymnasts follow a daily routine of cleansing and moisturizing their hands and controlling calluses. To keep rips to a minimum, a gymnast changes apparatus if his or her hands begin to feel hot from friction. If the hands begin to feel hot while working on parallel bars, for example, he or she may switch to floor exercises to rest his hands. After a workout, he washes his hands to remove the gym chalk, which would otherwise dry his skin and increase its susceptibility to blisters and rips. He also applies a hand cream or a glycerin-based massage lotion a few times daily.

A gymnast's hands need protection, but to perform well he must have a feel between his hands and the bar. A leather hand protector may be worn, or one may be fashioned out of tape. Holes are cut through the elastic tape for the index and middle fingers, and the tape is placed

---

BOX 2:
Rehabilitation Progression for the Fingers

OBJECTIVES

- To strengthen flexors and extensors to normal. Tone is more important than strength.
- *Flexibility:* Flexibility is more important than strength. The MP, PIP, and DIP joints should be worked individually.
- *Endurance:* Athletes should seek more synchronous motion.

STAGES

- Initial
    Ice and active range of motion in an ice cup. Splinting as necessary (Table 12.1).
- Intermediate
    Isolated active and passive joint motion with the uninvolved joints stabilized.
- Advanced
    Grip-strengthening exercises such as gathering and squeezing a bicycle inner tube, winding a wrist roller, or climbing a rope.

---

over his benzoin-coated palm. The elastic tape is anchored at the wrist with adhesive tape and can be chalked with magnesium carbonate.

If the skin rips, it should be cleaned and an antiseptic applied. The skin should then be kept clean and should be moistened with massage lotion to decrease the chance of the underlying skin's cracking.

Weight lifters suffer blisters, especially when they use a bar that has deep knurling. Blisters may also trouble baseball pitchers (75). A curve ball may cause a blister to form on a pitcher's thumb, and a fast ball may cause blistering on his fingertips. Although blisters on his fingertips indicate that the pitcher is releasing the ball correctly, they can certainly interfere with his throwing.

To prevent finger blisters, ballplayers can apply benzoin to their fingers, especially during layoffs from pitching. All players are advised to report blisters early because an ice cube applied to a hot spot or to a blister may reduce the formation of fluid. A blister may also be aspirated sterilely. If a blister tears, it is cleaned, and the shreds are removed. The main covering is then replaced and attached with benzoin adherent (61).

Gloves for Athletes

Gloves protect an athlete's hands. Lacrosse gloves have a flexible thumb and extra padding over the scaphoid. The palm is open so that the lacrosse player has a feel

TABLE 12.1. *Splinting of finger injuries*

Injury	Constant splinting (wk)	When to begin motion (wk)	Splinting during competition (wk)	Joint position
MP fractures	3	3	+4–6	30° flexion
Phalangeal fractures	4–6	4–6	+3	N/A
DIP, PIP fractures	9–11	3	+3	30° flexion
DIP and PIP dislocations	3	3	+3	30° flexion
Boutonnière deformity	6–8	6–8	+6–8	PIP in extension; DIP, MP not included
Volar plate injuries	5	3	+3	30° flexion
Collateral ligament	3	2	+4–6	30° flexion
FDP repair	3	3	+3	
Mallet finger	9	9	+3	Slight DIP hyperextension

From Gieck JH, McCue FC III. Splinting of finger injuries. *Athletic Training* 1978;17:215.

for the stick. To gain an even better feel for the stick, some players cut out the fingers of their gloves up to their fingertips, but a finger may then slip out and be injured.

The baseball catcher's mitt is now flexible so that the catcher may catch one-handed, thus protecting his ungloved hand from damage. The catcher may wear a pad inside his mitt to absorb shocks and to help prevent thromboses or aneurysms of the radial and ulnar arteries. An aneurysm occurs most commonly at the hook of the hamate where the vessels are least protected.

The boxer's glove is actually a mitten, since the thumb is separated from the other fingers. An extra pad guards the thumb, and a firm leather pad in the palm of the glove supports all four finger metacarpals. Football linemen wear boxing gloves and linebackers wear gloves that leave their fingers free so they can intercept passes. Skiers should *not* wear short gloves. A young skier's gloves should be checked to be sure that he or she has not outgrown them, leaving the wrists susceptible to a sharp ski edge. Long ski gloves protect a skier's wrists from cuts from a ski edge.

Platform tennis enthusiasts, who play in cold weather, may wear a mitten or a wool sock that has a hole cut in it to receive the handle of the paddle. While wearing this ingenious glove, the player's hand stays warm, yet he or she retains a feel for the paddle.

Still other athletes use gloves. Cyclists may use cycling gloves or, alternatively, pad their handlebars to avoid pressure on the ulnar nerve as it passes through the canal of Guyon. Fencers use a gauntlet to protect their wrists from blows. Wheelchair racers wear gloves to prevent possible damage to hands that have impaired sensations. Tennis or racketball players may wear light, cotton gloves inside outer gloves to prevent skin irritation when the player sweats. They should carry a number of these as replacements when one pair becomes wet.

REFERENCES

1. Adams JE. Injury to the throwing arm: a study of traumatic changes in the elbow joints of boy baseball players. *Calif Med* 1965;102:127–132.
2. Albright JA. Clinical study of baseball pitchers: correlation of injury to the throwing arm with method of delivery. *Am J Sports Med* 1978;6:15–21.
3. Bassett FH, Malone T, Gilchrist RA. A protective splint of silicone rubber. *Am J Sports Med* 1979;7:358–360.
4. Bennett GE. Shoulder and elbow lesions of the professional baseball pitcher. *JAMA* 1941;117:510–514.
5. Berg K. Prevention of tennis elbow through conditioning. *Phys Sportsmed* 1977;5(2):110.
6. Black SA. Blistered and torn hands disrupt gymnast's straining. *First Aider, Cramer* 1979;48(6):10–11.
7. Blazina ME, Lane C. Rupture of the insertion of the flexor digitorum profundus tendon in student athletes. *J Am Coll Health Assoc* 1966;14:248,249.
8. Brogdon BG, Crow NE. Little Leaguer's elbow. *Am J Roentgenol* 1960;83:671–675.
9. Browne EZ Jr, Dunn HK, Snyder CC. Ski pole thumb injury. *Plast Reconst Surg* 1976;58:17–23.
10. Brown R, Blazina ME, Kerlan RK, et al. Osteochondritis of the capitellum. *Am J Sports Med* 1974;2:27–46.
11. Buckhout BC, Warner MA. Digital perfusion of handball players: effects of repeated ball impact on structures of the hand. *Am J Sports Med* 1980;8:206,207.
12. Burton RI, Eaton RG. Common hand injuries in the athlete. *Orthop Clin North Am* 1973;4:809–838.
13. Carroll RE, Match RM. Avulsion of the flexor profundus tendon insertion. *J Trauma* 1970;10:1109–1118.
14. Commandre F, Viani JL. The football keeper's thumb. *J Sport Med Phys Fitness* 1976;16:121,122.
15. Curtin J, Kay NR. Hand injuries due to soccer. *Hand* 1976;8:93–95.
16. Danek E. Martial arts: the sound of one hand chopping. *Phys Sportsmed* 1979;7(3):140,141.
17. Dangles CJ, Bilos ZJ. Ulnar nerve neuritis in a world champion weightlifter. a case report. *Am J Sports Med* 1980;8:443–445.
18. DeHaven KE, Evarts CM. Throwing injuries of the elbow in athletes. *Orthop Clin North Am* 1973;4:801–808.
19. Dobyns JH, O'Brien ET, Linscheid RL, Farrow GM. Bowler's thumb: diagnosis and treatment: a review of seventeen cases. *J Bone Joint Surg (Am)* 1972;54:751–755.
20. Dunham W, Haines G, Spring JW. Bowler's thumb. *Clin Orthop* 1972;83:99–101.
21. Ellsasser JC, Stein AH. Management of hand injuries in a professional football team. *Am J Sports Med* 1979;7:178–182.
22. Farnum S. Traumatic bursitis. *Phys Sportsmed* 1978;6(5):147.
23. Francis R, Bunch T, Chandler B. Little League elbow: a decade later. *Phys Sportsmed* 1978;6(4):88–94.
24. Froimson AI. Treatment of tennis elbow with forearm support band. *J Bone Joint Surg (Am)* 1971;53:183,184.
25. Gamekeeper's thumb on the ski slopes (editorial). *Br Med* 1974;1:213–214.
26. Ganel A, Aharonson Z, Engel J. Gamekeeper's thumb: injuries of the ulnar collateral ligament of the metacarpophalangeal joint. *Br J Sports Med* 1980;14(2–3):92–96.

27. Gardner RC. Hypertrophic infiltrative tendinitis (HIT syndrome) of the long extensor. The abused karate hand. *JAMA* 1970;211:1009–1010.

28. Grana WA, Rashkin A. Pitcher's elbow in adolescents. *Am J Sports Med* 1980;8:333–336.

29. Grenier R, Rouleau C. Boxer's elbow: an extension and hyperextension injury. *Am J Sports Med* 1976;3:282–287.

30. Gruchow HW, Pelletier D. An epidemiologic study of tennis elbow: incidence, recurrence and effectiveness of prevention strategies. *Am J Sports Med* 1979;7:234–238.

31. Gugenheim JJ, Stanley RF, Woods GW, Tullos HS. Little League survey: the Houston study. *Am J Sports Med* 1976;4:189–200.

32. Gunn CC, Milbrandt WE. Tennis elbow and the cervical spine. *Can Med Assoc J* 1976;114:803–809.

33. Harris G. Elbow flexion strap for dislocated elbows. *Athletic Training* 1978;13(1):12.

34. Indelicato PA, Jobe FW, Kerlan RK. Correctable elbow lesions in professional baseball players: a review of 25 cases. *Am J Sports Med* 1979;7:72–75.

35. Kelly DW, Pitt MJ, Mayer DA. Index metacarpal fractures in karate. *Phys Sportmed* 1980;8(3):103–106.

36. King JW, Brelsford HJ, Tullos HS. Analysis of the pitching arm of the professional baseball pitcher. *Clin Orthop* 1969;67:116–123.

37. Kisner WH. Thumb neuroma: a hazard of ten pin bowling. *Br J Plast Surg* 1976;29:225,226.

38. Kulund DN, Brubaker CE. Injuries in the Bikecentennial Tour. *Phys Sportsmed* 1978;6(6):74–78.

39. Kulund DN, Rockwell DA, Brubaker CE. The long term effects of playing tennis. *Phys Sportsmed* 1979;7(4):87–94.

40. Kulund DN, McCue FC, Rockwell DA, Gieck JH. Tennis injuries: prevention and treatment. *Am J Sports Med* 1979;7:749–753.

41. Larose JH, Sik KD. Karate hand-conditioning. *Med Sci Sports* 1969;1(2):95–98.

42. Larson RL, Singer KM, Bergstrom R, Thomas S. Little League survey: the Eugene study. *Am J Sports Med* 1976;4:201–209.

43. Leach RE, Wasilewski S. Olecranon bursitis (dart thrower's elbow): a case report illustrating overuse/abuse in the sport of darts. *Am J Sports Med* 1979;7:299.

44. Leddy JP, Packer JW. Avulsion of the profundus tendon insertion in athletes. *J Hand Surg* 1977;2:66–69.

45. Linscheid RL, Dobyns JH. Athletic injuries of the wrist. *Clin Ortho* December 1985;198:141.

46. Lipscomb AB. Baseball pitching injuries in growing athletes. *Am J Sports Med* 1975;3:25–34.

47. Marmor L. Bowler's thumb. *J Trauma* 1966;6:282–284.

48. Marmor LL. Bowler's thumb. *J Bone Joint Surg (Am)* 1970;52:379–381.

49. McCue FC III, Abbott JL. The treatment of mallet finger and boutonniere deformities. *Va Med Monthly* 1967;94:623.

50. McCue FC III, Honner R, Johnson MC, Gieck JH. Athletic injuries of the promixal interphalangeal joint requiring surgical treatment. *J Bone Joint Surg (Am)* 1970;52:937–956.

51. McCue FC III, Hakala MW, Andrews JR, Gieck JH. Ulnar collateral ligament of the thumb in athletes. *Am J Sports Med* 1974;2:270.

52. McCue FC III, Hakala MW, Andrews JR, Gieck JH. Ulnar collateral ligament of the thumb in athletics. *Am J Sports Med* 1975;2:70–80.

53. McCue FC III, Baugher WH, Kulund DN, Gieck JH. Hand injuries in athletics. *Am J Sports Med* 1979;7:275–286.

54. Menon J, Wood VE, Schoene HR, Frykman GK, Hohl JC, Bestard EA. Isolated tears of the triangular fibrocartilage of the wrist: results of partial excision. *J Hand Surg* 1984;9A(4):527–530.

55. Miller JE. Javelin thrower's elbow. *J Bone Joint Surg (Br)* 1960;42:788–792.

56. Nagle DJ. Arthroscopic treatment of degenerative tears of the triangular fibrocartilage. *Basic Wrist Arthros and Endos* 1994;10(4):615–624.

57. Norell HG. Roentgenologic visualization of the extracapsular fat: its importance in the diagnosis of traumatic injuries to the elbow. *Acta Radiol* 1954;42:205–210.

58. North ER. An anatomic guide for arthroscopic visualization of the wrist capsular ligaments. *J Hand Surg* 1988;13:815–820.

59. Palmieri TJ. Pisiform area pain treated by pisiform excision. *J Hand Surg* 1982;7:477–480.

60. Priest JD, Jones HH, Nagel DA. Elbow injuries in highly skilled tennis players. *Am J Sports Med* 1974;2:137–149.

61. Raymond P. Care of the hands. *Oarsman* 1977;9(2):40–41.

62. Reef TC. Avulsion of the flexor digitorum profundus: an athletic injury. *Am J Sports Med* 1977;5:281–285.

63. Reichelderfer TE, et al. Skateboard policy statement. *Pediatrics* 1979;63:924–925.

64. Roles NC, Maridsley RH. Radial tunnel syndrome: resistant tennis elbow as a nerve entrapment. *J Bone Joint Surg (Br)* 1972;54:499–508.

65. Rovere GD, Gristina AG, Stolzer WA, Garver EM. Treatment of gamekeeper's thumb in hockey players. *Am J Sports Med* 1975;3:147–151.

66. Ryan AJ (moderator). Round table: prevention and treatment of tennis elbow. *Phys Sportsmed* 1977;5(2):33–54.

67. Savastano AA, Kamionek S, Knowles K, Gibson T. Treatment of resistant tennis elbow by a combined surgical procedure. *Int Surg* 1972;57:470–474.

68. Siegel IM. Bowling thumb neuroma. *JAMA* 1965;192:163.

69. Stolle F. How to put topspin on your backhand. *World Tennis* 1980;27:85–88.

70. Steetong JA. Traumatic hemoglobinurina caused by karate exercises. *Lancet* 1967;2:191.

71. Terrill RQ. Use of arthroscopy in the evaluation and treatment of chronic wrist pain. *Basix Wrist Arthr and Endos* 1994;10(4):593–603.

72. Torg JS, Pollack H, Sweterlitsch P. The effect of competitive pitching on the shoulders and elbows of preadolescent baseball players. *Pediatrics* 1972;49:267–272.

73. Torisu T. Fracture of the hook of the hamate by a golfswing. *Clin Orthop* 1972;83:91–94.

74. Tullos HS. Unusual lesions of the pitching arm. *Clin Orthop* 1972;88:169–182.

75. Vere-Hodge N. Injuries in cricket. In: Armstrong JR, Tuckers WE eds. *Injury in sport.* Springfield, IL: Charles C Thomas, 1964:168–171.

76. Waris W. Elbow injuries of javelin throwers. *Acta Chir Scand* 1946;93:563–575.

77. Whipple TL. The role of arthroscopy in the treatment of wrist injuries in the athlete. *Clin Sports Med* 1992;11(1):227–238.

78. Williams JGP. Surgical management of traumatic common noninfective tenosynovitis of the wrist extensors. *J Bone Joint Surg (Br)* 1977;59:408–412.

79. Wilson FD, Andrews JR, Blackburn TA, McCluskey G. Valgus extension overload in the pitching elbow. *Am J Sports Med* 1983;2(2):83–88.

80. Woods W, Tullos HS. Elbow instability and medial epicondyle fractures. *Am J Sports Med* 1977;5:23–30.

81. Zlatkin MB, Chao PC, Osterman AL, Schnall MD, Dalinka MK, Kressel HY. Chronic wrist pain: evaluation with high-resolution MR imaging. *Radiology* 1989;173:723–726.

The Injured Athlete, Third Edition,
edited by D. H. Perrin.
Lippincott–Raven Publishers, Philadelphia © 1999.

CHAPTER 13

The Back

David M. Kahler

The five vertebrae of the lumbar spine must transmit all of the compressive, bending, and twisting forces generated between the upper and lower body. Modern sporting activities often generate forces of sufficient magnitude to injure the normal lumbar spine and its supporting structures. For this reason, back pain is an exceedingly common complaint among athletes. Episodes of back pain are usually related to an acute traumatic event or to overuse, and ordinarily resolve within a few days or weeks, with or without treatment. Athletes with persistent low back pain, however, will usually be found to have an acquired condition or structural problem that accounts for their pain. As with all other medical conditions, effective treatment relies on first obtaining an accurate diagnosis. Certain sporting activities are associated with characteristic acquired lesions; this knowledge, when combined with a thorough history and physical examination, will often dictate when to refer an athlete for further testing. Most causes of back pain in athletes can be treated nonsurgically if they are identified early and treated appropriately.

Back pain is an extremely common cause of disability in the modern world. About 80% of all Americans will experience an episode of low back pain severe enough to cause them to seek treatment. Four percent of all laborers will miss more than 6 months of work during their careers because of disabling back pain. In 1980, back pain accounted for 123 million lost days of work in the United States (2).

One of the most frustrating aspects in treating back pain is the difficulty in arriving at an accurate diagnosis. Historically, it has been possible to positively identify an anatomic cause of pain in about only 10% to 20% of adult patients with job-related low back pain. Although modern imaging modalities such as magnetic resonance imaging (MRI) have greatly improved our ability to iden-

tify abnormalities such as degenerative disks, we still have difficulty in determining whether the abnormality found on the imaging study is truly the source of the pain. A great many of the surgical procedures performed for excision of herniated or bulging intervertebral disks fail to relieve the patient's back pain, and this often leads to subsequent operations in search of the actual source of pain. A variety of social and psychological factors invariably come into play in the assessment of back pain; in the work force, workers' compensation insurance may make it possible for the back pain sufferer to potentially benefit from his disability. These confounding issues have given some clinicians a defeatist and cynical attitude in the treatment of low back pain.

The situation is much different in the athletic population. Athletes generally have little incentive to stay injured; on the contrary, they will often continue to participate in sporting events despite significant pain, and will frequently ignore recommendations to decrease activity while injured. The combination of a delay in diagnosis with an athlete who refuses to restrict activity may result in permanent structural damage in certain conditions. For this reason, the complaint of persistent back pain in an athlete must always be taken seriously. It will be possible to identify an anatomic cause of back pain in a very high percentage of these individuals.

A corollary can be drawn to the treatment of back pain in children. The complaint of back pain in a child is rarely a manifestation of a psychological problem, and is usually related to an identifiable structural disorder. The clinician must therefore be alert to the possibility of a potentially serious underlying condition, such as an infection, tumor, or congenital anomaly. It has been suggested that all prepubertal patients with back pain be subjected to a complete diagnostic workup. This will allow accurate diagnosis in 80% to 90% of subjects (as opposed to 10% to 20% of laborers with chronic back pain), and will prevent a delay in the diagnosis of the more serious conditions (3,6,11,24).

D. M. Kahler: Department of Orthopaedic Surgery, University of Virginia, Charlottesville, Virginia 22908

Careful physical examination and the use of appropriate diagnostic testing will identify the cause of persistent back pain in most athletes. Certain sports and activities are associated with typical injuries. Knowledge of these conditions will allow directed physical examination of the athlete, and selection of appropriate diagnostic studies. Most of the conditions causing back pain in athletes can be treated nonsurgically. Nonetheless, accurate diagnosis allows initiation of specific treatment directed at the actual cause of the pain. The common congenital abnormalities, acquired conditions, and overuse syndromes causing back pain in athletes will be discussed, along with appropriate diagnostic tests and treatment regimens.

ANATOMY AND PATHOGENESIS OF BACK PAIN

The lumbar spine consists of a mobile segment of five vertebrae with the relatively immobile thoracic and sacral segments at either end. The thoracic spine is stabilized by the attached rib cage and intercostal musculature, whereas the sacral segments are fused, providing a stable articulation with the ilium. Thus, the lumbar spine sees a great deal of stress in transmitting loads between the upper body and lower extremities (5). The erect posture assumed by modern man appears to have increased the amount of stress borne by the lumbar spine beyond what it can tolerate over the course of a lifetime. We may not be as highly evolved as we would like to think.

The static stabilizers of the lumbar spine are the soft tissue interconnections between adjacent vertebrae. These specialized structures include the longitudinal ligaments and intervertebral disks between the vertebral bodies, and the facet joint capsules connecting the posterior elements of the spine. The weak spots in these interconnections appear to be the intervertebral disk itself, and a frail portion of the posterior arch known as the pars interarticularis.

The intervertebral disk is made up of two components, the annulus fibrosus and the nucleus pulposus. The annulus is a dense fibrous ring at the periphery of the disk, which has strong attachments to the vertebrae and serves to confine the gelatinous nucleus pulposus. The annulus is a richly innervated structure. Stimulation of the annulus fibrosus through stretching or tearing has been shown to play a large role in the generation of back pain (16,26). During the aging process, the water content of the nucleus pulposus gradually decreases. In childhood, the nucleus pulposus is 88% water, compared with 69% hydration by the eighth decade of life (22). This degenerative process diminishes the cushioning function of the nucleus, and may result in increased transmission of stress to the annulus fibrosus during activity. Degenerative disk disease is presumably the etiology of much of the activity-related back pain experienced by older athletes. Although disk degeneration is inevitable during the aging process, it may be completely asymptomatic.

The pars interarticularis is a relatively weak portion of the posterior vertebral arch. The pars is found bilaterally just inferior to the superior articular facets, and superior to the spinous process. This small area has received a great deal of attention because it is well recognized as a weak area in the axial skeleton. When a defect is found in the pars interarticularis bilaterally, the condition is known as spondylolysis. About 5.8% of the adult population of the United States has such a defect in one of the lower lumbar vertebrae, usually at L-5. The defect is usually fibrocartilage, and is radiolucent, making it visible on plain x-ray studies. There has been some controversy concerning whether spondylolysis represents a congenital or an acquired defect. As the pars interarticularis and posterior spinal elements arise from a single ossification center, it is hard to imagine how a congenital pars defect could occur. Wiltse has presented evidence that isthmic spondylolysis is an acquired lesion secondary to fatigue fracture of the pars interarticularis (32). The incidence of these defects increases precipitously between the ages of 5.5 and 6.5 years of age, and only about 0.8% of the population will acquire a pars defect after this time. There appears to be a genetic predisposition toward acquiring a spondylolytic defect. The defect occurs in response to repetitive stressful activity, particularly hyperextension of the spine (Fig. 13.1). Rarely, a single episode of trauma causes a fracture and subsequent nonunion of the pars interarticularis.

A defect in the pars interarticularis decreases the resistance to shearing forces between adjacent vertebrae. Spondylolisthesis occurs when a vertebral body slips forward relative to the adjacent inferior vertebra. This condition does not occur in everyone who has spondylolysis. It always represents some degree of spinal instability, but does not necessarily preclude participation in sports. The forward slipping of the superior vertebrae (usually L-5 on S-1) is a slow chronic process, and is most likely to progress during the adolescent growth spurt, if at all.

The lumbar spine is essentially surrounded by powerful musculature, which dynamically stabilizes this relatively mobile area of the skeleton. The abdominal musculature can act in concert with the paraspinous muscles to increase the intraabdominal pressure, lending further stability to the spine. The musculature surrounding the lumbar spine effectively prevents direct palpation of the spine during attempted diagnosis of painful conditions. For this reason, physical examination of the painful lower back relies primarily on indirect maneuvers.

The sacroiliac joints are the primary junction between the lower end of the spine and the lower extremities and are a potential source of low back pain. These joints are spanned by the strongest ligaments in the human body, and are rarely sprained despite the heavy loads placed across them. The sacroiliac joints allow a small but sig-

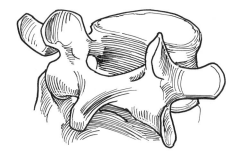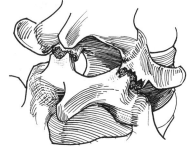

FIG. 13.1. Spondylolysis (*shown at right*) is a nondisplaced fatigue fracture occurring through the relatively weak pars interarticularis. This acquired lesion is more common in athletes subjected to repeated hyperextension of the lumbar spine, such as football linemen. (Adapted from Kuland, DN. *The Injured Athlete,* 1st ed. Philadelphia: JB Lippincott, 1982.)

nificant amount of motion in the first few decades of life, but are essentially immobile in most individuals beyond that time. Athletes with excessive motion in the sacroiliac joints may be prone to sporadic episodes of pain related to heavy activity or overuse. In addition, these joints are particularly susceptible to the inflammatory arthritides that sometimes affect young athletes; symmetrical involvement of the sacroiliac joints should prompt evaluation for an inflammatory condition such as Reiter's syndrome or ankylosing spondylitis. Although many physical therapists focus on the sacroiliac joints during treatment of low back pain, it should be remembered that many conditions cause poorly localized pain in this region.

A variety of intraabdominal processes can cause pain that radiates to the back. Blood or air in the peritoneal cavity from a ruptured abdominal organ causes pain, which typically radiates to the interscapular region. Urinary tract obstruction or infection causes unilateral back or flank pain that radiates to the groin.

Sciatica is caused by irritation of a lumbar or sacral nerve root. Although the pain of sciatica is perceived in the leg, the actual cause of the condition is usually in the back. As the nerve roots exit the spinal canal, they are susceptible to compression by a variety of anatomic structures. A herniated nucleus pulposus or hypertrophied facet joint is the most common culprit. Studies have shown that traction on a normal nerve root is painless, whereas a chronically compressed or inflamed nerve root is very painful when put under stretch (16,26). Although the strict definition of sciatica is pain along the course of the sciatic nerve, the condition is often accompanied by low back pain. The nerve roots and sciatic nerve may also be compressed by muscles, ligaments, or growths distant from the spine.

EVALUATION OF THE ATHLETE WITH LOW BACK PAIN

A thorough history is often more useful than the physical examination in evaluating the athlete with low back

pain. The following should be determined in taking the history:

1. Mechanism of injury and/or sport involved.
2. Duration and severity of symptoms.
3. Aggravating factors (especially hyperextension versus flexion).
4. Radiation of pain into shoulders, groin, buttocks, or legs.
5. Presence of normal bowel, bladder, and sexual function.
6. Numbness or weakness in the lower extremities.
7. Family history of rheumatic conditions.

A careful history helps to direct physical examination and later diagnostic testing. Physical examination of the spine itself is limited to strength and range of motion testing, inspection for asymmetry and spinal alignment, and palpation for spasm or tenderness. Beyond this, the physical exam is used to rule out or confirm the presence of signs indicative of other system involvement. Nerve root impingement is tested for by using the straight leg raising test, which puts traction on the nerve roots. A careful neurologic examination of the lower extremities is performed to rule out neurologic deficits. The hamstrings should be assessed for abnormal tightness. The sacroiliac joint may be stressed through the "FABER" maneuver (flexion, abduction, and external rotation) in an attempt to elicit pain. Palpation of the abdomen is done to search for a possible visceral cause of back pain. The patient should be observed during forward bending to look for the characteristic rib hump of scoliosis. And finally, the patient should be assessed for subtle leg-length discrepancy by ensuring that the pelvis is level during stance.

Diagnostic Testing

Plain x-rays are best used in looking for acute fractures, pars defects, arthritic changes, and congenital or neoplastic processes involving the bony portion of the spine. Radiography of the spine requires a substantial amount of radiation in order to penetrate the surrounding soft tissues. It is not cost effective to initially obtain plain x-rays on every patient who complains of back pain, unless an acute fracture is suspected. If the pain is severe, well localized, and interfering with ambulation, or if a neurologic deficit is present, then a lumbar spine series should be obtained acutely. Back pain that is consistent and persists for several weeks should almost always be evaluated with x-rays.

The Technetium bone scan may assist in localizing a painful lesion. There are two situations in which the bone scan is extremely useful. First, when plain x-rays initially appear normal, the bone scan may identify a stress reaction or a subtle lesion that was not visible or obvious on screening radiographs. Second, when a skeletal abnormality is seen on plain films, a ''hot'' bone scan serves to confirm that the lesion is acute or active, and a likely cause for the pain.

Computed tomography (CT) is an excellent modality for evaluating the bony skeleton. Although CT has also been used for evaluating soft tissues, the CT scan has been largely replaced by MRI for visualization of disks, neural structures, and other soft tissues. MRI utilizes a strong electromagnetic field for imaging, and this is felt to be safer than the ionizing radiation used for x-rays and CT. The widespread availability of MRI has greatly decreased the use of myelography in the evaluation of nerve root impingement. In the athlete with significant back pain but with normal x-rays and bone scan, our current policy is to proceed with MRI scanning.

There is now good evidence that the stress of athletic participation may cause significant changes in the immature lumbar spine. Using MRI, it is possible to demonstrate anatomic changes in the spine in both athletes and nonathletes during terminal skeletal growth, and most of these changes are demonstrated following injury or athletic participation (15). It has been suggested that excessive loading that puts the back at risk of acute injury during the pubertal growth spurt may be harmful. The significance of the changes seen on routine MRI surveillance remains to be determined.

When nerve root impingement is suspected, electromyography (EMG) is sometimes helpful in confirming the level of nerve compression. EMG can differentiate between compression of the nerve root itself and more distal compression of a peripheral nerve, and may also give information regarding the chronicity of the condition.

COMMON CAUSES OF BACK PAIN IN ATHLETES

The following is by no means an exhaustive listing of all of the possible causes of back pain in athletes. Most of the treatable causes of back pain occur in young athletes, particularly during the adolescent growth spurt. As athletes age, the natural process of disk degeneration becomes more and more prominent in the etiology of back pain, and transient pain is often seen in response to overuse and poor conditioning. For this reason, much of the discussion to follow will deal with back pain in young athletes. This is not to suggest that the older athlete be denied the same care in diagnosis and treatment afforded to the young athlete with back pain.

Acute Fractures

The common acute spinal fractures seen in athletes are compression or vertebral end-plate fractures because of sudden axial loading, transverse process avulsion by the origin of the psoas major, spinous process avulsions, and acute fracture of the pars interarticularis from hyperextension. Radiography is the best method for diagnosis of these injuries; more expensive diagnostic testing is reserved for those cases in which the chronicity of the lesion is in question, or when nerve root impingement is suspected based on physical examination.

Vertebral body compression fractures are more common in athletes with decreased bone density because of disease, exercise-associated amenorrhea, or advanced age. This type of injury generally requires only bracing or rest if the angulation is minimal, but may cause spinal cord or cauda equina compression if the posterior aspect of the vertebral body is driven into the spinal canal. These more serious burst fractures demand cross-sectional diagnostic imaging, and may require surgery for decompression of neural structures and stabilization of the involved levels. The adolescent athlete with a vertebral end-plate fracture (Schmorl's node) or apophyseal avulsion fracture usually requires only accurate diagnosis and a period of rest.

The relatively innocuous appearance of the transverse process avulsion fracture may be misleading. These fractures may cause significant bleeding into the retroperitoneal space, resulting in decreased hematocrit, ileus (cessation of intestinal motility), and in rare cases hypotension and shock. A blood count should be obtained at the time of diagnosis, and repeated if the athlete shows any signs of retroperitoneal bleeding (tachycardia, orthostasis, or a silent abdomen).

Spinous process avulsion fractures are most common in the cervical spine (clay shoveler's fracture), but may also occur in the lumbar spine. They occasionally result from direct trauma, but are most commonly the result of forcible flexion and rotation. These injuries are not associated with neurologic dysfunction unless the posterior neural arch is involved.

Stress reactions and fractures of the pars interarticularis will be discussed in the next section.

Stress Reaction of the Pars Interarticularis

The growing athlete is particularly susceptible to a variety of conditions that result in the perception of back pain. Micheli feels that a majority of adolescents with back pain are suffering from traction injuries to the muscles and ligaments surrounding the spine (18). During periods of rapid growth, the skeleton may grow faster than the soft tissues, resulting in relative inflexibility and increased susceptibility to injury. A similar situation is seen in the poorly conditioned older athlete who has not maintained flexibility. These conditions usually cause sporadic pain that does not generally prevent participation in sports.

Although soft tissue injuries are a common cause of transient pain, they should not be automatically blamed for chronic pain in the young athlete. This age group is more susceptible to rare but serious conditions such as disk space infection and skeletal neoplasia. The most common significant cause of back pain in the skeletally immature athlete is related to the relative weakness of the pars interarticularis of L-5 (19). Knowledge of this simple fact will enable early diagnosis and treatment of the athlete with a stress reaction or fatigue fracture of the pars, and may potentially prevent the development of spinal instability and its attendant sequelae.

Sports that cause frequent hyperextension of the lumbar spine place undue stresses on the pars interarticularis. Jackson et al. published a well-known study that showed that female gymnasts have an incidence of pars defects four times greater than the general population (13). This is presumably the result of gymnastic maneuvers that load the spine in hyperextension (dismounts, back walkovers, and aerials). Three of 100 patients who requested treatment in the above series had negative x-rays initially, but went on to develop frank defects of the pars interarticularis following continued participation in gymnastics. It is quite likely that the initial cause of pain in these athletes was a stress reaction of the pars.

The stress reaction of the pars interarticularis should be thought of as an impending stress fracture; it is a treatable condition, and proper treatment may allow healing of the lesion and prevent progression to spondylolysis or spondylolisthesis. The longer the condition goes without accurate diagnosis, the less likely it is to respond to treatment. No competent clinician would allow an impending stress fracture of the femoral neck to become a complete fracture prior to initiating treatment; the stress reaction of the pars should be treated just as aggressively.

When a pars stress reaction is suspected, and plain x-rays of the lumbar spine are negative, the next diagnostic step is radionuclide bone scanning. The Technetium bone scan is minimally invasive, and exposes the patient to a very small dose of radiation. Any area of increased bone turnover is identified by bone scanning, and for this reason, the test is relatively nonspecific. This is particularly true in the growing skeleton, in which normal intense uptake in growth plates may obscure the abnormal uptake of a pathologic process. A diagnosis is rarely made on the basis of a bone scan alone, but a positive scan often helps to direct further evaluation of a specific area of the skeleton. In a patient with normal lumbar spine radiographs, a focal area of increased tracer uptake in the posterior elements of a lower lumbar vertebrae is consistent with a stress reaction of the pars interarticularis.

Computed tomographic bone scintigraphy (SPECT) has gained popularity in diagnosing stress reactions. This modality allows better localization of uptake in the posterior elements. A recent study showed that SPECT was almost twice as sensitive as conventional bone scanning in identifying focal abnormalities of the lumbar spine, especially stress injury to the pars (1). The extra cost of SPECT scanning, where available, may be justified in light of this improved sensitivity.

Treatment of stress reaction of the pars interarticularis consists of application of a custom molded rigid antilordotic brace, designed to hold the lumbar spine in slight flexion. During the period of brace wear, special attention is directed toward stretching the hamstrings, which are invariably tight in this condition. Bracing is usually continued for a minimum of 3 months; the earlier a stress reaction is detected, the shorter the treatment period that is required. All activities that cause pain should initially be eliminated, but the athlete is later allowed to resume conditioning. In some cases, the compliant, honest young athlete may be allowed to resume competition in certain sports while still wearing the brace. Follow-up bone scanning or SPECT may be used to insure that healing of the stress reaction has taken place. Following removal of the brace, the athlete should undergo a course of supervised therapy to restore flexibility and strengthen the abdominal musculature.

Spondylolysis (Defects in the Pars Interarticularis)

As stated previously, a frank defect in the pars interarticularis is an acquired lesion caused by fatigue fracture (32). The lesion is usually acquired while the athlete is skeletally immature, but may not become symptomatic until adulthood. This lesion may be painless, and a significant proportion of the population presumably goes through life with an undiagnosed spondylolysis or spondylolisthesis. In families with a congenital predisposition to spondylolysis, the demands of everyday life are presumably enough to cause this stress fracture early in life. The defect is seen in competitors in many sports that require repetitive or prolonged hyperextension of the spine; the tennis serve, the volleyball spike, hiking out in sailing, reaching to correct over-rotation in diving, pole vault, and high jump may all place the spine at risk. In Jackson's study group of 100 female gymnasts, 11 had a pars defect with or without spondylolisthesis; five of these 11 had no prior history of back pain (13). Ferguson's study of college football interior linemen showed that 50% of his subjects with back pain had a pars defect; the incidence in the entire study group, including those without back pain, was 24% (8). Because spondylolysis is not always painful, mere identification of a pars defect in an athlete with back pain does not confirm the cause of the pain, and other potential causes should be ruled out.

Athletes with back pain and spondylolysis fall into two main groups: those with acute or subacute lesions, and those with a well-established, chronic spondylolysis. The acute/subacute group may have a single precipitating episode of hyperextension trauma, and the bone scan will be positive. It may take 72 hours for a bone scan to become positive following an acute fracture. In this group, casting or bracing is indicated to relieve symptoms, and potentially to allow the injury to heal. Micheli documented a 32% healing rate in his series of patients with acute spondylolysis who were treated in an antilordotic brace for 6 months (18).

In chronic spondylolysis the bone scan is usually negative, and the bone adjacent to the defect appears sclerotic and rounded off. Back pain in these patients may be related to overuse or to early segmental instability. Bracing may be indicated in this group as well, if the back pain does not respond to the usual conservative modalities. Lateral flexion/extension radiographs are traditionally used to detect spinal instability.

In the skeletally immature athlete, back pain associated with spondylolysis may be indicative of a ''preslip'' condition, where a growth spurt is causing progression to early spondylolisthesis with resultant pain. All growing athletes with spondylolysis should be followed with x-rays at 6-month intervals to detect progression to spondy-lolisthesis. In the presence of symptoms, a hot bone scan in association with spondylolysis or spondylolisthesis denotes an active process, and mandates a period of restricted activity. Bracing is definitely indicated in those patients with a clinical picture characteristic of a preslip condition.

Asymptomatic spondylolysis should not exclude any athlete from participation. Once skeletal maturity is reached, there is minimal risk of progression of a simple pars defect to spondylolisthesis. The most common symptom in spondylolysis is intermittent pain associated with hyperextension activities. Semon and Spengler compared two groups of college football players with back pain—one group with documented spondylolysis, and one group with normal x-rays. There was no significant difference in time lost from participation during the college careers of both groups (25).

Unilateral spondylolysis is a perplexing condition. We have seen a young football player with an acute unilateral pars interarticularis fracture at L-5 that healed following a short period of bracing. However, most of these lesions are probably bilateral pars fractures in which one side has healed and the other has failed to unite. Figure 13.2 shows the CT scan of a skeletally mature female softball/volleyball player with consistent pain in the left gluteal region when hyperextending to spike the ball. Two years prior to this scan, she had a 1-month period of similar back pain after hyperextending her low back during a headfirst slide. In retrospect, the x-rays taken at that time showed a possible acute bilateral pars defect at L-5, which was not appreciated. When her pain recurred, a bone scan was obtained that showed increased uptake in the left posterior elements of L-5. Her CT scan shows a characteristic unilateral spondylolysis, with hypertrophy of the contralateral pars and adjacent facet joints. CT-guided injection

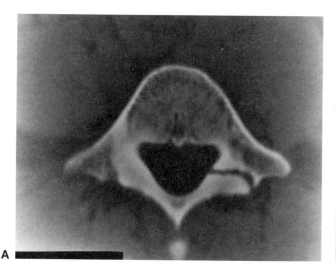

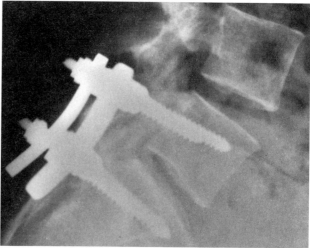

FIG. 13.2. A: Axial CT reveals a symptomatic unilateral spondylolysis at L-5 that may have resulted from an acute fracture two years prior to this study. There is hypertrophy of the pars and pedicle on the right as a result of increased stress. **B:** Failure of conservative treatment eventually led to a posterior L-5—S-1 spinal fusion with instrumentation, allowing unrestricted activity without pain.

of the pars defect with local anesthetic gave the patient transient relief of her symptoms, confirming that the defect was the cause of her pain. After failure of conservative treatment, she elected to undergo a posterior spinal fusion. She remains active in sports and coaching.

Spondylolisthesis

Defects in the pars interarticularis may allow forward slipping of one vertebrae on top of another, resulting in isthmic spondylolisthesis (see Fig. 13.1). Rarely, an elongated but intact pars allows spondylolisthesis; this dysplastic condition may be the result of malunion of an acute fracture or fatigue fracture.

Any degree of slippage in spondylolisthesis implies instability of that segment of the lumbar spine. This instability does not necessarily preclude participation, however. The most important factors in evaluating spondylolisthesis are the degree of symptoms, the age of the patient, the amount of slippage, and evidence of progression of the slip.

Spondylolisthesis is graded in severity by the amount of slippage, expressed as a percentage of the width of the vertebral body as seen on the lateral x-ray. Grade I (25%) and early grade II (up to 50%) slips are considered mild and generally require only symptomatic treatment and observation for progression. Figure 13.3 shows the lateral lumbar spine films of an 18-year-old high school football

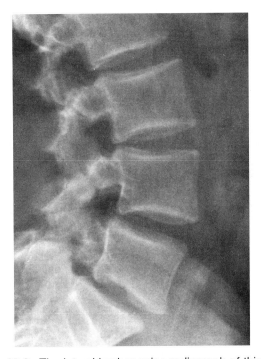

FIG. 13.3. The lateral lumbar spine radiograph of this high school football lineman reveals defects of the pars interarticularis (spondylolysis) at L-3 and L-4, with a stable grade I spondylolisthesis at the lowest segment (L-5–S-1).

defensive lineman. His spine showed no instability on flexion and extension, despite spondylolysis at L-3, trace spondylolisthesis at L-4, and grade I spondylolisthesis at L-5. He was intermittently kept from competition because of symptoms of low back pain, but was able to continue playing without progression of his disorder. Slips of 50% or greater are more severe, and may require spinal fusion to arrest progression.

The highest risk of progression occurs in the 9 to 14 year age group, during the terminal growth spurt (32). Athletes with mild spondylolisthesis in this age group should be allowed unrestricted participation only if they are asymptomatic. Lateral x-rays should be obtained twice a year in order to detect possible progression of the slip (14). A recent retrospective study involving 86 child and adolescent athletes with L-5 spondylolysis or spondylolisthesis revealed that very few athletes had significant progression of their disorder over a 4-year period. Although the spondylolisthesis increased by an average of 10.5% in about one-half of the subjects, very few had progression of greater than 10%, and these progressions were not clinically significant (23). Symptomatic young athletes, or those with a slip approaching 50%, should be restricted from sports requiring forcible hyperextension of the spine, such as football, gymnastics, and wrestling. Documented progression of a slip from grade I to grade II is an indication for full-time bracing until skeletal maturity. The immature athlete with a slip of grade II or greater should be barred from contact sports, skiing, and gymnastics, and spinal fusion should be considered. It is not advisable to allow athletes to return to these strenuous sports even if a successful spinal fusion has been performed.

Spondylolisthesis in the mature athlete rarely progresses, if at all. The degree of symptoms, however, frequently increases over time. Symptoms may be caused by degenerative changes in the disk at the involved level or by nerve root impingement. The presence of L-5 or S-1 nerve root symptoms should probably warrant restriction from contact sports and hyperextension activities. Severe slips may gradually progress to an advanced osteoarthritic condition because of loss of the disk space. Mature athletes with high-grade slips are usually unable to routinely participate in strenuous sports. Spinal fusion with or without laminectomy is sometimes required for relief of symptoms in the mature athlete.

The Scapulothoracic Articulation

There is normally a great deal of motion between the scapulae and the underlying rib cage. Anything that interferes with this motion can result in upper back pain. The large bursa between the intrinsic muscles of the shoulder and the chest wall may become inflamed and act as a source of pain. Healed fractures of the scapula or underlying ribs may restrict scapulothoracic motion and cause symptoms during specific maneuvers. Occasionally, benign tumors such as osteochondroma or elastofibroma may arise from the scapula and cause deep pain. Physical examination and radiography are usually sufficient to localize the source of pain, but MRI is occasionally indicated. Arthroscopy of the scapulothoracic bursa as a diagnostic and therapeutic modality is in its infancy.

Scheuermann's Kyphosis

Scheuermann's disease consists of a progressive kyphosis of the thoracic spine with characteristic radiographic features. In the immature athlete, Scheuermann's disease is the most common cause of symptoms in the thoracic spine, whereas the pars interarticularis is the most likely source of symptoms in the lumbar spine. The humpback deformity seen in this disorder appears to be more common in weight lifters and swimmers who specialize in the butterfly stroke. Irregularities of the vertebral endplates and Schmorl's nodes (intravertebral disk herniations) are seen on lateral spine films. As the deformity progresses, the increased pressure on the anterior vertebral bodies may lead to necrosis of the growth centers and further progression of the deformity. Symptoms are similar to other stress fractures and stress reactions, with pain at night and at rest, relief of pain with modest activity, and increased pain with more strenuous activity. The stress-related radiographic changes generally cease to progress and may resolve if activity is restricted appropriately. Athletes with symptomatic kyphosis and radiographic changes should be restricted from forceful axial loading of the spine as in weight lifting, and should also avoid the butterfly stroke and exercises that isolate the pectoralis major. Progressive Scheuermann's kyphosis may require bracing, and in rare cases anterior and posterior spinal fusion to halt progression of the disorder. Mild cases cause cosmetic deformity but little dysfunction or pain, leading some to question whether the treatment is worse than the disease itself.

Scoliosis

Up to 12% of school children seen in screening programs have some degree of scoliosis (7). Scoliosis is defined as a lateral curvature of the spine, and about 75% to 80% of all scoliosis is the idiopathic type occurring during the adolescent growth spurt. Scoliosis is diagnosed by the presence of a unilateral rib hump that is seen during forward bending on physical examination. In cases of mild scoliosis, the spine may appear completely straight when the athlete is sitting or standing erect. In the skeletally immature athlete, the scoliotic curve must be followed closely to watch for progression. A mild, fixed scoliosis is generally of little significance in the mature athlete.

The important thing to remember about idiopathic scoliosis is that it is usually painless. The curve is generally a disorder of growth, and is usually discovered because of visible asymmetry, not because it interferes with function or causes pain. An athlete who presents with a painful scoliosis must be assumed to have an underlying cause for this condition; in other words, the scoliosis is a result of the pain, rather than the cause of the pain.

The most common cause of symptomatic scoliosis in athletes appears to be leg-length discrepancy. In order to stand, run, and walk erect, the athlete with unequal leg lengths must have a compensatory spinal curve to accommodate their tilted pelvis. This may lead to painful muscle imbalance or chronic spasm secondary to asymmetric loading of the facet joints. A mild discrepancy of less than 2 cm is easily treated with a heel lift or built-up shoe. About one-half of the total discrepancy should be corrected initially in an attempt to relieve symptoms. Discrepancies greater than 2 cm require further investigation and may require surgical treatment.

Other causes of painful scoliosis include benign or malignant soft tissue or bone tumors, spinal infection, tethering of the spinal cord during growth, and various intraabdominal problems. The athlete with an unexplained painful scoliosis should undergo a complete diagnostic evaluation to ascertain the cause of the pain.

Congenital Anomalies

There are several common congenital anomalies of the lumbosacral region that can cause low back pain. The major congenital anomalies, such as spina bifida and congenital scoliosis, usually become apparent early in life and rarely surface during athletic participation. The lesser deformities, however, may not cause problems until secondary degenerative changes occur later in life.

Spina bifida occulta is a partial failure of the posterior vertebral elements to close during embryonic growth. The lesion is visible as a vertical cleft in the spinous process of L-5 or S-1 on the anteroposterior (AP) spine x-ray. In the absence of neurologic problems, this is an incidental finding; the only clinical significance of spina bifida occulta is that patients with this condition have a higher incidence of pars defects than the general population.

Partial or complete sacralization of the lower lumbar vertebra occurs frequently. Its true incidence is unknown, since it is often asymptomatic and therefore undetected until x-rays are taken for another reason. In this anomaly, an articulation or complete fusion occurs between the transverse processes of L-5 and the adjacent sacrum or ilium. If this articulation is fused, or large enough to significantly limit motion at L-5–S-1, it is usually asymptomatic. If the pseudoarticulation is small and unilateral, however, early degenerative changes may occur. Figure

13.4 shows the AP pelvis radiograph of a 28-year-old recreational athlete who had been troubled by right gluteal pain for over a year. She had failed to consistently respond to sacroiliac joint manipulations over the course of a year. Routine radiography revealed partial sacralization of the lowest lumbar vertebra with false articulation between the lumbar transverse processes and the sacrum and ilium, causing early degenerative changes. She has declined invasive treatment of this lesion, which might have included corticosteroid injection or surgical excision of the pseudoarticulation.

Lumbar Disk Disease in Athletes

The importance of intervertebral disk disease in young athletes has finally been appreciated in recent years. Although not as big a problem as the pars interarticularis, disk disease is no longer diagnosed only in the mature athlete. Jackson states that 50% of the young athletes he sees with back pain have a problem related to the pars interarticularis (stress reaction, spondylolysis, or spondylolisthesis); a full 10%, however, have pain referable to an intervertebral disk (12). This number does not include athletes with disk-related problems such as vertebral end-plate fractures, apophyseal ring avulsions, and lumbar Scheuermann's disease. These disorders may make up a significant portion of the remaining patients.

Lumbar disk degeneration occurs as the nucleus pulposus gradually loses its water content. This results in a loss of resistance to compression, with axial loads then being

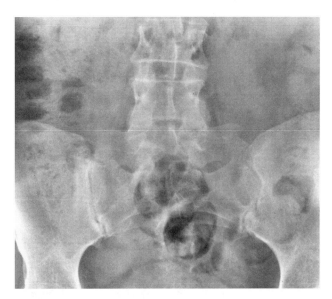

FIG. 13.4. The enlarged transverse processes of L5 form a painful articulation with the ilium in this female athlete. Although the congenital partial sacralization is relatively symmetrical in this case, the symptoms were confined to the right side. Diagnostic injections confirmed that the false articulation was the source of pain.

transmitted to the richly innervated annulus fibrosus. Disk degeneration is a normal process of aging; 99% of adults will have degenerated disks by the sixth decade of life, most commonly at the L-3 to L-4 and L-4 to L-5 levels (22). Males are more prone to disk degeneration than females. Cadaver studies have shown that mild disk degeneration can be identified in about one third of males by age 20 (22). It should be remembered that degenerated disks are not necessarily painful.

MRI allows noninvasive assessment of the water content of the nucleus pulposus. A recent MRI study compared 15-year-olds with and without back pain; degenerated disks were found in 38% of children with back pain, and in 26% of control subjects. The difference between the two groups was not statistically significant (31). A similar MRI study looked at gymnasts with back pain, and found that only 3 of 35 gymnasts had degenerated disks; in each case, the degeneration was associated with another pathologic process (spondylolysis or Scheuermann's disease). The MRI added nothing to plain lumbar radiography in terms of diagnosis (30). These findings show that although symptomatic disk degeneration can occur in the young athlete, it is of minimal significance compared to the other common causes of back pain. It should also be remembered that a large proportion of degenerated disks are incidental findings, and are not associated with back pain.

The mature athlete with degenerative disk disease will have intermittent bouts of pain following periods of heavy activity. The pain is usually localized in the low back, is worsened by lifting, and may radiate to the buttocks. A regular exercise program consisting of abdominal strengthening and flexibility exercises may be of benefit to the occasional athlete.

Disk Herniation

The classic posterior or posterolateral disk herniation with nerve root impingement has been well described. Herniation of a lumbar disk may occur in athletes of any age, and few clinicians would miss the characteristic findings of back pain, sciatica, and positive nerve root stretch signs. Thoracic disk herniation is relatively rare, but does not generally cause sciatica and may therefore be difficult to diagnose. Confirmation of disk herniation no longer requires invasive tests such as myelography. Figure 13.5 is the sagittal MRI scan of a college offensive lineman with a large posterolateral disk herniation. The acute herniation occurred early in the football season, and was initially very symptomatic. He was treated with an epidural corticosteroid injection and his symptoms rapidly abated. He was able to return to competition after missing two games, and opted to undergo laminectomy and disk excision after his final college season.

In the skeletally immature athlete, such a classic picture

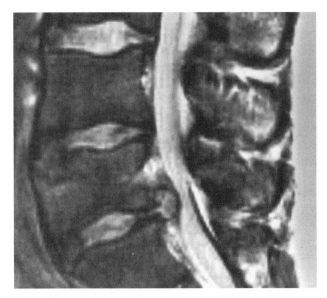

FIG. 13.5. MRI is now the procedure of choice for diagnosis of disk disease, such as this large L-5–S-1 disk herniation. Note also the dark signal in the adjacent L-4–L-5 disk, indicating degeneration (loss of water content).

is rare. The typical herniation of the nucleus pulposus is unlikely to occur unless there is a predisposing condition, such as spondylolisthesis or partial sacralization. Disk herniations in this group usually occur through the apophyseal growth plate or the superior end-plate of the vertebral body, as these areas are weaker than the annulus fibrosus during growth. An adolescent with classic symptoms of sciatica may be found to have herniated a small fragment of the ring apophysis into the spinal canal along with the disk material. More frequently, apophyseal avulsion and disk

herniation occur anteriorly in this age group. Disk herniation through the superior end-plate causes the formation of a Schmorl's node, which is a characteristic radiolucency within the vertebral body. An intravertebral disk herniation occurring at the anterior radial margin of the vertebral body is seen in lumbar Scheuermann's disease. Scheuermann's disease can be the result of chronic overuse activity, or it may be caused by a single violent flexion-compression injury. A hyperextension thoraco-lumbo-sacral orthosis (TLSO) may be required for treatment of the more acute variety. Although these variants of disk herniation do not cause sciatica, they can cause acute pain. The x-ray changes will persist into adulthood, but these conditions will not require surgical intervention.

The symptomatic posterior or posterolateral disk herniation, whether associated with an apophyseal fracture or not, frequently improves with nonsurgical treatment. Conservative treatment modalities include epidural steroid injections and physical therapy. Nonetheless, surgery may be required in up to 30% of athletes with a persistently symptomatic disk herniation (12). Surgical intervention in the young patient involves only a small laminectomy with removal of the offending disk fragment; a spinal fusion is not performed. There has been recent interest in percutaneous diskectomy in the treatment of this condition, and return to activity within 4 to 6 weeks following this procedure has been reported in college football players (4). Young athletes with disk herniations can generally expect to return to activity, whether or not they undergo surgery (20,27). One should be careful not to prolong conservative treatment in the face of continued severe symptoms. Athletes who have experienced prolonged irritation of neural structures may not experience com-

Line Spcg: 2.0 mm
Raw Beam: 19078, 12447

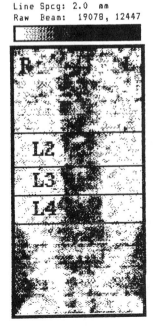

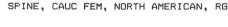

SPINE, CAUC FEM, NORTH AMERICAN, RG

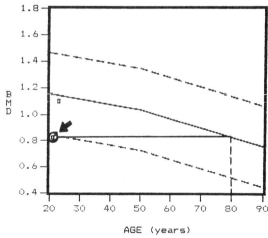

FIG. 13.6. This bone mineral density study of a 20-year-old amenorrheic cross-country runner is markedly abnormal (arrow). Extrapolation to the mean bone density curve plotted on the study shows that her bone density would be considered normal only in an 80-year-old woman.

plete relief of symptoms even after adequate surgical decompression.

Metabolic Bone Disease

Decreased bone density, because of metabolic or endocrine imbalance, causes increased susceptibility to fracture. In severe osteoporosis, the lumbar vertebral bodies may sustain compression fractures following minimal axial loads. Although this syndrome is frequently seen in postmenopausal women, it is unusual to see decreased bone density in the athletic population. One exception is the young female distance runner who has become amenorrheic because of frequent sustained exertion, decreased body fat percentage, and low estrogen stores. These athletes may have surprisingly low bone densities for their age group. Figure 13.6 is the bone density study of a nationally ranked 20-year-old cross-country runner with low back and gluteal pain. She had been amenorrheic since becoming competitive in high school 3 years previously. The x-ray and a bone scan confirmed a sacral insufficiency fracture of the type usually seen only in elderly osteoporotic women. This would be an unusual injury in an active young female, were it not for the fact that her bone density would have been normal only for an 80-year-old woman. With appropriate estrogen supplementation and dietary counseling, her bone density returned to near normal for her age.

THE MATURE ATHLETE

Back pain in the skeletally mature or middle-aged athlete is often the result of poor physical conditioning. With the exception of elite and professional athletes, a relatively sedentary lifestyle during the week with excessive activity over the weekend is the rule. Poor posture significantly increases the risk of back pain; weak abdominal muscles and a hyperlordotic posture predispose the patient to arthrosis of the facet joints. As disk degeneration becomes more prominent with advancing age, activity-related symptoms are likely to increase.

The clinician who diagnoses every case of acute low back pain as a lumbosacral strain will be right most of the time, regardless of the age of the athlete. Unfortunately, this diagnosis is overused, particularly when applied to chronic back pain. The routine strains of muscle, musculotendinous junctions, fascia, and ligaments that occur commonly in athletic competition should resolve relatively rapidly with local treatment and rest. This diagnosis should be questioned in any athlete whose back pain fails to resolve in a reasonable amount of time. Although chronic strain of the iliolumbar ligament has been implicated as a cause of low back pain, this diagnosis should be confirmed with diagnostic injections of local anesthetic mixed with corticosteroids. Making an erroneous diagnosis may delay the identification and treatment of a more serious condition.

Disk degeneration probably accounts for about 50% of the chronic low back pain seen in the mature athlete. The loss of water content in the nucleus pulposus associated with aging results in transmission of greater compressive and torsional stresses to the richly innervated annulus fibrosus. The annulus has been identified as one of the major anatomic locations in the spine for perception of pain. Although diskogenic pain is common during competition in football and soccer players, it becomes common in all sports with advancing age. Back pain secondary to disk degeneration and arthritic changes is almost endemic in older golfers. In general, pain caused by disk degeneration should be treated symptomatically, with appropriate restriction of activity and rehabilitation modalities during flare-ups. This is in contrast to the back pain seen in younger athletes, particularly in hyperextension sports, in which about 50% of symptomatic athletes will be suffering from pain related to the pars interarticularis (21). It has been suggested that back pain in the young athlete be treated diagnostically, whereas the older athlete should be treated symptomatically (28,29). Any athlete with persistent undiagnosed pain despite adequate treatment should of course undergo a thorough diagnostic evaluation (10,17).

As nearly every mature athlete will experience back pain at some time, there is a tendency to approach this complaint with a somewhat cavalier attitude. Although most back pain in this age group will result from degenerative disorders or lumbosacral strain, it is important to rule out intraabdominal problems as the source of the back pain. Abdominal aortic aneurysm, uterine fibroids, and malignancies such as multiple myeloma and cancer of the rectosigmoid are all seen predominantly in the older population. Figure 13.7 is the bone scan and abdominal CT of a 40-year-old marathon runner who did not seek treatment for her low back and right groin pain until 6 months after the onset of symptoms. Her plain x-rays were normal (see Fig. 13.7C), but the bone scan showed vaguely increased uptake in the right femoral neck that could have been interpreted as a stress fracture of the femoral neck. The abdominal CT revealed a large liver metastasis from what proved to be ovarian carcinoma. She died of her disease 3 months later.

Arthrosis of the facet joints causes spinal stenosis. The osteophytes and thickened capsules about the joints impinge upon the nerve roots as they exit the spinal canal. Levels with a degenerated disk are more likely to exhibit the changes of spinal stenosis. An athlete with spinal stenosis experiences back and leg pain during activities that cause hyperextension of the spine. This pain is typically relieved only by a period of sitting with the lumbar lordosis reduced. Conservative treatment of spinal stenosis involves flexion and abdominal strengthening exercises, and in some cases antilordotic bracing for activity.

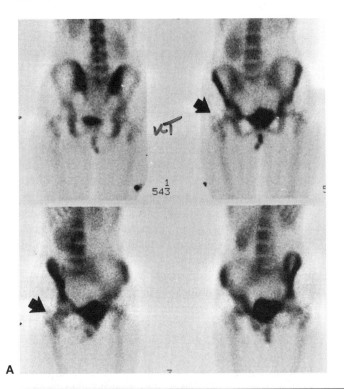

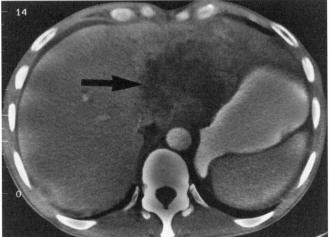

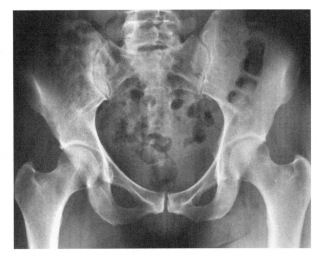

FIG. 13.7. A: A Technetium bone scan of the pelvis in a 40-year-old long-distance runner reveals diffuse uptake in the right hip *(arrows)*. This uptake is not as focal as that seen in a stress fracture of the femoral neck. **B:** Her abdominal CT scan shows a large liver lesion from metastatic ovarian carcinoma, which also proved to be responsible for the hip lesion. **C:** The normal x-ray.

Severe cases with neurologic deficits may require surgical decompression.

A variant of facet joint arthrosis is degenerative spondylolisthesis. In this condition, spondylolisthesis occurs when the support of the normal facet joints is lost because of arthritic changes, allowing slippage of one vertebrae on another. This most commonly occurs at the L4-5 level. In contrast to the more typical isthmic spondylolisthesis, there is no defect of the pars interarticularis. Although degenerative spondylolisthesis implies a degree of segmental instability, appropriate restriction of activity during flares may be all that is necessary for treatment. In chronic cases with evidence of nerve root impingement, spinal fusion may become necessary.

There has been some controversy concerning whether or not heavy athletic activity will predispose the athlete to back pain in later life. There appears to be little question that certain sports produce acquired lesions that can result in chronic back pain. Retired top-ranked wrestlers have been found to have a higher-than-normal incidence of back pain and also frequently have evidence of old fractures of the lumbar spine. Weight lifters have a high incidence of disk-space narrowing and spondylolisthesis, but appear to have no more back pain than the general population (9). Retired athletes may have a higher tolerance for back pain because of better overall conditioning.

CONCLUSION

The etiology and prognosis of back pain in athletes differs greatly from the situation in the work force at large. The clinician can arrive at an accurate diagnosis in a high percentage of cases, allowing initiation of a rational treatment protocol. Modern imaging techniques have made it easier to make a diagnosis early in the course of a disorder. Most of the conditions causing back pain in athletes can be treated without surgery.

REFERENCES

1. Bellah RD, Summerville DA, Treves ST, Micheli LJ. Low-back pain in adolescent athletes: detection of stress injury to the pars interarticularis with SPECT. *Radiology* 1991;180:509–512.
2. Bonica JJ. The nature of the problem. In: Carron H, McLaughlin RE, eds. *Management of low back pain.* Boston: John Wright-PSG, 1982:1–15.
3. Bunnel WP. Back pain in children. *Orthoped Clin North Am* 1982; 13(3):587–604.
4. Day AL, Friedman WA, Indelicato PA. Observations on the treatment of lumbar disk disease in college football players. *Am J Sports Med* 1987;15(1):72–75.
5. Deusinger RH. Biomechanical considerations for clinical application in athletes with low back pain. *Clin Sports Med* 1989;8(4): 703–715.
6. Dyment PG. Low back pain in adolescents. *Ped Ann* 1991;20(4): 170–178.
7. Edmonson AS. Scoliosis. In: Crenshaw AH ed. *Campbell's operative orthopaedics.* St. Louis: Mosby, 1987:3167–3236.
8. Ferguson RJ, McMasters MC, Stanitski CL. Low-back pain in college football linemen. In: *Proceedings of the American Academy of Orthopaedic Surgeons. J Bone Joint Surg* 1974;56A:1300.
9. Granhed H, Morelli B. Low back pain among retired wrestlers and heavyweight lifters. *Am J Sports Med* 1988;16(5):530–533.
10. Halpern BC, Smith AD. Catching the cause of low-back pain. *Phys Sportsmed* 1991;19(6):71–79.
11. Hensinger RN. Back pain in children. In: Bradford DS, Hensinger RN, eds. *The pediatric spine.* New York: Thieme, 1985:41–60.
12. Jackson DW. Low back pain in young athletes: evaluation of stress reaction and diskogenic problems. *Am J Sports Med* 1979;7(6): 364–366.
13. Jackson DW, Wiltse LL, Cirincione RJ. Spondylolysis in the female gymnast. *Clin Orthop Rel Res* 1976;117:68–73.
14. Kraus DR, Shapiro D. The symptomatic lumbar spine in the athlete. *Clin Sports Med* 1989;8(1):59–69.
15. Kujala UM, Taimela S, Erkintalo M, et al. Low back pain in adolescent athletes. *Med Sci Sports Exerc* 1996;28(2):165–170.
16. Kuslich SD, Ulstrom CL, Michael CJ. A report of pain response to tissue stimulation during operations on the lumbar spine using local anesthesia. *Orthop Clin North Am* 1991;22(2):181–187.
17. Marks MR, Haas SS, Wiesel SW. Low back pain in the competitive tennis player. *Clin Sports Med* 1988;7(2):277–287.
18. Micheli LJ. Back injuries in gymnastics. *Clin Sports Med* 1985;4: 85–93.
19. Micheli LJ. Low back pain in the adolescent: differential diagnosis. *Am J Sports Med* 1979;7(6):362–364.
20. Micheli LJ. Sports following spinal surgery in the young athlete. *Clin Orthop Rel Res* 1985:152–157.
21. Micheli L, Wood R. Back pain in young athletes: significant differences from adults in causes and patterns. *Arch Pediatr Adolesc Med* 1995;149:15–18.
22. Miller JAA, Schmatz C, Schultz AB. Lumbar disk degeneration: correlation with age, sex, and spine level in 600 autopsy specimens. *Spine* 1988;13(2):173–178.
23. Muschik M, Hahnel H, Robinson PN, et al. Competitive sports and the progression of spondylolisthesis. *J Pediatr Orthop* 1996;16(3): 364–369.
24. Rosenblum BR, Rothman AS. Low back pain in children. *Mount Sinai J Med* 1991;58(2):115–120.
25. Semon RL, Spengler D. Significance of lumbar spondylolysis in college football players. *Spine* 1981;6(2):172–174.
26. Smith MJ, Wright V. Sciatica and the intervertebral disk. An experimental study. *J Bone Joint Surg* 1958;40A:1401–1418.
27. Snyder-Mackler L. Rehabilitation of the athlete with low back dysfunction. *Clin Sports Med* 1989;8(4):717–729.
28. Stanish W. Low back pain in athletes: an overuse syndrome. *Clin Sports Med* 1987;6(2):321–344.
29. Stanish W. Low back pain in middle-aged athletes. *Am J Sports Med* 1979;7(6):367–369.
30. Tertti M, Paajanen H, Kujala UM, et al. Disk degeneration in young gymnasts: a magnetic resonance imaging study. *Am J Sports Med* 1990;8(2):206–208.
31. Tertti MO, Salminen JJ, Paajanen HEK, et al. Low-back pain and disk degeneration in children: a case-control MR imaging study. *Radiology* 1991;180:503–507.
32. Wiltse LL, Widell EH, Jackson DW. Fatigue fracture: the basic lesion in isthmic spondylolisthesis. *J Bone Joint Surg* 1975;57A: 17–22.

The Injured Athlete, Third Edition,
edited by D. H. Perrin.
Lippincott–Raven Publishers, Philadelphia © 1999.

CHAPTER 14

The Torso, Pelvis, Hip, and Thigh

Henry T. Goitz, S. D. Steen Johnsen, and Lorraine J. Armstrong

CHEST INJURIES

Ribcage Injuries

Most athletic injuries to the chest result from direct blunt trauma to the ribs, resulting in either contusion or fracture. These occurrences are sport specific; they usually involve the equipment (such as balls and sticks) and/or the direct contact of the athletes. For example, a tackle or fall onto a ball or player in football, a line drive to the chest in baseball, or a stick to the ribs in hockey or lacrosse, can all result in injury to the chest wall and/or underlying viscera.

Ribcage trauma has also been implicated in rib injury from either repetitive activity or from a sudden, singular muscular contraction. The site of injury (i.e., upper versus lower ribs) appears to be sport specific. Repetitive overhead sporting activities such as serving in tennis and clean jerks in weight lifting can be associated with first rib stress fractures as well as complete fractures. In throwers, these fractures have been seen in both the dominant (throwing) and nondominant (nonthrowing) extremity. First rib fractures were also reported in basketball players and are associated with rebounding. This has been referred to as rebound rib. A mechanism for an indirect first rib fracture is theorized from opposing muscle forces between the scalenes and upper part of the serratus anterior. In contrast, lower rib fractures have been reported in golfers; these fractures have been identified on the side contralateral to the golfers' handedness. Lower rib fractures have also been seen in the overhead throwing athlete, as well.

H. T. Goitz: Department of Orthopaedic Surgery, Athletic Medicine, Henry Ford Medical Center—Lakeside, Sterling Heights, Michigan 48313-2195

S. D. S. Johnsen: Institute for Bone and Joint Disorders, Phoenix, Arizona 85012

L. J. Armstrong: Department of Pediatrics, Henry Ford Medical Center—Pierson, Grosse Pointe, Michigan 48236

An athlete with a rib fracture will usually give a history of a recallable single, traumatic event resulting in significant, acute pain at the fracture site; an individual usually exhibits pain to direct palpation and with deep inspiration. Ununited fractures might result in a click with respiration.

An upright plain anterior posterior (AP) chest radiograph is recommended for suspected anterior or posterior fractures; lateral fractures require oblique radiographs to visualize the fracture site. More importantly, a pneumothorax should be ruled out, both radiographically and clinically, as a patient may exhibit subcutaneous emphysema in the latter. Moreover, one must keep in mind that lower rib fractures could injure abdominal viscera such as liver, spleen, or kidney. If a stress fracture is suspected, a bone scan can be used to confirm the diagnosis.

Isolated rib fractures are treated symptomatically. Athletes are encouraged to breath deeply and avoid splinting in order to minimize the risk of atelectasis. An athlete can return to sport when the discomfort from the activity is tolerable and respirations are full without splinting, usually within 2 to 3 weeks. The chest can be protected initially with taping to reduce motion to the injured segments (except in older athletes with obstructive lung disease, as taping can restrict total volume). Intercostal nerve block can be used for markedly severe pain. Protective equipment including a rubber chest protector, blocking vests, and flack vest (inflatable bladder with a plastic shield) can also be used, particularly with initial return to sport.

Costochondral Injury

A separation of a costocartilage from the sternum can result from a direct blow to the chest or from a twisting injury such as commonly encountered in wrestling. As in rib fractures, the injured costocartilage can be exquisitely painful in the acute setting and the athlete might note a snapping or popping sensation. Here, the athlete is treated symptomatically; protective gear can be utilized on initial return to sport. Deep breathing is encouraged to minimize risk of atelectosis.

Pectoralis Major Rupture

The muscle of the pectoralis major arises from the medial clavicle, sternum, first six ribs, and aponeurosis of the external oblique. It inserts into the proximal humerus and functions to adduct, flex, and internally rotate the humerus.

A rupture of the pectoralis major results from excessive tension in a contracted muscle. It is seen in weight lifters, particularly in bench pressing. The tear may be within the muscle itself, at the musculotendinous junction, or at the tendon insertion to bone. Symptoms can involve a snap or pop, sudden sharp pain in the proximal arm, chest ecchymosis, and swelling. Abduction, flexion, and internal rotation of the arm is weakened; the pectoralis muscle belly bulges on the chest with resisted adduction. With resisted adduction, a defect can usually be palpated in the anterior axillary fold and an asymmetry is visualized with complete injury.

An injured person can resume activity after a pectoralis major tendon rupture but has much less strength for strenuous activity. Surgery is advised for professional athletes or young athletes in strenuous sports to restore full strength and function. A good result with a predictable outcome is greatest with tendon avulsion injury. Surgical repair involves a deltopectoral incision, and tendon reattachment with sutures through bone. The athlete then wears a sling for several weeks, gradually increases range of motion and begins progressive resistance exercises. A power lifter should be restricted from heavy training for 3 to 6 months from surgery.

Latissimus Dorsi

Rupture of the latissimus dorsi is rare. The muscle originates from the lower six thoracic vertebrae, the thoracolumbar fascia, and the upper crest of the posterior pelvis and inserts into the proximal humerus. It functions to adduct, extend, and internally rotate the humerus.

The contracted muscle can rupture when the tension of internal rotation, extension, and adduction is excessive and the limit of muscle resistance is exceeded. Few athletic activities require such motion other than isolated football drills for linemen. The symptoms include a snap or pop, sudden onset of pain, ecchymosis, and swelling. Resisted adduction, extension, and internal rotation is weakened with a latissimus dorsi rupture, and a defect is expected in the posterior axillary fold. Although surgery is suggested for professional athletes, particularly linemen, when such injury occurs by bony avulsion, nonoperative treatment in a professional football player was reported with a return to full strength and full activity

without deficit when the rupture occurred at the musculotendinous junction (22). In short, this injury should be treated on a case-to-case basis.

Pulmonary Injury

Traumatic injury to the chest can affect pulmonary function. It is important to recognize the spectrum of treatment of these injuries and treat them appropriately to reduce resultant morbidity. These conditions include pulmonary contusion (bruise to the lung parynchema with parynchemal bleeding), tension pneumothorax (lung collapse), hemothorax (lung compression by chest cavity blood), or a combination of these. Nontraumatic spontaneous pneumothorax has been described in otherwise healthy, young muscular athletes. In severe traumatic cases, these injuries can be life-threatening. Once the level of consciousness is assessed, the ABCs (airway, breathing, circulation) of emergency care should be instituted.

Pulmonary Contusion

In pulmonary contusion, blood escapes from injured pulmonary blood vessels into the lungs; this can compromise usual respiration. It can occur from blunt trauma resulting in rib fracture(s) and is manifested by shortness of breath with a rapid inspiratory rate (Figs. 14.1 and 14.2). Pulmonary contusion might not develop until sev-

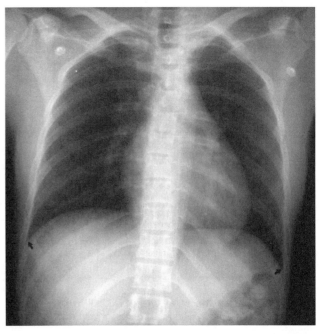

FIG. 14.1. Normal chest PA radiograph with *arrows* showing sharp costophrenic angles (i.e., no abnormal fluid accumulation) with lung marking to periphery of rib cage cavity (i.e., no collapse of lung).

Pneumothorax

A pneumothorax, or collapsed lung, occurs when air leaks from within the lung parenchyma to a pleural space just outside of it. This can occur from closed, blunt chest trauma in which a subsequent rib fracture lacerates the lung. It can also occur from open, penetrating trauma in which the lung is lacerated with concomitant communication to the outside air. A pneumothorax associated with blood accumulation is known as a hemopneumothorax (Fig. 14.3).

Tension Pneumothorax

In a closed pneumothorax, if the lacerated lung fails to seal off, a tension pneumothorax will develop. In this condition, air is constantly forced out of the lung into the surrounding pleural space with each inspiration. If allowed to progress, the entire lacerated lung will collapse from the increased surrounding pressure. The air pressure within the thorax will continue to rise and the contralateral lung will eventually be compressed from increased tension (Fig. 14.4). This increased pressure can exceed normal venous pressure and prevent normal blood return to the heart. Failure to relieve this pressure will result in a rapid cardiopulmonary shut-down and death.

Clinically, the athlete with a tension pneumothorax presents with rapidly progressive respiratory distress, a weak pulse, decreased blood pressure, with congested and distended veins in the neck and upper body. These individuals require emergent decompression of air from the

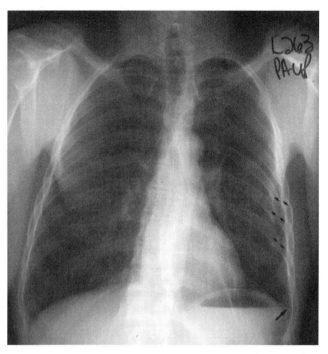

FIG. 14.2. Upright chest PA radiograph illustrating multiple left rib fractures. Several displaced fractures identified by *pairs of arrows*. Small fluid accumulation (pleural effusion) noted at base of left lung field *(thicker single arrow)* identified by blunting of costophrenic angle. This patient suffered a pulmonary contusion.

eral hours after injury. A thorough evaluation is required to determine the extent of injury. Arterial blood gases and chest x-ray should be obtained as well as cardiac isoenzymes and electrocardiograph (EKG) to rule out associated events.

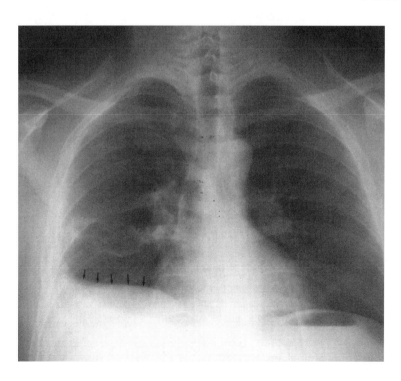

FIG.14.3. Hemopneumothorax with contour loss of both normal costophrenic angle and right hemi-diagram *(arrows).*

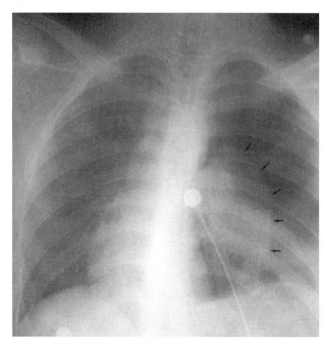

FIG. 14.4. Tension pneumothorax with collapsed left lung *(arrows)* and loss of lung markings in most of lung field. Note shift of heart to right lung field.

chest. This can be done by placing a large bore needle into the second intercostal space.

Open Pneumothorax

A penetrating trauma in which a lacerated lung communicates with the outside air is known as an open pneumothorax. Initial treatment is immediate application of a sterile occlusive dressing. With such a dressing in place, if the lacerated lung fails to seal off, a tension pneumothorax can result by the same mechanism as described earlier. If this occurs, simple release of the dressing usually decreases thoracic pressure.

Spontaneous Pneumothorax

A spontaneous pneumothorax is known to occur as a noncontact event—even at rest—in young, otherwise healthy athletes. This can occur when a lung bleb or congenitally weak area of the lung ruptures, allowing air from within the lung to leak into the pleural space. All degrees of this condition can exist from no clinical symptoms to respiratory distress. This is directly dependent upon the ability of the compromised lung tissues to seal off. If it fails to do so, a tension pneumothorax will result.

Myocardial Injury

Traumatic injury to the chest can affect cardiac function, which includes myocardial contusion (bruise to the myocardium) and pericardial tamponade (abnormal blood or fluid collection in the pericardial space that compresses the myocardium). These injuries, particularly pericardial tamponade, can be life threatening. Once the level of consciousness is assessed, the ABCs of emergency care should be instituted.

Myocardial Contusion

These injuries are usually the result of blunt chest wall trauma. Resultant sternal fractures require a full cardiac workup (Fig. 14.5). Myocardial compromise might present as an arrhythmia and the athlete should be checked for a rapid or irregular pulse. One should keep in mind, however, that these injuries could initially be clinically silent. If such an injury is suspected, therefore, the athlete should be removed from the field and undergo a thorough medical evaluation including cardiac isoenzymes, EKG, chest x-ray and arterial blood gases, as well as an echocardiogram.

Pericardial Tamponade

This condition results from penetrating trauma to the heart in which blood leaks from the heart's chamber(s) with each beat and rapidly accumulates in the surrounding pericardial sac. This collection of blood compresses the heart in its chambers and prevents normal blood return to the heart. This is a medical emergency. Failure to reduce this fluid accumulation and relieve this pressure around the heart will result in death.

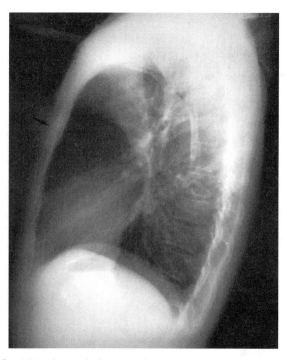

FIG. 14.5. Lateral chest radiograph illustrating displaced sternal fracture *(arrow)*.

Clinically, the athlete will exhibit a weak pulse, decreased/faint heart sounds and decreased blood pressure with congested and distended veins in the neck and upper body. These individuals require emergent decompression of this pericardial fluid.

ABDOMINAL INJURIES

Abdominal Muscle Injury

Although direct blunt contusion to the muscle wall of the abdomen is common in athletics, abdominal muscle tears can occur from abrupt twisting and contractions associated with athletic play. Early treatment includes ice and a compressive elastic wrap as well as appropriate stretching and strengthening. It must be emphasized that although an athlete's pain might not resolve in the short run (particularly an injury to the rectus abdominus muscle), it is important to employ proper therapeutic modalities to minimize extended morbidity.

Abdominal Visceral Injury

In most sports, the athlete's abdomen is usually not covered by protective gear, and, therefore, is susceptible to injury. Fortunately, the lower ribs and strong abdominal and back muscles help to protect the abdominal contents from injurious blows. Although an alert athlete will tense abdominal musculature to guard the underlying viscera, internal damage can still occur when a player reaches overhead for a pass or is tackled, as in football.

Apparent rapid recovery in a healthy young athlete after an abdominal blow does not exclude internal injury. Even a small laceration within the abdominal cavity may lead to considerable intraperitoneal bleeding, as resistance to blood flow in the abdominal cavity is very low. A high index of suspicion with careful, repeat examinations will ensure early diagnosis. These injuries can be either closed (blunt) or open (penetrating), with the former being far more common in sports.

Lower right and left rib fractures have been associated with hepatic and splenic injury, respectively. These organs, together with the intestines, mesenteric vessels, kidney, and bladder can all be injured without an associated fracture.

Clinically, an athlete with internal abdominal injury presents with a variable amount of abdominal pain, nausea, and vomiting. On examination, the athlete should lie supine with bent knees to relax the abdominal musculature. The abdomen can then more accurately be evaluated for guarding, tenderness, bowel sounds, rigidity, and rebound.

Ruptured viscus spills digestive enzyes and undigested food and/or bowel contents into the abdomen resulting in an inflammatory peritonitis. This would present as severe abdominal pain, a rigid abdomen, guarding, rebound, absent bowel sounds, and abdominal distension. Rupture of a hollow viscus could result in intraabdominal air (pneumoperitoneum) that could be identified radiographically (Fig. 14.6). Splenic and other solid organ injury can cause significant hemorrhage from their rich vascularity. Such bleeding could result in a decrease in systemic blood pressure with a resultant rapid pulse and rapid, shallow respirations which are systemic signs of shock. In short, trauma to the abdomen can be life threatening. As with any signficant trauma, the ABCs of emergency care should be employed.

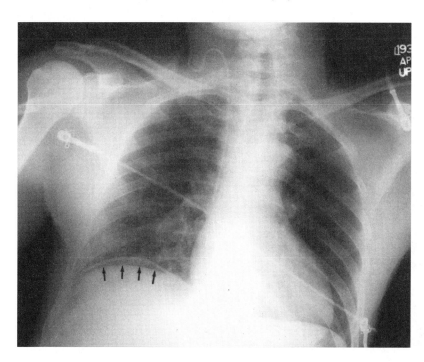

FIG. 14.6. Pneumoperitoneum illustrating air under right hemidiagram (arrows).

GENITOURINARY INJURIES

Renal Contusion

A blow from a helmet or knee or a tackle to the flank or abdomen can result in a varying degree of renal injury. Injuries can range from mild and intracapsular (intracapsular bleed) to severe and extracapsular (capsular rupture with intraperitoneal bleeding). The injured athlete usually relates resultant flank pain with or without gross hematuria. Clinical suspicion of injury should necessitate a urinalysis. Workup includes a radiographic flat plate of the abdomen in which extracapsular bleeding is implied with obliteration of the psoas margin. Persistent flank pain with a negative urinalysis (i.e., no hematuria) requires repeat examination and repeat urinalysis. Pain with hematuria and/or a strong suspicion for renal damage requires an IVP (intravenous pyelogram).

Exercise-Induced Hematuria

Hematuria can accompany or follow vigorous athletic activity without direct trauma. During intensive exercise, blood is shunted into active muscle and renal blood flow can be significantly decreased. This leads to relative renal ischemia and hematuria. Erythrocytes, albumin, and erythrocyte casts have all been found in urine specimens of athletes of a number of particularly exertional sports with distance swimmers and long-distance runners showing the greatest abnormality. However, this usually clears within 48 hours. The frequency of abnormal urine parallels the

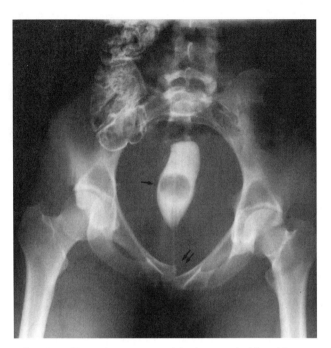

FIG. 14.7. Normal cystogram *(single arrow)* with pubic symphysis diastasis *(double arrow)*. Catheter is placed into bladder, dye is injected and no extravasation of dye is noted.

severity of exertion, and the abnormality usually disappears with the reduction of the athlete's daily exercise load.

Bladder/Urethral Injury

Although unusual, injury to the bladder and urethra can occur. A full bladder is more susceptible to injury, as it

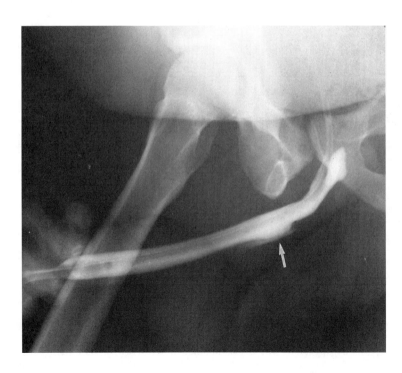

FIG. 14.8. Abnormal urethrogram in which dye extravasation is noted *(arrow).*

can rise above protection of the bony anterior pelvic brim, whereas an empty bladder is less susceptible. A retrograde cystogram will indicate injury with dye leakage (Fig. 14.7). A catheter is not to be passed into the urethra if urethral injury is suspected as this can result in further damage. A retrograde urethrogram is performed first (Fig. 14.8).

Genital Injury

The external male genitalia results in more frequent injury than seen with a female. Protective devices are used in those sports that place the male at a particular risk such as a catcher in baseball or a goalkeeper in hockey.

PELVIC INJURIES

Hip Pointer

A hip pointer is caused by a direct blow to the crest of the ileum. The crest of the ileum is subcutaneous and vulnerable at the anterior superior iliac spine and the abdominal muscles. The anterior superior iliac spine is the insertion site of the sartorius, external oblique, transverse abdominus, and tensor fascia lata muscles. The posterior superior iliac spine is an insertion site for the internal oblique as well as the aponeurosis of the latissimus dorsi and paraspinous muscles. At these locations, the iliac crest is so superficial that dimpling of the skin can be seen in lean, athletic individuals. The skin, tendon, aponeurosis, peritenon, and bone are very susceptible to direct contusion and avulsion.

Hip pointers are more common in sports involving sig-nificant contact between players, such as football or ice hockey. A traumatic event in a low or noncontact sport, such as a fall while roller-blading, can also cause this problem and must not be overlooked. In contact sports, this injury is most frequently incurred because of inadequate protection. In sports such as football or ice hockey, hip pads must be used to protect the iliac crest.

When an athlete complains of anterior or posterior iliac crest pain and has a history of a traumatic blow to the region or is involved in a contact sport, a hip pointer must be considered. The pain from the hip pointer may increase in severity several days prior to the patient's clinic visit. Therefore, a patient may present subacutely. Some patients may not initially be able to give a history of trauma because of the delayed presentation of symptoms.

Clinically, the athlete is usually tender on direct palpation of the anterior or posterior iliac spine. Many patients will have obvious swelling and ecchymosis acutely. This may be caused by contusion or subcutaneous hematoma formation. Patients with delayed presentation may give a history of continued pain in the area with pain on direct palpation and abdominal movement. This may be caused by tendinitis, periostitis, bone contusion, or unrecognized iliac crest or spine avulsion.

After taking a careful history and performing a thorough examination, radiographs are useful to rule out a fracture of the iliac crest or iliac wing as well as an avulsion of the iliac spine or apophysis (in the skeletally immature). After these entities are ruled out, the diagnosis of hip pointer may be considered. It is important to remember that the term hip pointer includes both the acute swelling, ecchymosis, and possible subcutaneous hematoma as well as the subacute or chronic periostitis and tendinitis.

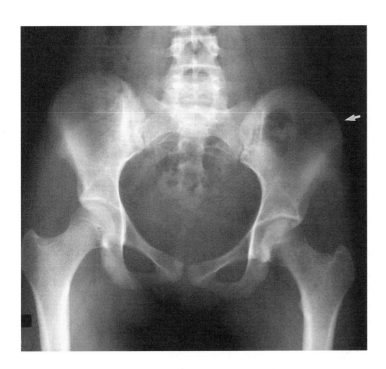

FIG. 14.9. Acute, unilateral pelvic crest pain *(arrow)* in high school track runner during race. History, clinical exam, and anteroposterior (AP) pelvis radiograph shown here suggests avulsion.

Early treatment can decrease the severe pain that can be associated with a hip pointer. Ice should be applied to the area as soon as possible. Although some physicians advocate aspiration of the subcutaneous hematoma, the majority feel that aspirated subcutaneous hematomas will not only reaccumulate, but will increase the risk of infection. Such hematomas, therefore, should be left alone. Ice and compression should be used for at least 48 hours after injury. Nonsteroidal antiinflammatory drugs (NSAIDs) can be started at initial presentation. As the acute symptoms resolve, many athletes will experience ongoing tenderness and pain with motion.

This may be especially noticeable as the individual restarts exercise or training. This may represent ongoing periostitis or tendinitis and NSAIDs and icing should be continued. Heat or ultrasound therapy can be used prior to exercise, while icing should be used after exercise. Contact avoidance will encourage healing, and patients should consider future padding to prevent reinjury (8).

Iliac Apophysitis

The iliac apophysis begins as a cartilaginous rim on the iliac crest. With maturation, ossification occurs within the

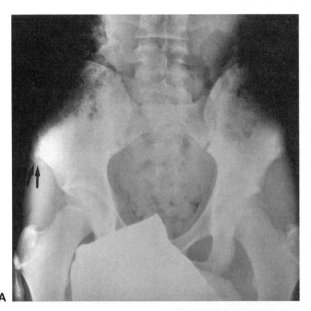

A

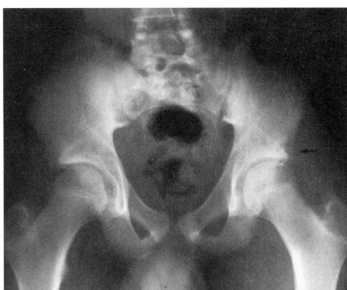

B

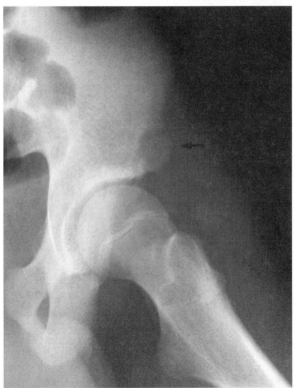

C

FIG. 14.10. Pelvic and proximal femoral apophysis avulsion of athletes in their early teens: anterior superior iliac spine (**A**), anterior inferior iliac spine (**B, C**) ischial tuberosity (**D,E**), and lesser trochanter (**F,G**).

apophysis. The ossification center is separated from the ileum by a physeal plate. With repeated muscle traction overuse, microtrauma to the physis occurs. This can lead to inflammation of the apophysis. A violent muscle contraction can lead to avulsion (Fig. 14.9). This condition can affect either the anterior or posterior apophyses. It typically occurs in the young athlete between 9 and 17 years of age and is associated with muscle-tendon imbalance and growth spurts (13,47). It is commonly associated with running sports and can be confused with a hip pointer (21,38).

Anterior iliac apophysitis can be demonstrated by tenderness on direct palpation and with resisted hip abduction (tensor fascia lata, gluteus medius, and abdominal obliques). Posterior iliac apophysitis can be demonstrated by tenderness on direct palpation and with resisted hip abduction with the hip in flexion (12). All anterior iliac apophysitis patients were symptom free after 4 to 6 weeks

of rest. All athletes had no return of symptoms after resuming training.

Radiographs of an individual with iliac apophysitis may be normal, exhibit discontinuity of the apophysis without displacement or show avulsion of the apophysis with displacement. The iliac crests begin to ossify around 13 to 15 years of age (53). Fusion of the iliac apophyses occur around 15 to 17 years of age (68). Apophyseal fusion can occur, however, during the late teens and early twenties. The symptoms of most young athletes with this condition resolve with 4 to 6 weeks of restricted activity.

Avulsion Fractures of the Pelvis

An avulsion fracture of an apophysis occurs as a result of a sudden muscle contraction, or through excessive pas-

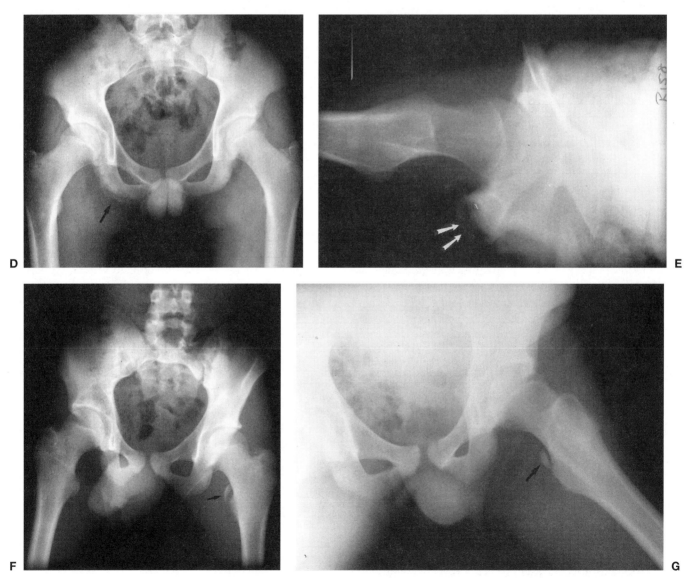

FIG. 14.10. (*Continued.*)

sive stretching of a musculotendinous group that inserts on the pelvis (Fig. 14.10). Avulsion fractures of the pelvis usually occur in the immature pelvis at apophyses. The most common locations in the pelvis are the anterior superior iliac spine (sartorius, abdominal muscles), ischial tuberosity (hamstrings) (24,41), anterior inferior iliac spine, and less commonly the iliac crest (15) and the acetabular margin. Also in this region, the lesser trochanter can be avulsed (iliopsoas) (11). Occasionally, iliac crest avulsions will be found in the evaluation of a hip pointer.

These injuries have been described in patients in running and kicking sports as a result of sudden muscle contraction. They have also been described in dancers and cheerleaders as a result of excessive passive stretch. At the time of injury, most patients will experience a sudden and severely painful popping sensation. Some patients will have a prelude of localized pain (incomplete avulsion) followed by a sudden popping sensation (total avulsion). Patients complain of localized pain at the avulsion site. Pain can be elicited with contraction of the avulsed muscle group. Some patients will position their leg and thigh to decrease tension on the avulsed musculotendinous group. Patients with avulsed anterior superior iliac spine (ASIS) or anterior inferior iliac spine (AIIS) will be more comfortable keeping their hip in flexion. Patients with an ischial tuberosity avulsion will keep their knee in flexion. Some patients will have a palpable defect at the insertion site of the muscle group with resulting weakness and pain. Radiographs can usually confirm the diagnosis (see Fig. 14.10). It is important to note that malignancy (especially Ewing's sarcoma) or osteomyelitis can occasionally resemble a healing avulsion fracture in some patients. Many of these patients will give nondescriptive histories.

Treatment is usually nonoperative (40). The athlete is allowed to return to sport when a full, pain-free range of hip motion and near full muscle strength is achieved.

Osteitis Pubis

Osteitis pubis is caused by inflammation of the symphysis pubis. In the past, this term had been used to include osteomyelitis of the pubic bones, gracilis syndrome, and avulsion fractures of the gracilis insertion site on the medial pubic bone. Most authors, however, now view osteitis pubis as a separate pathologic entity. Osteitis pubis should be distinguished from these clinically similar entities.

Individuals with osteitis pubis may present with a variety of complaints. Most will complain of pain localized to the pubic region. Some will also complain of radiation of pain into the abdomen, scrotum, or proximal thigh. Many patients will also have a classic waddling gait. Trendelenberg and antalgic gaits have also been described. Some patients will give a history of overuse or sudden increase in use. Others will complain of a groin

pull or a muscle spasm that has not improved with initial conservative therapy. Pain may be exacerbated by kicking, running, or abrupt pivoting. On exam it can sometimes be elicited with direct palpation (external, vaginal exam, or rectal exam), restricted active adduction of the thigh, or with passive abduction of the thigh.

Osteitis pubis is most commonly seen as an athletic injury. Its most common presentation is in sports that involve kicking, cutting, twisting, and running. This includes soccer, rugby, football, ice hockey, tennis, basketball, running, and race walking. Most authors feel that these actions create repetitive shearing forces across the pubic symphysis especially during the kick or stride. These motions allow simultaneous pulling of the abdominal muscles and thigh adductor muscles. This creates opposing forces and shear across the symphysis pubis. Repetitive and violent contraction leads to local microtrauma and inflammation of the periosteum, bone, cartilage, and ligamentous structures in the region of the pubic symphysis.

Osteitis pubis is not necessarily easy to diagnose. On initial presentation, it is necessary to rule out an infectious process. Patients with a recent history of urologic, obstetric, or gynecologic procedures in the area should be considered to have infectious pathology until proven otherwise. Also, some patients may give no history of trauma or overuse. In these patients, rheumatologic disorders must be considered. Osteitis pubis occurs frequently in women with ankylosing spondylitis and can also be seen in rheumatic arthritis and Reiter's syndrome. Inguinal hernia, radiculopathy, prostatitis and orchitis can also present with similar symptoms.

Early roentgenograms may be negative. It may take up to 4 weeks after the start of symptoms before characteristic changes of sclerosis and margin irregularity are seen on x-ray. Instability of the pubic ramus may sometimes be demonstrated with the classic flamingo views (AP pelvis while patient lifts one leg and puts weight on opposite leg). A bone scan is also often used in the diagnosis of osteitis pubis (Fig. 14.11). It often shows bilateral, symmetrical increased activity in the area of the pubic bones that abuts the pubic symphysis. Computed tomography (CT) scans, CT-guided biopsies, and magnetic resonance imaging (MRI) have also been used; however, many times the diagnosis can be made without these studies.

In 90% to 95% of patients with osteitis pubis, symptoms will resolve with conservative therapy. Conservative therapy consists of rest, oral NSAIDs, local modalities, adductor stretching, and hydrotherapy. Bicycling and light running have also been advocated. Progression of therapy should be limited by pain. Under a closely supervised conservative therapy program, most patients will exhibit full recovery within 7 to 9 months.

Local hydrocortisone injection into the site of maximal tenderness has been described for those who do not respond to initial conservative therapy and for athletes who need symptomatic relief for fast and temporary return to

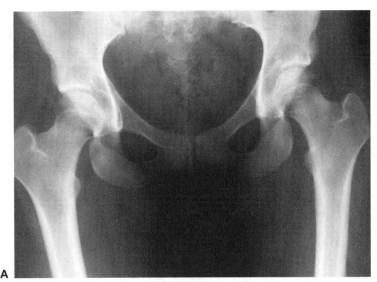

A

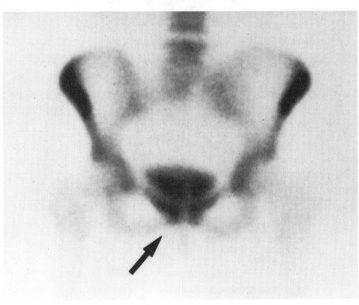

B

FIG. 14.11. Normal plain pelvic anteroposterior (AP) radiograph in division I college crew athlete (**A**) with pain localized to pubic symphysis. Bone scan (**B**) reveals increased uptake in region of pubic symphysis *(arrow)*, consistent with osteitis pubis.

their sport. Cortisone injections for osteitis pubis, however, are controversial. There is no good long-term study describing its benefits.

For athletes who do not respond to conservative therapy, wedge resection can be considered. It should be noted wedge resection involves a long postoperative recovery period before patients become asymptomatic and that many patients may be unsatisfied with the long-term results of the procedure. Debridement of the symphysis pubis and arthrodesis has also been described. Once again, no prospective, randomized double-blinded scientific study of these surgical options has been performed.

Pelvic Ring Fracture

Pelvic ring fractures can also occur in virtually any sport (Fig. 14.12). They are more common in sports

involving increased contact, such as football and ice hockey. While a further discussion of pelvis ring fractures is beyond the context of this chapter, it is important to note that many ring fractures are orthopaedic emergencies and can signify other intrapelvic injuries (iliac artery, iliac vein, or bladder laceration).

Sacral Stress Fractures

Sacral stress fractures resulting from athletics are rare. In the literature, sacral stress fractures are most commonly associated with runners who suddenly increase their training distance as well as in military recruits (1–4). Patients with sacral stress fractures complain of pain in the lower back, gluteal region, or in the posterior thigh. Many will complain of worsening pain with increased activity. Some will demonstrate an antalgic gait and some will have a

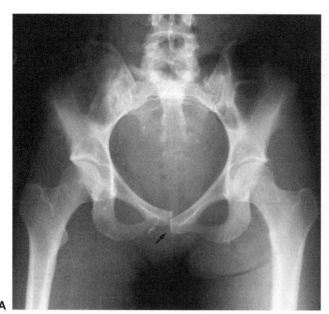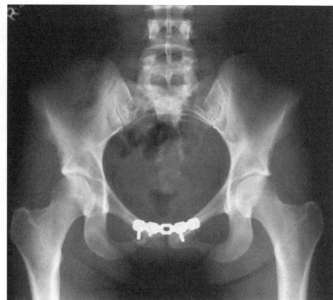

A   B

FIG. 14.12. Pelvic ring fracture (**A**) with plate fixation (**B**).

positive ''figure-of-four test'' (Patrick test). Sacral stress fractures should be considered in the differential diagnosis of a competitive athlete who is being evaluated for low back pain. Sacroiliac joint septic arthritis, sacral osteomyelitis, and malignancy must be considered in the differential diagnosis of sacral stress fractures.

Sacral stress fractures are not commonly seen on plain radiographs. Bone scan, CT, and MRI have all been used in the evaluation of sacral stress fractures (1–4). Treatment usually consists of bed rest and non–weight-bearing on the affected side, with slow and gradual return to activity.

Piriformis Syndrome

The piriformis is a weak external hip rotator when the thigh is extended and a weak abductor when the thigh is flexed. Piriformis syndrome is a rare condition that causes thigh and buttock pain through compression and irritation of the sciatic nerve. It remains a disputed entity that is difficult to diagnose (4,9).

The anatomy of the piriformis muscle and its relationship to the sciatic nerve is important in the understanding of piriformis syndrome. The sciatic nerve exits the pelvis adjacent to the bony edge of the sciatic notch and enters the hip region after passing under the edge of the piriformis. Any condition affecting the piriformis muscle can alter this relationship and irritate the sciatic nerve. This includes direct trauma (47,54), spasticity (9), hypertrophy or contracture (54), as well as prolonged intraoperative compression while under anesthesia (7). Aberrant anatomy has also been implicated (66).

There is no diagnostic test that is accurate in the diagno-

sis of piriformis syndrome. The diagnosis is made after exclusion of other causes of sciatica and is usually based on clinical findings. Electrodiagnostic studies (17,61), bone scan (33), CT, and MRI (29) have detected abnormalities in patients with piriformis syndrome, but have not been proven to be consistent in the diagnosis of this condition. Lumbar or sacral radiculopathy, lumbar facet syndromes, soft tissue injuries to other hip structures and other myofascial conditions can mimic or overlap with piriformis syndrome (4).

On physical examination, patients with piriformis syndrome frequently complain of buttock pain with or without buttock tenderness to direct palpation. Some patients will have tenderness on deep palpation of the sciatic notch. Some patients may have pain that radiates to the thigh or leg. Symptoms are usually aggravated by prolonged sitting or activities involving use of the lower extremities. Straight (Laseque's sign) leg raising is usually positive. Pain with forced internal rotation of the extended thigh (Freiberg's sign) may also be present. On rectal or vaginal exam, palpation of the pirformis at the sciatic notch may produce pain. Pain can also be reproduced with prolonged hip flexion, adduction, and internal rotation. Some patients may also have pain on resisted hip abduction while sitting. With long-standing piriformis syndrome, some may also show gluteal atrophy and weakness of hip abductors.

Piriformis syndrome is difficult to treat because it is a diagnosis of exclusion and is often present with other conditions. Other conditions that may present should be identified and addressed. Initial treatment consists of a piriformis stretching program and ultrasound treatment. NSAIDs, transrectal massage, and transvaginal ultrasound have also been described in initial conservative management of this problem. Corticosteroid injection with local anesthetic has been described and recommended for use up to three times (46). This can be done with radiopaque dye under fluoroscopic guidance and can include neuromuscular blocking agents (4). No study has shown the long-term effectiveness of nonsurgical versus surgical management.

Surgical release of the piriformis tendon at its origin, release or resection of fibrous bands or compressing vessels, and external neurolysis have been well described (18,42,58). The piriformis is a weak short external rotator of the hip and its release has minimal implication to hip strength. Surgical release has been shown to give good results with appropriate patient selection.

Adductor Muscle Strain

Injury to the adductor longus muscle is the most common cause of groin strain. This occurs when excessive stretch is placed on the adductor muscles past their elastic limit. This generally occurs after the thigh is violently externally rotated with excessive abduction. It can also occur with resisted adduction and internal rotation, such as a block while kicking a soccer ball.

Groin strain can also occur as the result of injury to the iliopsoas muscle. This injury usually occurs as the result of resisted hip flexion, and is less common than adductor longus injury. A severe injury can result in avulsion of the lesser trochanter. The rectus abdominis muscle can also be involved in groin strain. It also gives pain with resisted hip flexion.

Many patients with groin strain are able to give a history of an acute event with a pulling sensation followed by immediate or gradual onset of groin pain. Others will give a history of involvement in a sport with ongoing groin pain that persists for weeks and is exacerbated by increased involvement or usage.

On physical exam, many patients with adductor strain will have pain with resisted adduction or pain with passive abduction of the thigh. Some patients may also have pain with direct palpation of the adductor muscles. Iliopsoas strains will often be tender on palpation of the anterior thigh and will be painful with resisted hip flexion or passive hip extension. Patients who have pain with abdominal muscle contraction may have associated abdominal muscle strain.

Radiographs in muscle strain are usually negative; however, radiographs can rule out avulsion fracture, myositis ossificans, osteitis pubis, and hip joint disease. Musculoskeletal ultrasound can be very helpful in diagnosing groin strain (32,34). CT and MRI have been used in the acute setting when the diagnosis is difficult or in the chronic setting when infection or tumor is suspected. These imaging modalities, however, are often not needed

when the history and physical exam enable a reliable diagnosis (59).

Groin strain is initially managed conservatively through avoidance of aggravating activity and physical therapy. Therapy should include local modalities and NSAIDs; stretching and strengthening of the adductor muscles is very important (52).

An approach to chronic groin pain might include a multidisciplinary approach involving general surgeons, urologists, and radiologists (16,62).

Operative treatment of chronic groin strain unresponsive to physical therapy is controversial. Some advocate subcutaneous adductor tenotomy with debridement of granulation tissue (1). Most groin strains, however, do not require surgical intervention and can be managed conservatively.

HIP INJURIES

Stress Fractures of the Femur

Stress fractures of the femur are relatively uncommon injuries in healthy athletes (23,36,44). A high incidence, however, has been noted in runners, especially long-distance runners. Stress fractures of the femur are most common in the femoral neck. Subtrochanteric fractures and femoral shaft fractures can occur, but are less common.

The most common and earliest symptom of a femoral neck stress fracture is groin pain (20). Athletes may also complain of persistent hip, thigh, or knee pain. This pain will improve in some with activity; however, after continued activity, individuals will claim that the pain becomes worse. Older individuals may not give a history of excessive exercise; weaker, osteoporotic bone is more susceptible to these injuries.

Roentgenograms and bone scan are the mainstay for the radiographic diagnosis of a stress fracture. Femoral neck fractures may not be detected on plain radiographs, but are frequently discovered on bone scan and give confirmation to a clinically suspected femoral neck stress fracture.

Femoral neck stress fractures have been classified by Fullerton and Snowdy in terms of the biomechanics and degree of displacement (20). A type I stress fracture occurs on the tension side (superior) of the nondisplaced femoral neck, and on radiograph can show callus or a fracture line. A type II stress fracture occurs on the "compression side" (inferior) of the nondisplaced femoral neck and can show evidence of callus or a fracture line. A type III stress fracture exhibits displacement. Nondisplaced type I and type II fractures can be treated conservatively. Type I or type II fractures that show disruption of both cortices or fracture-gap widening should be considered for prophylactic internal fixation (Fig. 14.13). Type III

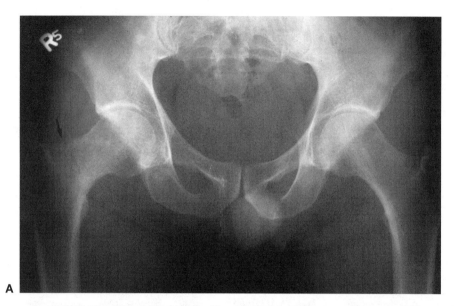

FIG. 14.13. Pelvis (AP) (**A**) and cross table lateral right hip (**B**) radiographs of femoral neck stress fracture (Type I- compression) in a 31-year-old long-distance runner with complaints of persistent right groin pain of insidious onset. Compression hip screw used for internal fixation (**C**).

A

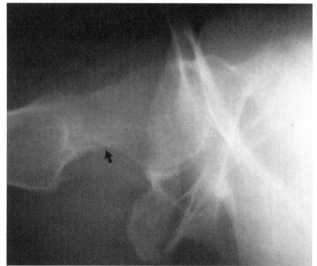

B

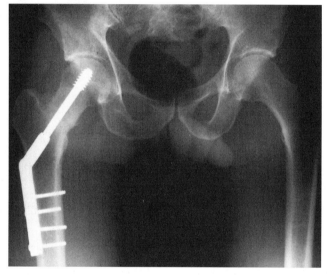

C

fracture treatment requires immediate reduction and internal fixation.

Subtrochanteric stress fractures are similar in etiology to femoral neck stress fractures. They have been associated with running and the pathogenesis is thought to be similar. Patients with subtrochanteric stress fractures will often complain of persistent thigh pain. Some authors feel that if a subtrochanteric stress fracture is suspected, treatment should begin with two weeks of conservative therapy. If symptoms do not resolve, a bone scan should then be used to aid in the diagnosis. Displaced subtrochanteric stress fractures should be treated with internal fixation.

Stress fractures of the femoral shaft are uncommon in athletes (44,45,60). They are thought to occur most frequently in the proximal one-third of the shaft of the femur (23). Few studies have evaluated femoral shaft fractures in athletes. Most of the initial studies describing femoral shaft stress fractures involve military recruits

(51). Some feel that most femoral shaft stress fractures in athletes go undiagnosed, and many note the difficulty in diagnosis. Most of these fractures are nondisplaced and can be treated with a conservative therapy program including rest and initial non–weight-bearing, followed by bicycling and swimming. Gradually, patients are then returned to sport. Most athletes will be able to return to sport in 8 to 14 weeks. Operative treatment should be reserved for displaced or complete fractures.

Hip Dislocation

Dislocation of the hip is a rare but significant athletic injury (Fig. 14.14). Most hip dislocations occur posteriorly. A posterior hip dislocation in athletics is caused by a violent force, usually directed posteriorly on the knee with a flexed hip. This force can occur during collisions, such as a tackle in football or a check in hockey. Patients

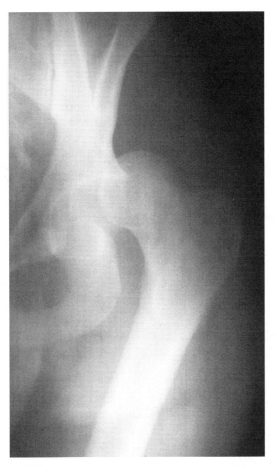

FIG. 14.14. Plain anteroposterior (AP) left hip radiograph illustrating a hip dislocation in a 21-year-old that occurred while skiing.

with a posterior hip dislocation will hold their thigh in a classic flexion, adduction, and internal rotation position. A hip dislocation is extremely painful and represents a true orthopaedic emergency.

The blood supply to the femoral head pierces the femoral capsule. A hip dislocation can interrupt the blood supply to the femoral head and result in avascular necrosis. Hip fractures reduced within 6 hours of their occurrence have a significantly lower incidence of avascular necrosis (27).

All hip dislocations should be reduced as soon as possible and in the correct medical environment (70). Radiographs should be taken to determine the position of the femoral head and if other fractures are present. These should be closely evaluated for proximal femur and acetabular rim fractures (Fig. 14.15). Sedation should then be used for adequate muscle relaxation and pain relief prior to an attempt at reduction. Some advocate general anesthesia.

Several reduction techniques have been recommended (5,35). For posterior dislocations, the patient is placed in a supine position, and the pelvis is stabilized. The hip is then flexed to 90 degrees and axial traction is applied to the distal thigh. This manuever will sometimes immedi-

ately reduce a posterior dislocation. Several other similar reduction techniques have been described. If closed reduction is not possible after one or two attempts and under adequate sedation, any further attempts should be made under general anesthesia. Failure of a closed reduction usually occurs from pieces of torn acetabular labrum or osteochondral fragments of the acetabular wall or femoral head becoming interposed in the joint. In patients in which closed reduction is not possible, or in which fragments are noted in the joint prior to reduction, open reduction is employed (28). A CT scan should be done after reduction of all closed hip dislocations to rule out intraarticular loose bodies and fractures of the femoral head and acetabular wall.

After closed reduction has been performed, bedrest and gentle passive range-of-motion exercises are employed. Patients gradually progress to weight bearing as tolerated. A period of non–weight-bearing is recommended by some, but is controversial. Some suggest that traction be used if the relocated hip is suspected to be unstable (27).

Even after uncomplicated reduction, simple hip dislocations can be a cause of significant morbidity. The long-term incidence of avascular necrosis of the femoral head after a simple hip dislocation has been reported at 8% to 15% (10,64). The incidence of avascular necrosis (AVN) is most likely related to the time interval between the dislocation and the reduction—the greater the time interval, the greater the incidence of AVN (27). In a 15-year follow-up study, the incidence of osteoarthrosis was found to be as high as 24%. This incidence was noted to be significantly higher in fracture dislocations (27,28, 30,64,65). It is important to follow patients with a hip dislocation for several years to observe for AVN, and patients should be made aware that they may eventually develop osteoarthrosis in the hip that was dislocated. Hip dislocation with spontanous reduction, although uncommon, has been identified in the more violent sports such as football (Fig. 14.16). The management of these injuries is no different than outlined above for the frank hip dislocation that requires manual reduction.

Greater Trochanteric Bursitis

Greater trochanteric bursitis is an entity that is becoming more identifiable. The trochanteric bursa rests between the bony greater trochanter of the femur and the iliotibial band. The greater trochanter, trochanteric bursa, and iliotibial band are subcutaneous and chronic inflammation of the bursa can be caused by direct contusion to the area. This can be seen in contact sports, such as football and ice hockey. Trochanteric bursitis is also commonly seen in running sports. This occurs as the result of excessive friction between the iliotibial band and the greater trochanteric structures as they pass over each other in hip flexion and extension. This is seen particularly in runners who run on

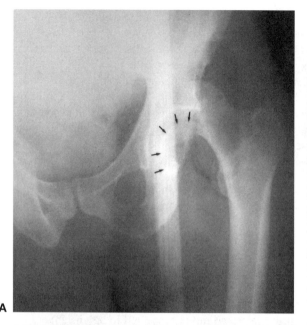

A

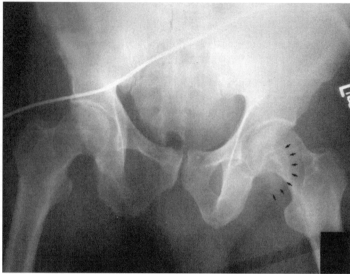

B

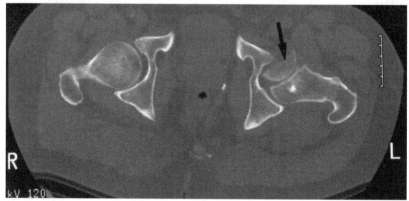

C

FIG. 14.15. Plain left hip radiograph in a 39-year-old race car driver illustrating a hip fracture dislocation (**A**) with arrows suggesting a femoral head fracture subsequent to a crash. Anteroposterior (AP) pelvis radiograph shows the hip reduced (**B**) with a persistent shadow consistent with a femoral head fracture *(arrows)*. Computed tomography (CT) scan (**C**) clearly illustrates the fractured femoral head *(arrows)*.

curved roadsides or on short-distance, non-banked indoor tracks. It is also seen in female runners with wide hips and in runners whose feet cross the midline.

Patients with trochanteric bursitis will often have localized pain over the greater trochanter to direct palpation. Some patients will also complain of pain that radiates into their buttock or lateral thigh. Pain may also be exacerbated when pressure is applied to the greater trochanter as the hip is brought from flexion into full extension (13).

The majority of greater trochanteric bursitis is successfully treated with rest, ice, antiinflammatory medication, iliotibial band stretching and hip muscle strengthening. Some patients may require lidocaine and cortisone injections, and severe cases may require resection of the trochanteric bursa with partial resection of the iliotibial band.

Snapping Hip Syndrome

Various anatomic problems have been attributed to the cause of a snapping sensation in the hip region. The most common is believed to be the result of movement of the iliotibial band over the greater trochanter. Other causes include snapping of the iliopsoas tendon over the iliopectineal eminence, the iliofemoral ligaments over the femoral head, and the tendinous origin of the long head of the biceps femoris muscle over the ischial tuberosity. Also, intraarticular causes such as loose bodies, synovial chondromatosis, osteocartilaginous exostosis, and hip subluxation can produce a snapping sensation.

In patients with snapping of the iliotibial band over the greater trochanter, treatment is initially conservative and includes rest, ice, antiinflammatory drugs, and iliotibial band stretching. Some patients will develop significant trochanteric bursitis and may require corticosteroid injections. Although infrequent and uncommon, some may require excision of the trochanteric bursa and partial iliotibial band resection.

Hip Injury in the Skeletally Immature

In any child or adolescent with hip pain, the diagnoses of Legg-Calvé-Perthes disease, slipped capital femoral

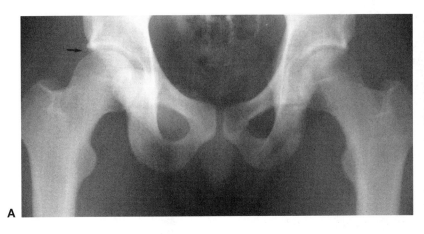

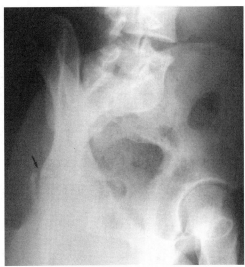

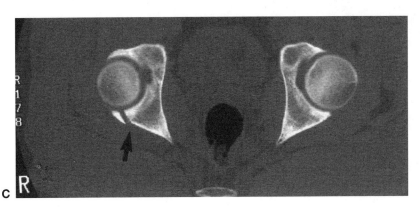

FIG. 14.16. Right hip subluxation with spontaneous resorption in professional football player. Pelvic AP radiograph (**A**) only suggests injury with small bone avulsion *(arrow)*. Oblique radiograph (**B**) illustrates posterior acetabular wall fracture, with computed tomography (CT) scan (**C**) best identifying the fracture *(arrow)*.

epiphysis, transient synovitis, osteomyelitis and septic hip should be considered.

Legg-Calvé-Perthes Disease

Legg-Calvé-Perthes disease is a potentially devastating condition. The etiology is unknown. Proposed theories suggest a disruption in the blood supply to the developing femoral head. Growth hormone abnormalities and transient synovitis have been suggested to be contributing factors (26). Pathologically, either all or a portion of the femoral head undergoes infarction, resorption, collapse and reossification and can be followed radiographically (Fig. 14.17). In the early stages of the disease, cartilage proliferation and hyperplastic synovitis also occurs. The disease is self-limiting and many patients will eventually develop the classic flattening of the weight-bearing surface of the femoral head.

Although this condition is most commonly seen in patients from 4 to 8 years of age, it should be considered in all athletic patients up to 12 years old. Of the few prognostic determinants, the most important is age. Patients who are younger at the onset of the disease seem to do better, particularly those less than 6 years of age.

Also, those with less than 50% of femoral head involvement also appear to have a better prognosis.

This disease is often not identifiable by plain radiographs in the early stages (first 3 to 6 weeks) of the disease (14). Bone scan or MRI is often used as the most sensitive early indicators of the disease, with MRI the most sensitive in identifying the disease in its earliest stages—prior to plain radiographic changes.

Containment of the femoral head within the acetabulum is the current strategy of treatment. This involves nonsurgical and surgical approaches toward keeping the healing and deformable femoral head within the dome of the acetabulum. Both approaches are best instituted prior to advanced femoral head collapse and prior to epiphyseal extrusion (6).

Nonsurgical approaches involve abduction (Petrie), casting (48), or bracing (e.g., Scottish Rite brace, abduction hinged brace). Most patients can be managed nonoperatively. For pain-free individuals, weight bearing in a brace can be employed; however, the benefit of this treatment has not been proven statistically.

Surgery is used late in the disease to optimize femoral head coverage of a deformed head. Surgical indications are controversial. Salter innominate and femoral osteotomies are commonly used (Fig. 14.18). High-impact load-

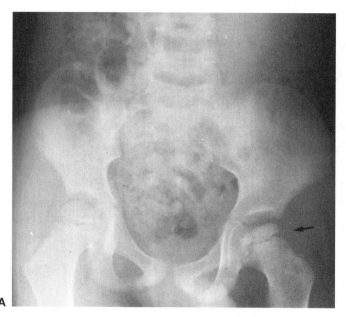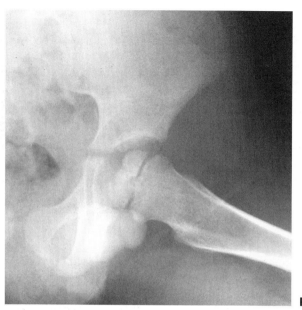

A   **B**

FIG. 14.17. Pelvis AP (**A**) and frog-leg lateral (**B**) radiographs of Legg-Calvé-Perthes disease in a 5-year-old soccer player with left hip pain that is exacerbated with activity. Note the infarction, resorption and collapse of the left femoral head *(arrow)*.

ing at the hip (which is required of most sports other than biking and swimming) is not recommended until the healing phase of the disease is reached, unless the disease is mild and involves less than 50% of the femoral head.

Treatment should be individualized; yet, nonsurgical and surgical approaches have been known to have similar outcomes (14,19,49).

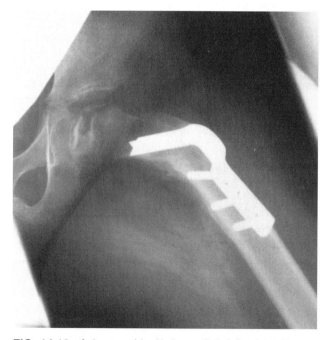

FIG. 14.18. A 9-year-old with Legg-Calvé-Perthes disease showing resorption, collapse, and reossification of the femoral head. This individual had undergone a proximal femoral osteotomy with internal fixation.

Slipped Capital Femoral Epiphysis

A slipped capital femoral epiphysis is the most common hip disorder seen in adolescents. It is noted to have a higher incidence in black youths. It is also more common in males than in females. Many patients with slipped capital femoral epiphysis are noticeably obese or tall and lanky. The average age at the time of initial diagnosis is approximately 13 years and is usually thought to occur between 10 and 15 years of age. Approximately 37% to 40% of adolescents will develop a slipped capital femoral epiphysis on the contralateral side (37).

This condition is defined as acute, chronic, or acute on chronic. A patient with a sudden onset of symptoms of less than 3 weeks' duration is described as ''acute'' (some authors make this cutoff at 2 weeks). A patient with a gradual onset of pain that is greater than 3 weeks' duration is described as a ''chronic slip.'' A patient with symptoms greater than 3 weeks, who then has a sudden exacerbation of symptoms is described as an acute on chronic slip.

The major complaint in a patient with a slipped capital femoral epiphysis is pain. Most patients will localize this pain to the groin region. Some will complain of pain radiation in the anterior or medial thigh, or even the knee (Fig. 14.19). Most patients will demonstrate an antalgic gait, and some (especially in acute slips) will refuse to place weight on the affected extremity.

Radiographic views include an AP pelvis and frog leg lateral of both hips, taking care to compare and evaluate both hips. Some patients may have bilateral slipped capital femoral epiphyses. On radiographs, the head slips posteromedially on the neck. Some describe this as the

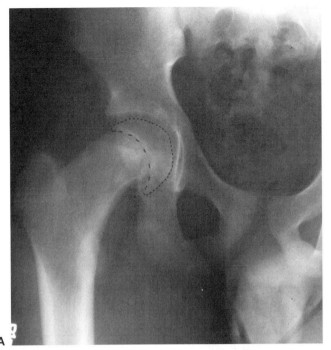

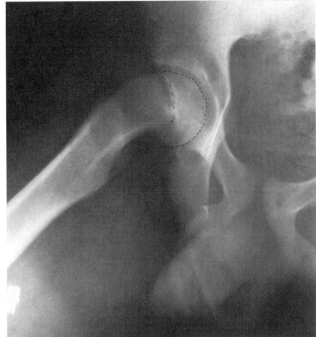

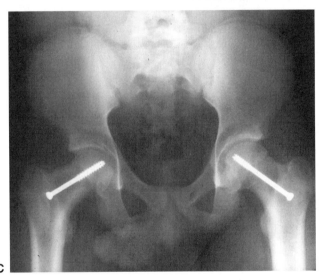

FIG. 14.19. Slipped capital femoral epiphysis in an obese 13-year-old. Dotted lines on plain AP of the right hip (**A**) and frog-leg lateral (**B**) radiographs evidence slipped epiphysis. A single internal fixation screw to fixate bilateral slips as seen on the AP pelvis radiograph (**C**).

neck slipping anterolaterally on the head. Many patients with a slipped capital femoral epiphysis will also show physeal widening. In addition, some patients with a chronic slip may show periosteal calcification (2).

The degree of the slip can be determined using the epiphyseal line—femoral shaft angle. This is performed on the AP and frog-leg lateral views and is compared to the contralateral limb. A slip of less than 30 degrees is mild. A moderate slip is considered between 30 and 60 degrees and a severe slip is greater than 60 degrees (10).

Operative fixation is the basis of treatment for most patients with slipped capital femoral epiphyses. The goal is to stabilize the epiphysis and promote physeal fusion. This can be accomplished through threaded pins, or more recently, cannulated screws. Bone graft epiphyseodesis

has also been used (69). In patients with large "acute" or "acute on chronic" slips, perioperative gentle traction with internal rotation, although controversial, has been used to reduce the slip. Excessive traction and traction in patients with a "chronic" slipped capital femoral epiphysis are contraindicated as a high incidence of aseptic necrosis has been noted (28).

Avascular necrosis, chrondrolysis, and early osteoarthrosis are the potential long-term complications of slipped capital femoral epiphysis. Also, patients may develop a contralateral slipped capital femoral epiphysis, and therefore, should be followed until skeletal maturity. Patients with more severe slips may require an osteotomy to restore alignment, improve acetabular coverage of their femoral head and improve hip motion.

THIGH INJURY

Quadriceps Contusion

A quadriceps contusion is usually caused by a strong external blow to the anterior, medial, or lateral thigh. This causes disruption of muscle fibers, capillaries, and sometimes veins and arteries. The most severe damage is caused by transmission of force to the layer of quadriceps that interfaces with the anterior femur. Intramuscular bleeding and hematoma formation can occur. This can sometimes lead to the formation of heterotopic bone, called myositis ossificans.

The patient with a quadriceps contusion will give a history of trauma. This injury is common in contact sports such as football. Athletes who receive trauma to the thigh and are suspected to have a quadriceps contusion should be removed from further competition. Continued activity can lead to increased blood flow to the area and cause increased thigh compartment pressures.

Patients with a quadriceps contusion have thigh pain with active and passive motion of the knee. Thigh swelling may also be prominent in moderate and severe cases. Thigh girth should be measured on initial presentation and compared to the contralateral thigh, and should be monitored. Increased swelling and tightness of the thigh warrants compartment pressure measurements. Other compartment syndrome signs such as pain out of proportion to the injury, paresthesias, pallor, and pulselessness are less reliable in the thigh (55,61,67). In moderate and severe cases, continued swelling and thigh enlargement after 48 hours may indicate arterial bleeding and the need for an arteriogram.

In a patient with suspected quadriceps contusion, radiographs are taken to rule out a femur fracture. Also, care should be taken to evaluate the knee extensor mechanism and rule out quadriceps tendon or muscle rupture.

The treatment protocol for thigh contusions consists of three phases (57). The first phase involves rest, ice, compression, and an evaluation of the thigh. Rest should occur with flexion of the knee and hip to patient pain tolerance. This phase usually lasts for 24 hours in mild contusions and 48 hours in moderate and severe contusions. Phase II involves restoring knee mobility. Weight bearing should occur with the assistance of crutches until the patient is able to flex the knee to 90 degrees and ambulate with good control and without pain. When the patient is able to actively flex to 120 degrees without pain, they advance to the next phase of treatment. Phase III involves restoring full strength, motion, and endurance. It also involves gradual return to contact sports after these objectives are reached. Thigh pads should be worn in contact sports such as football because of the high risk of such an injury.

Myositis Ossificans

Myositis ossificans is a benign condition caused by the formation of heterotopic bone. In the thigh, most patients will give a history of trauma. It is thought to occur as the result of hematoma formation that leads to granulation tissue formation, and then heterotopic endochondral ossification (Fig. 14.20). When myositis ossificans is suspected from bone formation on plain radiographs, it is always necessary to rule out parosteal and periosteal osteosarcoma. Radiographs, ultrasound, contrast angiography, bone scans, and CT scans have been used to evaluate myositis ossificans. Myositis ossificans can be connected to the femur by a stalk, can appear to have a large base connected to the femur, or may be entirely separated (63). The bony mass usually becomes apparent radiographically 2 to 4 weeks after trauma to the thigh and continues to enlarge and ossify for up to 3 to 6 months. Surgical excision of the ossified mass in myositis ossificans is unusual and should only be performed after conservative measures have failed to treat the symptomatic patient. If surgically excised, it is only after the lesion has ''matured,'' which is usually not earlier than 18 months post injury. A cold bone scan can be used preoperatively to confirm maturation.

Thigh Compartment Syndrome

A thigh compartment syndrome is rare. It can be caused by a femur fracture, a thigh tourniquet, a thigh contusion, arthroscopy, and exercise. A thigh compartment syndrome can occur in any of the three compartments of the thigh including the anterior, medial, or posterior. Patients may have a tense thigh on palpation. Pain with passive stretch and pain out of proportion to the injury are not often accurate indicators as many patients will experience these with any significant thigh or femur injury. Pulselessness and paresthesias may sometimes be present, but their absence does not rule out a compartment syndrome (55,67). If compartment syndrome is suspected, compartment pressures should be checked and monitored. The threshold for suspicion should be low in a patient with a history of significant trauma.

Any patient with suspected increased thigh compartment pressure should be initially treated with rest, ice, and elevation until compartment pressures can be evaluated. Some advocate close monitoring and nonoperative treatment in patients with an isolated thigh compartment syndrome (55). Most, however, advocate surgical fasciotomies (50,56,67). The compartment pressure threshold for surgical intervention is also contested. Some suggest 30 mm Hg (43), while others use 40 mm Hg (39), and some use arterial pressure (56). The consequences of not effectively treating a compartment syndrome of the thigh

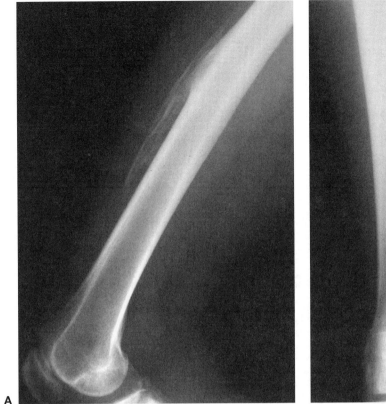
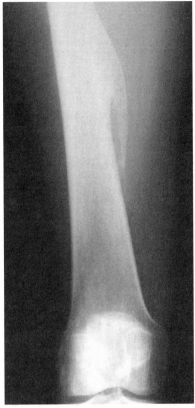

FIG. 14.20. Myositis ossificans can occur subsequent to a blow such as a helmet in football to the thigh that produces a hematoma and ossifies. Typical AP (**A**) and lateral (**B**) radiographic finding.

can be disastrous. Patients suspected of developing or having this problem should be treated emergently and aggressively.

Hamstring Strain

A hamstring strain is the most common muscle injury in the thigh. The most common hamstring injured is the short head of the biceps femoris (25). A hamstring strain occurs when excessive passive stretch occurs or when excessive load is placed on the hamstrings during muscle contraction. The injury usually occurs at the myotendinous junction. Tearing of the myotendious unit or muscle fibers can lead to inflammation, edema, hemorrhage, or muscle rupture.

Hamstring strains typically occur during acceleration-deceleration and high-speed running activities (31). The athlete usually experiences immediate pain. Some athletes experience a popping or snapping sensation. Pain occurs in the posterior thigh with ambulation. Most athletes will have tenderness on palpation of the posterior thigh and some may have a palpable mass or defect. Weakness and pain can be elicited with resisted flexion of the knee. Some athletes may also have swelling, poor flexibility, tight hamstrings, hamstring-quadricep

strength imbalance, muscle fatigue, and inadequate hamstring strength.

Hamstring strains can be graded. Grade I involves mild overstretching and minimal changes in the musculotendinous continuity. Grade II is a moderate injury causing an incomplete tear of the muscle. Grade III is a complete rupture of the muscle. Grade I and II injuries are treated conservatively. Grade III injuries are also usually treated conservatively; yet, some promote surgical repair. Ultrasound, CT scan, and MRI have all been described to evaluate the extent of injury to the hamstrings.

Most hamstring injuries can be treated acutely with NSAIDs, ice, an elastic wrap, and rest. Ambulation may be initially difficult. Crutches may be required in more severe cases. Initially, gentle passive range-of-motion exercises and stretching should be used. Athletes are then progressed to muscle strengthening and hamstring endurance and flexibility (12,31). Athletes also work on running coordination prior to return to sport.

Strains of the hamstring muscles tend to recur. This may be caused by inadequate or less than complete rehabilitation. In an athlete's rehabilitation and return to sport, special attention should be taken to maintain adequate strength of the hamstrings. Adequate warm-up and passive stretching can also help to decrease the risk of reinjury.

REFERENCES

1. Akermark C, Johansson C. Tenotomy of the adductor longus tendon in the treatment of chronic groin pain athletes. *Am J Sports Med* 1992;20(6):640–643.
2. Aronson D, Carlson W. Slipped capital femoral epiphysis: a prospective study of fixation with a single screw. *J Bone Joint Surg* 1992;74A(6):810–819.
3. Atwell A, Jackson D. Stress fractures of the sacrum in runners: two case reports. *Am J Sports Med* 1991;19(5):531–533.
4. Barton P. Piriformis syndrome: a rational approach to management. *Pain* 1991;47:345–352.
5. Bassi J, Ahuja SC, Singh H. A flexion adduction method for the reduction of posterior dislocation of the hip. *J Bone Joint Surg* 1992;74B:157–158.
6. Beaty J. Legg-Calvé-Perthes disease: diagnostic and prognostic techniques. *Instr Course Lectures* 1989;Chap 24:291–296.
7. Brown J, Braun M, Namey T. Pyriformis syndrome in a 10-year-old boy as a complication of operation in a sitting position. *Neurosurgery* 1988;23:117–119.
8. Butler W, Allen W. Fracture of the iliac crest apophysis: an unusual hip pointer. *Am J Sports Med* 1975;3:192–193.
9. Cameron H. The piriformis syndrome. *Can J Surg* 1988;31(4):210–212.
10. Canale T. Problems and complications of slipped capital femoral epiphysis. *Instr Course Lect* 1989;Chap 23:281–290.
11. Caudle R, Craford A. Avulsion fracture of the lateral acetabular margin. A case report. *J Bone Joint Surg* 1988;70A:1568–1570.
12. Cibulka M. Rehabilitation of the pelvis, hip, and thigh. *Clin Sports Med* 1989;8(4):777–803.
13. Clancy W. Runners injuries part two. Evaluation and treatment of specific injuries. *Am J Sports Med* 1980;8(4):287–289.
14. Cooperman D, Stulberg S. Ambulatory containment in Perthes disease. *CORR* 1986;203:289–300.
15. Draper D, Dustman A. Avulsion fracture of the anterior superior iliac spine in a collegiate distance runner. *Arch Phys Med Rehab* 1992;73:881–882.
16. Ekberg O, Persson NH, Abrahamsson PA, Westlin NE, Lilja B. Longstanding groin pain in athletes—a multidisciplinary approach. *Sports Med* 1988;6:56–61.
17. Fishman L, Zybert PA. Electrophysiologic evidence of piriformis syndrome. *Arch Phys Med Rehabil* 1992;73:359–364.
18. Freiberg A. Sciatic pain and its relief by operations on muscles and fascia. *Arch Surg* 1937;34:337–350.
19. Fulford G, Lunn PG, Macnicol M. A prospective study of nonoperative and operative management for Perthes' disease. *J Pediatr Orthop* 1993;13(3):281–285.
20. Fullerton L, Snowdy H. Femoral neck stress fractures. *Am J Sports Med* 1988;16(4):365–377.
21. Godshall R, Hansen CA. Incomplete avulsion of a portion of the iliac epiphysis. *J Bone Joint Surg* 1973;55A:1301–1302.
22. Goitz HT. Upper extremity tendon rupture in professional football. [Paper presentation] *NFL Team Physician's Soc.* Indianapolis: February 1996.
23. Hajek M. Stress fractures of the femoral neck in joggers: case report and review of the literature. *Am J Sports Med* 1982;10(2):110–116.
24. Hamada G, Rida A. Ischial apophysiolysis. Report of a case and review of the literature. *CORR* 1963;31:117–130.
25. Heiser T, Weber J, Sullivan G, Clare P, Jacobs RR. Prophylaxis and management of hamstring muscle injuries in intercollegiate football players. *Am J Sports Med* 1984;12(5):368–370.
26. Herring J. The treatment of Legg-Calvé-Perthes disease. *J Bone Joint Surg* 1994;76A(3):448–458.
27. Hougaard K, Thompson P. Coxarthrosis following traumatic posterior dislocation of the hips. *J Bone Joint Surg* 1987;69A(5):679–683.
28. Jacob JR, Rao JP, Ciccarelli C. Traumatic dislocation and fracture dislocation of the hip. *CORR* 1987;214:249–263.
29. Jankiewicz JJ, Hennrikus WL, Houkom JA. The appearance of the piriformis muscle syndrome in computed tomography and magnetic resonance imaging. *CORR* 1991;2 62:205–209.
30. Jaskulka RA, Fischer G, Fenzl G. Dislocation and fracture dislocation of the hip. *J Bone Joint Surg* 1991;73B(3):465–469.
31. Jonhagen S, Nemeth G, Eriksson E. Hamstring injuries in sprinters. The role of concentric and eccentric hamstring muscle strength and flexibility. *Am J Sports Med* 1994;22(2):262–266.
32. Kalebo P, Karlsson J, Sward L, Peterson L. Ultrasonography of chronic tendon injuries in the groin. *Am J Sports Med* 1993;21(1):634–639.
33. Karl RD Jr, Yedinak MA, Hartshorne MF, Cawthon MA, Bauman JM, Howard WH, Bunker SR. Scintigraphic appearance of the piriformis muscle syndrome. *Clin Nuc Med* 1985;10:361–363.
34. Karlsson J, Sward L, Kalebo P, Thomee R. Chronic groin injuries in athletes: recommendations for treatment and rehabilitation. *Sports Med* 1994;17(2):141–148.
35. Lefkowitz M. A new method for reduction of hip dislocations. *Orth Rev* February 1993:253–254.
36. Leinberry CF, McShane RB, Stewart WG Jr, Hume EL. A displaced subtrochanteric stress fracture in a young amenorrheic athlete. *Am J Sports Med* 1992;20(4):485–487.
37. Loder R, Aaronson DD, Greenfield ML. The epidemiology of bilateral slipped capital femoral epiphysis. A study of children in Michigan. *J Bone Joint Surg* 1993;75A(8):1114–1147.
38. Lombardo SJ, Retting AC, Kerlan RK. Radiographic abnormalities of the iliac apophysis in adolescent athletes. *J Bone Joint Surg* 1983;65A:444–446.
39. Matsen F, Winquist R, Krugmire R. Diagnosis and management of compartmental syndromes. *J Bone Joint Surg* 1980;62A:286–291.
40. Metzmaker N, Pappas A. Avulsion fractures of the pelvis. *Am J Sports Med* 1985;13(5):349–358.
41. Milch H. Ischial apophysiolysis. A new syndrome. *CORR* 1953;2:184,185.
42. Mizuguchi T. Division of the piriformis muscle for the treatment of sciatica. Postlaminectomy syndrome and osteoarthrosis of the spine. *Arch Surg* 1976;111:719–722
43. Murbarak SJ, Owen CA, Hargens AR, Garetto LP, Akeson WH. Acute compartment syndromes: diagnosis and treatment with the aid of a wick catheter. *J Bone Joint Surg* 1978;60A: 1091–1095.
44. Orava S. Stress fracture. *Br J Sports Med* 1980;14:40–44.
45. Orava S, Puranen J, Ala-Ketola L. Stress fractures caused by physical exercise. *Acta Orthop Scan* 1978;49:19–27.
46. Pace S, Nagle D. Piriformis syndrome. *West J Med* 1976;124:435–439.
47. Peck D. Apophyseal injuries in the young athlete. *Am F Phys* 1995;51(8):1891–1895.
48. Petrie JG, Bitenc I. The abduction weight bearing treatment in Legg-Perthes disease. *J Bone Joint Surg* 1971;53B:54–62.
49. Poussa M, Yrjonen T, Hoikka V, Osterman K. Prognosis after conservative and operative treatment in Perthes disease. *CORR* 1993;297:82–86.
50. Presnal B, Hearilon J. Exercise induced acute compartment syndrome of the thigh: case report. *Am J Knee Surg* 1995;8(2):77–79.
51. Provost R, Morris J. Fatigue fractures of the femoral shaft. *J Bone Joint Surg* 1969;51A:487–498.
52. Renstrom A. Tendon and muscle injuries in the groin area. *Clin Sports Med* 1992;11(4):815–831.
53. Risser J. The iliac apophysis: an invaluable sign in the management of scoliosis. *CORR* 1958;11:111–119.
54. Robinson D. The piriformis syndrome in relation to sciatic pain. *Am J Surg* 1947;73:355–358.
55. Robinson D, On E, Halperin N. Anterior compartment syndrome of the thigh in athletes: indication for conservative treatment. *J Trauma* 1992;32:183–186.
56. Rooser B. Acute compartment syndromes from anterior thigh muscle contusion. Report of eight cases. *J Ortho Trauma* 1991;5:55–59.
57. Ryan J, Wheeler JH, Hopkinson WJ, Arciero JA, Kolakowski KR. Quadriceps contusions. West Point update. *Am J Sports Med* 1991;19(3):299–304.
58. Solheim LF, Siewers P, Paus B. The piriformis muscle syndrome: sciatic nerve entrapment treated section of the piriformis muscle. *Acta Orth Scan* 1981;52:73–75.
59. Speer KP, Lohnes J, Garrett WE Jr. Radiographic imaging of muscle strain injury. *Am J Sports Med* 1993;21(1):89–96.

60. Sullivan D, Warren RF, Pavlov H, Kelman G. Stress fractures in 51 runners. *CORR* 1984; 187:188–192.
61. Synek V. The piriformis syndrome: review and case presentation. *Clin Exp Neurol* 1987;23:31–37.
62. Taylor D, Meyers W, Moylan J, Lohnes J, Bassett F. Abdominal musculature abnormalities as a cause of groin pain in athletes: inguinal hernias and pubalgia. *Am J Sports Med* 1991;19(3):239–242.
63. Tredget T, Godberson CV, Bose B. Myositis ossificans due to hockey injury. *CMAJ* 1977;116:65–66.
64. Upadhyay S, Moulton A. The long term results of traumatic posterior dislocation of the hip. *J Bone Joint Surg* 1981;63B(4):548–551.
65. Upadhyay S, Moulton A, Srikrishnamurthy K. An analysis of the late effects of traumatic posterior dislocation of the hip without fractures. *J Bone Joint Surg* 1983;65B(2):150–152.
66. Vandertop WP, Bosma NJ. The piriformis syndrome. *J Bone Joint Surg* 1991;73(A):1095–1096.
67. Viegas SF, Rimoldi R, Scarborough M, Ballantyne GM. Acute compartment syndrome of the thigh. *CORR* 1988;234:232–234.
68. Wang L, Bowen JR, Puniak MA, Guille JT, Glutting J. An evaulation of various methods of treatment in Perthes disease. *CORR* 1993;297:82–86.
69. Weiner D. Bone graft epiphysiodesis in the treatment of slipped capital femoral epiphysis. *Instr Course Lect* 1989;Chap 21:281–290.
70. Yang R, Tsuang YH, Hang YS, Liu TK. Traumatic dislocation of the hip. *CORR* 1991;265:218–226.

The Injured Athlete, Third Edition,
edited by D. H. Perrin.
Lippincott–Raven Publishers, Philadelphia © 1999.

CHAPTER **15**

The Knee

Mary Lloyd Ireland, Mark R. Hutchinson, Richard I. Williams,
and Michael Gaudette

THE KNEE

With advances in technology, more experience, and basic research, our understanding of knee injuries has reached a new level. Procedures once considered uncharted, radical, and dangerous are now the "gold standard." An open meniscectomy is unusual. Repairing and saving the meniscus is routine. The goal is to restore normal homeostasis of the knee (61).

Technologic advances in fiberoptics, computerized video data transmission, and the development of specialized instrumentation have resulted in the acceptance of arthroscopy and arthroscopically assisted procedures by an overwhelming majority of orthopaedic surgeons. New hopes for restoring "normal knee function" include articular surface reimplantation and meniscal allograft. Once reserved for only the most elite athletes, anterior cruciate ligament (ACL) reconstruction is commonplace among even middle-aged weekend warriors who enjoy and want to continue an active lifestyle.

Careful objective reporting of clinical results has provided an opportunity to reevaluate the earlier surgical procedures such as lateral retinacular release for "chondromalacia patella" or "diagnostic" arthroscopy. With the climate of health care reform, questions regarding access to specialty care have placed scrutiny on the results of our therapies, and "outcomes research" has become mandatory in the 21st century.

M. L. Ireland: Kentucky Sports Medicine Clinic, Lexington, Kentucky 40517

M. R. Hutchinson: Department of Orthopaedics and Sports Medicine, University of Illinois at Chicago, Chicago, Illinois 60612-7342

R. I. Williams: Upper Cumberland Orthopaedics and Sports Medicine, Cookeville, Tennessee 38501

M. Gaudette: Joyner Sportsmedicine Institute, Lexington, Kentucky 40517

A growing trend can be seen away from "emergent" and "urgent" operative intervention in most types of knee injuries. Studies documenting increased complications from stiffness following ACL reconstruction results in reconsideration of taking the athlete from the football field or ski slope directly to the operating room. After the acute knee injury, careful repeated examinations will establish the correct diagnosis. Prior to surgery, the goal is a normal-appearing knee—no swelling, normal range of motion, and good lower extremity muscle function. The physician should carefully stress to the athlete, however, that nonoperative treatment is not the same as "no treatment." The athlete must participate in his/her own care. Imagine the emotions involved when an urgent surgical procedure is performed for an acutely unstable knee and the result is less than satisfactory: the athlete did not have an opportunity to experience the consequences of the injury—perhaps it barely hurt at all—but he/she can certainly see the effects of the surgical intervention! The unfortunate consequence is the shifting of anger by the athlete from the injury itself to the treating physician, physical therapist, or athletic trainer.

Progress in other areas, including the advent of magnetic resonance imaging (MRI) for diagnostic use in selected cases, and rehabilitation protocols emphasizing closed chain activities and rapid return to play, have facilitated a more comprehensive and directed approach to therapy. The accuracy of MRI has revealed interesting injury patterns, such as "bone bruises" associated with ligament tears. The specificity of such diagnostic exams has rendered the old, nonspecific terminology "internal derangement of the knee" an historic footnote. Conversely, the fiscal and market separation of orthopaedist and physical therapist, brought about in the United States by ethical concerns regarding overutilization and self-referral, have caused a rethinking of protocols.

Indeed, controversy remains in almost every realm of

treating knee injuries. Operative versus nonoperative treatment of complete medial collateral ligament (MCL) tears, appropriate graft material choice and fixation in ACL surgery, treatment of combined instabilities, and indications for meniscal repair are currently hot topics for debate. Therefore, it is even more imperative that clinicians be systematic and thorough in all phases of diagnosis and treatment. Documentation of findings and therapies is of paramount importance, not only for future research but in a litigious climate to protect caregivers from frivolous attack. Always remember to examine the contralateral extremity, perform a systematic, complete exam, and record the findings in a medical record.

The importance of ongoing research, both on a basic science/biomechanical level, and solid clinical research (case series, prospective and well-defined retrospective studies) cannot be overemphasized. The health-care professional must remain current and well-read. New advances should be examined critically. Anecdotal experience should be viewed skeptically. Informed, thoughtful decisions should be made regarding ''advances'' in treatment and technology. Beware of the new technologic advance, which is not backed by solid clinical and basic research. Newer is not *always* better. Similarly, one must be careful not to hang on to outmoded concepts and therapies. A given technique or procedure should remain a viable alternative if it yields objectively acceptable results, and does not involve undue limitations or negative long-term consequences for the athlete. It may be better to stick with a tested remedy than switch to one involving a long learning curve and technical pitfalls that might jeopardize the ultimate outcome.

Finally, in order to apply the most effective treatment program, the correct diagnosis must be made. The basic requirement is a complete knowledge of the normal knee anatomy. Differential diagnosis is made easy by correlating the mechanism of injury with the physical exam.

ANATOMY

Understanding knee anatomy provides the basis for diagnosis and treatment of knee injuries. Knee anatomy has been well described in textbooks (16,57,69,94,114,134, 175,178,200,210,221,234). Indeed, some textbooks are dedicated to a single component of knee anatomy such as the patellofemoral articulation (68,77) or the ACL (49,123). Surgical textbooks also provide detail of knee anatomy (49,96,104,114,123,175,221). Advances in arthroscopic techniques help to correlate anatomy, mechanism of injury, operative findings and treatment (9,126, 166). This anatomy section will review bony anatomy, extensor mechanism, ligaments and capsule, (medial side lateral side) menisci, and cruciate ligaments.

Bony Anatomy

The knee joint is the largest and one of the most complex joints in the human body. There are three independent articulations. The patella and trochlear groove of the femur or patellofemoral (PF) articulation is anterior. The two weight-bearing compartments are the medial or inner compartment and the lateral or outer compartment. Each is composed of the tibial plateau, the femoral condyle and the meniscus with capsuloligamentous attachments. Each compartment is unique anatomically. The PF articulation can be compared to a train on a track. The patella (train) is more stable on a well-formed deep trochlear groove (track). The medial compartment has more compression forces and stronger capsuloligamentous attachments to the meniscus. The lateral compartment has a more convex lateral tibial plateau, more movement, distraction, and rotation (Fig. 15.1).

The distal femur forms two large, curved knuckles, or condyles, with a sulcus or depression in between. The distal portions of the condyles articulate with the tibial plateau, whereas the anterior sulcus or trochlea provides the contact surface for the patella, a floating sesamoid bone, embedded within the anterior quadriceps ''extensor'' mechanism. The lateral ridge of the trochlea is more anterior and wider than its medial counterpart and resists lateral translation of the patella (Fig. 15.2).

The condyles have a different shape and radius of curvature. The medial condyle is elliptical, larger, more distal, and a factor in the normal 5 to 9 degrees of valgus alignment. The lateral condyle is shorter and more spheroid (234). The differential sizes of the condyles result in a phenomenon known as the ''screw-home'' mechanism,

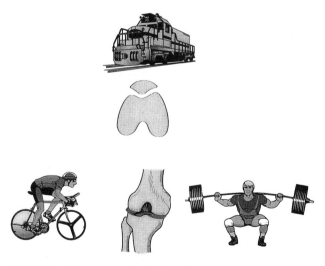

FIG. 15.1. Diagrammatically, the three compartments of the knee can be compared to a train (patella) on a track (trochlear groove). Medial compartment has more stability and compressive forces similar to a weight lifter and the lateral compartment has more mobility and rotation, compared to a bicyclist in a velodome.

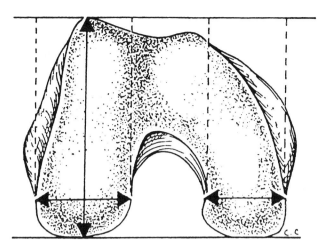

FIG. 15.2. A comparison of the medial and lateral femoral condyles shows that the lateral condyle is broader in the transverse plane. (Reprinted with permission from ref. 16.)

whereby the tibia subtly rotates externally on the femur slightly as the knee comes into full extension (234). Between the femoral condyles distally is a recessed area referred to as the intercondylar notch where the cruciate ligaments attach. The intercondylar notch size, width, and shape forms in relation to the size of the ACL. If the ligament is small, the notch will accordingly be small. On the tibial surface opposing the notch are two raised areas known as the medial and lateral tibial spines or eminences. These spines reduce rotational forces and serve as anatomic landmarks for the surgeon.

The tibia also serves as the insertion point of multiple muscles and ligaments that control knee function. These structures include: the tibial tubercle for the patellar tendon/ligament; Gerdy's tubercle—for the iliotibial tract; and the proximal fibula—for biceps femoris and lateral collateral ligament.

The patella is a sesamoid bone that functions as a fulcrum to improve the efficiency of the quadriceps mechanism. The undersurface of the patella consists of the following facets: medial, lateral, odd, and nonarticulating (77) (Fig. 15.3). The patella functions to increase the lever arm of the quadriceps and to shield and protect the femoral condyles. The articulating surface is covered with the thickest layer of hyaline cartilage in the body. Patellar

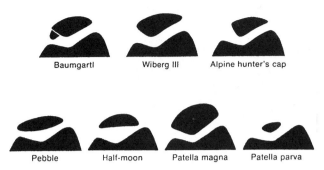

FIG. 15.4. Variations in patella form considered dysplastic. (Reprinted with permission from ref. 77.)

stability is enhanced by a deeper trochlear groove, less valgus alignment, and quadriceps balance between the vastus lateralis and vastus medialis obliquus. Wiberg and Baumgartl have described seven different types of patellar shape depth of the sulcus, including Baumgartl, Wiberg III, Alpine hunter's cap, Pebble, Half-moon, Patella magna, and Patella parva (Fig. 15.4) (19,221,253).

Patellar contact increases and moves more proximally throughout knee flexion. Early flexion at 30 degrees has contact at the superior trochlear groove (1) (Fig. 15.5). Also, with increasing knee flexion angle, there is increased tension in the quadriceps and patellar tendon (32,77,97). Excessive lateral pressure will cause a bony response with direct radiologic signs (77) (Fig. 15.6A). Patients with excessive lateral patellar syndrome (ELPS) have a very long patellar facet, an acute osteopenic medial patellar facet, and a long, flattened lateral trochlear groove. The result is thickening of the patellar subchondral plate, increased density of the lateral facet and cancellous bone, and lateralization of trabecula (see Fig. 15.6B). More localized problems of ELPS are lateral retinacular fibrosis and calcification, lateral osteophyte of the patella and sometime matching osteophyte of the femur, lateral facet hyperplasia and medial side hypoplasia.

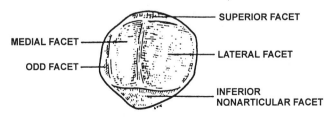

FIG. 15.3. Patellar articular surface consists of odd, medial, and lateral facets. Superior and inferior nonarticular facets are shown.

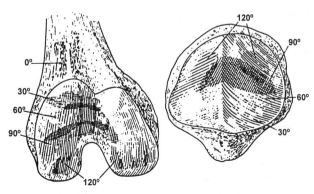

FIG 15.5. Patellofemoral contact areas are shaded at 0, 30, 60, 90, 120 degrees flexion in this right-knee diagram. Femur (*lateral to left and medial to right*) and patella (*lateral to right and medial to left*) are shown. (Reprinted with permission from ref. 1.)

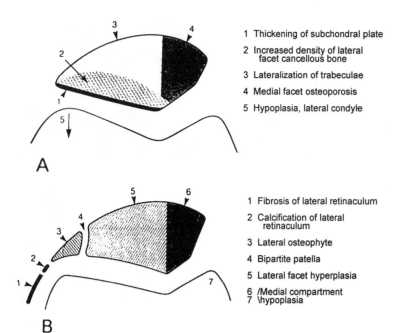

A.

1 Thickening of subchondral plate

2 Increased density of lateral facet cancellous bone

3 Lateralization of trabeculae

4 Medial facet osteoporosis

5 Hypoplasia, lateral condyle

B.

1 Fibrosis of lateral retinaculum

2 Calcification of lateral retinaculum

3 Lateral osteophyte

4 Bipartite patella

5 Lateral facet hyperplasia

6 /Medial compartment
7 \hypoplasia

FIG. 15.6. A. Indirect radiologic signs of excessive lateral pressure. **B.** Indirect radiologic signs of excessive lateral ligamentous tension. (Reprinted with permission from ref. 77.)

The Extensor Mechanism

The quadriceps muscle group originates from the proximal femur and anterior hip capsule/pelvis. Muscular components include the rectus femoris, vastus lateralis, vastus intermedius, vastus medialis, and vastus medialis obliquus (VMO). The rectus femoris crosses the hip and knee joint, acting in hip flexion and knee extension. During a normal gait cycle, momentum and gravity actually allow for knee extension during the swing phase without significant quadriceps activity. The quadriceps eccentrically decelerates the flexed knee following heel strike (147). Walking creates patellofemoral force of one-half body weight, stair climbing 3.3 times body weight and with activities such as landing, forces approach seven to eight times body weight (208).

The four quadriceps muscles blend together in the distal thigh to form the quadriceps tendon, which subsequently envelops the patella. Two subspecialized portions of the quadriceps arise distally. The articularis genu comes from the deep vastus medialis and serves to retract the suprapatellar pouch from beneath the patella during extension. Although the vastus medialis obliquus (VMO) does not provide extension force, it stabilizes the patella medially (146). The VMO inserts on the proximal half of the medial patella at a 65-degree angle from its origin on the intermuscular septum and adductor magnus (Fig. 15.7). The appearance of the VMO reflects the overall health of the quadriceps. With its thinner fascia, the VMO is the first muscle to atrophy with injury and the last to return with full recovery.

The various anatomic structures in the knee act in concert. No one structure performs a particular function by itself. The terminal 15 degrees of knee extension requires 60% more force by the quads than is needed up to that point; however, when the VMO effectively centers the patella, this force is decreased by 13% (146). Electromyographic (EMG) analysis has confirmed the medialization role of the VMO (147,159,207). Medially and laterally the extensor mechanism is stabilized by sheets of expanded fascia called the "retinaculum."

The quadriceps tendon/expansion narrows considerably

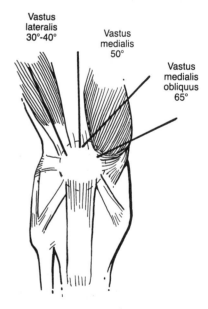

FIG. 15.7. Various muscular elements of the quadriceps. Different portions attach at different angles to the long axis of the thigh, creating various vectors of force. (Reprinted with permission from ref. 57.)

as it traverses the patella, tapering into the patellar tendon or more correctly a "ligament" in that it connects bone to bone. The average patellar tendon is between 30 to 40 mm in width and 40 to 50 mm in length.

Biomechanics

The knee joint functions to absorb the shock of weight bearing, and maintain the height of the body's center of gravity along a gentle, sinusoidal line. As the link between hip and ankle, the knee possesses great flexibility and durability, and protects the important neurovascular structures of the limb while transmitting them from the thigh to the foot.

The bony anatomy of the knee provides very little inherent stability. Of the three rotational and three translational degrees of freedom that the knee joint is subject to, only rotation in the coronal plane and translation vertically are significantly limited by the bony anatomy of the knee (23,67,89,181) (Fig. 15.8).

The movements about the knee are around three planes—axial, coronal, and sagittal. The movements in the axial plane are rotational—internal (compression) and external (distraction); in the coronal plane, movements are flexion and extension; and in the sagittal plane, movements are adduction (varus) and abduction (valgus). To stabilize the knee in all other planes and directions, the knee depends on its capsule, menisci, ligaments, and muscle tendons. Although the patellofemoral joint contains some inherent stability relating to the depth of the patellofemoral groove, the height of the median ridge of the patella and lateral femoral condyle, it too depends on musculotendinous units, ligaments, and capsule for stability.

Ligaments and Capsule

The bony anatomy of the knee joint does provide some static stability to the knee, especially in extension, whereas the muscle groups (quads, hamstrings, gastrocsoleus) crossing the knee lend dynamic control. However, the four major ligaments of the knee are of utmost importance in maintaining knee kinematics throughout the vigorous acts of running, cutting, pivoting, and traveling on inclined surfaces. The functions of the ligaments are integrated and interdependent. Stability must exist in extension allowing a solid platform, yet great flexibility and rotational capacity must occur to dissipate anterotibial-directed tibial kinetic energy when "cutting" and shifting body momentum. The structures of the knee will be divided into sections: medial side (29,88,125,148,217), lateral side (86,88,223,242,243, 247), menisci (135), and the cruciate ligaments—anterior (52,83), and posterior (34,45,57a,90).

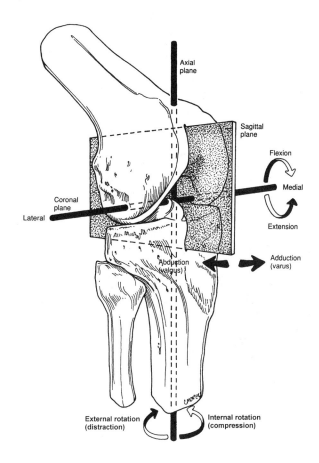

FIG. 15.8. A six-degrees-of-freedom model illustrates all possible rotations and translations about the knee. (Reprinted with permission from ref. 16.)

The Medial Side of the Knee

It is helpful to think of the medial anatomy in three "layers"—discussing the various structures in relation to their depths (251) (Fig. 15.9). The most superficial layer (layer 1) contains the deep or crural fascia of the leg and the pes anserinus. In layer 2 are the superficial medial collateral ligament (SMCL), vertical fibers of the superficial medial collateral ligament, which have been termed the posterior oblique ligament. Layer 3 is the knee-joint capsule, deep medial ligament, and oblique popliteal ligament (98,104,217,251). The pes anserine tendon consists of three tendons shaped as a "goose's foot." It inserts into the tibia 3 cm. distal to the joint over the superficial tibial collateral ligament (Fig. 15.10). Each contributing muscle is innervated differently (sartorius—extensor group/femoral nerve; gracilis—adductors/obturator nerve; semitendinosus—hamstrings/sciatic nerve). The pes anserine serves to rotate the tibia internally and flex the knee. The sartorius, also known as the tailor's muscle, is the longest muscle in the body. The semimembranosus has multiple insertions onto the posterior tibia

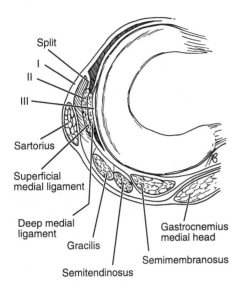

Split

I

II

III

Sartorius

Superficial
medial ligament

Deep medial
ligament

Gracilis

Semitendinosus

Semimembranosus

Gastrocnemius
medial head

FIG. 15.9. A bird's-eye view of the three layers of the medial structures, deep or crural fascia, sartorial fascia, superficial tibial collateral ligament and posteromedial corner, and layer III, joint capsule. The area labeled split denotes where the retinacular fibers anterior to the SML leave layer II and the SMA 3 to join layer I. (Reprinted with permission from ref. 217.)

(217,246). The medial head of the gastrocnemius is located posteromedially and can be used as an anatomic landmark for approaches to the posterior cruciate ligament (PCL) and posterior capsule. The plantaris originates from the linea aspera of the lateral femoral condyle proximal and superficially to the origin of the lateral head of the gastrocnemius. It inserts on the medial calcaneus. It does not appear to have any significant function at the knee.

Layers two and three merge posteriorly. The posterior oblique ligament forms a sling around the medial femoral condyle (37). The posteromedial complex (PMC) includes the posterior deep capsular ligament, which runs obliquely. The oblique popliteal ligament (OPL) and part of the semimembranosus expansion blend to insert into the posterior capsule (Fig. 15.11). In flexion, the medial hamstring dynamically tightens the posteromedial capsule and retracts the posterior horn of the medial meniscus. The remaining components of the semimembranosus insertion include a slip to the medial meniscus, one blending with the MCL, and a direct tibial attachment.

The deepest layer (layer 3) is the joint capsule itself. The capsular attachments to the medial meniscus have been named coronary ligament, deep capsular medial ligaments and deep MCL (29,99). The meniscal attachments to the capsule are described as the meniscotibial and me-

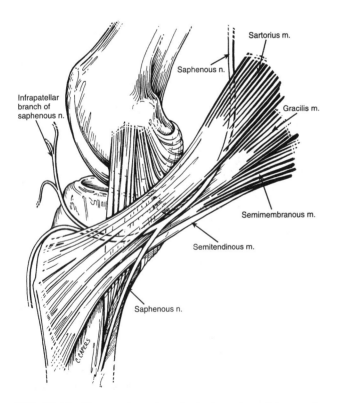

FIG. 15.10. The pes anserinus is the insertion of the tendinous expansions of the sartorius, the gracilis, and the semimembranosus muscles. (Reprinted with permission from ref. 16.)

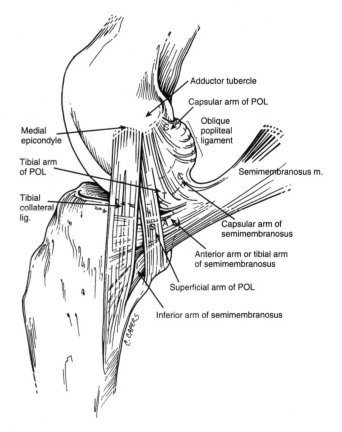

FIG. 15.11. The medial ligaments of the knee: medial view side. (Reprinted with permission from ref. 16.)

niscofemoral ligaments (Fig. 15.12). The ''menisco-femoral ligament'' is more stout and especially thick in the region just deep to the tibial collateral ligament.

The Lateral Side of the Knee

Excellent descriptions of the lateral structures have been published (45,86,90,223,242,243). Correlation of injured structures to physical exam and injury mechanism is often helpful (57,104,175,247).

The iliotibial band (ITB) originates at the pelvis with contribution from gluteus maximus and tensor fascia latae. The iliotibial band is a fascial covering attaching to the lateral intermuscular septum at the level of the lateral femoral condyle, running over the lateral femoral epicondyle and blending anteriorly with the lateral patellar retinaculum. The iliotibial tract tapers distally, converging to insert on the proximal tibia at Gerdy's tubercle. Primarily a static stabilizer, some dynamic function occurs because of its proximal muscular connections. The biceps femoris inserts primarily at the fibular head, but also sends fibers to the posterolateral tibia, the joint capsule, and the iliotibial tract (Fig. 15.13). Both resist posterolateral tibial rotation.

The lateral side of the knee is also described in three layers (86,175,223,247) (Fig. 15.14). Layer 1 consists of the iliotibial tract, and deep fascia of the thigh and calf. The biceps expansion and lateral insertion sites are also in this most superficial layer. The peroneal nerve is posterior to the biceps and classified in a knee layer. Layer 2 is formed by the quadriceps retinaculum confluent with the patella and the two patellofemoral ligaments. Layer 3, the deepest layer, is comprised of the lateral collateral

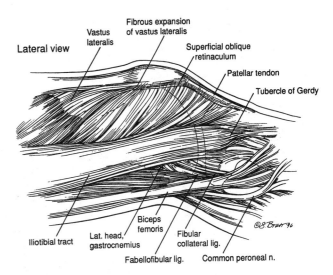

FIG. 15.13. Line drawing of the anatomy of the superficial portion of the lateral retinaculum and iliotibial tract of the knee. (Reprinted with permission from Greenleaf JE. The anatomy and biomechanics of the lateral aspect of the knee, *Operative Tech Sports Med* 1996;4(3):141.)

ligament (LCL), lateral capsule, fabellofibular ligament, short lateral ligament, lateral head of the gastrocnemius, popliteus tendon and coronary ligament, and the arcuate ligament. The Y-shaped arcuate ligament has two limbs—medial from proximal capsule to popliteus terminating in the oblique popliteal ligament and lateral from the posterior capsule to popliteus and fibular head. The LCL is a well-defined, pencil-shaped structure originating from the lateral epicondyle of the femur, inserting onto the fibular head. The LCL is tight in extension but relaxes in flexion. The arcuate complex is a triangular sheet of fibers diverging from the fibular head—the stronger lateral limb courses obliquely to the posterior femur, while the weaker medial limb attaches to the tibia posteriorly, crossing over the belly of the popliteus muscle. The fabellofibular complex is somewhat variable, arising from the fabella (itself variably present) on the deep aspect of the lateral head of the gastrocnemius muscle.

Recent interest in posterolateral knee instabilities has sparked a number of anatomic studies of the complex anatomy in this region (45,247). The posterolateral corner anatomy is key to understanding complex knee instabilities (223) (Fig. 15.15). Compared to the medial capsule, there is no distinct thickening of the capsule and less meniscal attachment. The lateral meniscus is much more mobile. An intraarticular structure, the popliteus tendon varies in its attachment to the meniscus and is a landmark for arthroscopic orientation much like the biceps of the shoulder. The popliteus originates on the tibia and inserts on the femur, which is opposite from all other muscles with origins proximal and insertions distal. The popliteus attaches to the distal and posterior aspect of the lateral condyle, and courses obliquely through an opening be-

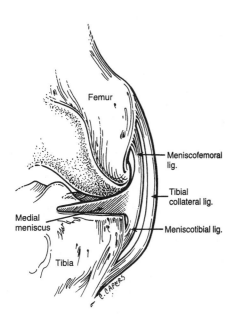

FIG. 15.12. The medial ligaments of the knee: anteroposterior view. (Reprinted with permission from ref. 16.)

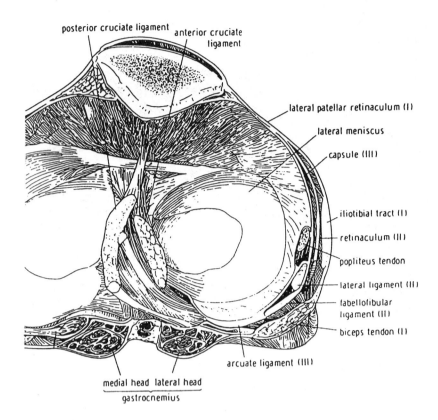

FIG. 15.14. Cross section demonstrating the layered approach to anatomy of the lateral aspect of the knee. Numerals I, II, and III designate layers 1, 2, and 3. (Reprinted with permission from ref. 223.)

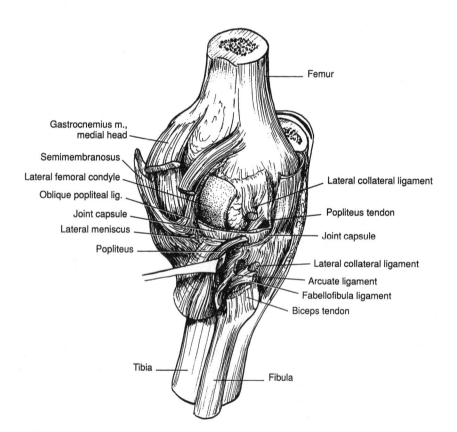

FIG. 15.15. The posterolateral corner of the knee. (Reprinted with permission from ref. 223.)

tween the lateral meniscus and the capsule. Fibers may originate from the posterior meniscus and fibula. The popliteus functions to stabilize the posterolateral corner in flexion and govern the movement of the lateral meniscus.

Menisci

The menisci are semicircular fibrocartilaginous structures between the tibia and the femur (16,146). Meniscal shapes and attachments to PCL and medial capsule are shown by bird's eye view (Fig. 15.16). The functions of the menisci are to increase conformity and transfer stresses between tibia and femur, increase stability, provide shock absorption and cartilage nutrition, and reduce articular cartilage wear (248). The importance of load transmission has been demonstrated in follow-up in patients who have had an arthrotomy and total meniscectomy (63,230,239). Following subtotal medial meniscectomy, radiographs show progressive joint narrowing, sclerosis and progressive varus deformity over time. In the ACL deficient knee, the medial meniscus does provide stability. The medial meniscus reduces anterior displacement of the tibia on the femur (64). The lateral meniscus covers a large portion of the lateral compartments. Meniscectomy changes these forces (127).

Made of type I collagen and fibrocartilage, the menisci are wedge-shaped in cross section and wider at the periphery, which allows the curved femoral surface to better conform to the flat tibia. The menisci are not rigidly fixed to the tibia, which allows them to conform to the different surfaces and varying radius of curvature of the femoral surfaces at varying angles of flexion (12).

The medial meniscus is more tightly attached than the lateral meniscus, which may be a factor in the increased incidence of isolated medial meniscus tears. It is "C" shaped and covers the concave plateau. The lateral meniscus is more oval or "O" or "U" shaped and covers a larger area of the more convex lateral plateau. The lateral meniscus is more mobile with less peripheral attachment and variable anatomy at the popliteus hiatus.

The primary nutrition for the menisci comes from the synovial fluid by diffusion. The cyclical compression and decompression of the meniscal fibrocartilage causes the synovial fluid to flow in and out of the meniscus. Peripheral vascularity is present only in the outer 25% to 30% of the meniscus (12). Blood supply is from the periphery through the medial and lateral geniculate arteries, which supply radial branches from the capsule. In fetal development, the blood supply extends more centrally but with aging is peripheral only. Therefore, only tears in the peripheral third or vascular red/white junction are most amenable to surgical repair.

Cruciate Ligaments

Crossing in the intercondylar notch, the anterior cruciate ligament (ACL) and posterior cruciate ligament (PCL) are intraarticular and extrasynovial. The tibial and femoral attachments of the ACL and PCL are important for understanding function and principles of surgical reconstruction. The ACL and PCL attachment points on the tibia and femur have been well described by Girgis (81). The ACL is divided into two bundles based on location on the tibia, the anterior medial bundle (A-A') and posterior

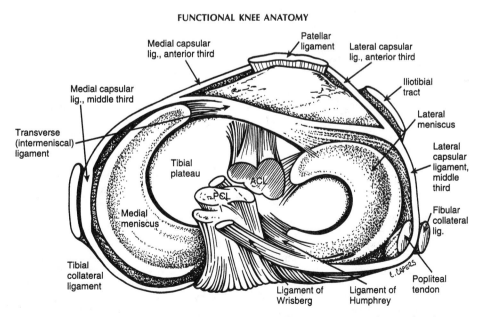

FUNCTIONAL KNEE ANATOMY

FIG. 15.16. An overhead view of the menisci shows the ligamentous attachment by the transverse ligament and the ligaments of Humphrey and Wrisberg. (Reprinted with permission from ref. 16.)

lateral bundle (B-B'). In extension, the intraarticular length is 30 mm and attachment on the femur is in a 4 × 23 mm area, just 4 mm anterior to the posterior wall of the lateral femur. Both bundles are tight in extension (Fig. 15.17A) but only the anteromedial bundle is tight in flexion (see Fig. 15.17B).

The PCL is much broader than the ACL, attaches on the tibia in an "over-the-bottom" position 13 mm below the articular level on the posterior tibia in the fovea. Bundles have been described based on naming attachments on the tibia and the femur. Girgis described the attachments on the tibia as the anterior or bulk bundle, the small or posterior bundle, and ligaments of Humphrey and Wrisberg (see Fig. 15.17C,D). In extension, the small bundle is taut and the bulk bundle is loose. The bulk of

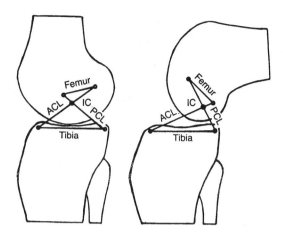

FIG. 15.18. The four-bar cruciate linkage model. The model includes two *crossed bars*, which represent the anterior and posterior cruciate ligaments (ACL; PCL). The remaining two *bars* represent the tibial and femoral attachments of the ligaments. IC, instantaneous center of joint rotation. (Reprinted with permission from Hefzy MS, Grood ES. Review of knee models. *Appl Mech Rev* 188;41:1–13.)

the PCL is loose in extension and becomes tight at 30 degrees flexion (see Fig. 15.17C). Newer anatomic definitions label the bands off of the femur. The PCL attachment to the femur measures 30 mm (81,90). The bands based on names from the femur are anterolateral and posteromedial. The posteromedial band tightens in knee extension, and the anterolateral band tightens in knee

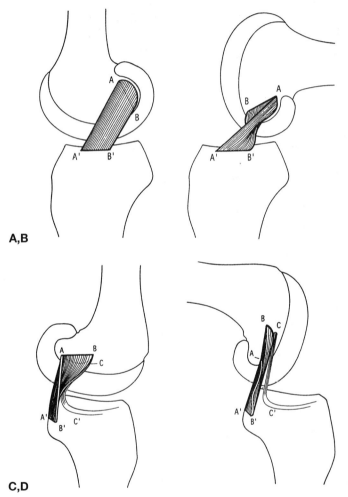

FIG. 15.17. A,B. Schematic drawing representing changes in the shape and tension of the anterior cruciate components in extension and flexion. In flexion lengthening of small medial band (A-A') and shortening of the bulk of the ligament (B-B'). **C,D:** Schematic drawing representing changes in the shape and tension of the posterior cruciate components in extension and flexion. In flexion lengthening of the bulk of the ligament (B-B') and shortening of small band (A-A'). C-C' is the ligament of Humphrey attached to the lateral meniscus. (Reprinted with permission from ref. 81.)

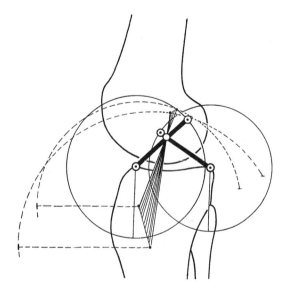

FIG. 15.19. The circular paths of motion of the anterior cruciate ligament are indicated by solid lines. The smaller circle is traced out by the shorter posterior cruciate ligament, and the larger circle by the longer anterior cruciate. The broken lines show the paths of the anterior and posterior edges of the medial collateral ligament and indicate a smaller circle for the fibers that insert anteriorly on the tibia and a larger circle for those that insert posteriorly. (Reprinted with permission from ref. 175.)

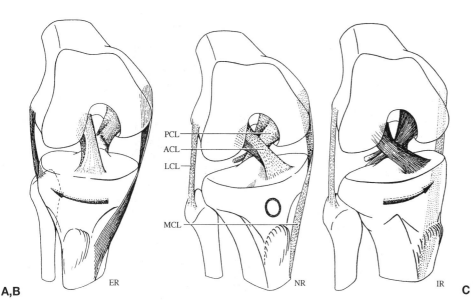

PCL
ACL
LCL

MCL

A,B   ER   NR   IR   C

FIG. 15.20. Besides their synergistic functions, the cruciate and collateral ligaments also exercise a basic antagonistic function during rotation. **A.** In ER it is the collateral ligaments which tighten and inhibit excessive rotation by becoming crossed in space. **B.** In NR none of the four ligamentous structures is under unusual tension. **C.** In IR the collateral ligaments become more vertical and so are lax, while the cruciate ligaments become coiled round each other and come under strong tension. (Reprinted with permission from ref. 175.)

flexion. The anatomic sites on the femur have been described arthroscopically (174). The anterolateral band attaches on the femur 13 mm posterior and 13 mm inferior the articular surface. The posteromedial band attaches 8 mm posterior and 20 mm inferior to the articular surface of the femur. The importance of these two femoral attachments is best appreciated by inability to successfully reduce all posterior translation by the present ''single tunnel'' reconstruction techniques (90,174).

A four-bar linkage system is formed by the ACL, PCL, femur, and tibia (23,52,175,191) (Fig. 15.18). The intersection centrally represents the instant center of the joint in the sagittal plane. The cruciate ligaments and fibers change shape during flexion and extension. With rotation, the bony femoral and tibial lengths change. Reconstructive surgery must restore this four bar linkage system with appropriate tunnel placement on the femur and tibia and ligament tautness. All ligamentous elements contribute to the principles of the Burmester curve, a model for describing the complex kinematics of the knee joint (175). Numerous reviews of the principles of the Burmester curve are necessary for a full understanding. This complex model emphasizes the importance of a thorough knowledge of basic anatomy and restoration of normal instant centers, in an attempt to recreate normal knee function. During rotation, the cruciate and collateral ligaments act antagonistically. With tibial external rotation, the collateral ligaments tighten to prevent excessive rotation (Fig. 15.19). In neutral tibial rotation, none of the four ligamentous structures are under excessive tension. In internal rotation, the cruciate ligaments become coiled around each other and are under significant tension (Fig. 15.20). When analyzing mechanisms of injury such as a noncontact ACL tear, many factors should be viewed. With internal rotation of the tibia, the ACL is under significant tension. If weight bearing has occurred, there is compression under tension, which will result in potential failure. If the joint is loaded, there are significant compression forces in the medial and lateral compartments, resulting in meniscal or articular surface injury (Fig. 15.21).

The menisci move posteriorly in flexion and anteriorly in extension. There is more movement of the lateral meniscus. The menisci also move with rotation as the knee flexes (175). During external rotation, the femoral condyle moves the medial meniscus posteriorly and the lateral meniscus anteriorly at a much greater distance. During femoral condyle internal rotation, the medial meniscus is displaced anteriorly and the lateral meniscus is displaced posteriorly at a much greater distance. Because of the

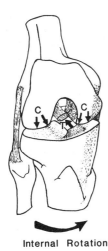

Internal Rotation

FIG. 15.21. Internal rotation of the tibia relative to the femur. The internal rotation causes the femoral condyles to ride up on the tibial spine, producing tension in the cruciate ligaments and a compressive force across the articular surfaces. *C*, the compressive force produced between the tibiofemoral articular surfaces; *T*, the tensile load developed along the anterior cruciate ligament. (Reprinted with permission from ref. 57.)

meniscal role as a stabilizer and shock absorber, restoration of these particular movements during surgical reconstruction with attempts to save the meniscus must be performed.

Principles of restoring the knee to its normal function are based on anatomic reattachments of all ligaments and preserving the menisci. If ligaments are not anatomically positioned, risks of abnormal joint kinematics and stretching out of the reconstruction exist.

NEUROVASCULAR STRUCTURES

The Popliteal Fossa

The structures in the popliteal fossa include the popliteal artery and vein, tibial nerve, and common peroneal nerve (Fig. 15.22) (224). A branch of the femoral artery, the popliteal artery lies directly on the posterior capsule, secured proximally at the adductor hiatus. In knee dislocations, careful neurovascular assessment must be done. There is risk of inimal arterial or venous injury (by stretch or puncture) or deep venous thrombosis. The blood supply to the ACL, PCL, and posterior capsule is the middle genicular artery, a branch of the popliteal artery. The

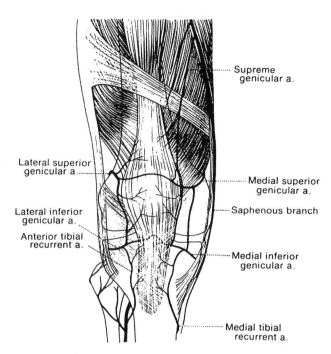

FIG. 15.23. The branches of genicular arteries provide the blood supply of the patellofemoral joint. The lateral genicular artery is at risk when a lateral release is performed. (Reprinted with permission from ref. 77.)

anastomosis of genicular arteries (medial superior, medial inferior, lateral superior, and lateral inferior provide the blood supply to the patella (77) (Fig. 15.23). The lateral superior genicular artery is usually sacrificed during a lateral release. Four nerves cross the knee joint: saphenous, peroneal, tibial, and sural. The saphenous nerve pierces through the medial hamstrings and branches into the infrapatellar branch, as it becomes more superficial, emerging through the semimembranosus. Branches of the saphenous nerve can be injured during medial meniscal repairs, resulting in reduced sensation from the medial calf to the ankle (see Fig. 15.10). The peroneal nerve is at the most risk with lateral meniscal repairs and injuries involving the proximal fibula and posterolateral corner of the knee. Pre- and postoperative assessment of peroneal nerve function including assessment of dorsiflexion strength and sensation on the dorsum of the foot should be standard practice.

PHYSICAL EXAMINATION OF THE KNEE

The examiner must develop a systematic and routine approach to a knee evaluation (16,69,235). After a detailed history has been obtained, one should have several specific diagnoses in mind. Allow the patient to demonstrate the functional problem. If pain is caused by the patient, it is much more easily accepted by them. If you anticipate a potentially painful test, that test should be

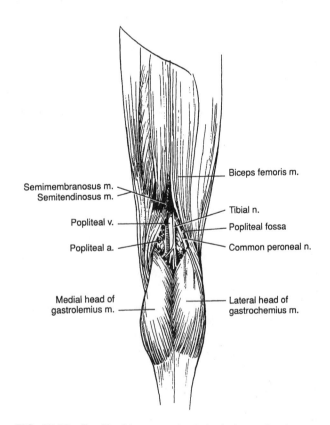

FIG. 15.22. Popliteal fossa contents include popliteal artery and vein, tibial and common peroneal nerves. The borders are bone and capsule anteriorly, medial hamstring and medial gastrocnemius and laterally biceps femoris and lateral gastrocnemius. (Reprinted with permission from ref. 57.)

performed at the end of your exam. For example, if the patient has a potential meniscus tear, then the provocative meniscal tests should be performed after ligamentous testing. Observation of gait, standing alignment, documentation of active and passive range of motion, particularly any differences in extension, should be routinely performed.

Physical Examination—Normal Knee

Have the patient stand to observe his or her natural alignment, muscle definition, knee joint position, and ankle and foot flexibility and position (Fig. 15.24). In the "feet together" stance, better assessment of the femoral anteversion, patellar orientation, and alignment is shown (Fig. 15.25).

Assessment of the posterior tibialis function and foot alignment should routinely be performed. As the patient rises up on his or her toes, the heel should naturally invert (Fig. 15.26). Posterior tibialis tendon rupture is rare in the young athlete; however, posterior tibialis dysfunction is common secondary to painful inhibition.

With the patient standing, observation of squatting maneuvers is helpful in assessment of patellar tracking and meniscal function. Squatting in hyperflexion with the feet

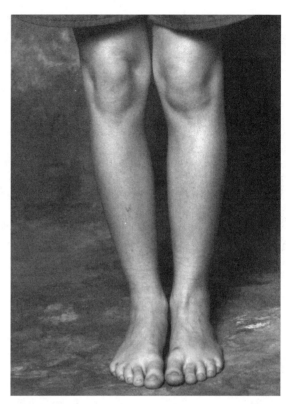

FIG. 15.25. In the foot-together stance, better assessment of the femoral anteversion, patellar orientation, and alignment is shown.

pointed straight can help localize the pain, specifically to anterior, medial, or lateral aspect of the knee (Fig. 15.27).

Assessment of the medial meniscus is best done with the feet and tibia externally rotated while palpating the medial joint line (Fig. 15.28, *arrows*). If there is pain in this position, specifically over the medial joint line, this is indicative of a medial meniscus tear. In the "snow-

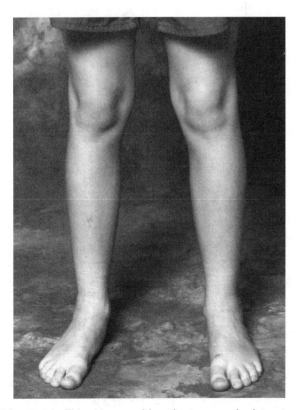

FIG. 15.24. This 10-year-old patient was asked to stand naturally. He demonstrates a valgus attitude, feet apart for balance, hindfoot in valgus, forefoot pronation.

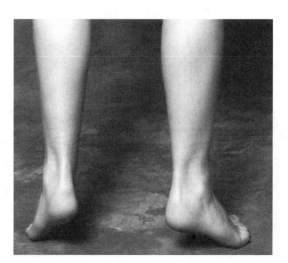

FIG. 15.26. As the patient goes up on his toes, the heel should naturally invert, indicative of normal posterior tibialis tendon function.

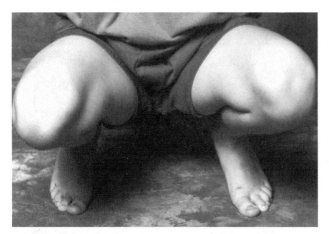

FIG. 15.27. Squatting in hyperflexion with the feet pointed straight can help localize the pain, whether it is anterior, medial, or lateral.

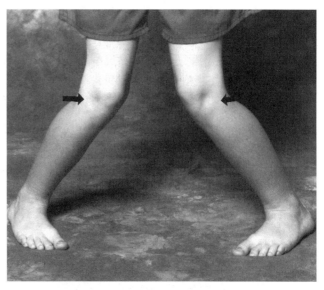

FIG. 15.29. Snowplow or internally rotated position with the feet maximally apart loads the lateral joint line (*arrows*).

plow'' or internally rotated position with the feet maximally apart, the lateral compartment is loaded and painful popping may indicate a lateral meniscus tear (Fig. 15.29, *arrows*).

With the patient sitting on the table, Q angle measurements, palpation of the patella, and observation of patellar tracking with resistive testing of active extension should be performed (Fig. 15.30). The Q angle is measured from the anterior superior iliac spine to the center of the patella—to the center of the tibial tubercle. A Q angle measurement can be performed in several positions—standing, 30 degrees flexed, supine 0 degree, and 90 degrees flexion. A ''J'' sign indicates patellar maltracking. This occurs at about 30 degrees when the patella is centralized in the trochlear groove, then incongruently jumps laterally

as the knee goes into further extension. This is best observed when having the patient actively extend against the examiner's hand. Always compare to the opposite, normal knee.

After comparing range of motion, palpation of the joint

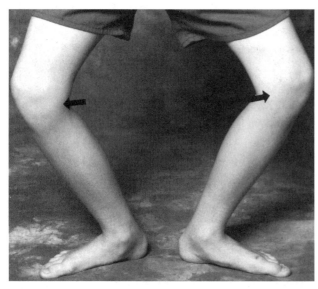

FIG. 15.28. Assessment of the medial meniscus is best done with the feet and tibia externally rotated and palpating the medial joint line (*arrows*).

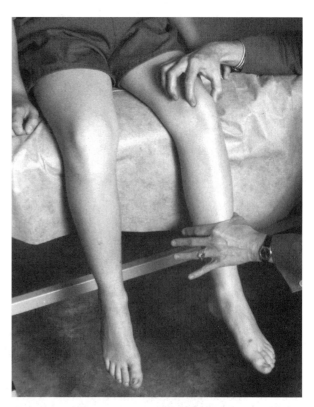

FIG. 15.30. Patient sitting on the table, Q angle measurements, palpation of the patella, observation of patellar tracking with resistive testing of active extension should be performed.

line, tibial tubercle, inferior pole of the patella, quadriceps insertion, medial, and lateral patellar facet should be done. The apprehension test for patellar subluxation is performed with the knee at 30 degrees of flexion (Fig. 15.31). Assessment of lateral retinacular tightness should also be done. Move the patella to estimate quadrants of movement medially and laterally.

The medial tibial plateau is usually 5 to 8 mm anterior to the medial femoral condyle. Palpation of this should be done to determine integrity of the PCL (Fig. 15.32). If the PCL is involved, the medial tibial plateau will be in a more posterior position compared to the normal 5 to 8 mm anterior location. Anterior drawer test is performed in neutral, internal, and external rotation with positive pulling of the tibia forward (Fig. 15.33). Palpate the hamstrings to make sure they are relaxed. Perform a drawer test with rotation, pushing the tibia posterior in an externally rotated position to assess the laxity of the posterolateral corner. Always compare both sides starting with the uninjured site. In the 90-degree knee-flexed position, there is often significant "normal" physiologic movement of the lateral tibial plateau both posterolaterally and anterolaterally. The Lachman test is performed with the knee in 30 degrees flexion pulling the tibia forward and keeping the femur stationary. The Lachman test is more reliable, especially in the acute setting because the hamstrings are in a less favorable position to resist anterior and directed force than the 90 degree flexed anterior drawer position.

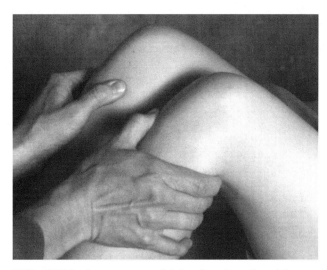

FIG. 15.32. Assessment of lateral retinacular tightness should also be done and the estimate based on quadrants of movement. The medial tibial plateau is usually 5–8 mm anterior to the medial femoral condyle. Palpation of this should be done to determine integrity of the posterior cruciate ligament (PCL).

There are many variations of the pivot shift maneuver. Descriptions of various pivot shift maneuvers have been described by numerous authors (78,99,131). The flexion rotation drawer, or reduction, test is performed from extension to flexion (179,232). The subluxation test is performed from flexion to extension (152). The most comfortable way to stabilize the leg to perform a pivot shift is by letting the patient's calf rest on the forearm and apply an axial load along with gentle tibial internal rotation using that arm. The opposite hand pushes the proximal tibia forward with the forces directed more anteriorly than toward internal rotation. If the ACL is injured, a shifting is felt at 40 degrees as the lateral tibial plateau

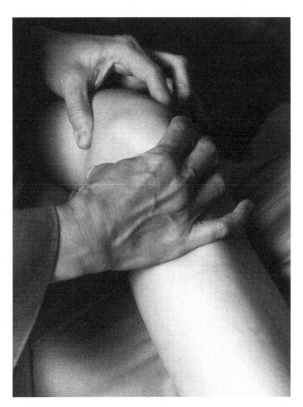

FIG. 15.31. Apprehension test for patellar subluxation is performed with the knee at 30 degrees of flexion.

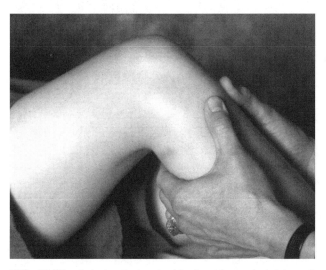

FIG. 15.33. Anterior drawer test is done in neutral, internal, and external rotation.

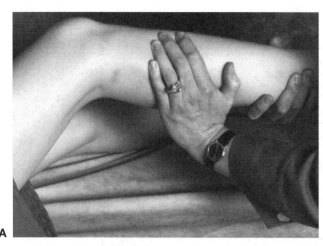

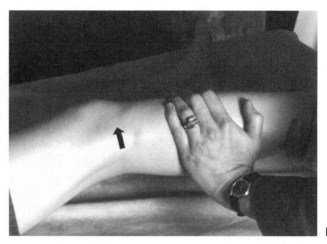

FIG. 15.34. In a subluxation test, the knee is taken from flexion to extension. **A:** At 30–40 degrees if the anterior cruciate ligament (ACL) is injured, a clunk or shifting is felt. **B:** The lateral tibial plateau (*arrow*) is shown subluxing in physiologically pivot glide.

subluxes (Fig. 15.34A). A physiologically normal pivot glide is shown in this subluxation pivot shift test (see Fig. 15.34A). The lateral tibial plateau is reduced at 60 degrees flexion and glides forward at 30 degrees flexion (see Fig. 15.34B, *arrows*).

McMurray's test is performed by rotating the tibia externally in hyperflexion for medial meniscus tear and internal rotation for lateral meniscus tear. Palpate the joint line for popping (168) (Fig. 15.35). If pain and popping over the joint line is reproducible, particularly in hyperflexion with an axial load, the exam indicates a probable meniscal tear. A bounce home test is performed by grab-

bing the heel and gently extending the knee. A positive test will result in pain if there is a posterior horn tear in the medial meniscus. The more common location for a lateral meniscus tear is within mid-third. With the knee flexed, a small localized cyst associated with pain on palpation is often seen (Fig. 15.36).

Apley's compression test is performed with the patient prone, applying axial or compressive load and external rotation, while palpating the medial joint line (Fig. 15.37A). A distraction test will help identify more capsular and medial collateral ligament sprains by stabilizing the thigh and pulling up on the foot and palpating the ligament (see Fig. 15.37B).

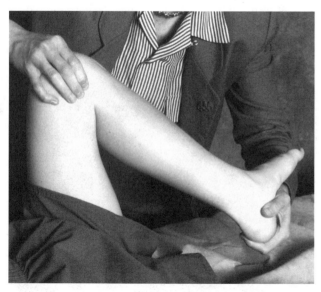

FIG. 15.35. McMurray's test is performed hyperflexing the knee while palpating the joint line being stressed for medial hyperflexion external rotation, and for lateral hyperflexion internal rotation.

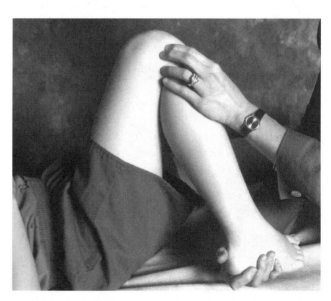

FIG. 15.36. Apley's compression test with palpation of the lateral joint line for a cyst.

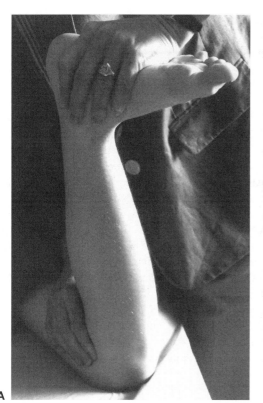 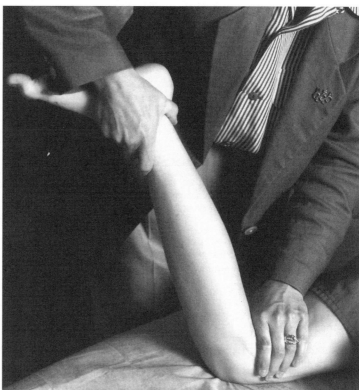

A   B

FIG. 37. A: Apley's compression test is performed with the patient prone, applying axial load and external rotation, while palpating the medial joint line. **B:** Palpation of the medial joint line while loading the foot in external rotation. Distraction tests will help identify more capsular and medial collateral ligament sprains by stabilizing the thigh and pulling up on the foot and palpating the ligament.

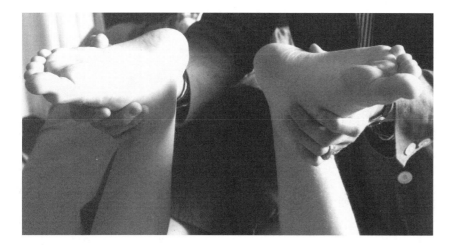

FIG. 15.38. While supine, any excessive rotation of the feet or an asymmetry will identify posterolateral corner injury.

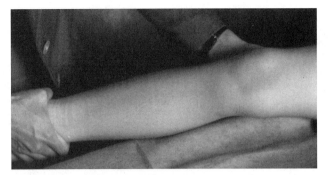

FIG. 15.39. With Lachman or varus-valgus, the leg can be rested on the examiner's leg or held over the side of the table testing the medial side at 30 degrees for medial opening.

A prone comparison is done to look for any excessive rotation of the feet or asymmetry that could identify a posterolateral corner injury (Fig. 15.38). Varus-valgus testing for ligamentous stability is performed at both 0 degrees and 30 degrees. Varus-valgus testing is done with the leg resting on the examiner's leg or held over the side of the table testing the medial side at 30 degrees by abduction/adduction forces (Fig. 15.39).

DISORDERS AND INJURIES

Epidemiology of Injury

The National Collegiate Athletic Association (NCAA) runs an injury surveillance system where 18% of member institutions, division I, II, and III, are polled (176). The athletic training staff completes an injury questionnaire for 16 sports—spring football, wrestling, women's soccer, women's gymnastics, football, men's soccer, women's basketball, ice hockey, men's basketball, women's field hockey, men's lacrosse, women's volleyball, women's lacrosse, women's softball, men's gymnastics, and baseball. The injury rates are reported as the number of injuries per 1,000 athletic exposures. The averages over a three-year period, beginning 1993 to 1994, ending in 1995 to 1996 are shown (Table 15.1). For overall knee injury rates, spring football is the highest at 2.06, then wrestling (1.99), women's soccer (1.68), women's gymnastics (1.45), and football (1.22). Statistics are completed in different categories. ACL and meniscus injuries rates are shown (Table 15.2). No determination of contact versus noncontact is made in this initial format. The top six ACL injury sports were

TABLE 15.1 *NCAA injury rates: knee*

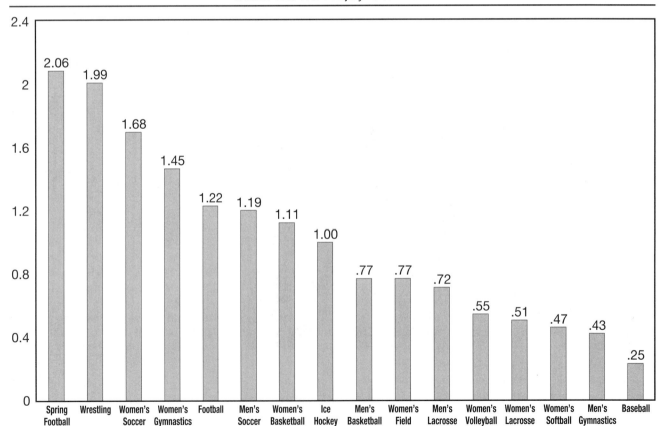

Average injury rates per 1,000 athletic exposures, 1993–1994 through 1995–1996 seasons.
Data from NCAA Injury Surveillance System. Graphic © 1997, Mary Lloyd Ireland, M.D.

TABLE 15.2 *NCAA injury rates: ACL, meniscus*

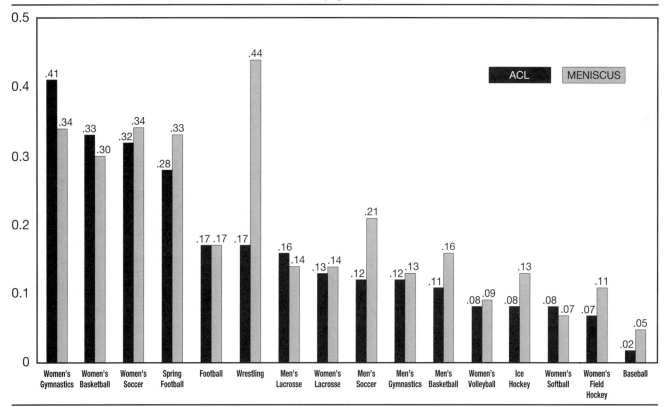

Average injury rates per 1,000 athletic exposures, 1993–1994 through 1995–1996 seasons.
Data from NCAA Injury Surveillance System. Graphic © 1997, Mary Lloyd Ireland, M.D.

women's gymnastics (.41), women's basketball (.33), women's soccer (.32), spring football (.28), football (.17), and wrestling (.17). The top five sports rates for meniscal injury were wrestling (.44), women's gymnastics (.34), women's soccer (.34), spring football (.33), women's basketball (.30) (176). An NCAA study comparing men's and women's soccer and basketball divided the mechanism of contact, noncontact, collision of ACL injuries over five years, 1989 to 1993. The ACL injury rate in women was 4.1 times greater in basketball and 2.4 times greater in soccer compared with men (11).

Three high school level epidemiology studies from the San Antonio area have been done for the three sports of girls' basketball, boys' basketball, and boys' football. The need for knee surgery was greater and injury rates greater in girls' basketball than boys' football or boys' basketball (26,56,82,83,109,116,265) (personal communication— DeLee J).

An assessment of knee injuries was performed at the Olympic Trials in 1988 (109). Eighty male and 64 female elite athletes tried out for the U.S. team. Female athletes had a statistically significant increase in both knee injuries and the need for surgery in comparison to their male counterparts. Twenty female athletes underwent 25 knee surgeries with 13 of the surgeries be-

ing for the ACL. Six male athletes underwent six knee surgeries with three of the surgeries being for the ACL. Other operative findings are shown (Table 15.3). Male and female injury rates in the military are equalizing (47). Injury rates of the knee comparing genders have been published for flag football (42), basketball (11,82,

TABLE 15.3. *Injuries sustained during 1988 Olympic basketball trial*

Parameter	Males	Females	Total
Number of participants	80	64	144
Athletes with knee injuries	11[a]	34	45
ACL injuries	3	13	16
Number of athletes requiring surgery	6[b]	20	26
Number of procedures	6	25	31
Type of procedure			
Arthroscopy	3	17	20
ACL reconstruction	3	8	11

a Statistically significant $p < 0.0001$.
b Statistically significant $p < 0.0007$.
Abbreviations and symbols: ACL, anterior cruciate ligament; [a,b] indicate a statistically significant difference between male and female athletes ([a] = $p < 0.0001$, [b] $p < 0.0007$).
Reprinted with permission from Adis International Limited, Auckland, New Zealand.

83,91,116,156,176,266), and other sports (56,252). Comparisons of many sports with regard to injuries and contributing factors have been explored (55,87, 107,117,205) (Fig. 15.40).

Anatomical differences between males and females may contribute to increased ACL injury rates. Differences can be divided into intrinsic–nonchangeable, extrinsic–changeable, or combinations of both. Alignment factors are intrinsic and not significantly changeable. The female lower extremity alignment typically has a wider pelvis, increased femoral anteversion, genu valgus, narrower notch, and external tibial torsion relative to the increased femoral internal rotation, and pronation (see Fig. 15.40A). This compares to the male alignment typically shown with a narrow pelvis, wider notch, neutral or varus knee, and internal or neutral tibial torsion (see Fig. 15.40B). From the muscular standpoint, the female has less muscular development, less developed vastus medialis obliquus, increased flexibility and hyperextension in valgus (see Fig.

15.40A) compared to the male with more developed thigh musculature, tight hamstrings, less overall flexibility and genu varum (see Fig. 15.40B). With malalignment, injury to the retinacular nerve has been documented histologically (72).

Intrinsic or not changeable differences are physiologic rotatory laxity, the size of the ACL, alignment, and hormonal influences. Extrinsic or potentially controllable factors include strength, conditioning, motivation, and shoe choices. Other factors include skill, coordination, position sense, neuromuscular firing order, and patterns-order of activation (119,120).

Differences in females that have been reported as a possible contributing factor in ACL injuries include later firing of the hamstrings and a different order of muscle component activation with quadriceps activity (108,109,119,120,149,150,260). Fatigue has also been shown to change the forces across the joints (43,189).

Measurement of the width of the notch is done routinely. The ratio of notch width at the popliteal hiatus

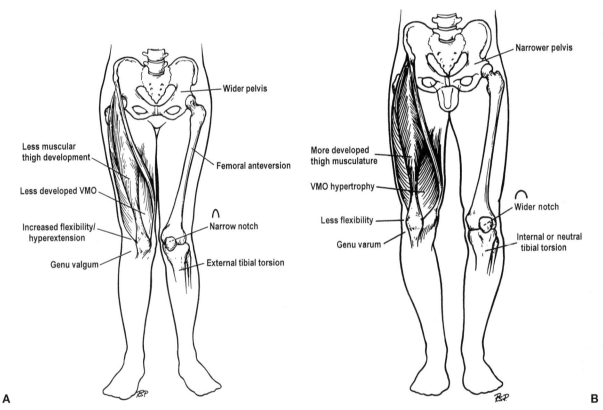

A

B

FIG. 15.40. A: Lower extremity anatomic alignment in female, showing wider pelvis, femoral anteversion, internal rotation, narrow femoral notch, genu valgum, less muscular development, increased flexibility, hyperextension, external tibial torsion, and pronated foot. **B:** Male lower extremity alignment is diagrammed with narrow pelvis, more developed thigh musculature, vastus medialis obliquus (VMO) hypertrophy, less flexibility, neutral genu varum, a wider femoral notch, and internal or neutral tibial torsion. (Reprinted with permission from ref. 69.)

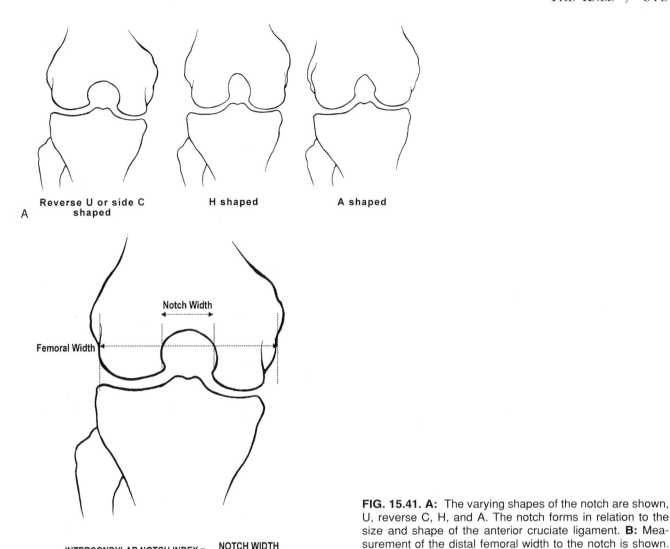

A: Reverse U or side C shaped

H shaped

A shaped

Notch Width

Femoral Width

B INTERCONDYLAR NOTCH INDEX = $\dfrac{\text{NOTCH WIDTH}}{\text{FEMORAL WIDTH}}$

FIG. 15.41. A: The varying shapes of the notch are shown, U, reverse C, H, and A. The notch forms in relation to the size and shape of the anterior cruciate ligament. **B:** Measurement of the distal femoral width to the notch is shown. This ratio is routinely measured.

to the width of the condyles is the notch width ratio (Fig. 15.41B). A ratio of less than 0.2 is indicative of a stenotic notch (237). With a stenotic notch, increased incidence of noncontact ACL injuries has been shown (136,237). The notch develops in relation to the ACL. Differing shapes, like C, or reverse U, H, and A are also seen (69,136,236,237) (see Fig. 15.41A). Absolute measurements of notch width in men show higher risk for ACL tear if less than or equal to 15 mm (228). Assessment by CT scan gives a more three-dimensional view (6). Hormonal influences are also a factor. Estrogen receptors are present on the ACL (149,150). The levels of estrogen vary during the cycle surging from day 6 and peaking at day 12 during the follicular phase. The menses are day 1 to 5. In a study of 28 females, ACL injuries were more likely to occur during days 10 to 14 (262).

Classification of Instability

Instability classification patterns have been discussed by many prominent individuals (8,99,138,153,175,182, 184,233). Classification of knee instabilities is based on the degree, direction and duration of the injury. The grades are 1 to 4 when estimated by millimeters of opening: 1, less than 5 mm; 2, 5 to 10 mm; 3, 10 to 15 mm; 4, greater than 15 mm (3). Some degree of physiologic rotatory laxity, such as a pivot glide, is a normal variant; therefore, the pivot shift test is more difficult to grade in millimeters. The pivot shift is described as negative or positive. The Lachman test at 30 degrees flexion is graded as negative, positive with a soft end point, or positive with no end point. The medial and lateral joint line opening can be documented more easily with millimeters of joint opening. If one correlates the mechanism of injury with the involved anatomic structures and the physical findings, it is much easier to describe the instability. The number of months from the time of injury is used to determine chronicity. Acute is less than three months and chronic is greater than three months from injury (183).

The term "ACL deficient knee" describes the ligament's absence; however, the functional disability that results from this injury is anterolateral rotatory instability and better describes the functional complaints. Excellent articles exist correlating the biomechanical principles of injury and anatomic cutting sections with the resultant instability (8,34,89,181).

Classification of knee instability is based on dividing the tibia into four quadrants and describing the motion of the tibia on the femur. For example, a torn ACL is described as anterolateral rotatory instability, meaning the lateral tibial plateau moves anteriorly. Instabilities are best understood when correlated with mechanism of injury, involved anatomic structure, and physical findings (175). The cruciates (ACL and PCL) are more central with axis of rotation more medial. The ligaments of Wrisberg and Humphrey attach the lateral meniscus to the PCL (Fig. 15.42). The knee is divided into quadrants—anteromedial quadrant (medial meniscus); anterolateral quadrant (lateral meniscus); posterolateral quadrant [lateral collateral ligament (LCL), popliteus, posterolateral complex (PLC), ligament of Humphrey, and ligament of Wrisberg]; and posteromedial quadrant [posterior cruciate ligament (PCL), posteromedial complex (PMC), and superficial medial collateral ligament (SMCL)]. The posteromedial complex (PMC) refers to the thickened medial capsular ligament, including the posterior oblique ligament, the capsular arm of the semimembranosus, the oblique popliteal ligament and deep medial capsule, meniscofemoral, and meniscotibial ligaments. The superficial medial collateral ligament (SMCL) lies anterior and superficial. The posterolateral complex (PLC) includes the arcuate ligament, fabellofibular ligament, popliteus tendon, popliteal fibular ligament, popliteal meniscal vesicles and thinner meniscofemoral ligaments (PLC).

Correlating and understanding the anatomy to the mechanism of injury will give the language of classifying the functional instability of the knee. Instability is rotatory, straight or combined. The direction of movement of the tibia on the femur is anteromedial, anterolateral, straight posterior, posterolateral, straight medial, straight lateral, and straight posteromedial. The direction of the tibia on the femur provides the language of instability (Table 15.4). The shaded areas represent the injured structures. The diagnosis and grade of instability, involved anatomic structure, physical findings and the usual mechanism and direction of forces are shown in columns. Combined instabilities are common. Anteromedial rotatory instability (AMRI) usually occurs from a lateral blow on the tibia with the foot planted. The anterior drawer is positive in external rotation if the meniscotibial attachment is injured but the ACL can be intact. As the valgus force continues in the extended knee, further injury to the posteromedial capsule and involvement of the ACL occurs in the classic triad of O'Donoghue (192) involving tears of the MCL, medial meniscus and ACL. An anterior drawer in external rotation occurs with 2+ AMRI. The pivot shift may not be as significant if the medial stabilizing structures are injured, in that there is no post around which to pivot (see Table 15.4, Section 2).

In noncontact ACL injuries, it is common to see a lateral capsular sprain, usually off of the tibia. Think about the mechanism in noncontact sports of basketball or gymnastics (Fig. 15.43). The lateral tibial plateau shifts anteriorly and rotation occurs (see Table 15.4, Section 3). The position of no return occurs and the ACL fails. The knee buckles, the patient is usually falling forward and toward the opposite side in a rapid distal deceleration mechanism. The usual observed position is body forward-flexed and rotated, hip in internal rotation and adduction, the knee slightly flexed and in valgus and tibia externally rotated and foot pronated. With more severe force, continued internal rotation of the tibia, and increasing medial contact, there will be a more severe instability, which involves the posterolateral complex (Table 15.4, Section 3).

PCL injuries are much less common than ACL injuries (176). Straight posterior instability indicates a tear of the PCL with or without involvement of the ligaments of Humphrey and Wrisberg attaching the posterior horn of the lateral meniscus to the PCL anteriorly and posteriorly respectively (see Table 15.4, Section 4) (175).

The "tetrad" injury and posterolateral instability includes injury to the popliteus corner, PCL, posterior

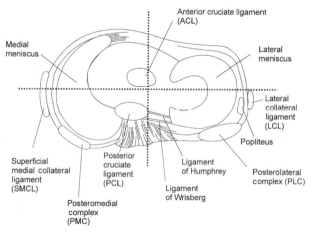

FIG. 15.42. Bird's-eye view of the tibia divides the tibia into four quadrants showing the important structures located in each quadrant: anteromedial (medial meniscus), anterolateral (lateral meniscus), posterolateral (lateral collateral ligament [LCL]), popliteus, posterolateral complex (PLC), ligament of Humphrey, and ligament of Wrisberg, and posteromedial (posterior cruciate ligament [PCL]), posteromedial complex (PMC), and superficial medial collateral ligament (SMCL). (Adapted and reprinted with permission from ref. 175.)

TABLE 15.4 *Classification of knee instabilities: rotatory, straight, or combined*

Section 1. Anteromedial rotatory instabilities (AMRI)

Diagnosis	Diagram	Involved anat. structure	Physical findings	Mechanism and forces
1+		PMC	1+ AD in ER	Contact: Lateral Force: Valgus
2+		PMC SMCL	1+ AD in ER 1+ — 2 + Valgus 30°	Contact: Lateral Anterior Forces: Valgus Extension Tibia ER

Section 2. Combined AMRI and ALRI

3+		PMC SMCL ACL	3+ AD in ER 2+ AD in N 2+ Valgus 30°	Contact: Lateral Forces: Valgus Extension Tibia ER
4+		PMC ACL PLC	3+ AD in ER 2+ AD in NR 2+ Valgus at 30° 1+ Recurvatum 1+ PS	Contact: Lateral Forces: Valgus Rotation Extension

Section 3. Anterolateral rotatory instabilities (ALRI)

1+		ACL Lateral Capsule	+ AD in N and Tibial IR PS	Noncontact Forces: Rotation Foot Planted
2+		ACL LCL PLC	+ AD + IR + Lachman + PS 1+ Varus 30°	Noncontact or Contact: Medial Forces: Varus Extension Tibia IR

Section 4. Straight posterior

Posterior		PCL ± Humphrey ± Wrisberg	PD 90° Neutral	Contact: Proximal Anterior Tibia Force: Posterior on Tibia Flexed or Hyperextension

Section 5. Posterolateral rotatory instabilities (PLRI)

1+		LCL PLC	ERR 2—3+ ADD at 30° PD Most 30° PLD 1+ RPS ER at 30° and 90°	Contact: Medial Forces: Varus Extension

TABLE 15.4 *Continued*.

Section 5. Posterolateral rotatory instabilities (PLRI)

Diagnosis	Diagram	Involved anat. structure	Physical findings	Mechanism and forces
2+		PCL PLC	PD increased 30° more than 90° Moderate ER at 30° and 90°	Contact: Medial Forces: Varus Extension
3+		LCL PLC PCL PMC	ERR 2—3+ VAR 0° PD in Neutral Severe Hyperextension Rotation at 30° and 90°	Contact: Medial Anterior Forces: Hyperextension Varus

Section 6. Combined ALRI and PLRI

| | | ACL
PLC
PCL
Lateral Capsule | PS
RPS
Lachman
ERR
PLD
PD Neutral
ER at 20°
Fx | Contact:
Anterior
Forces:
Valgus
Extension or
Hyperextension |

Section 7. Straight instabilities

Diagnosis	Diagram	Involved anat. structure	Physical findings	Mechanism and forces
1+ Lateral (rare)		Isolated LCL	1+ ADD 30°	Contact: Medial Force: Varus
3+ Lateral		LCL PLC PCL ±ACL	2—3+ ADD 0° ERR PD in N AD in IR Hyperextension with ACL Injury	Contact: Medial Anteromedial Tibia Forces: Extension Varus
1+ Medial		SMCL	ABDUCTION at 30°	Contact: Lateral Forces: Valgus
Posteromedial Instability (PMI) (rare)		SMCL PMC PCL	ABDUCTION 0° PD IR+ Neutral AD in ER 2+ Valgus at 30° and 0°	Contact: Anterior Forces: Valgus Extension

(Table adapted by ML Ireland from ref. 175.)

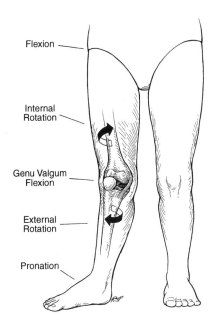

Flexion

Internal
Rotation

Genu Valgum
Flexion

External
Rotation

Pronation

FIG. 15.43. By videotape analysis this diagram shows the position of no return for the anterior cruciate ligament (ACL). The lower extremity position is one of body forward flexion, hip adduction, internal rotation, 20–30 degrees knee flexion, external rotation of the tibia and forefoot pronation. The knee will buckle, the patient is usually falling forward and toward the opposite side in a rapid distal deceleration mechanism.

oblique ligament, and lateral collateral ligament; this pattern of injury produces severe posterolateral rotatory instability, posterior drawer, and varus instability (see Table 15.4). Combined instabilities, particularly involving a complete tear of the PCL and capsular injury necessitate early surgical intervention, including ACL/PCL reconstructions and capsular repair.

Repeated exams for posterolateral rotatory instability should be meticulously performed (100) (see Table 15.4, Section 5). If the posterolateral corner and PCL are torn, acute repair of the posterolateral complex and PCL reconstruction or repair is indicated (see Table 15.4, Section 5, 2+,3+). Combined anterolateral rotatory instability and posterolateral rotatory instability also occurs (see Table 15.4, Section 6).

Straight instabilities are less common but do occur. With a medial blow severe straight lateral instability involves the lateral structures, ACL, and PCL (Table 15.4, Section 7). One must assess the peroneal nerve function. The posteromedial corner can rarely be injured in an isolated way. Because of the axis of the femur and the anatomy present, there is no true posteromedial rotatory instability (99). A consistent communication language regarding knee injuries by degrees of instability for treatment and follow-up purposes is necessary.

Ligament Rating Scales/Outcomes

Numerous knee ligament rating scales have been developed by many authors. These have been frequently revised, indicating the lack of overall acceptance of any single rating instrument (4,84,92,116,132,138,153,154, 180,182,184,186,199,226,241,250).

Outcome studies to assess knee ligament injuries treated operatively and nonoperatively are done by both subjective and objective measurements and most include a detailed patient questionnaire (unpublished data, N. Mohtadi University of Calgary, Alberta, Canada). Objectively, it is very important to have a standard classification so multicenter studies can be done. Comparisons of these knee-rating scales have been done (7,8,153,154,180,182,225,241). Prospective outcome studies on the ACL-injured patient have been published (53). This study does not support patients with ACL reconstruction having improved activity level and less arthritis. In this study, patients who underwent ACL reconstruction did not increase their activity level and developed arthritis.

PHYSICAL EXAMINATION

Abnormal Signs

A good physical exam should correlate the injured structures to the resultant instability patterns. The most painful test should be performed last. If ligaments are injured distraction forces cause pain. Compression causes pain if there is meniscal or articular surface injury.

Alignment

The line drawings compare normal (Fig. 15.44A) and "miserable malalignment" (see Fig. 15.44B) (117). Normal patella alignment is a Q angle measured from the anterior superior iliac spine to the center of the patella to the tibial tubercle of less than 15 degrees. Normal muscular activity with a well-developed vastus medialis obliquus creates forces to medialize the patella, resulting in central tracking (see Fig. 15.44A). Miserable malalignment syndrome with increased femoral anteversion, excessive Q angle, genu valgum, external tibial torsion, and foot pronation may result in lateral patellar subluxation (see Fig. 15.44B). Also seen with these patients is overall quadriceps weakness and VMO dysplasia. This male football athlete demonstrates excellent quadriceps development with hypertrophic vastus medialis, vastus lateralis, 10 degrees Q angle and straight alignment (Fig. 15.45). Another example is a cheerleader with rotational malalignment with relatively straight varus/valgus alignment but sig-

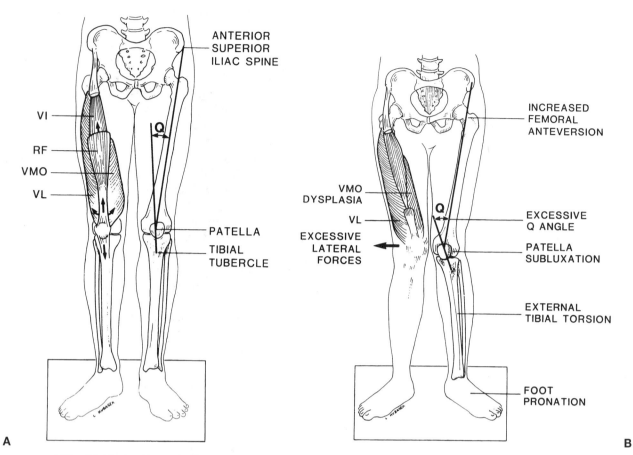

FIG. 15.44. A: Normal alignment with normal Q angle measured from anterosuperior iliac spine central portion of the patella, patella to tibial tubercle of less than 15 degrees, normal musculature of developed vastus medialis obliquus, create forces, which centralize the patella, resulting in normal patellofemoral tracking. **B:** Miserable malalignment syndrome consists of increased femoral anteversion, excessive Q angle, external tibial torsion, and foot pronation. All of these factors cause lateral patellar subluxation. This miserable malalignment syndrome is frequently seen in females (43B). (Reprinted with permission from ref. 69.)

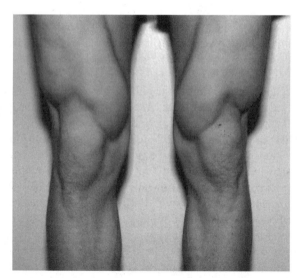

FIG. 15.45. Excellent normal alignment with legs essentially straight. Excellent quadriceps development including vastus medialis obliquus in male football athlete.

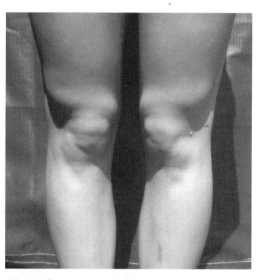

FIG. 15.46. Excessive femoral anteversion with patella pointed toward each other, hyperextension and internal rotation of the tibias. This cheerleader had anterior knee pain due to patellar tilt, rotation problems. She does have excellent vastus medialis obliquus development; however, her femoral anteversion is significantly causing abnormal patellofemoral biomechanics.

nificant femoral anteversion with internally rotated femur resulting in a patellar tilt and anterior knee pain (Fig. 15.46). The patellae pointing toward one another have been coined ''squinting'' or ''grasshopper'' eye patellae (Fig. 15.46). Note the excellent VMO development and overall quadriceps health in this female. This runner has had chronic problems with her left knee because of recurrent lateral patellar subluxation (Fig. 15.47). The normal right knee exhibits classic miserable malalignment signs of VMO dysplasia, external tibial torsion, genu valgum (see Fig. 15.47).

Differential Diagnosis

Anterior knee pain has been termed the ''low back pain'' of sports medicine (4). Differential diagnosis can be classified into three categories—mechanical, inflammatory, and other (Table 15.5). To help accurately monitor these problems, pain diagrams are helpful (203). In the adolescent athlete, hip problems such as Legg-Calvé-Perthes disease or slipped capital femoral epiphysis may cause pain referred to the knee. This football athlete noticed a different appearance of his left thigh but did not remember a specific injury. Note the asymmetry of the vastus lateralis (Fig. 15.48). Femoral nerve palsy was confirmed by EMG and spontaneous resolution occurred after six months.

If the origin of the pain is the patella, is it the soft

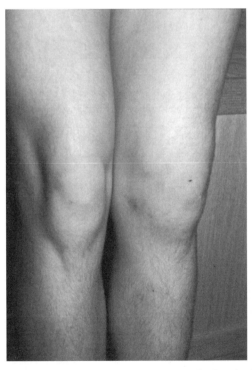

FIG. 15.47. Vastus medialis obliquus (VMO) dysplasia, left recurrent patellar subluxation with effusion. Absent vastus medialis obliquus (VMO).

tissue, articular surface, or subchondral bone? Can the pain be localized by clinical exam? Physical exam signs include pain on direct palpation, positive apprehension test, and a J sign with a jump as the knee is extended and the patella jumps laterally. One must not forget the importance of quadriceps flexibility as well as hamstring flexibility. Tight hamstrings tend to exacerbate anterior knee pain by accentuating the compressive joint reaction forces.

The correct diagnosis must be determined in the athlete who complains of pain in the anterior aspect of the knee (75,76). The classification of PF disorders has been well described (72,170). An algorithm for anterior knee pain is being developed by the American Academy of Orthopaedic Surgeons (AAOS) based on physical examination and plain radiographs (4).

Radiographic Assessment

Standard radiographic studies of the knee should always include an AP, lateral, and patellar sunrise view. The sunrise view provides a tangential view of the patella with its relationship to the femoral groove, and may show radiopaque loose bodies laterally or medial patella avulsion fractures. Views should be routinely done in a similar manner, bilateral, and consistent degree of flexion. Greater flexion may not show the subluxation. Cine CT and Cine MRI have been advocated to elucidate tracking in an active fashion. To date, these studies are quite expensive and may not provide additional information beyond standard radiography and a good clinical exam.

Many measurements can be made of different angles, tilts, or ratios for assessment of patellar height to tendon height (2,4,22,33,58,65,149,155,164,225). The plain radiographic measurements of angles for instability and the potential problematic patella are reported in detail (2,33,36,36a,44,57a,74,113,142,169). Testing with CT scan (158) MR (164) and bone scan (60) has been outlined. The patella at risk for having excessive lateral pressure syndrome is the one with a relatively flat trochlear groove, long lateral patellar facet and acutely angled medial patellar facet. Radiographs of sunrise view show this painfully subluxed patella (Fig. 15.49). The length ratio of the patella to the patellar tendon height is also important to note on the lateral view. A ratio greater than 1:1 means the patella is low-riding or patella infera (Fig. 15.50A). A ratio less than 1:1 means the patella is high-riding or patella alta (see Fig. 15.50B). The infera or low-riding position increases risk of articular cartilage damage from excessive contact pressure. The patient with patella alta is at risk for patellar instability and tracking problems.

TABLE 15.5. *Differential diagnosis: anterior knee pain*

Mechanical	Inflammatory	Other
Repetitive Microtraumatic	Bursitis	Referred Pain
• Patella	• Prepatellar	• Lumbar Disk Herniation
Stability	• Retropatellar	• Others
Subluxation	Semimembranosus	Reflex Sympathetic Dystrophy
Dislocation	Pes Anserinus	Tumors
Tilt	Tendinitis	• Benign
Rotation	• Quadriceps Patella	• Malignant
Malalignment	• Pes Anserinus	
Fracture	• Semimembranosus	
Stress	Pigmented Villonodular Synovitis	
Bipartite	Neuromata/Retinacular Pain	
Fibrous Union	Arthritis	
Acute Fracture	• Osteo	
• Pathologic Medial Plica	• Rheumatoid	
• Patellofemoral Stress Syndrome	• Psoriatic	
• Osteochondral Fracture	• Others	
Trochlear Groove	Syndromes	
Patella	• Reiter's	
• Loose Bodies		
Cartilaginous		
Osteochondral		
• Osteochondritis Dissecans		
Patella		
Trochlear Groove		
• Skeletally Immature		
Osgood-Schlatter's Disease		
Sinding-Larsen-Johansson Syndrome		
Acute Macrotraumatic Injury		
• Extensor Mechanism Disruption		
Quadriceps Rupture		
Patellar Tendon Rupture		
Inferior Avulsion Fracture		
Interstitial		
Skeletally Immature		
Tibial Tubercle Fracture		
• Patellar Fracture		
Transverse		
Displaced/Nondisplaced		
Comminuted		
Status Post ACL Reconstruction with Central Third Patellar		
Tendon Bone		

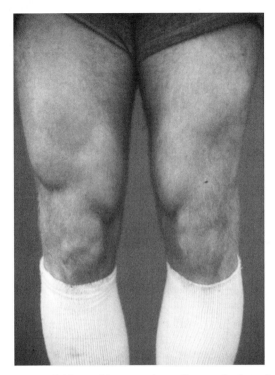

FIG. 15.48. Athlete with vastus lateralis atrophy from femoral nerve stretch or contusion.

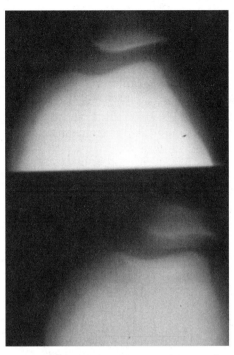

FIG. 15.49. The patella at risk for being painful and for chondromalacic change and excessive lateral pressure syndrome is the one with a relatively flat trochlear groove, long lateral patellar facet and acutely angled medial patellar facet. Radiographs of sunrise view show this problem patella.

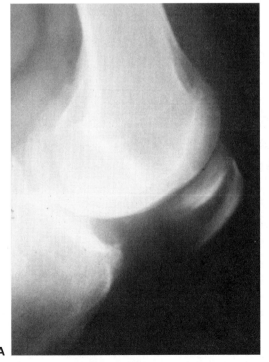

A

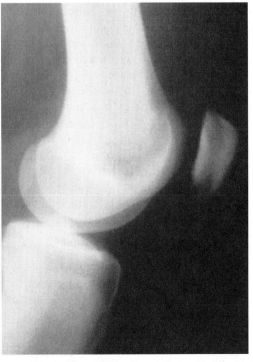

B

FIG. 15.50. A, B: These two lateral knee radiographs show very different orientations of the patella. In **A,** the patella is low-riding patella or patella infera. **B** shows a high-riding patella or patella alta, associated with hypermobility and instability. The patella infera is associated with patellar compression and pressure problems.

OVERUSE CONDITIONS

These entities to be discussed include patellar tendinitis, disruption of the extensor mechanism, quadriceps and patellar tendon ruptures, tibial tubercle avulsion, patellar fractures, bipartite patella, patellar instability, patellar subluxation, and patellar dislocation. A variety of overuse conditions from repetitive microtrauma can cause localized anterior knee pain.

Patellar Tendinitis

The patellar tendon transmits the combined forces of the ground reaction force proximally and the quadriceps muscle force distally. Repetitive loads can lead to inflammation and irritation at the proximal insertion of the tendon onto the patella (jumper's knee) or inflammation or degeneration of the tendon in its mid-substance. An association between patellar height and patellar tendinitis has been debated (65,264). Magnetic resonance imaging (MRI), however, can show focal inflammation and degeneration and provide a more complete delineation of the extent of the pathologic process.

Treatment is generally conservative but may be prolonged because of the resistant nature of the condition. The extent of treatment can be based on the level and degree of the patient's complaints (25). Does the athlete have pain during and/or following performance of his or her sport? Does it affect his or her ability to perform at a satisfactory level? The earliest phase can respond to eccentric quadriceps rehabilitation, hamstring stretching, ice massage, deep friction massage, antiinflammatory medications and a knee support with patellar tendon strapping or taping. If complaints have existed for an extended period of time or the athlete is having pain during the performance of his or her sport, reduced activity, extended rehabilitation, and additional therapeutic modalities are in order. Altering the athlete's activity to decrease the axial loading while maintaining cardiovascular fitness can be very beneficial during the period of therapeutic intervention (50). Others have emphasized the importance of rehabilitating the entire lower extremity, including hip muscles and the ankle dorsiflexors and invertors (24,238).

A steroid injection is not performed in most cases because of the risk of partial or complete rupture of the patellar tendon. In athletes not responding to a lengthy course of conservative treatment, surgical debridement of the necrotic site of the tendon with drilling of the patella to increase vascularity to the area can provide relief. Other authors would suggest a diagnostic arthroscopy prior to proceeding with patellar tendon debridement (249).

In the skeletally immature athlete, the transmitted loads can lead to a traction apophysis of the distal pole of the patella (Sinding-Larsen-Johansson syndrome) or the tibial tubercle (Osgood-Schlatter's syndrome) (194).

This gymnast had point tenderness at the inferior pole of the patella. Lateral radiograph shows elongation of the periosteal sleeve and sclerosis indicating Sinding-Larsen-Johansson syndrome (Fig. 15.51). Radiographically, in Osgood-Schlatter's disease there is fragmentation or separation of the tibial tubercle apophysis. Clinically, OSD is seen with a prominence of the bursa and tibial tubercle (Fig. 15.52). These conditions represent a growth imbalance—not a true disease. Rapid femoral growth results in hamstring tightness, relative quadriceps weakness and increasing distraction pressures on the extensor mechanism. Most of these patients are male and may have had Sever's disease (calcaneal apophysitis). Hamstring tightness is measured by the degree of knee flexion with the hip flexed to 90 degrees. Treatment begins with avoiding the repetitive eccentric quadriceps loading maneuvers that cause pain. Treatment may include patellar tendon taping, knee sleeves, closed chain strengthening and hamstring stretching, and quadriceps strengthening (194).

Disruption of the Extensor Mechanism

Displaced patella fracture, quadriceps tendon rupture, patellar tendon rupture, and tibial tubercle avulsion each interrupt the continuity of the extensor mechanism. The diagnosis is made by a palpable defect in the tendon or deformity from the fracture and inability to actively extend the knee.

Quadriceps and Patellar Tendon Ruptures

Extensor mechanism tendon disruption can occur at the quadriceps or patellar tendon level. Most authors believe

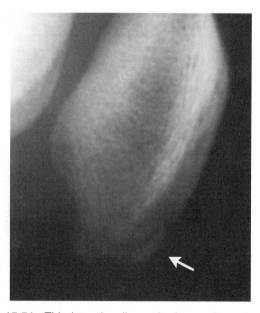

FIG. 15.51. This lateral radiograph shows elongation and periosteal sleeve and sclerosis indicating Sinding-Larsen-Johansson syndrome (*arrow*).

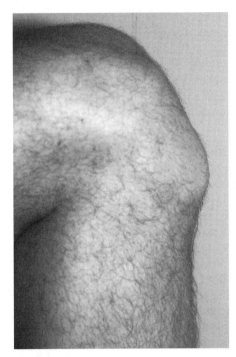

FIG. 15.52. Clinically, Osgood-Schlatter's disease (OSD) is shown with prominence of the bursa and tibial tubercle.

that normal tendons rarely rupture (50,130,167,238). There may be a previous history of chronic inflammatory complaints, systemic disease such as autoimmune disorders, or previous steroid injection into the tendon.

All displaced tendon ruptures should be urgently repaired. This individual with overdeveloped quadriceps slipped on a wet spot while walking and fell backwards (Fig. 15.53A). He felt a rip in his quadriceps and was

unable to extend his knee. He ruptured his quadriceps tendon from a violent eccentric quadriceps contraction in an off-balance position while flexing the knee. His surgical findings were an avulsion of the quadriceps mechanism from the patella extending into the VMO and lateral retinaculum (see Fig. 15.53B).

Rehabilitation of Quadriceps Tendon and Patella Tendon Ruptures

The two tenets of successful rehabilitation of quadriceps and patella tendon repairs are to minimize the effects of scarring and to maximize flexion. The period of immobilization and early range of motion is dictated by the surgeon. Ice, electrical stimulation, compression stockinette, and elevation are employed to reduce swelling. Transverse friction massage is initiated approximately 5 to 7 days postoperatively. The degree of pressure is dependent on the status of the incision and repair. Patella mobilizations are performed in the medial, lateral, inferior, and superior directions. Typically, this is done prior to stretching into flexion to facilitate the inferior patella glide. Stretching the quadriceps while holding the hip in an extended position assists in maximizing the quadriceps stretch and minimizing anterior knee discomfort (Fig. 15.54). Proprioceptive neuromuscular facilitation (PNF) techniques such as hold/relax and contract/relax are usually very beneficial therapeutic tools in gaining flexion. However, initially the patient must be instructed to provide a very minimal contraction so as not to stress the repair. Hold/relax is an isometric technique in all planes of motion applied to a restricted muscle and is most beneficial when there is a fair amount of pain present. Contract/relax is an isometric technique of the flexion/exten-

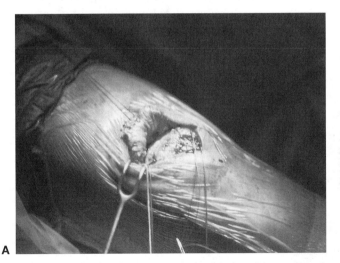

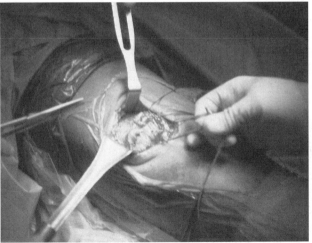

A   B

FIG. 15.53. A,B. This individual with overdeveloped quadriceps slipped on a wet spot in front of his washer/dryer and fell backwards. Repair is done by reattaching the quadriceps tendon back down to the patella, which can be done with suture anchors or through drill holes in the patella itself.

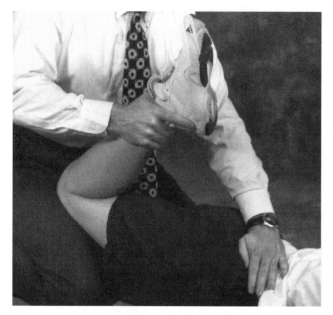

FIG. 15.54. Quadriceps stretch. Stretching the quadriceps while holding the hip in an extended position assists in maximizing the quadriceps stretch and minimizing anterior knee discomfort.

sion and abduction/adduction components but active in the rotation of the agonistic component. This technique is not as appropriate with pain. These techniques should only be employed when the clinician trusts that the patient understands the concepts and purpose for using them. Strengthening can begin in one week with three-way straight leg raises (abduction, adduction, extension). By week three, submaximal quadriceps setting, straight leg raises (flex) with immobilizer on, and terminal knee extension (both open and closed chain, with the amount of weight bearing dependent on the status of the repair) can be added (Figs. 15.55 and 15.56). The bicycle is an excellent exercise to promote quadriceps contraction and knee flexion. Generally, it takes approximately 95 degrees of knee flexion to perform a good revolution. As the strength of the repair improves, typical strengthening exercises are added, such as leg presses, hamstring curls, short arc

lunges, mini squats, step-ups/downs, and calf raises. Gait training exercises such as carioca, high knee, and line walking are also initiated once the patient is full weight-bearing (Fig. 15.57 to 15.59). It is important to emphasize eccentric control of the hip musculature, quadriceps, and gastroc, as deficits in these areas are often contributing factors in the initial injury.

Tibial Tubercle Avulsion

In the skeletally immature athlete, a violent eccentric quadriceps contraction during jumping is the typical mechanism resulting in tibial tubercle avulsion (204). There is no conclusive association between Osgood-Schlatter's disease (OSD) and tibial tubercle avulsion. One report stated 40% of athletes may have had preexistent OSD (257).

Classification is based on displacement and orientation of the avulsed fragment of the tibial tubercle (194). If displacement is minimal or reduction can be obtained with the knee in extension, the knee is casted in extension for 4 to 6 weeks. If the fragment is displaced or there is any physeal or articular surface offset, open reduction and internal fixation is indicated (194,204,257).

This 15-year-old came down from a jump playing basketball and felt severe pain and was unable to extend his knee. Clinical exam shows significant ecchymosis and swelling (Fig. 15.60A). Lateral radiograph shows the displaced fracture of the tibial tuberosity with extension intraarticularly posterior to the ACL attachment (see Fig. 15.60B). A CT scan was helpful to demonstrate the orientation of the fragment and to document only two pieces (see Fig. 15.60C). For this Ogden type 3A, arthroscopy and then open reduction internal fixation was performed. The lateral view shows anatomic reduction fixed with three screws (see Fig. 15.60D). He had a good result with eventual return to all activities, including basketball, by one year post-surgery. Rehabilitation of tibial tubercle avulsions mimics that of patella fractures. Typically, range of motion can be restored more quickly and exercises can progress more rapidly, particularly if internal fixation is used.

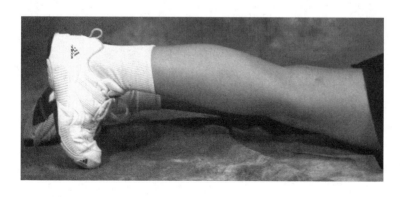

FIG. 15.55. Terminal knee extension. The foot is maintained in dorsiflexion to provide approximately 20 degrees of terminal knee extension range.

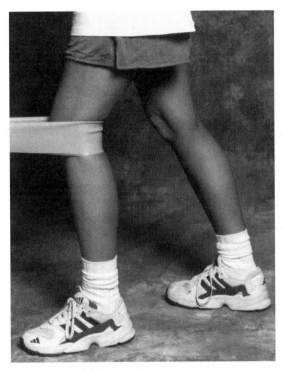

FIG. 15.56. Closed kinetic chain terminal knee extension. Weight-bearing stance, Theraband, or Theratubing providing resistance to terminal knee extension.

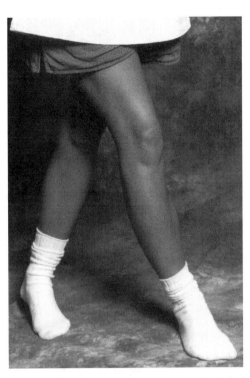

FIG. 15.57. Carioca or cross-over walks assist in improving balance and neuromuscular control.

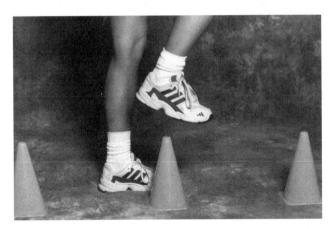

FIG. 15.58. Forward high-step walking. The patient ambulates over cones or other objects to accentuate normal knee bend.

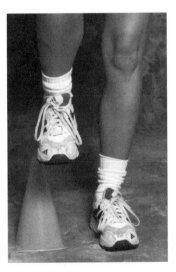

FIG. 15.59. Lateral high-step walks. Accentuates normal knee bend during gait and contributes lateral function of push-off and stance legs.

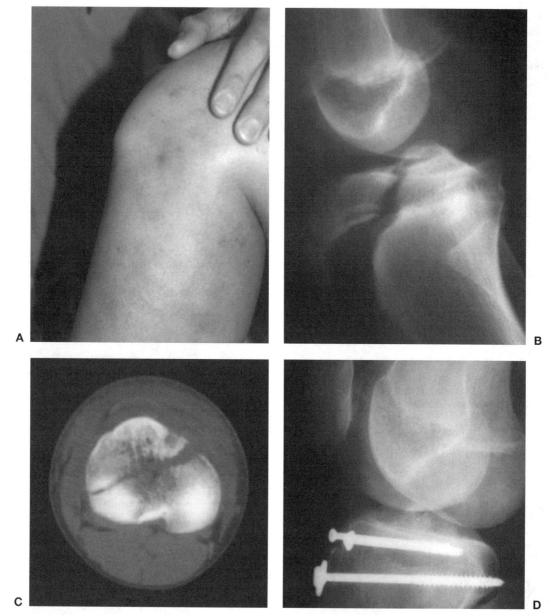

FIG. 15.60. A: This 15-year-old came down from a jump playing basketball and felt severe pain and was unable to extend his knee. Clinical exam shows significant ecchymosis consistent with a probable fracture and inability to extend his knee. **B:** Radiographs show the displaced fracture of the tibial tuberosity with involvement intraarticularly posterior to the anterior cruciate ligament (ACL) attachment. This is best seen on lateral view. **C:** A computed tomography (CT) scan was helpful to demonstrate the orientation of the fragment and the fact that there was a nondisplaced posterior portion. **D:** For this Ogden type III-A, arthroscopy and then open reduction, internal fixation was performed.

Patella Fractures

In athletes, fractures of the patella commonly occur from direct contact. The fracture pattern is generally stellate and rarely displaced (200). If nondisplaced, the fracture can be treated in knee extension and immobilized for 4 weeks with early weight bearing.

Transverse fractures of the patella occur more frequently in an older population from a direct blow or a fall onto the knee, hyperextension or violent quadriceps contraction. If there is displacement of the fragment with articular surface, angulation or step-off, then open reduction (151,218) with cerclage wiring is performed. If there is significant comminution, a partial or complete patellectomy is done. Rehabilitation begins with patella mobilizations and range of motion exercises. Strengthening exercises are advanced based on healing of the patella fracture. Open chain strengthening exercises are avoided because of the high patellofemoral forces they cause. Return to activity depends on the nature of the fracture, healing and sport.

Complication of a patellar fracture following bone-patellar tendon-bone (BPTB) can occur. There is temporary weakness and osteopenia of the patella following harvesting of the graft. A fracture at the patella harvest site is often in the orientation of a Mercedes emblem. This potential complication is of concern, particularly in patients who have early return to their sport prior to adequate bone healing. Taking a smaller patellar fragment bone and bone-grafting the patellar defect with cancellous bone reduces the risk of fracture.

Bipartite Patella

A bipartite patella has one or more unfused ossification centers. Bipartite patellas exist in 2% to 3% of the population. The finding will be unilateral in 57% and bilateral in 43% (85). Seventy-five percent of the fragments are in the superolateral quadrant, 10% in a vertical lateral position and 5% are at the inferior pole (121,219). Most bipartite patellae are incidental findings and are asymptomatic. Symptomatic patients typically are in a stop/cut repetitive load sport such as soccer. A stress fracture through the bipartite fibrous union can occur. This classically presents as pain directly over the bipartite area of the patella. Radiographs may show displacement but more commonly show only the bipartite patella. A bone scan can be done if there is confusion regarding the diagnosis. However, if there is pain directly over the patella and a bipartite is present, surgical excision of this is usually necessary. Displaced fractures of bipartite patella have been reported (62,118). This football place kicker had pain over his plant knee. He underwent arthroscopy and open excision of the fragment with reattachment of the quadriceps anterior posterior knee mechanism. Radiograph with the ex-

cised fragment is shown (Fig. 15.61). Postoperatively, after his rehabilitation program, he returned to kicking activities at three months.

Patellar Instability

Patellofemoral stability is a result of a complex series of interactions involving joint congruity, alignment, and static and dynamic patellar stabilizers (74,202). Bony factors that predispose to patellar instability include; a small, short lateral femoral condyle, a shallow femoral groove, a flat patella, femoral internal rotation or anteversion of the hip, and an increased valgus or Q angle. The most common direction of patellar instability is lateral. The previous factors can magnify the forces or reduce the resistance to lateral displacement of the patella. Medial instability is more commonly iatrogenically because of surgical overcorrection of lateral subluxation (103,209).

Surgical intervention for recurrent patella dislocation and instability is open realignment, which can include distal tibial tubercle transfer, proximal reefing, and lateral release (77,102,231). In the skeletally immature unstable patella, only soft tissue procedures are done.

Additional factors that can contribute include generalized ligamentous laxity, previous trauma, tight lateral retinaculum, and motor imbalance or weakness. Generalized ligamentous laxity implies that all static restraining forces about the knee including the medial retinaculum are loose

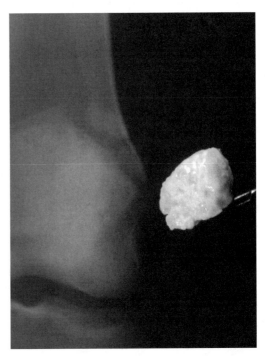

FIG. 15.61. This football place kicker had pain over his plant knee. He underwent arthroscopy and open excision of the fragment with reattachment of the quadriceps knee mechanism. Radiograph with excised fragment is shown.

and will not provide adequate resistance to patellar subluxation. Previous trauma with patellar dislocation is associated with tearing of the medial soft tissue structures including the patellofemoral and patellotibial ligaments, retinaculum and insertion of the vastus medialis obliquus (VMO). If these heal in a lengthened position, they will provide less resistance to lateral displacement. A tight or contracted lateral retinaculum can lead to patellar tilt or lateral subluxation. Finally, since the VMO is the only dynamic structure preventing lateral displacement, weakness or imbalance will lead to lateral instability.

Female athletes are at particular risk of patellofemoral problems including instabilities. The causes are multifactorial and include slight increased ligamentous laxity compared to males, a naturally increased valgus angle at the knee, dysplasia and VMO weakness, and muscular imbalance of the entire lower extremity. All female athletes should be aware of these risks as well as the techniques and exercises that can minimize their risk by maximizing the strength and neuromuscular control of their lower extremity, particularly the VMO.

Patellar Subluxation

The athlete with patellar subluxation will complain of anterior knee pain and may note a feeling of "giving way." In general, no true patellar dislocation has occurred. In moderate to severe cases, it may be apparent by inspection in the standing or seated position that the patellae point laterally. As the knee is passed through a range of motion against resistance, the patella may quickly shift from a medial position in flexion to laterally subluxed around 30 degrees of flexion. This is called "the J-sign." The examiner must consider the contributing causes including miserable malalignment syndrome, valgus alignment, genu valgum, femoral anteversion, generalized ligamentous laxity, VMO dysplasia, external tibial torsion and pes planus and pronation (Fig. 15.62). Similar complaints may be seen in other knee conditions such as plica syndrome, loose body, or osteochondral defect.

Treatment of patellar subluxation ranges from exercises, taping, orthotics, and braces to operative releases and reconstructions. Most athletes respond to conservative, nonoperative treatment. Careful identification of contributing factors guide the choice of treatment. Children may improve their VMO strength, reduce their valgus alignment angle, and increase the size of the lateral femoral condyle, thereby deepening their femoral groove—literally outgrowing the problem.

Patellar Dislocation

Patellar dislocations may be preceded by a prodrome of patellar subluxation. More frequently, the dislocation occurs because of a single isolated event. The mechanism

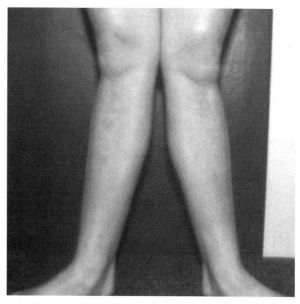

FIG. 15.62. Miserable malalignment syndrome is shown in this female patient. Valgus alignment of genu valgum, femoral anteversion, generalized ligamentous laxity, vastus medialis obliquus (VMO) dysplasia, external tibial torsion and pes planus and pronation are components of miserable malalignment syndrome.

of dislocation is from a twisting/cutting knee motion while the knee is in a valgus and flexed position. It may be associated with a particularly violent contraction of the quadriceps. Less common is a direct blow to the medial patella. The patella usually spontaneously reduces as the knee extends. An acute, tense hemarthrosis is common. Localized tenderness is at the VMO and medial retinaculum of the patella. Pain on the lateral aspect of the lateral femoral condyle indicates a lateral femoral impaction lesion. Osteochondral fractures and loose bodies complicate approximately 5% to 30% of acute patellar dislocations and frequently require surgical removal if present (110).

The sunrise or merchant patellar view is best to see a loose fragment, seen laterally, usually originating from the medial aspect of the patella (110) (Fig. 15.63A). Views of the radiographs of patellar view shows the fragment lying in the lateral gutter (see Fig. 15.63B). This 17-year-old sustained a lateral patellar dislocation during a baseball game. The most common location of osteochondral loose body is the medial patellar facet shown by diagram and arthroscopy. The loose fragment was found in the notch, located anterior to the ACL. A lateral impaction lesion is also seen correlated by diagram and arthroscopic finding. Diagrammatically, the fragment usually comes off at the area labeled *1C* and there is a lateral impaction lesion where the patella abutts on the lateral non−weight-bearing area of the femoral condyle (*2C*) (169) (Fig. 15.64). Diagrammatically, the patellar dislocation dislodged the medial patellar facet and the loose

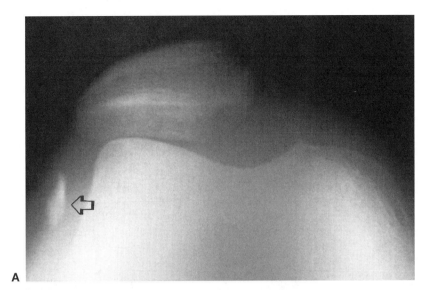

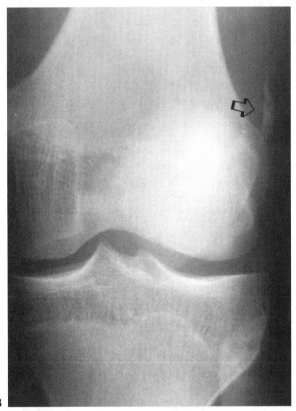

FIG. 15.63. A: Sunrise view showing location of the radiopaque loose body in the lateral compartment the source of the medial patella corresponds to the a and d, in Fig. 2 from ref. 110. **B:** Anteroposterior (AP) view with arrow showing radiopaque loose body. (Reprinted with permission from ref. 110.)

body was found lying just anterior to the ACL. The loose body was removed, and the patella and lateral femoral gutter were debrided. If the fragment has enough cancellous bone to successfully internally fix, this should be done.

Treatment in the case of an acute patella dislocation with no associated osteochondral fragments should be based on the presence or absence of predisposing factors for recurrent dislocation. Without predisposing factors, a conservative approach may be attempted with the knee

immobilized in extension with a lateral knee pad or taping to maintain reduction of the patella for 4 to 6 weeks. Institution of range of motion activities with the knee taped to medialize the patella can begin even earlier in compliant patients. The rehabilitation program addresses the trunk, hip, knee, and lower leg to assure that normal lower extremity kinetic chain function and balance is restored.

Some authors advocate surgical repair in most patients

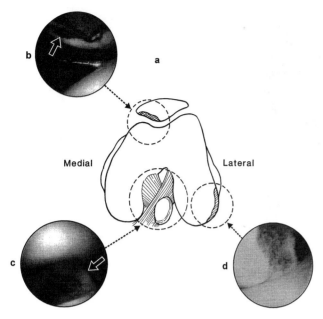

FIG. 15.64. This 17-year-old male sustained lateral dislocated patella with osteochondral loose body. Correlation of arthroscopic findings with diagram puts the mechanism of injury with arthroscopic findings. The patellar fracture and origin of loose body is usually the medial patellar facet, diagrammatically (*a*), and arthroscopically (*b*) (*arrow*). The fragment can be knocked off during dislocation or relocation. When the patella is dislocated, a lateral impaction lesion occurs (*d*). The loose body is seen diagrammatically lying anterior to the anterior cruciate ligament and the articular cartilage with underlying cancellous bone is shown (*c*) (*arrow*). (Reprinted with permission from ref. 110.)

and all athletes with an acute patellar dislocation regardless of predisposing factors (27,28,51,244). One series noted that the preoperative examination yielded the correct diagnosis of an osteochondral fracture in only 17% of patients (193). If osteochondral loose bodies are present, surgery is indicated. If the osteochondral fracture is large enough it can be fixed. Usually the fragment is articular cartilage only and requires removal. Arthroscopic debridement of the donor base is done. Arthroscopy is an excellent adjunct in identifying all loose fragments. A primary repair of the torn medial retinaculum and VMO can be performed through a small medial parapatellar approach. Postoperatively, surgically repaired patients are treated similarly to the nonoperative approach to protect the repair.

Rehabilitation of Excessive Lateral Facet Pressure/Patella Subluxations/Dislocations

Intrinsic rehabilitation of a patellofemoral problem is directed toward the identified causative factors. Control of the lower extremity starts with having a stable "core" or trunk. Once that has been established, muscles control-

ling the lower extremity can effectively do their job. Weakness in the hip can lead to too much internal rotation of the lower extremity with resultant excessive lateral pressure, subluxation, or dislocation of the patella. The hip extensors, abductors, and external rotators need to be rehabilitated with adequate strengthening and neuromuscular reeducation (Figs. 15.65 to 15.70) (263). The iliotibial band and lateral retinaculum should be aggressively stretched to prevent a lateral pull (Fig. 15.71 and 15.72). Stretching tight hamstrings will decrease patellofemoral joint compression (Fig. 15.73). Both open and closed chain exercises are effective in developing strength and neuromuscular control. A weak or dystrophic VMO will result in a muscular imbalance favoring a lateral pull of the patella. Strengthening the quadriceps throughout the full range of motion (or at least through the functional range relative to the sport) while emphasizing an isometric adduction of the hip can often be more effective in rehabilitating the dystrophic VMO because of the dual innervation from the femoral and obturator nerves (Fig. 15.74). Electromyographic biofeedback has been helpful in training the athlete to fire the VMO appropriately (258). The foot and ankle need to be assessed from a structural and functional standpoint. Structurally, excessive rearfoot

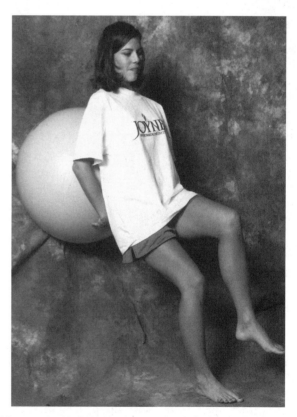

FIG. 15.65. Unilateral ball squats. Leaning against a ball allows for easy rolling down a wall when performing unilateral ball squats. Emphasis is placed on depth of squat and in lower extremity control during the squat.

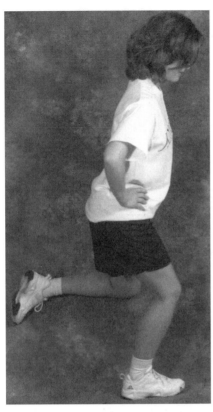

FIG. 15.66. Unilateral squat with contralateral hip abduction. The patient performs unilateral squat while abducting the contralateral hip into a wall to increase ipsilateral gluteus medius activity.

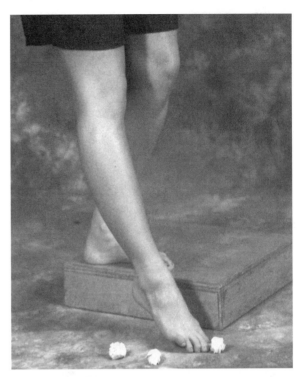

FIG. 15.67. Mini-squat with ball pick-up. The patient performs mini-squat at a variety of depths while performing ball pick-up with contralateral toes to provide challenge in balance and stability.

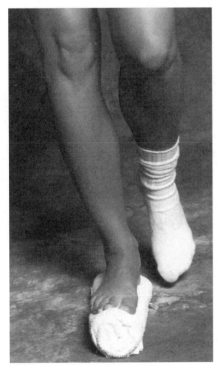

FIG. 15.68. Balance exercises. The patient performs a variety of activities while in unilateral stance on a towel roll to provide an unstable base.

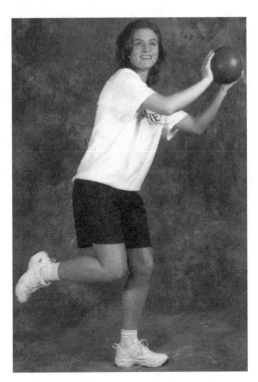

FIG. 15.69. Unilateral stance ball toss. The patient performs ball-catching activities at a variety of speeds and positions while in unilateral stance to challenge the balance and neuromuscular function of the lower extremity.

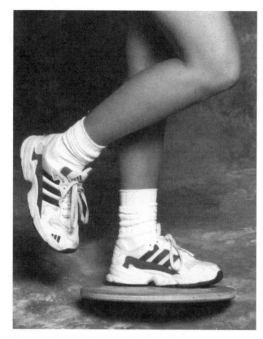

FIG. 15.70. Wobble board. Work on balance, not letting the rim of the board touch the floor. Can also work on full range of motion, riding the entire rim of the board around, touching the floor at all times.

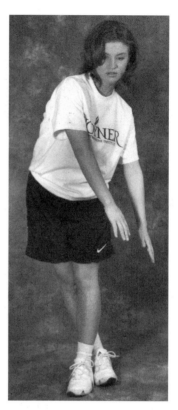

FIG. 15.71. ITB stretch. Place involved limb behind stance leg while going through a side stretch to the opposite side.

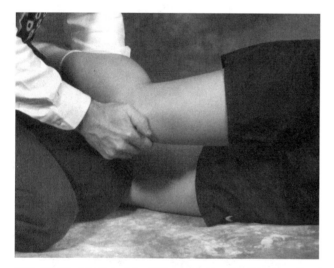

FIG. 15.72. Medial glide. With patient in side-lying, involved side up, clinician maintains a fixed knee angle while performing medial glides of the patella. Knee angle should correspond to the angle at which the patient experiences pain. This mobilization should not be painful.

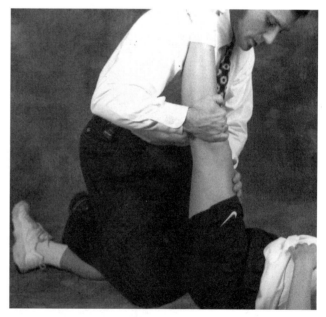

FIG. 15.73. Hamstring stretch. Maintain knee extension and stabilize the contralateral limb against the floor. It is helpful to utilize an active phase of resistance and perform the stretch during the relaxation phase.

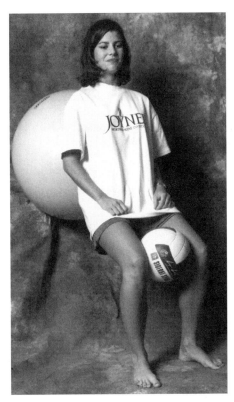

FIG. 15.74. Ball squats with adduction squeeze. The patient performs a ball squat in bilateral stance with adduction squeeze against a ball for resistance. Works to improve VMO activity through the origin of the vastus medialis obliquus (VMO) on the adductor magnus.

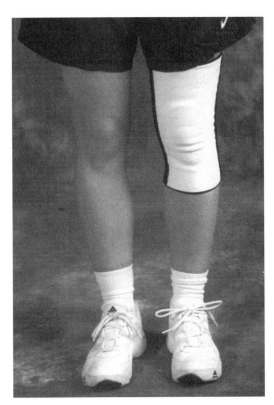

FIG. 15.75. Elastic support with a donut gel pad.

or forefoot varus can cause excessive pronation with resultant lower extremity internal rotation, again causing a lateral tracking, subluxation, or dislocation. Functionally, decreased strength and neuromuscular control of the anterior and posterior tibialis muscles can also lead to an excessive amount and speed of pronation and lower extremity internal rotation. Whether a structural or functional problem, orthotics that are properly measured and fitted can be a great benefit in the rehabilitation program. All of the previous areas need to be addressed in order to minimize the chance of recurrence.

Extrinsically, bracing and/or taping can be utilized to control the patella. Bracing ranges from a donut pad to a lateral buttress, depending on the severity of the symptoms (Fig. 15.75 to 15.77). Taping attempts to provide external control of the patella for lateral glide, lateral tilt, and rotational dysfunctions (Fig. 15.78). The soft tissue is stretched and the patella is taped to relieve the pain and further relax the offending pathology. The technique can work very well as a long-term solution if the patient actively works on VMO strengthening with the tape in place (165). A dynamic patellar stabilizing brace can serve a similar function (196). The brace consists of an elastic neoprene sleeve with a patella cutout, a lateral pad, and two circumferentially wrapped rubber arms that can

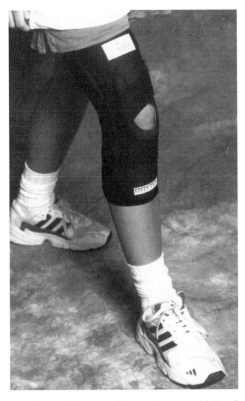

FIG. 15.76. Lateral buttress brace to prevent lateral subluxation/dislocation.

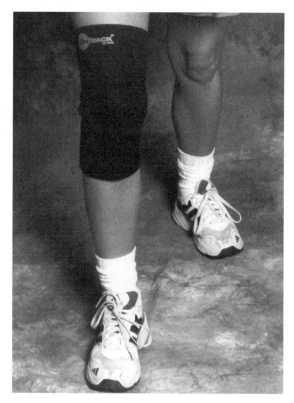

FIG. 15.77. On track patellofemoral brace to control patellofemoral malalignment and subluxation.

provide dynamic resistance to lateral patellar displacement (Fig. 15.79).

For resistant or severe cases, operative intervention may be indicated. Athletes with significant lateral patellar tilt and who cannot be rotated past a neutral position are excellent candidates for isolated lateral retinacular release arthroscopically or through a mini-open approach (77,133). All other athletes will probably require a more extensive realignment procedure.

Rehabilitation After a Lateral Retinacular Release

The immediate postoperative goal is to reduce swelling and limit the scarring of the lateral retinaculum. A foam or felt compression pad is used over the lateral aspect of the knee with overlying ace wrap or compression stockinette. This acts to force swelling out of the immediate wound area and decrease hypertrophic scarring. The use of electrical stimulation for its antiinflammatory effects and also for muscle reeducation after surgery can assist greatly in the rehabilitation process. The application of cold combined with elevation periodically throughout the day can help keep swelling to a minimum. Ice should be used no more than 20 minutes at a time, leaving enough time in between applications for the skin to warm to room temperature. Care should be taken to keep the ice more

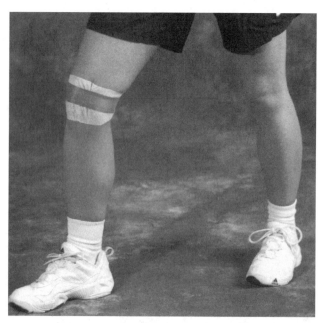

FIG. 15.78. McConnell taping technique is utilized to medially glide and tilt the patella. Also works with rotational components. Note the bunched-up skin under the tape to provide sufficient tension against the patella.

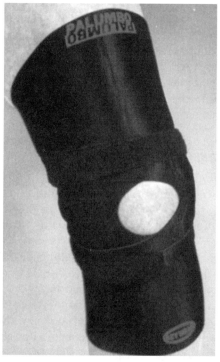

FIG. 15.79. The Palumbo patella stabilizer places medially directed force on the lateral border of the patella to resist patellar displacement.

proximal and avoid resting it on the common peroneal nerve.

The patient is allowed full weight bearing and is weaned off the immobilizer over a 1- to 2-week period. Active range of motion is begun on postoperative day 1 with heel slides and standing knee flexion. Quadriceps setting and four-way straight leg raises are also initiated at this time. Passively, knee flexion is gently pushed toward full flexion over the first two to three weeks.

Caution should be taken with stretching too aggressively when significant swelling is still present as repetitive tearing at the surgical site will perpetuate scar tissue formation. Once approximately 95 degrees of flexion has been obtained, the bicycle is added to the program, as are closed kinetic chain lower-extremity, strengthening exercises. The trunk, hip, knee, and lower leg are all included in the rehabilitation program to assure that normal mechanics have been restored and to maximize the chances for surgical success. A brace that has a lateral buttress can serve two functions. First, it can maintain compression over the release and, second, it can provide lateral stability and a medial glide to the patella.

Many authors have discussed a myriad of techniques to address recurrent patellar instability including soft tissue procedures proximal and distal to the patella, and distal bony realignment procedures with successes ranging from 30% to 90% (39,46,71,158,196,212). A successful result depends on proper diagnosis, identification of associated pathologies such as arthritis, meticulous surgical technique, and appropriate postoperative rehabilitation. For skeletally immature athletes, it is best to attempt to use a brace or taping until skeletal maturity is achieved. If necessary, a soft tissue only procedure is indicated with lateral retinacular release, VMO advancement, and occasionally a distal realignment as described by Roux-Goldthwaite (77). For mature athletes all procedures are preceded by diagnostic arthroscopy to assess the presence of degenerative changes of the patella. If the athlete has normal Q angles (less than 20 degrees), mild to no degenerative changes, and no ligamentous laxity, a proximal soft tissue realignment is indicated with lateral release and VMO advancement. If moderate to severe arthritic changes are present a tibial tubercle elevation may be indicated. For athletes with elevated Q angles or increased ligamentous laxity, distal bony realignment should be included with the proximal soft tissue reconstruction. The technique developed by Fulkerson (71,73,114,201) of anteromedialization of the tibial tubercle via an oblique osteotomy has distinct advantages. After diagnostic arthroscopy, the surgeon can adjust the amount of anterior displacement of the tibial tubercle required in relation to the amount of arthritic changes by changing the obliquity of the osteotomy and medialization to unload the damaged cartilage. A significant potential complication following realignment is medial instability (66,99,103).

Patellofemoral Articular Cartilage Involvement

The articular surface of the patella is the thickest in the body and is divided into medial and lateral facets by the median ridge or crest. With repeated wear or contact, the cartilage will begin to soften and progress through a sequence of degeneration that includes fibrillation, fissuring, thinning, fragmentation and finally complete cartilage loss. The athlete will frequently complain of pain when going up stairs or when sitting with the knees flexed for an extended period of time. There will be pain on palpation of the facets and crepitus with range of motion of the knee. Quadriceps atrophy and hamstring tendon tightness are commonly seen.

There can be chondral defects, osteochondral fractures, or varying grades of degeneration of the articular cartilage of the patella or trochlear groove. In the past, chondromalacia patella has been used as a "wastebasket" term for most anterior knee pain (21,195,197). The diagnosis is based on the pathology of articular cartilage involvement, and should be made only with visual inspection of the articular surface by open or arthroscopic means. Clinical

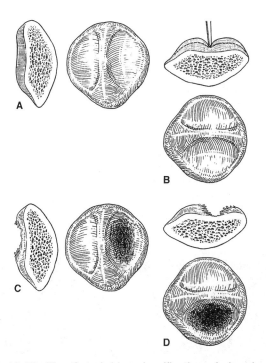

FIG. 15.80. The Outerbridge classification of chondromalacic change is shown diagrammatically. **A:** Normal articular cartilage of the patella is depicted. **B:** Grade I is softening only, without fragmentation or fissuring. **C:** Grades II and III are fissuring and fragmentation, with II being less than 1 inch and III being more than 1 inch. There is no exposed subchondral bone. **D:** Grade IV is down to subchondral bone. Documentation of the grade and size of the arthritic change is helpful, particularly in the patellofemoral articulation, in predicting success and outlining a rehabilitation program. (Reprinted with permission from ref. 9.)

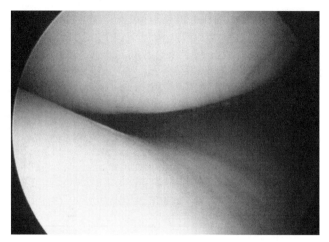

FIG. 15.81. Normal patellofemoral articulation is shown in patient undergoing anterior cruciate ligament (ACL) reconstruction with normal articular surface and tracking.

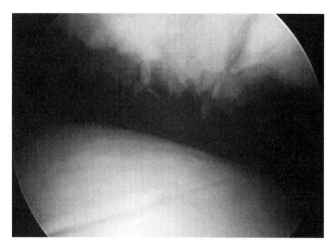

FIG. 15.82. Grade III lesion, chondromalacia patella shown arthroscopically.

descriptions should be used for the diagnosis, not the pathologic term "chondromalacia."

The grades (I to IV) of articular cartilage damage have been described by Outerbridge (Fig. 15.80). Grade I is softening. Grade II is fissuring and fragmentation with II being less than 1/2 inch, III being greater than 1/2 inch, and IV to exposed bone. Classification includes size and depth (185). Comparisons of classifications of chondral lesions exist (121). Normal patellofemoral articulation is shown in patient undergoing ACL reconstruction with normal articular surface and tracking (Fig. 15.81). Grade III lesion, chondromalacia patella is shown arthroscopically (Fig. 15.82). This patient had osteochondritis dissecans (OCD) of the patella. Sunrise views show lesion (Fig. 15.82) area measured 1 × 2 cm. These lesions are particularly troublesome for healing. Treatment for focal grade III and IV lesions arthroscopically include micropick, drilling, or abrasion (see Fig. 15.83B). These take a long time to heal, up to a year, and can significantly delay

functional return. Chondrocyte transplantation and allograft reconstruction have not been done long enough or in this age group to be performed routinely. Initially, treatment for articular cartilage problems is conservative and a majority of athletes will respond well. Treatment is focused on optimizing the knee function by improving the muscular balance from a strength and flexibility standpoint. Quadriceps strengthening improves patellar tracking and provides an active shock absorber to share the load of landing. Exercises should be performed in a pain-free arc of motion based on the angle at which the involved area comes in contact with the trochlear groove. Hungerford (105) has shown that contact stresses of different regions of the patella vary with the angle of knee flexion. Hamstring stretching reduces the forces that the quadriceps must overcome to attain extension, thereby reducing the patellofemoral joint reaction force. Occasionally, cushioned shoe inserts or encouraging the use of cushioned running shoes will further share the load of impact and reduce the patient's complaints. Adjuvant

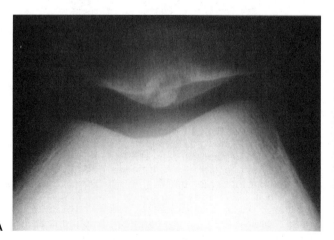

A

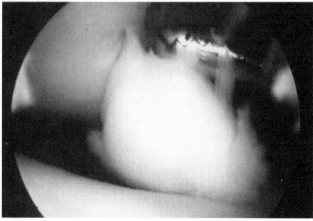

B

FIG. 15.83. A,B: This patient had OCD of the patella. Sunrise views shows lesion area measured 1 × 2 cm. Arthroscopic debridement of the loose osteochondral patellar fragment is shown.

treatment including ice and antiinflammatories can reduce pain to allow the athlete to participate in rehabilitation.

Resistant cases may require surgical intervention. Arthroscopy is an excellent tool that can confirm the diagnosis and provide initial treatment. Unstable cartilaginous fragments or loose bodies can be removed with excellent results. The cartilaginous defects are debrided and saucerized. Abrasion chondroplasty, microfracture with arthroscopic awls, or drilling has shown limited success on the femoral condyles but has had uniformly poorer results when used on the patellofemoral joint. Debridement of the lesion can reduce the chance for occurrence of loose bodies. Tibial tubercle transfer or elevation can be performed to reduce the stress on articular cartilage and improve tracking. In the most resistant and severe cases, patellectomy can be performed; however, significant functional weakness will invariably occur and complete pain relief is rare.

At the time of arthroscopy, documentation of the patella or trochlear groove articular surface defects with size and depth and contact areas by degrees of flexion should be performed (77) (Fig. 15.84). A rehabilitation program can then be outlined in the arc of motion that does not cause direct pressure and is not under the greatest contact. If surgical intervention is required, the surgeon must transfer the forces from the damaged tissues and also restore stability of the patellofemoral articulation. The PF articulation will deteriorate at an accelerated pace if pressure is increased (4).

Plicae

A synovial plica is a fold in the synovium, which is a residual of an embryologic synovial septum. The knee may have up to four plicae named by location—the suprapatellar, infrapatellar, lateral, and medial. Most synovial plica are asymptomatic but occasionally a plica can become inflamed from direct contact or overuse. The medial plica can be associated with chondral injury to the medial patella or defect in the nonarticulating medial femur.

The athlete complains of pain aggravated by activity or prolonged sitting. Some athletes complain of snapping, clicking, or the sensation of giving way on physical exam. Repetitive squatting and deep flexion often exacerbate the athlete's complaints. Symptomatic plica syndrome is more common in females and sports like gymnastics, cheerleading, and running. The thickened band is painful just superior to the medial femoral condyle and medial patellar facet.

Initial treatment is aimed at decreasing inflammation by using ice, local modalities, topical nonsteroidals, oral antiinflammatories and activity modification. Rehabilitation includes quadriceps strengthening, hamstring stretching, and correcting any weakness at the trunk, hip, and ankle that may be affecting normal knee function. Rovere

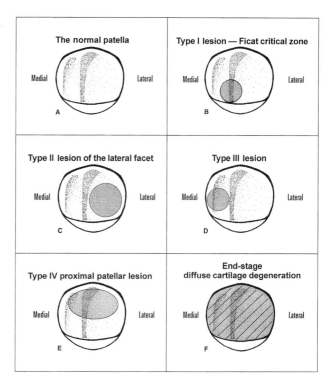

FIG. 15.84. A. A representation of the normal patella (medial left; lateral right). **B.** A type I lesion (Ficat critical zone) at the distal central ridge. **C.** A type II lesion of the lateral facet is usually related to excessive lateral pressure with tilt. This lesion is often associated with a type I lesion, and the two lesions may connect, particularly in a patient with longstanding lateral patellar tilt and subluxation. **D.** A type III lesion will occur related to relocation of a patella following dislocation, with shearing off of the medial facet. Lesions of the medial facet also occur from excessive medial overload (overzealous medial imbrication or Hauser transfer of the tibial tubercle). **E.** The proximal patellar lesion (type IV) that spans the facets is most often related to a crush, knee flexion injury (dashboard type) in which the proximal patella is articulating (knee flexed) at the time of impact. **F.** End-stage diffuse patella articular cartilage degeneration. (Adapted from and reprinted with permission from ref. 16.)

and Adar (213) suggested intraplical steroid and lidocaine injection. In 73% of patients lasting relief and return to sport was achieved. In cases not responding to rehabilitation and activity modification, arthroscopic resection of the symptomatic plica is indicated. At the time of arthroscopy, associated disorders such as chondral injuries or meniscal tears can be addressed.

Bursitis

Bursae are fluid-filled sacs that function to reduce friction and protect structures from pressure. The subcutaneous locations are shown (257) (Fig. 15.85). Bursal tissue becomes thicker and painful with increased blood flow from inflammation or contusion. Irritation and accompanying bursitis can result from acute or chronic trauma,

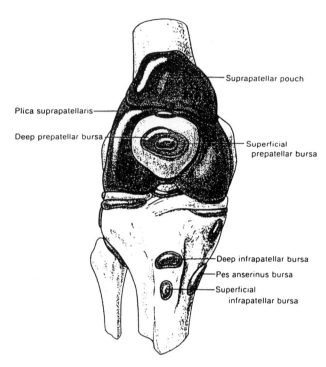

FIG. 15.85. Bursae in the front of the knee can mimic many knee disorders. These bursae should be examined in the evaluation of patients with anterior knee pain. (Reprinted with permission from ref. 77.)

inflammatory processes with metabolic deposits, or acute or chronic infection (48). Wrestlers, gymnasts, and football players are at increased risk of bursitis, particularly in the prepatellar bursa, from repeated contact. Acute hemorrhagic bursitis caused by small vessel rupture should be differentiated from inflammatory bursitis. The pes anserine bursa lies proximal to the insertion of the sartorius, gracilis, and semitendinosus tendons (the pes anserinus). The bursa lies between the aponeurosis of these tendons and the medial collateral ligament about 2 inches below the anteromedial joint line. Pes bursitis is more commonly caused by repeated friction rather than direct contusion (193).

Treatment is symptomatic with ice therapy, compression wraps, and antiinflammatories. Early motion, strengthening exercises, and even muscle stimulation can prevent muscle atrophy and enhance the athlete's early return to sport. Steroid injections in the pes anserine bursa can relieve the inflammatory process. Aspiration of the prepatellar bursa without steroid injection has also been recommended. Indications for surgical excision in athletes include multiple recurrences or an extremely large, chronically inflamed bursa extending beyond the diameter of the patella (193). Septic bursitis is treated by aspiration, culture, and appropriate surgical debridement.

Iliotibial Band Syndrome (ITB)

The iliotibial band originates from the gluteus maximus and tensor fascia latae. ITB syndrome is especially preva-

lent in joggers and cyclists. In jogging, there is a flight phase with no support. Upon impact, the hip and thigh must provide a significant contraction to stabilize the pelvis in a horizontal fashion against the ground reaction force. These strong, repetitive contractions typically result in decreased flexibility in the hip abductors and iliotibial band. The ITB moves over the femoral epicondyle anteriorly in extension and posteriorly in flexion. Direct tenderness over the ITB band is common. The patient's knee is flexed to 90 degrees and supported. Palpation of the ITB on the femur just proximal to the epicondyle is done and the knee is slowly extended. At 30 degrees of flexion, the patient complains of pain as the inflamed portion of the ITB is compressed between the examiner's thumb and the femoral epicondyle.

Primary treatment should be directed toward improving flexibility in the shortened tissues of the gluteus maximus, tensor fascia latae, and iliotibial band. The ITB can be stretched in standing or kneeling. In the kneeling position, one can often get a medial glide of the patella as well. Bringing in hip extension and adduction with the lean of the body allows for a good proximal quadriceps, gluteus medius, tensor fascia latae, and ITB stretch (Fig. 15.86).

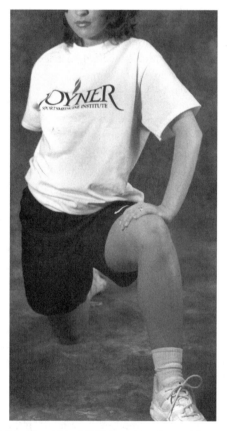

FIG. 15.86. Combined ITB band and quadriceps stretch. With patellofemoral pain, something soft may need to be placed under the knee. Keeping the stomach tight, forward lean to gain stretch in the quadriceps proximally followed by a slight lateral shift to change the emphasis to the superior lateral thigh.

Gaining flexibility in these tissues takes time and can be aided by the use of ultrasound and moist heat to improve tissue extensibility prior to stretching and iontophoresis, electrical stimulation, and ice to decrease inflammation after treatment. A thorough biomechanical evaluation should be completed to address any causative factors present at the hip, knee, and ankle. Taking a detailed history to determine training-factor influence such as road surface, mileage, and shoe wear is also helpful. Addressing weakness in the trunk, hip, knee, and lower leg can improve mechanics and efficiency as well as prevent further injury.

MENISCAL TEARS

Meniscal Tear Patterns

The classification of the tear pattern is described by location within the substance of the meniscus and the tear pattern. Types include radial, horizontal, longitudinal, degenerative, flap, or combinations of these (70) (Fig. 15.87). Meniscal tears are one of the most common knee injuries in the athletic population. Typically, the athlete presents with swelling, pain along the medial or lateral joint line, locking, and/or popping. Locking and inability to extend the knee after rising from a crouched position is present in 81% of patients with a bucket handle tear of the meniscus (229).

The most common finding on physical examination is pain with palpation or associated with provocative maneuvers. Bounce home, McMurray's, Apley's grind (10), and pain with varus or valgus stress all attempt to trap the torn meniscus between the tibial plateau and ipsilateral femoral condyle to elicit a diagnostic pain and pop. If pain alone is present, degenerative articular changes may also be the source of pain. Clinical squatting maneuvers with weight bearing or "standing McMurray's" are ex-

cellent added tests to discover subtle tears that may have evaded diagnosis with the other exams (5).

Routine radiographs include anterior-posterior, lateral, notch view, and bilateral patellar sunrise views. If the athlete is greater than age 50, standing 30 degrees flexed posteroanterior (PA) views are done to assess the joint space for degenerative arthritis. Magnetic resonance imaging is indicated if there are other intraarticular problems, associated ligament problems or confusion about the diagnosis (80,137,211). The majority of meniscus tears can be diagnosed by history and physical exam (80,95,124,173). Accuracy, sensitivity and specificity are extremely high for meniscal tears, better with the medial than lateral meniscus. A discoid lateral meniscus is a congenitally large meniscus that may occupy the entire articulating surface between the lateral femoral condyle and tibia. Symptoms of pain and clunking in the lateral compartment in adolescents is the common presentation. MRI scans can visualize these nicely aiding in the decision between surgical or nonsurgical treatment.

Treatment

Initial conservative management of relative rest, strengthening, compression, and decreasing joint effusion is performed. If recurrent mechanical signs and symptoms are present, arthroscopic intervention is indicated. At the time of surgery, a decision must be made regarding removal or repair of the torn meniscus. Attempt is made to repair menisci in the peripheral third or vascular zone. Central tears are avascular and have little ability to heal. If partial meniscectomy is required, removing as little of the meniscus as needed is the rule. Meniscus repair has a greater success rate in association with ligamentous reconstruction than in the cases of isolated meniscal surgery. There have been advances in meniscal transplantation with allografts. Initial reports of cryopreserved allograft transplantation in dogs were published in 1984 (13).

Meniscal tear patterns vary but principles of removal of the unstable fragments and restoring a balanced rim are followed routinely. A bucket handle tear of the meniscus or vertical pattern in orientation can displace into the notch (Fig. 15.88). Partial meniscectomy was performed.

The posterior horn flap tear was displacing in the medial gutter causing symptoms and mimicking a loose body (Fig. 15.89). This complex tear of the medial meniscus was resected with a handheld punch (Fig. 15.90).

Meniscal repair is done when the tear is in the red-white zone or peripheral third, usually vertical, and in a younger patient. Probing of the tear and repair with inside to outside techniques placing sutures arthroscopically is performed (Fig. 15.91A). The sutures are placed with a long needle, which can also be used for trephination to increase blood supply (see Fig. 15.91B).

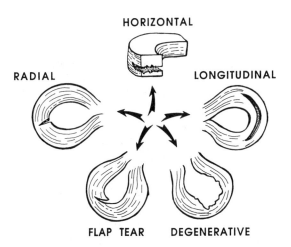

FIG. 15.87. Schematic illustration of the five main types of meniscal tears. (Reprinted with permission from ref. 57.)

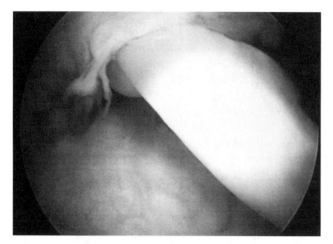

FIG. 15.88. In this left knee, arthroscopically, a vertical bucket handle tear is shown displaced into the notch. The anterior cruciate ligament is absent in the notch in this chronically injured anterior cruciate ligament (ACL) patient.

Rehabilitation of Meniscal Repairs

Communication between the surgeon and the rehabilitation team is critical with meniscal repairs (see Fig. 15.91). The site of the repair makes a big difference in the course of rehabilitation. If the tear is in the vascular zone, healing is better and the patient may be allowed to progress to touch down weight bearing earlier. If the

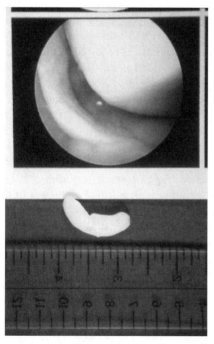

FIG. 15.89. View of posterior horn flap tear, view of anterior horn flap tear of the meniscus medially. The flap was in the medial gutter causing symptoms and mimicking a loose body. Shown is the medial femoral condyle, the displaced meniscal fragment and excised piece itself.

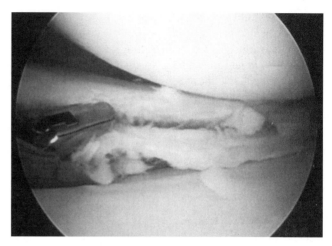

FIG. 15.90. A complex tear of the medial meniscus with more unstable tibial side is resected using a handheld punch.

vascularity of the repaired tissue is in question, the repair must be protected for a longer period of time. The patient should be toe touch to foot flat at 10% to 20% weight bearing for 2 to 4 weeks with range of motion limited to avoid hyperextension and flexion greater than 90 degrees. Extreme range of motion may cause increased strain on the repair. Isometrics and mid-range exercises in an open kinetic chain are initiated along with active range of motion in the prescribed range. Utilization of a stationary bicycle with no resistance can be effective for range of motion and to stimulate healing of the meniscus. The bicycle should be used in a rocking fashion; that is, forward and backward without a complete revolution, unless the complete revolution can be accomplished pain-free and with ease. When weight bearing is allowed, the exercise regimen is adjusted to include closed kinetic chain exercises, avoiding motions that bring the knee into greater than 90 degrees of flexion. Once again, the rehabilitation includes strengthening the trunk, hip, knee, and lower leg to control abnormal forces.

Articular Surface Injuries

Historically articular cartilage defects have been difficult to treat and an ulcerated cartilage will not heal (106). Genetics, alignment and the nature of the sport are contributing factors to articular cartilage health. Chondral and osteochondral fractures can occur and can be confused with meniscal injuries. If there is an effusion, increased crepitus on exam, history of axial loading in an adolescent with possible osteochondritis dissecans, articular surface injury should be highly considered (222). In soccer athletes, articular cartilage delamination has been reported (145). This basketball player sustained a noncontact knee injury landing from a rebound. His complaints were popping, swelling, locking. Arthroscopy showed a lateral femoral osteochondral fracture measuring 2 × 2 cm (Fig. 15.92A). He

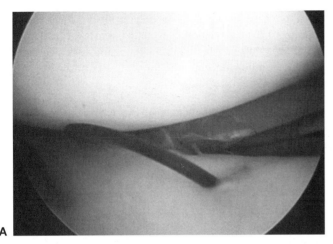
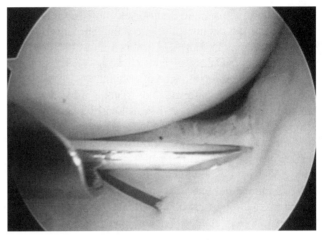

FIG. 15.91. A: Peripheral tear of the medial meniscus shown in the red/white zone with one suture placed and probe in tear. **B:** The needle through a cannula will introduce more anterior sutures to anchor the meniscus back to the capsule.

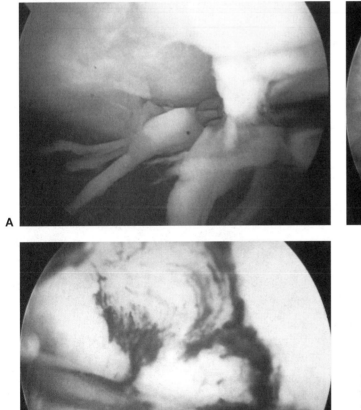
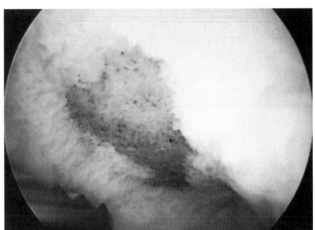

FIG. 15.92. A. This basketball player sustained a noncontact loading on his valgus knee injury. **B.** His complaints were popping, swelling, locking. Arthroscopy showed a lateral femoral osteochondral fracture with several loose bodies. **C.** He required removal of loose bodies and localized abrasion chondroplasty to stimulate bleeding of the bone and hopeful healing by fibrocartilage.

required removal of loose bodies, and unstable articular cartilage abrasion chondroplasty, to stimulate bleeding of the bone (see Fig. 15.92B). Documentation of bleeding is done by reducing inflow of fluid (see Fig. 15.92C). The hopeful result is fibrocartilage ingrowth.

This 16-year-old baseball and football athlete complained of pain, swelling, and occasional locking of his left knee. Clinically, he had tenderness on palpation over the medial femoral condyle, mild effusion, no medial or lateral joint line tenderness and stable ligaments. The notch view was most helpful to show osteochondritis dissecans of the medial femoral condyle (Fig. 15.93A). MRI scan after injection of gadolinium dye in the joint demonstrates the depth of the lesion and shows the defect in the medial femoral condyle in its typical location just lateral to the attachment of the PCL (see Fig. 15.93B, *arrow*). He underwent abrasion chondroplasty and at one year returned to football activities.

Counseling of athletes, particularly with lateral compartment involvement must be done early on. The likelihood of being able to play professional sports with a past history of arthroscopy and articular surface damage in the lateral compartment in a valgus knee is very small. Changing cardiovascular activities to reduce axial load is routinely discussed with the patient.

The future for treatment of articular surface defects is bright. Various techniques to stimulate blood supply exist. These include abrasion chondroplasty, microfracture techniques and drilling. Taking plugs of bone from a non–weight-bearing surface of the knee peripherally in the trochlear groove and transplanting this to the prepared condyle defect is now being done with the early results proving effective. Harvesting and culturing of articular cartilage and reimplantation of the cartilage is also being done in limited settings (30).

Rehabilitation of Injuries with Articular Surface Damage

Injuries involving damage to the articular surface can be very difficult to rehabilitate because of the nature of the injury: the damage to weight-bearing surface that has no inherent ability to ''protect itself.'' The surgeon must communicate to the rehabilitation team where the damage was found and the range of motion that has been affected by the damage. The rehabilitation professional then has the information to develop a plan of care that will effectively strengthen the lower extremity while avoiding any undue stress on the damaged articular surface. In general, bicycling is beneficial as it is a non–weight-bearing activity that promotes regrowth of articular cartilage. Use of modalities, particularly electrical stimulation for muscle contraction and work on decreasing inflammation, can be used effectively with ice to keep swelling down. Exercises that are isometric in nature, non–weight-bearing, or done through a limited, pain-free arc are most beneficial in the beginning stages of rehabilitation. After abrasion chondroplasty, the articular surface must be protected from repetitive axial loading. Patient education and activity modification are mandatory for the long-term success of these patients.

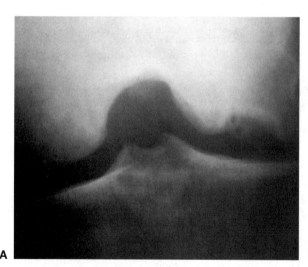
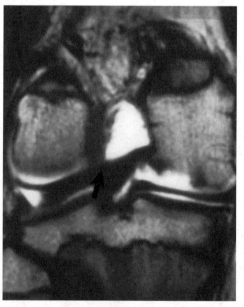

FIG. 15.93. A: Osteochondral dissecans of the medial femoral condyle shown on the right knee. Notch view is best to demonstrate this. The radiolucent area involving the entire medial femoral condyle is shown. Magnetic resonance imaging (MRI) scan (**B**) shows the extent of the lesion involvement into cancellous bone and location adjacent to the posterior cruciate ligament. Ligament of Wrisberg is also shown attaching the posterior cruciate ligament to the lateral meniscus (*arrow*).

Medial Collateral Ligament Injuries

Medial collateral ligament (MCL) sprains are very common in sports. MCL injuries typically occur when the foot is planted and the athlete sustains a blow to the lateral aspect of the knee. The treatment has evolved with increased knowledge obtained by arthroscopy and MRI. Grade I and II sprains and most isolated grade III MCL injuries can be treated nonoperatively. The more severe grade III MCL sprain is often associated with other ligamentous injuries. It is unusual to have an associated meniscal injury with an isolated MCL sprain since the mechanism is usually contact distracting the MCL. The pain is usually over the femoral attachment of the MCL. The "degree" of valgus opening should be established based on comparison with the other side and the knee should be stable and symmetrical in extension and different in 30 degrees of flexion.

In the 1980s surgical management of grade III MCL was commonplace (101,175,192). Now clinical diagnosis and nonoperative management is the rule for MCL sprains. We have seen treatment of medial injuries significantly change. There can be some problem from medial instability in ice hockey athletes (112,128), and these may require repair for an isolated grade III sprain. However, the current standard is nonoperative treatment and aggressive return to play. Grade I injuries involve initial rest and return to sport within a couple of weeks. Grade II may be slightly longer and grade III may require immobilization or protected weight bearing slowing their return for 6 to 8 weeks. Initial immobilization and non–weight-bearing may tighten up the medial structures more and result in less instability. However, healing generally occurs best with controlled mobility. Since isolated medial instability has not been shown to increase articular surface injury or knee problems, aggressive return to play and nonoperative treatment is presently the rule. Lateral knee braces have been used in hopes of preventing knee injuries, particularly in higher-risk positions in contact sports. These prophylactic or preventive braces attempt to protect the primary medial restraint that is the MCL. However, most scientific studies have yet to prove that lateral knee braces reduce the incidence of knee ligament injury (14,15,79,88,93,172,214,215,259,261). In controlled studies in the military, some reduction in the severity of injury with the brace has been shown (261). Indeed, in a survey of athletic traumas, a potential increase in injury, particularly fibular fracture and peroneal nerve injury secondary to the use of prophylactic braces has been reported (240). There are also questions as to whether braces preload the ligament. Certain criteria were set forward at the knee brace seminar report (59). A position statement from the AAOS states that "the routine use of prophylactic knee braces has not been proven effective in reducing the number or severity of knee injuries." In some circumstances, such braces may even potentially be a contributing factor to injury. Requiring players to use knee braces "just in case they might help" is not supported by the studies that have examined the effectiveness of such "braces."

If a brace is requested and the athlete is in a higher risk position, such as a football lineman, a thorough discussion with the athlete, his family, and his coach should be undertaken to assure the risks and benefits are understood. It should be stressed that there is still a chance for injury while wearing these braces.

Rehabilitation of Medial Collateral Ligament

Conservative treatment of medial collateral ligament (MCL) sprains has become more aggressive in recent years. Excellent results can be achieved if the rehabilitation program is approached in an aggressive, systematic manner, predicated on the attainment of milestones and healing time frames.

Grade I MCL Sprains

Grade I MCL sprains are treated with the knee immobilized for 1 week. Ice is used daily until pain and inflammation are under control. Quadriceps and hamstrings setting exercises (isometrics) may need to be done in 10 to 20 degrees of flexion to avoid pain in the end range of extension. Both open and closed chain exercises can be progressed as tolerated, as can range of motion. Achieving extension past 0 degrees extension (recurvatum) or 90 degrees flexion should be delayed until week two if still painful. Functional exercises and activities can be progressed aggressively as strength, neuromuscular control, and pain allow.

Grade II and III MCL Sprains

Grade II and III MCL sprains are treated in the initial 2 days with an emphasis on reducing pain and inflammation and protecting the MCL with an immobilizer or range of motion brace, limited to the pain-free range. The athlete will remain in a weight-bearing as tolerated status for 10 to 14 days. The doctor may order non–weight-bearing, depending on the severity of the sprain. Isometric quad sets and ham sets, straight leg raises in flexion, abduction and extension (avoiding the adduction motion), and PROM/AAROM to maintain range of motion are performed. Electrical stimulation for pain control, edema control, and muscle stimulation is utilized throughout the first week or two. Frequent application of ice will help reduce pain and swelling.

The tissue should warm and return to normal color before reapplying the ice. After the first 2 or 3 days, pain will be the limiting factor for weight bearing, range of motion, and exercise. The bicycle is used for gentle range

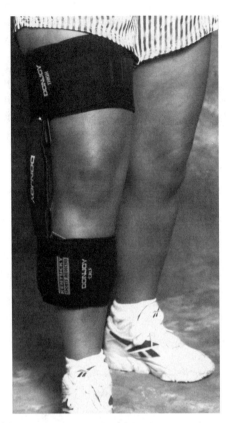

FIG. 15.94. Lateral knee bracing. Prophylactic knee bracing, primarily used for collision sports to prevent knee injury.

The focus of the second week is to progress strength and range of motion (ROM). Pool exercises can be advanced to weight bearing and jogging as tolerated. Bicycle work is increased for both time and resistance. Stretching exercises for the quads, hamstrings, ITB, and gastrocnemius are begun as long as the athlete remains pain-free. Proprioception exercises are advanced to facilitate full return of neuromuscular control. Closed kinetic chain exercises such as lunges, lateral step-ups, retro-walking, and stairmaster are advanced in duration and range of motion. When full pain-free flexion and extension have been achieved and strength and neuromuscular control are nearing 75% of the uninvolved side, a running progression can begin. The last step before a return to play is sports specific drills that are progressed slowly to allow the healing MCL to adapt to the new stresses. Lateral bracing may be needed to reduce medial stress and protect the healed tissue (Fig. 15.94). These types of braces can also be used prophylactically.

GROWTH PLATE INJURIES

In the skeletally immature athlete, the fracture about the knee with the most potential for complication is in the distal femur (31,167,177,198). The absolute number and percentage of all epiphyseal fractures for the distal femur, tibial tuberosity, proximal tibia, and proximal fibula are reported as shown (Table 15.6). In three series reporting the relative incidence of all physeal injuries, distal femur accounted for 5.0% (167), 5.5% (198), and 1.2% (177); proximal tibia 1.9% (167), 1.8% (198), and 0.7% (177); tibial tuberosity 3.1% (167), 0% (198), and 0% (177).

In 2,137 reported cases of athletic injuries in children, epiphyseal fractures involving the knee numbered 58 and the majority were Osgood-Schlatter's (41). There does not appear to be greater risk of growth plate injuries during competitive athletics than in other activities (139,140). If the athlete is hit about the knee and has pain over an epiphyseal plate, plain radiographs and stress views are indicated.

This skeletally immature football athlete sustained a blow to the outside of his left knee. The valgus, internal rotation deformity is shown (Fig. 15.95A). He sustained

of motion in a comfortable range. "Rocking" back and forth may be needed until a sufficient pain-free range is obtained. Swimming can begin with a gentle straight flutter kick only. Isometrics are performed at multiple angles, and gentle quadriceps exercises are begun through a pain-free range of motion. The brace is worn all the time at night and during the day as needed. Activity is immediately modified with any increase in pain, swelling, or instability. Well-leg exercises are performed during this period to maintain strength and endurance.

Once swelling and pain have stabilized with phase one activities and the athlete has a relatively pain-free range of motion from 100 degrees to 10 degrees, then they are ready to begin phase II. Goals for phase II include full, pain-free range of motion, normal gait, and restoring full lower extremity strength.

TABLE 15.6. *Lower extremity epiphyseal fractures*

Total # in Study:	Ogden 721		Peterson 330		Neer 2500	
	Number	Percent	Number	Percent	Number	Percent
Distal femur	36	5.0%	18	5.5%	28	1.1%
Proximal tibia	14	1.9%	6	1.8%	17	0.7%
Proximal fibula	4	0.6%			2	0.1%
Tibial tuberosity	22	3.1%				
Combined knee	76	10.5%	24	7.3%	47	1.9%

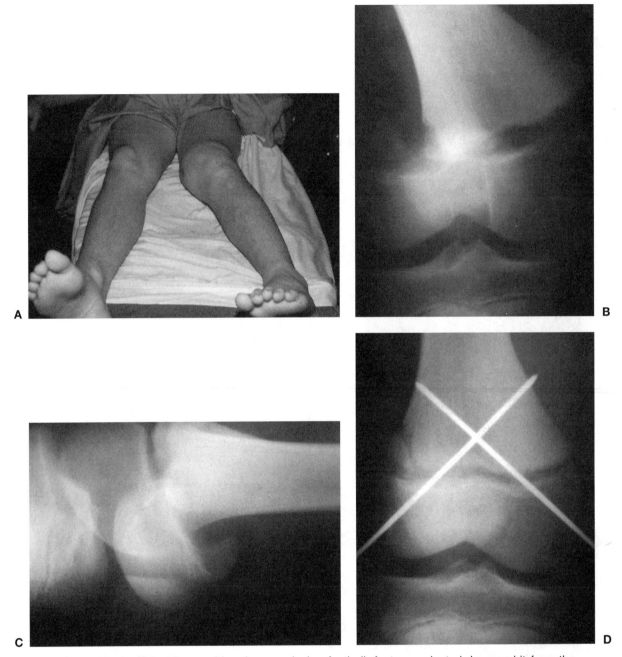

FIG. 15.95. A: This 14-year-old male was playing football, foot was planted, he was hit from the outside of his knee and had a Salter II fracture of the distal femur. **B,C:** Radiographs are shown. Emergency treatment is splinting the leg as it lies and transport to hospital. Treatment is with gentle reduction and internal fixation (**D**).

a Salter II fracture of the distal femur. Plain radiographs of AP (see Fig. 15.95B) and lateral views show the displaced distal femur fracture (see Fig. 15.95C). Emergency treatment includes splinting the leg as it lies and transport to hospital. Treatment is with gentle reduction and, in appropriate cases, internal fixation (see Fig. 15.95D). Potential complications from this fracture include leg-length discrepancy and angular deformity, usually in a progressive varus of the knee.

ANTERIOR CRUCIATE LIGAMENT (ACL) INJURIES

Skeletally Immature

In the skeletally immature patient, a tibial eminence avulsion fracture can occur rather than the typical mop end mid-substance tear of the ACL (162,167). A displaced McKeever type III tibial eminence fracture is shown in AP and lateral view (Fig. 15.96A, *arrow*). If the fragment does not reduce on extension, reduction and fixation is indicated.

An MRI scan was obtained (see Fig. 15.96B). On the lateral view the ACL can be seen to attach to the tibial eminence fragment, which is displaced. Oftentimes, the anterior horns of the medial and lateral menisci, or the intermeniscal ligament, can become interposed and pre-vent reduction. Arthroscopically aided internal fixation was done with two cannulated screws as shown in the lateral view (see Fig. 15.96C).

With a mop end ACL tear an extraarticular reconstruc-tion, using iliotibial band to avoid the epiphyseal plates, can be performed. With central plate closure, ACL recon-struction can be done with intraarticular reconstruction by femoral over the top and on the tibial above the epiphy-seal plate (139,163,227).

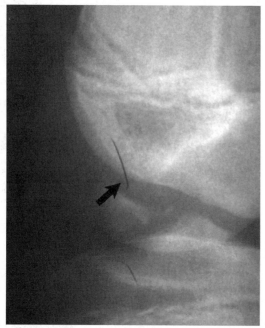

A

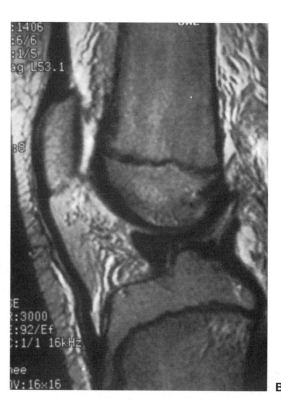

B

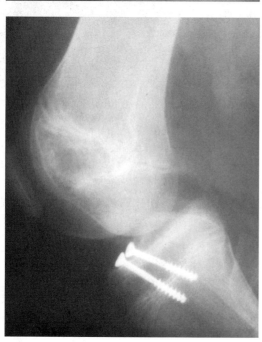

C

FIG. 15.96. A. (*arrow*) This skeletally immature male sustained a displaced McKeever type III tibial eminence fracture shown on lateral view in extension. **B.** Sagittal magnetic resonance imaging (MRI) scan shows the open epiphyseal plates and displaced tibial eminence. **C.** Lateral radiographs are shown following arthroscopically aided internal fixation with two cannulated screws with anatomic reduction of the tibial emi-nence fragment.

Skeletally Mature

The typical history for an ACL tear includes a noncontact mechanism, changing direction, feeling a shifting and ''pop,'' followed by swelling within a couple of hours. This left knee shows an acute hemarthrosis that occurred two hours after knee injury (Fig. 15.97).

Tests performed to diagnose an ACL tear include the Lachman, anterior drawer, and pivot shift. In the Lachman test, an anterior force is applied with the knee 30 degrees flexed and the proximal calf is supported by examiner's leg, pillow, or table (Fig. 15.98). The pivot shift maneuver has been described by various authors as going from flexion to extension and subluxating, or going from extension to flexion and relocating. A pivot shift is shown in the 30 degrees flexion position, applying internal rotation and anterior translation, a coupled movement of the tibia, with a clunk or shifting sensation being felt as the tibia subluxes. An MRI scan is performed if the diagnosis is unclear. There is need to document meniscal injury or bone bruise if surgery is not going to be performed. MRI scan shows a bone bruise in the middle portion of the distal femur and the posterior aspect of the tibia. When the tibial subluxation is in anterolateral rotatory direction, the bone bruise pattern can be easily understood (Fig. 15.99).

The treatment of ACL tears is by reconstruction, rather than primary repair. The complete midsubstance failure makes the ligament tissue abnormal and nonrepairable.

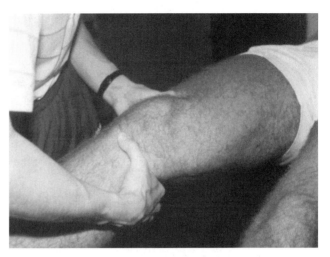

FIG. 15.98. Lachman test is performed with the knee at 30 degrees flexion, stabilizing the femur pulling forward on the tibia as the leg rests comfortably on a leg or pillow.

The choice of graft depends on availability, surgeon, and patient preference. Graft choices include the patellar tendon, hamstrings tendon, and allograft (57a,64,123,141, 188,245). Potential complications do exist from each procedure including graft failure, and are discussed in detail with the patient and family (188). Females and males do equally well following ACL reconstruction with bone-central third patellar tendon-bone (17,190). In the ACL deficient knee with severe varus alignment, combined or staged high tibial osteotomy may be necessary (187). Prosthetic ligaments have been tried but results have not been acceptable (129).

The typical tear pattern of the ACL is complete and midsubstance. A mop end tear (*arrow*) is seen superiorly

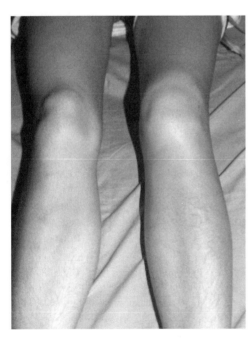

FIG 15.97. Acute anterior cruciate ligament injury caused this tense hemarthrosis from a mop end tear of this left anterior cruciate ligament. Note the normal patellar contour on the right and absence of patellar definition from the tense hemarthrosis.

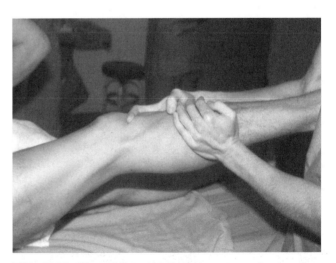

FIG. 15.99. Pivot shift test is shown in exam under anesthesia at the time of subluxation of the lateral tibial plateau anteriorly in this dislocation test going from flexion to extension. Anatomically, the IT band and hamstring spasticity in the acutely injured knee make this test more difficult to obtain and reproduce.

with the scope looking at the posterior horn of the medial meniscus (Fig. 15.100). In a chronic ACL tear, there is often associated meniscal injury (20,38,220) and articular surface injury. In the chronic ACL injury, one may see an empty notch sign, meaning that no ACL is present in the intercondylar notch (Fig. 15.101A). After tearing away from its origin, the ACL may scar down to the PCL but not back to the posterior femur. A meniscal tear can be repaired if it is in the vascular or red-white region in the peripheral third. A displaced bucket handle tear of the lateral meniscus is shown (see Fig. 15.101B). Sutures are being inserted in a modified inside-out technique to repair a peripheral tear of the lateral meniscus (see Figs. 15.101C and 15.101D). A bone-central third patellar tendon-bone ACL reconstruction is shown being inserted into the femur where a hole has been reamed (see Fig. 15.101E) and then the finished graft filling the notch (see Fig. 15.101F) with an interference screw in the femoral hole (see Fig. 15.101G) is shown.

The natural history of unreconstructed ACL injuries is such that there is progressive arthrosis, particularly in the lateral compartment in certain patients. This patient underwent partial lateral meniscectomy of his right knee in high school and elected not to have his knee reconstructed. Five years after his injury in his mid-20s, the lateral compartment narrowing is seen compared to his opposite normal side. Standing 30 degrees flexed PA views show narrowed lateral compartment (Fig. 15.102).

Rehabilitation of the Anterior Cruciate Ligament Reconstruction

Accelerated ACL rehabilitation programs have been well documented (54,111,122,157,256) as have injury prevention programs in skiing (160,216), basketball (87,119,120), and soccer (35).

There are two tenets upon which ACL rehabilitation is based: (1) the healing time of the graft and (2) reaching established performance goals.

Decisions about progression of rehabilitation rest mainly on these tenets. Other factors taken into account are pain, swelling, and increased laxity. Controlled stress acts as a physical stimulus to the formation and organization of collagen during the healing phase. Uncontrolled stress could lead to a strain and permanent mechanical deformation, or laxity, in the healing ligament.

The first postoperative 7 to 10 days comprise phase I. This phase includes attaining 90 degrees of flexion and having an independent straight leg raise with no extensor lag. Patella mobilizations are initiated to limit iatrogenic scarring in the patella tendon and bursae. Full passive range of the extension motion is critical in the early phase to ensure that the graft will sit fully in the intercondylar notch. Otherwise, notch stenosis will prevent the graft from seating properly and scar tissue will fill the notch. Pushing terminal extension after scar tissue has developed may stretch out the graft. The goal for extension is for the involved side to equal the uninvolved side or to be at least 0 degrees.

Weight bearing is increased until full weight bearing is achieved by one week postoperatively, depending on swelling and pain. The program includes full weight-bearing mini-squat exercises. Flexion range of motion activities should gradually address attaining 95 to 100 degrees of flexion by the end of phase I. Wall slides can gradually assist in increasing knee range of motion. Isometric quadriceps and hamstring setting exercises and resistive hamstring exercise can be performed throughout a comfortable range of motion and in high repetitions. Straight leg raise exercises are done in the abduction, adduction, and extension motions. The athlete maintains a stretching program for the hamstring, quadriceps, and gastrocnemius. Prone hangs help achieve terminal passive extension if the patient is having trouble with end range.

Phase II begins at about 2 weeks. The emphasis here is to resume a normal gait and to start increasing lower extremity strength. Exercises focus on strength and neuromuscular control of the lower extremity and are designed to be very functional. Knee extensions are avoided because of the anterior shear of the tibia on the femur, particularly in the terminal 30 degrees of extension. Phase II exercises are added on to Phase I exercises. Straight leg raise is added in the flexion motion. Calf raises are done with both a straight knee and in a seated, flexed knee position. Partial range of motion box lunges are limited to a comfortable range of motion. Proprioceptive exercises and balance training are begun in a weight-bearing as tolerated fashion. The degree of challenge with these exercises starts out relatively small and gradually increases as strength and ability allow. If a pool is avail-

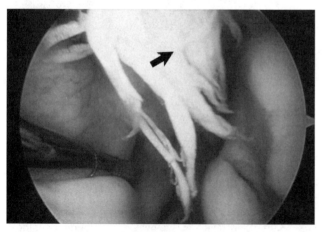

FIG. 15.100. The usual tear pattern for the anterior cruciate ligament is a mop-end complete failure as shown here. The scope is directed posteriorly in the posterior compartment at the posterior horn of the medial meniscus and the mop end tear is superior (*arrow*).

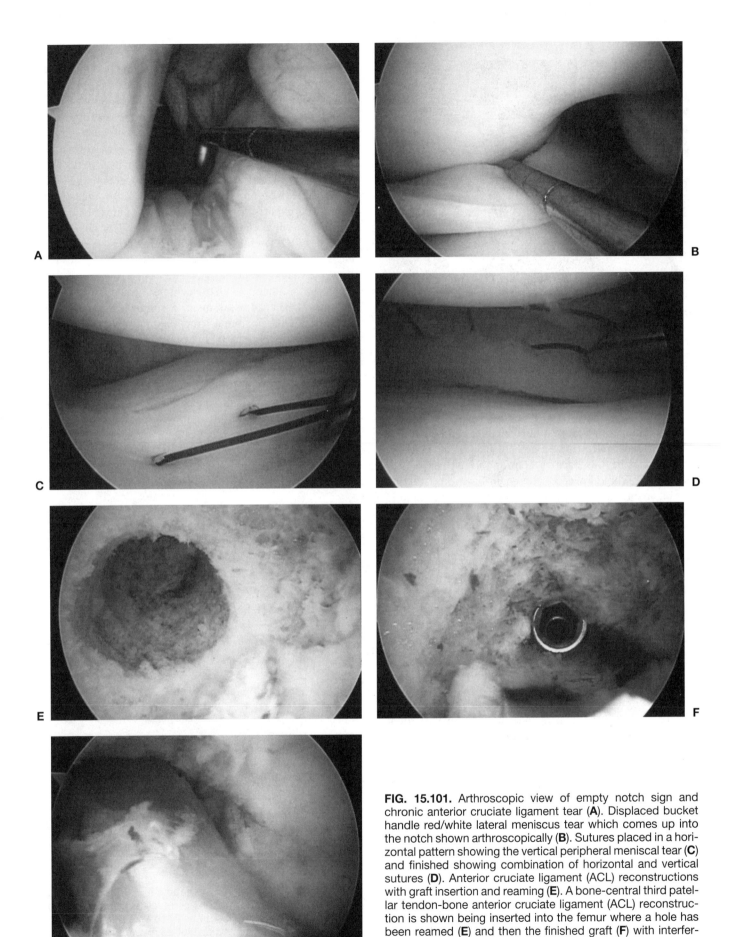

FIG. 15.101. Arthroscopic view of empty notch sign and chronic anterior cruciate ligament tear (**A**). Displaced bucket handle red/white lateral meniscus tear which comes up into the notch shown arthroscopically (**B**). Sutures placed in a horizontal pattern showing the vertical peripheral meniscal tear (**C**) and finished showing combination of horizontal and vertical sutures (**D**). Anterior cruciate ligament (ACL) reconstructions with graft insertion and reaming (**E**). A bone-central third patellar tendon-bone anterior cruciate ligament (ACL) reconstruction is shown being inserted into the femur where a hole has been reamed (**E**) and then the finished graft (**F**) with interference screw (**G**) is shown.

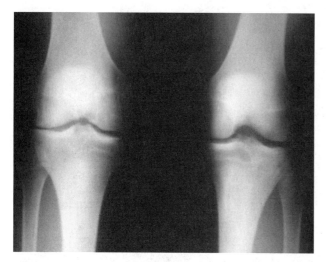

FIG. 15.102. Standing radiographs show degenerative joint disease of the lateral compartment and increased valgus in this patient who tore his anterior cruciate ligament in high school. Radiographs were obtained eight years later. He underwent partial lateral meniscectomy in high school and elected not to have his knee reconstructed.

able, walking and straight flutter kicking can begin. The Nordic Track and stair stepper are helpful as range of motion can be limited to a comfortable arc while still addressing whole lower kinetic chain function. Utilizing the bicycle to help maintain an increased range of motion and decreased stiffness and swelling will help in the athlete's progression. Criteria to advance to phase III are the ability to perform a 6-inch forward step-up, 0 degrees extension to 120 degrees flexion, and a normal gait.

Phase III lasts approximately 6 to 8 weeks. The emphasis at this stage is on progressive strengthening and neuromuscular reeducation exercises by repetition and time. The number and variety of closed chain exercises are increased as the patient tolerates. The graft is at its weakest point structurally at 8 to 10 weeks after surgery. Therefore, caution must be used in advancing the rehabilitation program only when the athlete demonstrates the appropriate strength and motor control to handle it. Goals for graduation from phase III include: bilateral quarter squat with 30% body weight, ten single leg quarter squats with good balance, controlled lateral step-up to a 6-inch height, single leg standing for 10 seconds with eyes closed, minimal swelling, and maintaining full passive knee extension.

Phase IV is a progression of phase III activities and leads up to testing the athlete's functional status. Emphasis is on easy plyometrics, control of jumping and soft landing as well as preparation for running. Depending on the patient's functional level, a functional assessment test is given during phase IV. This can be given anywhere from week 13 through week 16. The importance of functional testing is twofold: (1) to check the athlete's ability to initiate and control forces, and (2) obtain objective data regarding functional activities.

Functional tests are scored on two levels. Objective measures are taken for absolute values of weight lifted and centimeters jumped. More importantly, an observation of the activity is done to determine the neuromuscular control during landing activities, directional changes, and stopping. Points are assessed for poor performance in regards to quality of movement. An isokinetic test may be performed at 180 degrees per second and 300 degrees per second at 14 to 16 weeks to determine strength comparison of the involved to uninvolved leg. Once the athlete can perform 15 independent single leg squats, full bilateral squats with 50% body weight on each leg, and control the landing on jumps up to 12, they are ready for phase V.

The basic functional assessment performed in our clinic includes a balance assessment, a single leg squat at 45 degrees of knee flexion, a 1 rep maximum leg press from 60 degrees flexion to 0 degrees extension, and lastly, controlled landings up to both a 6-inch height and a 12-inch height. Three variations are tested for each height: the athlete starts with equal weight on both lower extremities, jumps up and lands on both feet; the athlete starts on both lower extremities, jumps up, and lands on the

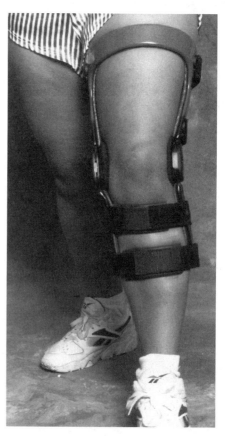

FIG. 15.103. Anterior cruciate ligament (ACL) derotational brace. Brace is used for anterior cruciate ligament (ACL) deficient and reconstructed athletes working primarily to decrease rotational instability, as well as anterior translation of the tibia on the femur.

uninvolved foot; the athlete starts on the involved foot, jumps up, and lands on the involved foot. After an assessment is made about his or her abilities with these four tests, the clinician can then more accurately assess the ability to perform advanced levels of exercise (143,206,255).

During phase V, the athlete's program is advanced in both the variety and difficulty of exercises through the four weeks following their achievement of a score on passing the basic functional assessment. Exercise incorporates lateral and turning movements with gradual increase to sport activities and forces. An advanced functional assessment is then given that includes a vertical jump test, a single leg long jump, a single leg triple jump, a single leg timed agility test over a 6-meter distance, a lateral shuffle test performed over a 5-meter distance, sports specific tests for stop, start, and cutting, and a 1 rep maximum leg press (143,206,255).

Running, agility training, and plyometric impact activity are progressed throughout phase V as the results of the functional tests dictate. Independent half speed running, both forward and backward, independent lateral hops, controlled landing down from a 12-inch height, control of rotational jumps and landings, and control of single leg landings during a 6-inch jump up to a mat are the milestones for passing phase V.

Phase VI is the final phase and focuses on a controlled return to actual sports activities at full speed. As the athlete tolerates these increases, plyometrics are increased and cutting motions are performed on the command of the therapist or athletic trainer. An isokinetic retest can be performed with the goal being 80% quadriceps and 100% hamstring strength of the involved side to the uninvolved side (254). Return to full activities is allowed after the athlete passes an advanced functional assessment, done at 4 to 6 months postoperatively.

While bracing following ACL reconstruction remains controversial, the risks and benefits of using the brace must be discussed. There still remain concerns regarding the specific effects of bracing on neuromuscular function

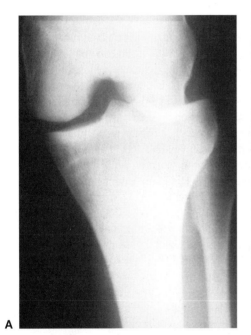

A

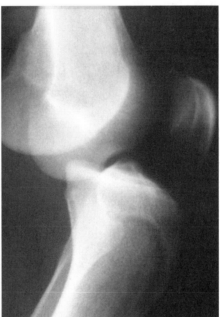

B

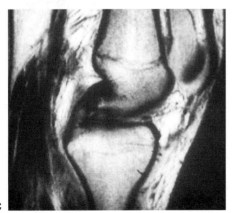

C

FIG. 15.104. This patient sustained an anterior knee dislocation. She was found to have anterior cruciate tears of both knees and it was suggested that she either stop cheerleading or have her knees reconstructed. She stopped cheerleading and while participating in a school play jumped from a 3 ft height. Radiographs of AP (**A**), lateral view (**B**) show anterior knee dislocation. **C.** The magnetic resonance imaging (MRI) scan shown on sagittal cut demonstrates an intact posterior cruciate ligament, absent anterior cruciate ligament.

(72,171,259,261,262) (Fig. 15.103). If an athlete is returning to a high-risk, highly competitive collegiate or high school sport, bracing is usually done the first year from the time of reconstruction. The most important brace is internal, musculoligamentous, and neurologic contribution. Restoration of proprioception and function are key after ACL reconstruction (18).

Anterior Knee Dislocation

When the tibia anteriorly moves from under the femur, an anterior dislocation can occur and is often associated with multiple ligament tears. In noncontact mechanisms, these injuries usually are self-reduced in the active individual. In a contact injury or unconscious patient, reduction is necessary. This patient with chronic bilateral ACL tears decided to stop cheerleading and did not want a reconstruction. She jumped from a 2-foot height during a play and sustained an anterior knee dislocation shown in radiographs of AP (Fig. 15.104A) and lateral view (see Fig. 15.104B). The MRI scan showed a complete ACL tear but an intact PCL (see Fig. 15.104C). After her dislocation, she developed a deep vein thrombosis. Assessment of vascularity must be done in severe knee injuries to assess arterial or venous injury. After a 4-month course of anticoagulant therapy, she underwent ACL reconstruction.

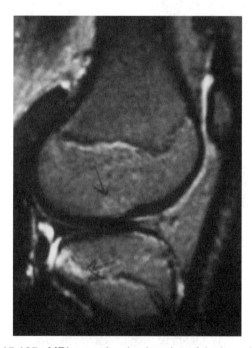

FIG. 15.105. MRI scan showing location of the bone bruise following anterior cruciate ligament (ACL) tear which is mid-third lateral femoral condyle and posterior third lateral tibial plateau in the skeletally immature athlete. Consider the status of the articular cartilage in between with bone bruises documented by MR like this.

Bone bruises are easily seen on MRI and are located on the posterior aspect of the lateral tibial plateau and the anterior aspect of the femur that can be correlated well with anterior knee dislocation (see Fig. 15.104B). The bone bruise location is shown on sagittal MRI (Fig. 15.105). The importance of bone bruises is unknown. A temporary anterior knee dislocation occurs when the ACL is torn. If one thinks about the contact pressures between these locations of the tibia and femur, the articular surface must have significant shear and compressive forces.

POSTERIOR CRUCIATE LIGAMENT (PCL) INSTABILITY

Classic mechanism of a PCL injury is a motor vehicle accident with the tibial tubercle hitting the dashboard providing a posterior force. In athletics, when someone falls, the foot classically is in a plantar flexed position so that the force of the fall is on the tibial tubercle. With the foot dorsiflexed, the blow would be to the patella and a patellar contusion or fracture would ensue (40). In the sport of tae kwon do, contact mechanisms with the opponent's foot can cause PCL injuries.

The clinical exam should include observation of any ecchymosis or abrasions on the tibial tubercle. The posterior drawer is done pushing the tibial posteriorly in neutral, internal, and external tibia rotation. The quads must be relaxed. With the knee at 90 degrees, the test is performed in neutral and then compared to the opposite side. A drop-back sign occurs when the tibial plateau is in a more posterior position relative to the femur.

This offensive lineman sustained a direct blow to the anterior tibial tubercle. His exam under anesthesia shows 4+ posterior drawer (Fig. 15.106A) with a posterolateral corner injury (see Fig. 15.106B). The injured capsule should be repaired acutely. His knee is also shown posteriorly dislocated (Fig. 15.106C). Vascular work-up was negative for deep venous thrombosis (DVT) or popliteal artery injury. Identification of a posterolateral injury is very important, as acutely, the posterolateral component should be addressed with the repair or reconstruction. Use of intraarticular grafts placed in an anatomically correct position and restoration of two bundles on the femur are done.

Rehabilitation of the Posterior Cruciate Ligament Reconstruction

Rehabilitation of the posterior cruciate ligament reconstruction presents many of the same problems as with rehabilitation of the ACL reconstruction. Reducing swelling, protecting the graft, and restoring normal strength and motor control are vital. Limitations of range of motion should be outlined by the surgeon. Electrical stimulation is used for muscle contraction of the quadriceps and for

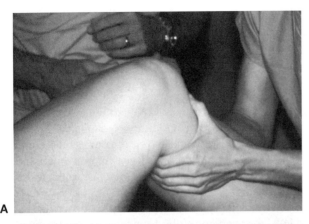

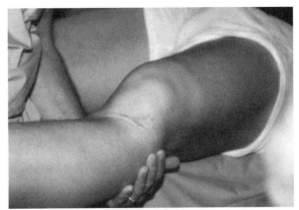

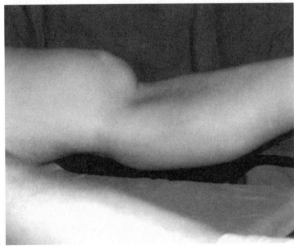

FIG. 15.106. A. Posterior drawer test done under exam under anesthesia with grossly positive posterior drawer. B. Posterolateral and posterior instability is demonstrated with this knee in a posterolateral dislocated position under anesthesia. C. Shows side view of the posterior dislocation.

decreasing inflammation in the knee. Ice and elevation are used frequently throughout the day, allowing enough time in between applications for the skin to resume its normal temperature and color. Exercises initiated on postoperative day 1 include ankle pumps with the leg elevated, quadriceps setting, and straight leg raises. Throughout the first week, multiple-angle isometrics, patellar mobilizations, and toe raises are added with the knee in full extension. Throughout the second week, week 1 exercises are continued, knee extension exercises are added from 0 to 60 degrees, proprioceptive training is initiated as tolerated and well-leg exercises are begun on the bicycle. Exercises are increased in the number of sets and repetitions all the way through to week 4. The addition of mini-squats, stationary bicycling, pool exercises, box lunges, and up to a 4-inch forward step-up all occur as the patient can tolerate and adequately perform these.

By week 7, passive range of motion should be approximately 120 to 125 degrees of flexion and 0 degrees of extension. There should be no changes in the KT-1000 arthrometer testing through this point in time. Submaximal hamstring isometrics can progress to short arc hamstring curls with minimal to no weight. A variety of closed chain exercises can be added and progressed all the way through to week 12. Pool exercises can be advanced to

light running. At approximately 3 to 4 months, pool running can advance to land running. Also, from the 3 to 4 months, isokinetic high speed can be initiated in an arc of motion from 40 degrees of flexion to 100 degrees of flexion. A basic functional test is performed in the 3.5- to 4-month time period prior to a formal running program being initiated. The functional test is described in detail under the rehabilitation of the ACL reconstruction section. Return to activity occurs at approximately 5 to 6 months. All the rehabilitation exercises during this phase are geared toward sports-specific activities, agility, balance, and plyometrics. Return to sport typically happens after 6 months postoperatively, once the athlete passes an advanced functional test.

ACL/MCL/PCL KNEE DISLOCATION

A knee dislocation requires hospitalization, radiographs, vascular assessment, and observation following reduction. This injury is potentially limb threatening. Exam under anesthesia shows gross 4+ opening on abduction stress testing at 0 and 30 degrees (Fig. 15.107A). The defect in the skin seen below the examiner's hand is the skin tissue that is entering the joint, since there is a

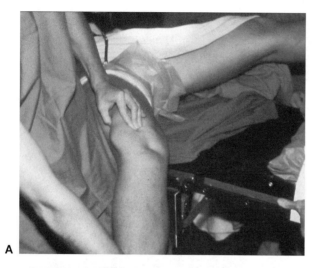

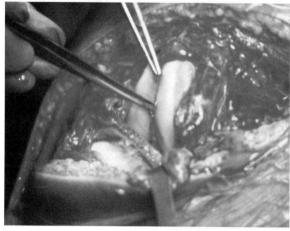

FIG. 15.107. Exam under anesthesia shows gross 4+ opening on abduction stress testing at 0 and 30 degrees (**A**). Reconstruction—open procedure (**B**) Exam showing instability to valgus stress testing at 0 and 30 degrees flexion, anterior posterior drawer, were grossly positive 4+ (A). The open shot shows the incision only being made (B).

complete tear of all intraarticular structures. This patient essentially had a knee dislocation with a laterally dislocated patella on the field. He had a complete tear of the ACL, PCL, and severe deep capsular injury with complete tears of the meniscofemoral and meniscotibial ligaments (see Fig. 15.107B). The meniscus is seen between the femur and tibia. Pickups are in the torn ACL that is mop end and above toward the PCL avulsion off of the femur. Although unusual, a knee dislocation with this severe medial instability will require a more open approach rather than the now more common arthroscopically aided approach.

CONCLUSIONS

Knowledge of knee anatomy is key in understanding diagnosis and treatment of knee injuries. Understanding basic anatomy allows development of a language that incorporates anatomy, mechanism of injury, and instability patterns. The healthcare providers can formulate the plan for the athlete—treatment, surgery, and rehabilitation. We must communicate in a common language.

Patterns of injury unique to the injured athlete's age, sport, and knee compartment—patellofemoral, medial, or lateral can be recognized. The exact diagnosis is made on the basis of history and physical exam. If the correct diagnosis is made early on, a successful outcome is predictably excellent in these highly motivated athletes. Be thorough and specific in the diagnosis.

Communication among health care providers must exist on a level to ensure the highest-quality care and treatment. Prospective outcome studies must be done. Standardized accepted knee-rating scales must be developed and revised.

ACKNOWLEDGMENTS

Thanks to Carolyn Large, transcriptionist; Rick Hood, photographer; Tom Adler, Ph.D., computer expert; and Sue Stanley, A.T.C., manuscript reviewer.

REFERENCES

1. Aglietti P, Insall JN, Walker PS. A new patellar prosthesis. *Clin Ortho* 1975;107:175–187.
2. Aglietti P, Insall J, Cerulli G. Patellar pain and incongruence. I. Measures of incongruence. *Clin Orthop* 1983;176:217–224.
3. American Medical Association. Standard Nomenclature of Athletic Injuries. Chicago: American Medical Association, 1966.
4. American Academy of Orthopaedic Surgeons, Dept. of Scientific and Research Affairs. Draft: knee pain—phase I, II; knee injury—phase I. Rosemont, IL, 1996.
5. Anderson AF, Lipscomb AB. Clinical diagnosis of meniscal tears. Description of a new manipulative test. *Am J Sports Med* 1986; 14:291–293.
6. Anderson AF, Lipscomb AB, Liudahl KJ, Addlestone RB. Analysis of the intercondylar notch by computed tomography. *Am J Sports Med* 1987;15(6):547–552.
7. Anderson AF, Snyder RB, Lipscomb AB. Evaluation of knee ligament rating systems. *Am J Knee Surg* 1993;6:67–73.
8. Andrews JR, Axe MJ. The classification of knee ligament instability. *Orthop Clin North Am* 1985;16:69.
9. Andrews JR, Timmerman LA. *Diagnostic and operative arthroscopy.* Philadelphia: WB Saunders, 1997.
10. Apley G. The diagnosis of meniscus injuries. *J Bone Joint Surg* 1947;29:78–84.
11. Arendt E, Dick R. Knee injury patterns among men and women in collegiate basketball and soccer: NCAA data and review of literature. *Am J Sports Med* 1995;23(6):694–701.
12. Arnoczky SP, Warren RF. Microvasculature of the human meniscus. *Am J Sports Med* 1982;10:90–95.
13. Arnoczky SP, Cuzzell JZ, McDevitt CA, Torzilli PA, Warren RF, Kristinicz TI. Meniscal replacement using a cryopreserved allograft—an experimental study in the dog. *Trans Orthop Res Soc* 1984;9:220.
14. Baker BE. The effect of bracing on the collateral ligaments of the knee. *Clin Sports Med* 1990;9(4):843–851.
15. Baker BE. Prevention of ligament injuries to the knee. *Exerc Sport Sci Rev* 1990;18:291–305.
16. Baker CL. *The Hughston Clinic sports medicine book.* Philadelphia: Williams & Wilkins, 1995.

17. Barber-Westin SD, Noyes FR, Andrews M. A rigorous comparison of results and complications between the sexes of results and complications after anterior cruciate ligament reconstruction. *Am J Sports Med* 1997;25(4):514–526.

18. Barrett DS. Proprioception and function after anterior cruciate reconstruction. *J Bone Joint Surg* 1991;73B:833–837.

19. Baumgartl F. *Das Kniegelenk*. Berlin: Springer-Verlag, 1944.

20. Bellabarba C, Bush-Joseph CA, Bach BR Jr. Patterns of meniscal injury in the anterior cruciate-deficient knee: a review of the literature. *Am J Orthop* 1997;26(1):18–23.

21. Bentley G, Dowd G. Current concepts of etiology and treatment of chondromalacia patellae. *Clin Orthop* 1984;189:209–228.

22. Berg EE, Mason SL, Lucas MJ. Patellar height ratios: a comparison of four measurement methods. *Am J Sports Med* 1996;24(2):218–221.

23. Beynnon BD, Johnson RJ. Relevant Biomechanics. In: DeLee JC, Drez D, eds. *Orthopaedic sports medicine: principles and practice*, vol. 2. Philadelphia: WB Saunders, 1994:1113–1133.

24. Black JE, Alten SR. How I manage infrapatellar tendinitis. *Phys Sportsmed* 1984;12:86–92.

25. Blazina ME, Kerlan RK, Jobe FW, Carter VS, Carlson GJ. Jumpers knee. *Orthop Clin North Am* 1973;4:665–678.

26. Boden BP, Garrett WE, Jr. Mechanisms of injuries to the anterior cruciate ligament. [Abstract] *Med Sci Sports Exerc Suppl* May, 1996;28(5):S26.

27. Bomberg BC, McGinty JB. Acute hemarthrosis of the knee: indications for diagnostic arthroscopy. *Arthroscopy* 1990;6(3):221–225.

28. Boring TH, O'Donoghue DH. Acute patellar dislocation: results of immediate surgical repair. *Clin Orthop* 1978;136:182.

29. Brantigan OC, Voshell AF. The tibial collateral ligament, its function, its bursae, and its relation to the medial meniscus. *J Bone Joint Surg* 1943;25A:121–131.

30. Brittberg M, Lindahl A, Nilsson A, et al. Treatment of deep cartilage defects in the knee with autologous chondrocyte transplantation. *N Engl J Med* 1994;331:889–895.

31. Buess-Watson E, Exner GU, Illi OE. Fractures about the knee: growth disturbances and problems of stability at long-term follow-up. *Eur J Pediatr Surg* 1994;4(4):218–224.

32. Buff HU, Jones LC, Hungerford DS. Experimental determination of forces transmitted through the patellofemoral joint. *J Biomech* 1988;21(1):17–23.

33. Busch MT, DeHaven KE. Pitfalls of the lateral retinacular release. *Clin Sports Med* 1989;18:279–290.

34. Butler DL, Noyes FR, Grood ES. Ligamentous restraints to anterior-posterior drawer in the human knee. A biomechanical study. *J Bone Joint Surg* 1980;62A:259–270.

35. Carraffa A, Gerulli G, Proietti M. Preview of ACL injuries: a control study or proprioceptive training. Knee surgery traumatology. *Arthroscopy* 1996;4:19–21.

36. Carson WG, James SL, Larson RL, Singer KM, Winternitz WW. Patellofemoral disorders: physical and radiographic evaluation. Part I: physical examination. *Clin Orthop Related Res* 1984;185:165–177.

36a. Carson WG, James SL, Larson RL, Singer KM, Winternitz WW. Patellofemoral disorders: physical and radiographic evaluation. Part II: radiographic examination. *Clin Ortho Related Res* 1984;185:178–186.

37. Casscells SW. The torn meniscus, the torn anterior cruciate ligament, and their relationship to degenerative joint disease. *Arthroscopy* 1985;1(1):28–32.

38. Cerabona F, Sherman MF, Bonamo JR, Sklar J. Patterns of meniscal injury with acute anterior cruciate ligament tears. *Am J Sports Med* 1988;16(6):603–609.

39. Chrisman OD, Snook GA, Wilson TC. A long-term prospective study of the Hauser and Roux-Goldthwaite procedures for recurrent patellar dislocation. *Clin Orthop* 1979;144:27.

40. Clancy WG, Shelbourne KD, Zoellner GB, et al. Treatment of knee joint instability secondary to rupture of the posterior cruciate ligament: report of a new procedure. *J Bone Joint Surg* 1983;65A:310–322.

41. Collins HR. Epiphyseal injuries in athletes. *Cleve Clin Q* 1975;42:285.

42. Collins RK. Injury patterns in women's flag football. *Am J Sports Med* 1984;15(3):238–242.

43. Colosimo AJ, Ireland ML, Horn T, Stine R, Shapiro R. Isokinetic peak torque and knee joint laxity comparison in female basketball and volleyball college athletes. (Abstract) *Med Sci Sports Exer* 1991;23(4):S135.

44. Cone RO. Imaging sports-related injuries of the knee. In: DeLee JC, Drez D, eds. *Orthopaedic sports medicine: principles and practice*, vol. 2. Philadelphia: WB Saunders, 1994:1549–1601.

45. Cooper DE, Warren RF, Warner JJP. The posterior cruciate ligament and posterolateral structures of the knee: Anatomy, function, and patterns of injury. In: Tullos HS, ed. *Instructional course lectures*, vol. XL. Rosemont, IL: AAOS, 1991:249–270.

46. Cox JS. An evaluation of the Elmslie-Trillat procedure for management of the patellar dislocations and subluxations. *Am J Sports Med* 1976;4:72.

47. Cox JS, Lenz HW. Women midshipmen in sports. *Am J Sports Med* 1984;12:241–243.

48. Cox JS, Blanda JB. Peripatellar pathologies. In: Delee JC, Drez D, eds. *Orthopaedic sports medicine: principles and practice*. Philadelphia: WB Saunders, 1994:1249–1260.

49. Crenshaw AH. *Campbell's operative orthopaedics*. St. Louis: Mosby-Year Book, 1992.

50. Curwin S, Stannish WD. *Tendinitis: its etiology and treatment*. Lexington, MA: DC Health, 1984.

51. Dainer RD, Barrack RL, Buckley SL, Alexander AH. Arthroscopic treatment of acute patellar dislocations. *Arthroscopy* 1988;4:267.

52. Daniel DM, Fritschy D. Anterior cruciate ligament injuries. In: DeLee JC, Drez D, eds. *Orthopaedic sports medicine: principles and practice*, vol. 2. Philadelphia: WB Saunders, 1994:1313–1361.

53. Daniel DM, Stone ML, Dobson BE, et al. Fate of the ACL-injured patient: a prospective outcome study. *Am J Sports Med* 1994;22(5):632–644.

54. De Carlo M, Klootwyk TE, Shelbourne KD. ACL surgery and accelerated rehabilitation: revisited. *J Sport Rehab* 1997;6(2):144–156.

55. DeHaven KE, Lintner DM. Athletic injuries: comparison by age sport, and gender. *Am J Sports Med* 1986;14(3):218–224.

56. DeLee JC, Farney WC. Incidence of injury in Texas high school football. *Am J Sports Med* 1992;20(5):575–580.

57. DeLee JC, Drez D, eds. *Orthopaedic sports medicine: principles and practice*, vol. 2. Philadelphia: WB Saunders, 1994.

57a. DeLee JC, Bergfeld JA, Drez D, Parker AW. The posterior cruciate ligament. In: DeLee JC, Drez D, eds. *Orthopaedic sports medicine: principles and practice*, vol. 2. Philadelphia: WB Saunders, 1994:1374–1400.

58. Dowd GSE, Bentley G. Radiographic assessment in patellar instability and chondromalacia patellae. *J Bone Joint Surg* 1986;68(2):297–300.

59. Drez D Jr. Symposium on knee braces. Am Acad Orthop Surg Annual Meeting, Las Vegas, January 1985.

60. Dye SF, Chew MH. The use of scintigraphy to detect increased osseous metabolic activity about the knee. *J Bone Joint Surg* 1993;(A) 75:1388.

61. Dye SF. The knee as a biologic transmission with an envelope of function: a theory. *Clin Orthop* 1996;Apr (325):10–18.

62. Echeverria TS, Bersani FA. Acute fracture simulating a symptomatic bipartite patella. *Am J Sports Med* 1980;8:48–50.

63. Fairbanks TJ. Knee joint changes after meniscectomy. *J Bone Joint Surg* 1948;30B:664–670.

64. Feagin JA. *The crucial ligaments*, 2nd ed. New York: Churchill Livingstone, 1994.

65. Feretti A, Ippolito E, Mariani P, Puddu G. Jumper's knee. *Am J Sports Med* 1983;11:58–62.

66. Flandry F, Hughston JC. Complications of extensor mechanism surgery for patellar malalignment. *Am J Orthop* 1995;24(7):534–543.

67. Flandry F. A classification of knee ligament instability. In: Baker CL, ed. *The Hughston Clinic sports medicine book*. Baltimore: Williams & Wilkins, 1995:481–493.

68. Fox JM, Del Pizzo W. *The patellofemoral joint*. New York: McGraw-Hill, 1993.

69. Fu FH, Stone DA, eds. *Sports injuries: mechanism, prevention, and treatment*, 2nd ed. Baltimore: Williams & Wilkins, 1994.

70. Fu FH, Baratz M. Meniscal injuries. In: DeLee JC, Drez D, eds.

Orthopaedic sports medicine: principles and practice, vol. 2. Philadelphia: WB Saunders, 1994:1146–1162.

71. Fulkerson JP. Anteromedialization of the tibial tuberosity for patellofemoral malalignment. *Clin Ortho* 1983;177:176–181.

72. Fulkerson JP, Tennant R, Jaivin JS, Grunnet M. Histologic evidence of retinacular nerve injury associated with patellofemoral malalignment. *Clin Orthop* 1985:187:196.

73. Fulkerson JP. Anteromedial tibial tubercle transfer without bone graft. *Am J Sports Med* 1990;18:490–497.

74. Fulkerson JP, Shea K. Current concepts: disorders of patellar alignment. *J Bone Joint Surg* 1990;72A:1424–1429.

75. Fulkerson JP, Kalenak A, Rosenberg T, Cox JS. Patellofemoral pain. In: *Instructional course lectures*, vol. XLI. Rosemont, IL: AAOS, 1992:57–71.

76. Fulkerson JP, Buuck DA. Patellofemoral disorders: biomechanics, diagnosis, nonoperative treatment, and arthroscopy. In: McGinty JB, ed. *Operative arthroscopy.* Lippincott-Raven, 2nd ed. 1996: 343–360.

77. Fulkerson JP. *Disorders of the patellofemoral joint*, 3rd ed. Philadelphia: Williams & Wilkins, 1997.

78. Galway R. Pivot-shift syndrome. *J Bone Joint Surg* 1972;54B: 558.

79. Garrick JG, Requa RK. Prophylactic knee bracing. *Am J Sports Med* 1987;15(5):471–476.

80. Gelb HJ, Glasgow SG, Sapega AA, Torg RS. Magnetic resonance imaging of knee disorders: clinical value and cost-effectiveness in a sports medicine practice. *Am J Sports Med* 1996;24(1):99–103.

81. Girgis FG, Marshall JL, Monajem ARS. The cruciate ligaments of the knee joint: anatomical, functional, and experimental analysis. *Clin Ortho Rel Res* 1975;Jan-Feb(105):216–231.

82. Gomez E, DeLee JC, Farney WC. Incidence of injury in Texas girls' high school basketball. *Am J Sports Med* 1996;24(5):684–687.

83. Gray J, Taunton JE, McKenzie DC, Clement DB, McConkey JP, Davidson RG. A survey of injuries to the anterior cruciate ligament of the knee in female basketball players. *Int J Sports Med* 1985; 6:314–316.

84. Green S, Clayton ML, Liedholt JD, et al. One-hundred point scale for assessment of knee disability, 1969. In: Smillie I, ed. *Diseases of the knee joint.* Edinburgh: Churchill Livingstone, 1974:28.

85. Green, WT Jr. Painful bipartite patella: a report of three cases. *Clin Orthop Related Res* 1975;110:177–200.

86. Greenleaf JE. The anatomy and biomechanics of the lateral aspect of the knee. *Operative Tech Sports Med* 1996;4(3):141–147.

87. Griffis ND, Vequist SW, Yearout KM, et al. Injury prevention of the anterior cruciate ligament. [Abstract] In: American Orthopaedic Society for Sports Medicine: meeting abstracts, symposia, and instructional courses, 15th annual meeting. June 19–22, 1989.

88. Grood SS, Noyes FR, Butler DL, Suntay WJ. Ligamentous and capsular retraints preventing straight medial and lateral laxity in intact human cadaver knees. *J Bone Joint Surg* 1981;63-A:1257–1269.

89. Grood ES, Noyes FR. Diagnosis of knee ligament injuries: biomechanical precepts. In: Feagin EJ, ed. *The crucial ligaments.* New York: Churchill Livingstone, 1988:245–260.

90. Harner CD, Xerogeanes JW, Livesay GA, et al. The human posterior cruciate ligament complex: an interdisciplinary study. *Am J Sports Med* 1995;23(6):736–745.

91. Harrer MF, Berson L, Hosea TM, Leddy TP. Lower extremity injuries: females vs. males in the sport of basketball. [Abstract] The AOSSM 22nd Annual Meeting, Lake Buena Vista, FL, June 16–20, 1996.

92. Hefti F, Muller W. Current state of evaluation of knee ligament lesions. The new IKDC knee evaluation form. *Orthopade* 1993; 22:351–362.

93. Hewson GF Jr, Mendini RA, Wang JB. Prophylactic knee bracing in college football. *Am J Sports Med* 1986;14(4):262–266.

94. Hollinshead WH. *Anatomy for surgeons, vol. 3: the back and limbs.* New York: Harper & Row, 1969.

95. Hoppenfeld S. *Physical exam of the spine and extremities.* Norwalk, CT: Appleton-Century-Crofts, 1976:171–196.

96. Hoppenfeld S, DeBoer P. *Surgical exposures in orthopaedics: the anatomic approach.* Philadelphia: JB Lippincott, 1984.

97. Huberti HH, Hayes WC, Stone WL, Shibut GT. Force ratios in quadriceps tendon and ligamentum patella. *J Orthop Res* 1984; 2(1):49–54.

98. Hughston JC, Eilers AF. The role of the POL in repairs of acute MCL tears of the knee. *J Bone Joint Surg* 1973;55A:923–940.

99. Hughston JC, Andrews JR, Cross MJ, Moschi A. Classification of knee ligament instabilities. Part I. The medial compartment and cruciate ligaments. *J Bone Joint Surg* 1976;58A:159–172, 173–179.

100. Hughston JC, Norwood LA. The posterolateral drawer test and external rotational recurvatum test for posterolateral rotatory instability of the knee. *Clin Ortho* 1980;147:82–87.

101. Hughston JC, Barrett GR. Acute anteromedial rotatory instability: long-term results of surgical repair. *J Bone Joint Surg* 1983;65-A(2):145–153.

102. Hughston JC, Walsh WM, Puddu G. *Patellar subluxation and dislocation.* Philadelphia: WB Saunders, 1984.

103. Hughston JC, Deese M. Medial subluxation of the patella as a complication of lateral retinacular release. *Am J Sports Med* 1988; 16(4):383–388.

104. Hughston JC. *Knee ligaments: injury and repair.* St. Louis: Mosby-Year Book, 1993.

105. Hungerford DS, Barry M. Biomechanics of the patellofemoral joint. *Clin Orthop* 1979;144:9.

106. Hunter W. On the structure and diseases of articulating cartilage. *Philos Trans R Soc Lond [Biol]* 1743;9:267.

107. Hunter LY, Andrews JR, Clancy WG, Funk JF Jr. Common orthopaedic problems in female athletes. In: *Instructional course lectures.* Rosemont, IL: AAOS 1982;31:126–151.

108. Huston LJ, Wojtys EM. Neuromuscular performance characteristics in elite female athletes. *Am J Sports Med* 1996;24:427–436.

109. Hutchinson MR, Ireland ML. Knee injuries in female athletes. *Sports Med* 1995;19(4):288–302.

110. Hutchinson MR, Ireland ML. Patella dislocation: Recognizing the injury and its complications. *Phys Sportsmed* 1995;23(10):53–60.

111. Hutchinson MR, Ireland ML. Special considerations: women. In: Hunter-Griffin LY, ed. *Rehabilitation of the injured knee.* Mosby-Year Book, 1995, 297–312.

112. Indelicato PA. Non-operative treatment of complete tears of the medial collateral ligament of the knee. *J Bone Joint Surg* 1983; 65A(3):323–329.

113. Insall JN, Aglietti P, Tria AJ. Patellar pain and incongruence. II. Clinical application. *Clin Orthop* 1983;176:225–232.

114. Insall JN. Anatomy of the knee. In: Insall JN, ed. *Surgery of the knee.* New York: Churchill Livingstone, 1984:1–20.

115. Insall JN. Disorders of the patella. In: Insall JN, ed. *Surgery of the knee.* New York: Churchill Livingston, 1984:191–260.

116. Ireland ML, Wall C. Epidemiology and comparison of knee injuries in elite male and female United States basketball athletes. *Med Sci Sports Exerc* [Abstract] 1990;14:S82.

117. Ireland ML. Special concerns of the female athlete. In: Fu FH, Stone DA, eds. *Sports injuries: mechanism, prevention, and treatment*, 2nd ed. Baltimore: Williams & Wilkins, 1994:153–187.

118. Ireland ML, Chang JL. Acute fracture bipartite patella: case report and literature review. *Med Science Sports Exerc* 1995;27(3):299–302.

119. Ireland ML. Anterior cruciate ligament injuries in young female athletes. *Your patient and fitness* 1996;10(5):26–30.

120. Ireland ML, Gaudette M, Crook S. ACL injuries in the female athlete. *J Sport Rehab* 1997;6:97–110.

121. Ireland ML, Williams RI. Degenerative arthritis of the knee. In: Andrews JR, Timmerman LA, eds. *Diagnostic and operative arthroscopy.* Philadelphia: WB Saunders, 1997:325–345.

122. Irrgang JJ, Harner CD. Recent advances in ACL rehabilitation: clinical factors that influence the program. *J Sport Rehab* 1997; 6(2):111–124.

123. Jackson DW. *The anterior cruciate ligament: current and future concepts.* New York: Raven Press, 1993.

124. Jackson RW. The painful knee: Arthroscopy or MR imaging? *J Am Acad Orthop Surg* 1996;4(2):93–99.

125. Jakob RP, Warner JP. Lateral and posterolateral rotatory instability of the knee. In: DeLee JC, Drez D, eds. *Orthopaedic sports medicine: principles and practice*, vol. 2. Philadelphia: WB Saunders, 1994:1275–1312.

126. Johnson LL. *Operative arthroscopy: principles and practice*. St. Louis: Mosby, 1986.

127. Jaureguito JW, Elliott JS, Lietner T, Dixon LB, Reider B. The effects of arthroscopic partial lateral meniscectomy in an otherwise normal knee: a retrospective reveiw of functional, clinical, and radiographic results. *Arthroscopy* 1995;11(1):29–36.

128. Kannus P. Long term results of conservative treated medial collateral ligament injury of the knee joint. *Clin Orthop* 1988;226:103–112.

129. Karzel, RP, Friedman MJ, Ferkel RD. Prosthetic ligament reconstruction of the knee. In: DeLee JC, Drez D, eds. *Orthopaedic sports medicine: principles and practice*, vol. 2. Philadelphia: WB Saunders, 1994, 1502–1527.

130. Kelly DW, Carter VS, Jobe FW, Kerlan RK. Patellar and quadriceps tendon ruptures: jumper's knee. *Am J Sports Med* 1984;12:375–380.

131. Kennedy JC, Fowler PJ. Medial and anterior instability of the knee: an anatomical and clinical study using stress machines. *J Bone Joint Surg* 1971;53A:1257–1270.

132. Kettelkamp D, Thompson C. Development of a knee scoring scale. *Clin Orthop* 1975;107:93–99.

133. Kolowich P, Paulos L, Rosenberg T, et al. Lateral release of the patella: indications and contraindications. *Am J Sports Med* 1990;18:(4):359–365.

134. Kulund DN. *The injured athlete*. Philadelphia: JB Lippincott, 1982.

135. Kusayama T, Harner CD, Carlin GJ, Xerogeanes JW, Smith BA. Anatomical and biomechanical characteristics of human meniscofemoral ligaments. *Knee Surg Sports Traumatol Arthrosc* 1994;2(4):234–237.

136. LaPrade RF, Burnett QM. Femoral intercondylar notch stenosis and correlation to anterior cruciate ligament injuries: a prospective study. *Am J Sports Med* 1994;22(2):198–203.

137. LaPrade RF, Burnett QM II, Veenstra MA, Hodgman CG. The prevalence of abnormal magnetic resonance imaging findings in asymptomatic knees: with correlation of magnetic resonance imaging to arthroscopic findings in symptomatic knees . . . including commentary by Curl WW. *Am J Sports Med* 1994;22(6):739–745.

138. Larson R. Rating sheet for knee function, 1972. In: Smillie I, ed. *Diseases of the knee joint*. Edinburgh: Churchill Livingstone, 1974:29,30.

139. Larson RL, McMahon RO. The epiphyses in the childhood athlete. *JAMA* 1966;196:607.

140. Larson RL. Epiphyseal injuries in the adolescent athlete. *Orthop Clin North Am* 1973;4:439.

141. Larson RV, Friedman MJ. Anterior cruciate ligament: injuries and treatment. In: Pritchard DJ, ed. *Instructional course lectures*, vol. 45. Rosemont, IL: AAOS, 1996;235–243.

142. Laurin CA, Dussault R, Levesque HP. The tangential x-ray investigation of the patellofemoral joint: x-ray technique, diagnostic criteria and their interpretation. *Clin Orthop* 1979;144:16–26

143. Lephart SM, Perrin DH, Fu FH, et al. Relationship between physical characteristics and functional capacity in the anterior cruciate ligament insufficient athlete. *JOSPT* 1992;16(4):174–181.

144. Levy IM, Torzilli PA, Warren RF. The effect of medial meniscectomy on anterior-posterior motion of the knee. *J Bone Joint Surg* 1982;64A:883–888.

145. Levy AS, Lohnes J, Sculley S, LeCroy M, Garrett W. Chondral delamination of the knee in soccer players. *Am J Sports Med* 1996;24(5):634–639.

146. Lieb FJ, Perry J. Quadriceps function: Anatomical and mechanical study using amputated limbs. *J Bone Joint Surg* 1968;50A:1535–1548.

147. Lieb FJ, Perry. Quadriceps function: an EMGic study under isometric conditions. *J Bone Joint Surg* 1971;53:749–758.

148. Linton RC, Indelicato PA. Medial ligament injuries. In: DeLee JC, Drez D, eds. *Orthopaedic sports medicine: principles and practice*, vol. 2. Philadelphia: WB Saunders, 1994:1261–1274.

149. Liu SH, Raad A-S, Lane J, Barber-Westin SD, Noyes FR. The estrogen-collagen interaction in the ACL: a potential explanation for female athletic injury. Presented AOSSM 22nd Annual Meeting, June 16–20, 1996, Lake Buena Vista, Florida.

150. Liu SH, Yu W, Hatch J, Panossian V, Finerman GAM. Estrogen affects the cellular metabolism of the female human anterior cruciate ligament: a potential explanation for female athletic injury. Book of abstracts & outlines, American Orthopaedic Society for Sports Medicine, 23rd Annual Meeting, Sun Valley, Idaho, June 22–25, 1997:805.

151. Lobenhoffer P, Tscherne H. Fractures of the patella. In Fu FH, Harner CD, Vince KG, eds. *Knee surgery*. Baltimore: Williams & Wilkins, 1994:1051–1057.

152. Losee RE, Johnson TR, Southwick WO. Anterior subluxation of the lateral tibial plateau. A diagnostic test and operative repair. *J Bone Joint Surg* 1978;60A:1015.

153. Lysholm J, Gillquist J. Evaluation of knee ligament surgery results with special emphasis on use of a scoring scale. *Am J Sports Med* 1982;10:150–154.

154. Lysholm J, Tegner Y, Gillquist J. Functional importance of different clinical findings in the unstable knee. *Acta Orthop Scan* 1984;55:471.

155. Malghem J, Maldague B. Depth insufficiency of the proximal trochlear groove on lateral radiographs of the knee: relation to patellar dislocation. *Radiology* 1989;170(2):507–510.

156. Malone TR, Hardaker WT, Garrett WE, et al. Relationship of gender to anterior cruciate ligament injuries in intercollegiate basketball participants. *J Sou Orth Ass* 1993;2(1):36–39.

157. Mangine RE, Kremchek. Evaluation-based protocol of the anterior cruciate ligament. *J Sport Rehab* 1997;6(2):157–181.

158. Maquet PGJ. Advancement of the tibial tuberosity. *Clin Orthop* 1976;115:225.

159. Mariani PP, Caruso I. An electromyographic investigation of subluxation of the patella. *J Bone Joint Surg* 1979;61B:169–171.

160. Marshall JL, Johnson RJ. Mechanisms of the most common ski injuries. *Phys Sportsmed* 1977;5(12):49–54.

161. Martinez S, Korobkin M, Fondren FB, Hedlund LW, and Goldner JL. Computed tomography of the normal patellofemoral joint. *Invest Radiol* 1983;18(3):249–253.

162. Matelic TM, Aronsson DD, Boyd DW Jr., LaMont RL. Acute hemarthrosis of the knee in children. *Am J Sports Med* 1995;23(6):668–671.

163. McCarroll JR, Shelbourne KD, Patel DV. Anterior cruciate ligament injuries in young athletes: Recommendations for treatment and rehabilitation. *Sports Med* 1995;20(2):117–127.

164. McCauley TR. Kier R, Lynch KJ, Jokl P. Chondromalacia patellae: diagnosis with MR imaging. *AJR* 1992;158(1):101–105.

165. McConnell J. The management of chondromalacia patella: a long term solution. *Aust J Physiother* 1986;2:215–223.

166. McGinty JB. *Operative arthroscopy*. Philadelphia: Lippincott-Raven, 1996.

167. McMaster PE. Tendon and muscle ruptures. Clinical and experimental studies on the causes of subcutaneous ruptures. *J Bone Joint Surg* 1933;15A:705–722.

168. McMurray TP. The semilunar cartilages. *Br J Surg* 1942;29:407–414.

169. Merchant AC, Mercer RL, Jacobsen RH, Cool CR. Roentgenographic analysis of patellofemoral congruence. *J Bone Joint Surg* 1974;56A:1391.

170. Merchant AC. Clinical classification of patellofemoral disorders. *Sports Med Arthroscopy Rev* 1994;2(3).

171. Millet CW, Drez DJ Jr. Principles of bracing for the anterior cruciate ligament-deficient knee. *Clin Sports Med* 1988;7(4):827–833.

172. Millet CW. Knee braces. In: DeLee JC, Drez D, eds. *Orthopaedic sports medicine: principles and practice*, vol. 2. Philadelphia: WB Saunders, 1994:1468–1474.

173. Miller GK. A prospective study comparing the accuracy of the clinical diagnosis of meniscus tear with magnetic resonance imaging and its effect on clinical outcome. *Arthroscopy* 1996;12(4):406–413.

174. Morgan CD, Kalman VR, Grawl DM. The anatomic origin of the posterior cruciate ligament: where is it? Reference landmarks for PCL reconstruction. *Arthroscopy* 1997;13(3):325–331.

175. Muller W. *The knee: form, function, and ligament reconstruction*. New York: Springer-Verlag, 1983.

176. National Collegiate Athletic Association. NCAA injury surveillance system. Overland Park, KS: NCAA, 1990–1996.

177. Neer CS II, Horwitz BS. Fractures of the epiphyseal plate. *Clin Orthop* 1965;41:24.

178. Nicholas JA. *The lower extremity and spine in sports medicine*, vol. 1, St. Louis: Mosby, 1986.

179. Noyes FR, Grood ES, Butler DS, et al. Clincal laxity tests and functional stability of the knee: biomechanical concepts. *Clin Orthop* 1980;146:84.

180. Noyes FR, Matthews DS, Mooar PA, et al. The symptomatic anterior cruciate deficient knee. Part II: The results of rehabilitation, activity modification and counseling on functional disability. *J Bone Joint Surg* 1983;65A:163–174.

181. Noyes FR, Grood ES. Diagnosis of knee ligament injuries: clinical concepts. In: Feagin EJ, ed. *The crucial ligaments*. New York: Churchill Livingstone, 1988:261–285.

182. Noyes FR, Barber SD, Mooar LA. A rationale for assessing sports activity levels and limitations in knee disorders. *Clin Orthop* 1989;246:238–249.

183. Noyes FR, Grood ES, Torzilli PA. Current concepts review: the definitions of terms for motion and position of the knee and injuries of the ligaments. *J Bone Joint Surg* 1989;71-A:(3)465–472.

184. Noyes FR. *The Noyes knee rating system*. Cincinnati: Cincinnati Sportsmedicine Research and Education Foundation, 1990.

185. Noyes FR. Stabler CL. A system for grading articular cartilage lesions at arthroscopy. *Am J Sports Med* 17(4):1989;505–513.

186. Noyes FR, Barber SD, Mangine RE. Abnormal lower limb symmetry determined by function hop tests after anterior cruciate ligament rupture. *Am J Sports Med* 1991;12:513–518.

187. Noyes RF, Simon R. The role of high tibial osteotomy in the anterior cruciate ligament-deficient knee with varus alignment. In: DeLee JC, Drez D, eds. *Orthopaedic sports medicine: principles and practice*, vol. 2. Philadelphia: WB Saunders, 1994:1401–1443.

188. Noyes FR, Barber-Westin SD. Reconstruction of the anterior cruciate ligament with human allograft: comparison of early and lateral results. *J Bone Joint Surg* 1996;78A(4):524–537.

189. Nyland JA, Shapiro R, Stine RL, Horn TS, Ireland ML. Relationship of fatigued run and rapid stop to ground reaction forces, lower extremity kinematics, and muscle activation. *JOSPT* 1994;20(3):132–137.

190. O'Brien SJ, Warren RF, Pavlov H, Panariello R, Wickiewicz TL. Reconstruction of the chronically insufficient anterior cruciate liagment with the central third of the patellar ligament. *J Bone Joint Surg* 1991;73-A(2):278–286.

191. O'Conner JJ, Shercliff T, Fitzpatrick D, et al. Geometry of the knee. In: Daniel DM, Akeson WH, O'Conner JJ, eds. *Knee ligaments: structure, function, injury and repair*. New York: Raven Press, 1990:163–199

192. O'Donoghue DH. Reconstruction for medial instability of the knee, techniques and results in 60 cases. *J Bone Joint Surg* 1973;55A:941–955.

193. O'Donoghue DH. Treatment of injuries to the knee. In: O'Donoghue DH, ed. *Treatment of injuries to athletes*, 4th ed. Philadelphia: WB Saunders, 1987:470–471.

194. Ogden JA. *Skeletal injury in the child*, 2nd ed. Philadelphia: WB Saunders, 1990:808.

195. Outerbridge RE. The etiology of chondromalacia patellae. *J Bone Joint Surg* 1961;43B(4):752–757.

196. Palumbo PM. Dynamic Patella brace: a new orthosis in the management of patellofemoral disorders: a preliminary report. *Am J Sports Med* 1081;9:1.

197. Parker RD, Calabrese GJ. Anterior knee pain. In: Fu FH, Harner CD, Vince KG, eds. *Knee surgery*. Baltimore: Williams & Wilkins, 1994:929–951.

198. Peterson CA, Peterson HA. Analysis of the incidence of injuries to the epiphyseal growth plate. *J Trauma* 1972;12:275.

199. Phillips B. Anterior cruciate ligament injuries. In: Andrews JR, Timmerman LA, eds. *Diagnostic and operative arthroscopy*. Philadelphia: WB Saunders, 1997, 355–390.

200. Pick TP, Howden R, eds. *Gray's anatomy*. Philadelphia: Running Press, 1974.

201. Post W, Fulkerson J. Distal realignment of the patellofemoral joint. *Orthop Clin of NA* October, 1992;23(4).

202. Post W. Surgical decison making in patellofemoral pain and instability. *Operative Tech Sports Med* 1994;2(4):273–284.

203. Post WR, Fulkerson J. Knee pain diagrams: correlation with physical examination findings in patients with anterior knee pain. *Arthroscopy* 1994;10(6):618–623.

204. Rask BP, Micheli LJ. Knee ligament injuries and associated derangements in children and adolescents. In: Fu FH, Harner CD, Vince KG, eds. *Knee surgery*. Baltimore: Williams & Wilkins: 1994;365–381.

205. Reider B, D'Agata SD. Factors predisposing to knee injury. In: DeLee JC, Drez D, eds. *Orthopaedic sports medicine: principles and practice*, vol. 2. Philadelphia: WB Saunders, 1994:1134–1145.

206. Risberg MA, Ekeland A. Assessment of functional tests after anterior cruciate ligament surgery. *JOSPT* 1994;19(4):212–217.

207. Reynolds L, Levin TA, Medeiros JM, Adler NS, Hallum A. EMG activity of the vastus medialis oblique and vastus lateralis muscles in their role of patellar alignment. *Am J Phys Med* 1983;62:61–70.

208. Rielly DJ, Martens M. Experimental analysis of the quadriceps force and patellofemoral joint reaction force for various activities. *Acta Orthop Scand* 1972;43:126–137.

209. Roberts TS, Terry GC. Complications of knee surgery. In: DeLee JC, Drez D, eds. *Orthopaedic sports medicine: principles and practice*, vol. 2. Philadelphia: WB Saunders, 1994, 1528–1548.

210. Rockwood CA Jr, Green DP, eds. *Fractures in adults*, vol. 2. Philadelphia: JB Lippincott, 1984.

211. Rose NE, Gold SM. A comparison of accuracy between clinical examination and magnetic resonance imaging in the diagnosis of meniscal and anterior cruciate ligament tears. *Arthroscopy* 1996;12(4):398–405.

212. Roux C. Recurrent dislocations of the patella: operative treatment. *Clin Orthop* 1979;144:4–8.

213. Rovere GD, Adar DM. Medial patellar shelf plica syndrome. Treatment by intraplical steroid injection. *Am J Sports Med* 1985;13:382–386.

214. Rovere GD, Haupt HA, Yates CS. Prophylactic knee bracing in college football. *Am J Sports Med* 1987;15(2):111–116.

215. Ryan JB. Prophylactic knee braces: the West Point experience. Book of abstracts and outlines, AOSSM 23rd Annual Meeting, Sun Valley, Idaho, June 22–25, 1997:696–697.

216. Ryder SH, Johnson RJ, Beynnon BD, Ettlinger CF. Prevention of ACL injuries. *J Sport Rehab* 1997;6(2):80–96.

217. Satterwhite YE. The anatomy and biomechanics of the medial structures of the knee. *Op Tech Sports Med* 1996;4(3):134–140.

218. Saltzman CL. Results of treatment of displaced patellar fractures by partial patellectomy. *J Bone Joint Surg* 1990;72A: 1279–1285.

219. Saupe H. Primare Knochemark Seilerung der Kniescheibe. *Deutsche Z Chir* 1943;258:386.

220. Schmitz MA, Rouse LM Jr, DeHaven KE. The management of meniscal tears in the ACL-deficient knee. *Clin Sports Med* 1996;15(3):573–593.

221. Scott WN. *The knee*. St. Louis: Mosby, 1994.

222. Sebastianelli WJ, DeHaven KE. Chondral fractures and intra-articular osteochondroses. In: DeLee JC, Drez D, eds. *Orthopaedic sports medicine: principles and practice*, vol. 2. Philadelphia: WB Saunders, 1994:1444–1467.

223. Seebacher JR, Inglis AE, Marshall JL, Warren RF. The structure of the posterolateral aspect of the knee. *J Bone Joint Surg* 1982;64A(4):536–541.

224. Silbey MB, Fu FH. Knee injuries. In: Fu FH, Stone DA, eds. *Sports injuries: mechanisms, prevention, treatment*. Baltimore: Williams & Wilkins, 1994:249–276.

225. Sgaglione NA, Del Pizzo W, Fox JM, Friedman MJ. Critical analysis of knee ligament rating systems. *Am J Sports Med* 1995;23(6):660–667.

226. Shapiro ET, Richmond JC, Rockett SE, McGrath MM, Donaldson WR. The use of a generic, patient-based health assessment (SF-36) for evaluation of patients with anterior cruciate ligament injuries. *Am J Sports Med* 1996;24(2):196–200.

227. Shelbourne KD, Patel DV, McCarroll Jr. Management of anterior cruciate ligament injuries in skeletally immature adolescents. *Knee Surg Sports Traumatol Arthrosc* 1996;4(2):68–74.

228. Shelbourne KD, Davis TJ, Klootwyk TE. The relationship between intercondylar notch width of the femur and the incidence of ante-

rior cruciate ligament tears. *Am J Sports Med* 1998;26(3):402–408.

229. Shoemaker SC, Markolf KL. The role of the meniscus in the A-P stability of the loaded anterior cruciate-deficient knee. *J Bone Joint Surg* 1986;68A:71–79.

230. Shrive NG, O'Connor JJ, Goodfellow JW. Load bearing in the knee joint. *Clin Orthop* 1978;131:279–281.

231. Sisk DT. Knee realignment and replacement in the recreational athlete. In: DeLee JC, Drez D, eds. *Orthopaedic sports medicine: principles and practice*, vol. 2. Philadelphia: WB Saunders, 1994:1475–1501.

232. Slocum DB, James SL, Larson RL, et al. Clinical test for anterolateral rotary instability of the knee. *Clin Orthop* 1976;118:63.

233. Slocum DB, Larson RL: Rotatory instability of the knee. *J Bone Joint Sur* 1968;50A:211–225.

234. Smillie IS. *Injuries of the knee joint*. 3rd ed. Baltimore: Williams & Wilkins, 1962.

235. Smith PA. Physical examination of the knee. In: *The Hughston Clinic sports medicine book*. Baltimore: Williams & Wilkins, 1995:416–425.

236. Souryal TO, Moore HA, Evans JP. Bilaterality in anterior cruciate ligament injuries: Associated intercondylar notch stenosis. *Am J Sports Med* 1980;8(3):449–454.

237. Souryal TO, Freeman TR. Intercondylar notch size and anterior cruciate ligament injuries in athletes: a prospective study. *Am J Sports Med* 1993;21(4):535–539.

238. Summer HM. Patellar chondropathy and apicitis, and muscle imbalances of the lower extremity in competitive sports. *Sports Med* 1988;5:386–394.

239. Tapper EM, Hoover NW. Late results after meniscectomy. *J Bone Joint Surg* 1969;51A:517–526.

240. Teitz CC, Hermanson EK, Kronmal RA, Diehr PH. Evaluation of the use of braces to prevent injury to the knee in collegiate football players. *J Bone Joint Surg* 1987;69(1):2–9.

241. Tegner Y, Lysholm J. Rating systems in the evaluation of knee ligament injuries. *Clin Orthop* 1985;198:43–49.

242. Terry GC, LaPrade RF. The biceps femoris muscle complex at the knee. Its anatomy and injury patterns associated with acute anterolateral rotatory instability. *Am J Sport Med* 1996;24(1):2–8.

243. Terry GC, LaPrade RF. The posterolateral aspect of the knee. Anatomy and surgical approach. *Am J Sport Med* 1996;24(6):732–739.

244. Vainionpaa S, Laasonen E, Silvennoinen T. Acute dislocation of the patella: a prospective review of operative treatment. *Acta Orthopaedica Scand* 1986;57:331–333.

245. Vangness CT Jr, Triffon MJ, Joyce MJ, Moore TM. Soft tissue for allograft reconstruction of the human knee: a survey of the American Association of Tissue Banks. *Am J Sports Med* 1996;24(5):705.

246. Vaupel G, Dye S. Functional knee anatomy. In: Baker CL, ed. *The Hughston Clinic sports medicine book*. Baltimore: Williams & Wilkins, 1995:403–405.

247. Veltri DM, Warren RF. Anatomy, biomechanics, and physical findings in posterolateral knee instability. *Clin Sports Med* 1994;13(3):599–614.

248. Walker P, Erkman M. The role of the menisci in force transmission across the knee. *Clin Orthop* 1975;109:184.

249. Walsh WM. Patellofemoral joint. In Delee JC, Drez D, eds. *Orthopaedic sports medicine: principles and practice*. Philadelphia: WB Saunders, 1994:1163–1248.

250. Ware JE Jr, Kosinski M, Keller SD. *SF-12: How to score the SF-12 physical and mental health summary scales*, 2nd ed. Boston: The Health Institute, New England Medical Center, 1995.

251. Warren LF, Marshall JL. The supporting structures and layers on the medial side of the knee: an anatomical analysis. *J Bone Joint Surg* 1979;61A:56–62

252. Whiteside PA. Men's and women's injuries in comparable sports. *Phys Sportsmed* 1980;8(3):130–140.

253. Wiberg G. Roentgenographic and anatomic studies of the femoro-patellar joint: with special reference to chondromalacia. *Acta Orthop Scand* 1941;12:319–410.

254. Wilk KE, Andrew JR. Current concepts in the treatment of atnerior cruciate ligament disuption. *JOSPT* 1992;15(6):279–293.

255. Wilk KE, Romaniello WT, Socia SM, Angio CA, Andrews JR. The relationship between subjective knee scores, isokinetic testing, and functional testing in the ACL-reconstructed knee. *JOSPT* 1994;20(2):60–73.

256. Wilk KE, Zheng N, Fleisig GS, Andrews JR, Clancy WG. Kinetic chain exercise: Implications for the anterior cruciate ligament patient. *J Sport Rehab* 1997;6(2):125–143.

257. Wiss DA, Schilz JL, Zionts L. Type III fractures of the tibial tubercle in adolescents. *J Orthop Trauma* 1991;7(3):591.

258. Wise HH, Fiebert IM, Kates JL. EMG biofeedback as treatment for patellofemoral pain syndrome. *J Orthop Sports Phys Ther* 1984;6:95–103.

259. Wojtys EM, Loubert PV, Samson SY, Viviano DM. Use of a knee brace for control of tibial translation and rotation. *J Bone Joint Surg* 1990;72-A:1323–1329.

260. Wojtys EM, Wylie BB, Huston LJ. The effects of muscle fatigue on neuromuscular function and anterior tibial translation in healthy knees. *Am J Sports Med* 1996;24(5):615–621.

261. Wojtys EM. The neuromuscular effects of functional bracing. Book of abstracts & outlines, AOSSM, 23rd Annual Meeting, Sun Valley, Idaho, June 22–25, 1997:699–700.

262. Wojtys EM, Huston LJ, Lindenfeld TN, Hewett TE, Greenfield MLVH. Correlation between the menstrual cycle and ACL injuries in female athletes. Book of abstracts & outlines, AOSSM, Sun Valley, Idaho, June 22–25, 1997.

263. Woodall W, Welsh J. A biomechanical basis for rehabilitation programs involving the patellofemoral joint. *J Orthop Sports Phys Ther* 1990;11:11.

264. Yamaguchi GT, Zajac FE. A planar model of the knee joint to characterize the knee extensor mechanism. *J Biomech* 1989;22:1–10.

265. Zelisko JA, Noble HB, Porter M. A comparison of men's and women's professional basketball injuries. *Am J Sports Med* 1982;10:297–299.

266. Zillmer DA, Powell JW, and Albright JP. Gender specific injury patterns in high school varsity basketball. *J Women's Health* 1992;1(1):69–76.

The Injured Athlete, Third Edition,
edited by D. H. Perrin.
Lippincott–Raven Publishers, Philadelphia © 1999.

CHAPTER 16

The Leg, Ankle, and Foot

Brian L. Fong and Michael E. Brunet

STRESS FRACTURES

Physical stress on bone causes osteoclastic reabsorption and subsequent osteoblastic new bone formation along the lines of stress. During the initial resorptive phase the bone is temporarily weakened. Overload stress at that point can cause plastic deformation, which with continued overload stress can progress to a frank fracture (63,71). In athletes, stress fractures are 10% of all sports injuries. The distribution of stress fractures is 49.1% tibia, 25.3% tarsal, 8.8% metatarsal, 7.2% femur, 6.6% fibula, 1.6% pelvis, 0.9% sesamoid, 0.6% spine. They are bilateral in 16.6%. Runners are the athletes most commonly affected, and the pattern of injury is different than seen in military recruits.

Many reasons account for stress fractures and predispose the injury. Training errors were found in 22.4% of athletes with stress fractures. Pronated feet had a higher incidence of tibia, tarsal and fibula fractures, and a lower incidence of metatarsal fractures. Cavus feet had a higher incidence of femur and metatarsal fractures (71). Women are 12 times more susceptible to developing stress fractures, all other factors being equal (44). Women with very irregular menses having a higher rate than those with normal menses (9).

The athlete presents with an insidious onset of a vague pain that occurs during and increases with activity. With the progression of the fracture, the pain occurs sooner and continues after activity has stopped. Tenderness and swelling are present in the area of fracture.

On initial presentation, only 9.8% of stress fractures will be radiographically evident. Radiographic changes may take 2 weeks to 3 months to occur (71). A bone scan, however, is diagnostic (Fig. 16.1).

There are essentially two classes of stress fractures.

Those in which the fracture occurs under tension and those that occur under compression.

Tension-related stress fractures appear radiographically as radiolucent lines in cortical bone. Because bone heals poorly under tension, these fractures, even after 6 weeks of cessation of training often fail to heal. Common examples of tension-related stress fractures are the diaphyseal tibia stress fracture and the fifth metatarsal diaphyseal stress fracture.

Compression-related stress fractures appear radiographically as fluffy lines of increased sclerosis within the cancellous bone. Buckling of the cortical margins may also be seen. These fractures heal readily and are treated symptomatically with a two-phase protocol (Table 16.1). Common examples of this fracture are the stress fracture of the metaphyseal tibia and the calcaneus.

Tibial Stress Fractures

Three types of tibial stress fractures occur; posterior medial metaphyseal, anterior diaphyseal, and medial malleolar.

The posterior medial metaphyseal stress fractures are found in both the proximal and distal metaphysis or metaphyseal-diaphyseal junction. It is commonly found in runners. This is a compression-type stress fracture and maximal tenderness is present posteriorly. Radiographs may show linear-increased sclerosis within the cancellous bone and periosteal new bone formation. Treatment is symptomatic (see Table 16.1).

The anterior diaphyseal stress fracture is a tension type stress fracture commonly found in jumping athletes. Well-localized tenderness and soft tissue thickening are present over the anterior crest of the tibia. Radiographs may show periosteal reaction anteriorly with a radiolucent fracture line starting anteriorly and extending posteriorly (Fig. 16.2). When a fracture line extends one-third or greater through the cortex, athletic activity must be stopped

B. L. Fong and M. E. Brunet: Department of Orthopaedics, Tulane University Medical Center, New Orleans, Louisiana 70112-2699

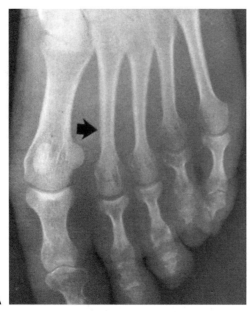
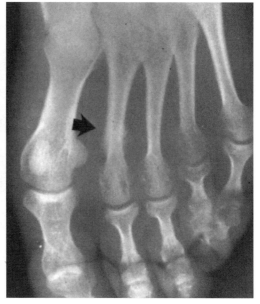

A   B

FIG. 16.1. A metatarsal stress fracture may not be visible for a few weeks on radiographs (**A**) and usually occurs through the very thin bone of the second metatarsal (**B**), which may be accompanied by early callus formation. (From ref. 47 with permission.)

immediately because of the significant risk of progression to a complete fracture. The athlete is placed in a non–weight-bearing short leg cast for 6 to 8 weeks. The average time to healing with casting alone is 8.7 months (44). Because of this, surgical treatment should be considered if significant healing has not taken place after 6 to 8 weeks of casting. The fracture is excised or drilled, then bone grafted. Reoccurrence or incomplete healing is common in athletes that play hard surface impact sports, that is, basketball and runners. In this situation, we are more likely to advise a reamed locked intramedullary rod. A well-fixed intramedullary rod allows aggressive rehabilitation and full weight bearing postoperatively. It has been reported an athlete may return to their sport as early as 6 weeks postoperatively, but more commonly at 3 months.

Medial Malleolar Stress Fractures

Medial malleolar stress fractures occur at the junction of the plafond and the medial malleolus and extend obliquely proximal. The medial pressure of the talus places tension on the medial malleolus causing the fracture. Nonoperative treatment is avoiding strenuous activity for 3 to 4 months. Orava in 1995 reported that recurrence is common if activity is resumed earlier than 4 to 5 months (81). If a fracture line is present on radiographs or computed tomography (CT) scan or an athlete desires to return to activity as soon as possible, primary surgical stabilization with one or two lag screws is recommended. Return to full participation in sports is allowed at 6 weeks (91,95).

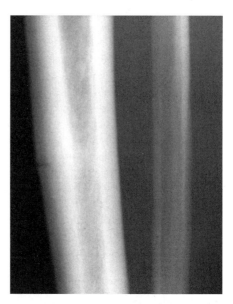

FIG. 16.2. The diaphyseal stress fracture is seen as a radiolucent line in the anterior cortex of the tibia.

TABLE 16.1. *Conservative stress fracture management*

Phase I—Symptomatic care
Stretching, isometrics, NSAID and ice massage. Full weight bearing for daily activities is allowed, but all running and jumping is stopped. Cycling, swimming, and water running are encouraged.
When the athlete is pain free for 10–14 days, Phase II is started.
Phase II—Return to activity
Previous training errors are identified and avoided. Shoes are evaluated and replaced as needed.
A gradual return to preinjury activity level is made over 4–6 weeks (2).

Fibular Stress Fractures

Fibular stress fractures are usually located just proximal to the distal tibia-fibular joint but may be found at any level of the fibula. It is more common in athletes with pronated feet, particularly if the hind foot is in valgus. Treatment is generally symptomatic (see Table 16.1). An orthotic is recommended if the heel is in excessive valgus (44).

Calcaneus Stress Fracture

Calcaneal stress fractures are a compression fracture that occurs at the junction between the body and the tuberosity and is perpendicular to the bony trabecula. This is the most common of the tarsal stress fractures. A lateral x-ray of the calcaneus will often demonstrate a fluffy linear density perpendicular to the trabecula. The treatment is symptomatic (see Table 16.1) (47).

NAVICULAR STRESS FRACTURES

Navicular stress fractures occur in the middle third of the navicular. The fracture line is in the sagittal plane. This fracture is found mostly in young male athletes. Radiographs often do not demonstrate the fracture and a bone scan, a CT scan or tomogram is needed to make the diagnosis. The treatment is a non–weight-bearing short leg cast for 6 to 8 weeks or until a CT scan or tomogram demonstrates a bony union. At an average of 5 to 6 months, 86% of athletes return to full activity (59). Surgical therapy is recommended for athletes that present with nonunion or have failed casting. Immediate internal fixation with screws and bone grafting returns 86% of athletes to full activity at 4 months (47,59).

Metatarsal Stress Fracture

Metatarsal stress fractures occur in the diaphysis, with the second metatarsal being the most commonly affected (see Fig. 16.1). Athletes with a short or hypermobile first metatarsal have an increased incidence of second metatarsal stress fractures because the percentage of body weight carried by that metatarsal is increased. Treatment for stress fractures of the second, third, and fourth metatarsals is symptomatic (see Table 16.1).

Stress Fracture of the Fifth Metatarsal Diaphysis

Diaphyseal stress fractures of the fifth metatarsal are clinically different from stress fractures of the metatarsals 2 through 4. Symptomatic treatment will lead to a nonunion. The fracture is classified radiographically (Table 16.2). Treatment for a type I fracture are a non–weight-bearing short leg cast, a stiff-soled shoe or a functional brace for 7 to 20 weeks (44). Primary placement of a single percutaneous 4.5-or 6.5-mm lag screw across the fracture should be considered in athletes. Operatively treated fractures will usually heal in 6 to 8 weeks, compared with the long period of immobilization and significant chance of progression that a nonunion conservative treatment entails. Type II fractures often require even longer periods of immobilization in a non–weight-bearing short leg cast and have an even lower chance of success. Primary curettage and bone grafting or percutaneous lag screw fixation should be encouraged. If conservative treatment is chosen, operative treatment should be strongly recommended if no radiographic improvement is seen after 6 to 8 weeks of casting. In type III fractures, conservative treatment is of no use and curettage of the sclerotic medullary canal with a sliding bone graft and screw fixation should be performed (29,47).

Medial Tibial Stress Syndrome

Medial tibial stress syndrome, commonly called shin splints, is caused by inflammation at the insertion of the soleus, not the posterior tibialis, on to the posterior medial border of the tibia (Fig. 16.3). Classically, it occurs in runners who increase the duration or intensity of their training. Changes in footwear and running surface have also been implicated. Pronated feet have a higher incidence because foot pronation increases the stress on the soleus, a supinator of the heel (76).

Posterior medial stress syndrome starts as pain along the posterior medial aspect of the tibia worsened with activity and improved with rest. With progression, the pain may become continuous. An increase in activity level or training environment can usually be elicited. Tenderness is palpable at the fascial-periosteal interface 5 to 7 cm proximal to the medial malleolus extending 13 cm proximally (2,32). Radiographs rarely demonstrate a periosteal reaction. Bone scans may show a diffuse uptake over the tender area or no change. A bone scan will differentiate posterior medial stress syndrome from a stress fracture (17,32,77).

Treatment consists of relative rest. Biking, swimming, and water running are initially substituted for running. Ice massage and Achilles stretching are performed 3 to

TABLE 16.2. *Classification of fifth metatarsal stress fractures*

Type I—Acute: fracture line present but no intramedullary sclerosis
Type II—Delayed union: widened fracture line and intramedullary sclerosis
Type III—Nonunion: complete obliteration of the medullary cavity (62).

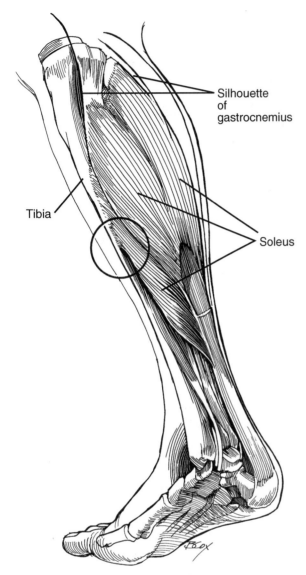

FIG. 16.3. The most common shin splints hurt posteromedially. To cure this condition, the surgeon may have to release the soleus fascia.

4 times per day and a nonsteroid antiinflammatory drug (NSAID) is prescribed. Training technique and equipment are evaluated. Athletes with pronated feet are fitted with semirigid orthotics. As the acute symptoms resolve, usually in 7 to 10 days, running is started on a soft surface in appropriate shoes (2). Shinsplint taping may be of benefit. Running starts at one-half the preinjury distance and pace and is increased over a 3- to 6-week period. Running distance is increased first, then the intensity. Recurrence is associated with resuming activity too quickly and usually occurs 1 to 3 weeks after resuming running.

Rarely, the symptoms become chronic, not resolving with long periods of rest or they recur with every attempt to increase activity. In these cases, a release of the symptomatic soleus attachment and cauterization of the underlying periosteum is indicated. Postoperatively, the patient ambulates as tolerated. Biking is started after 2 weeks and running after 3 weeks. At 3 months postoperatively, 93% will be improved and 78% completely cured (32).

COMPARTMENT SYNDROME

Compartment syndrome is a condition in which elevated interstitial pressure within a closed fascial compartment causes decreased tissue perfusion and neuromuscular compromise. A compartment syndrome can occur anywhere a muscle is surrounded by a noncompliant sheath.

In the leg, there are four fascial compartments. The anterior compartment contains the anterior tibialis, toe extensors, anterior tibial artery and vein, and the deep peroneal nerve. The lateral compartment contains the peroneal muscles and the superficial peroneal nerve. The deep posterior compartment contains the long toe flexors, posterior tibialis, posterior artery and vein, and the tibial nerve. The superficial posterior compartment contains the gastro-soleus complex (23). A fifth compartment containing only the posterior tibialis has also been proposed (30) (Fig. 16.4).

There are two types of compartment syndrome: acute and chronic. Acute compartment syndrome is most often caused by a tibia fracture. Revascularization, muscle rupture, blunt trauma, crush injuries, and circumferential burns are other etiologies. Swelling and/or intracompartmental bleeding increase the volume of the compartment because the compartment is relatively noncompliant. The interstitial pressure then rises. Casts and circumferential dressings increase the risk of compartment syndrome because they form an additional noncompliant sheath about the leg. When the interstitial pressure rises high enough, tissue perfusion is compromised and cellular death occurs.

An acute compartment syndrome presents with pain out of proportion to injury. The pain is exacerbated by passive stretch of the muscles traversing the compartment. There is swelling and palpable tenseness of the involved compartment. Paresthesia in the distribution of the nerve traversing the compartment and decreased 2-point discrimination are late findings. Pedal pulses are usually intact (4,84).

Chronic compartment syndrome is found in runners and military recruits. Eighty percent occur in the anterior or deep posterior compartments. With exercise, the muscles hypertrophy, decreasing the potential space within the compartment. Additionally, exercise can acutely increase muscle volume by 20%. The athlete will give a history of being completely asymptomatic during the off-season, but with training will develop a dull pain in the involved compartment toward the end of the run, which resolves within minutes or a few hours after activity has stopped. The symptoms are most commonly bilateral with

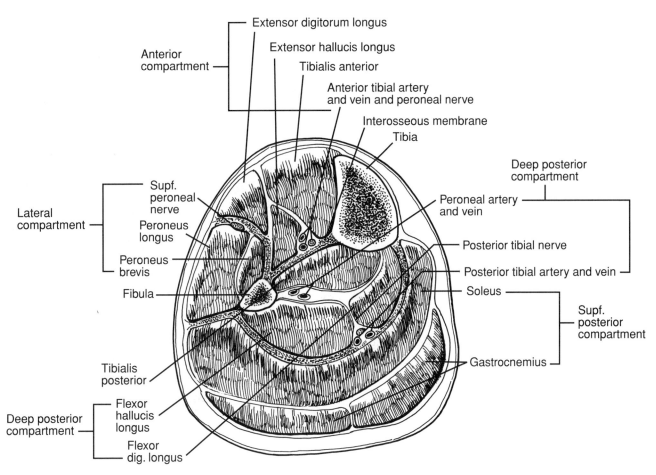

FIG. 16.4. Cross-sectional anatomy of the leg.

one side being worse than the other. With continued training, the symptoms start to begin earlier during running and last longer after running has stopped. Other symptoms are ankle weakness and paresthesia in the distribution of the nerve traversing the compartment (4,69). Muscle hernias are found in 40% of athletes with chronic compartment syndrome versus only 5% of normals (4).

In both acute and chronic cases, compartment pressure measurements are diagnostic. In acute cases, the resting compartment pressure is greater than 30 mm Hg and when found is a surgical emergency. Care must be taken to measure the intracompartmental pressure at the level of injury. Measuring the pressure distal to the level of injury can give an erroneously low value (49).

In chronic compartment syndrome, compartment pressure greater than 10 mm Hg at rest, greater than 30 mm Hg 1 minute postexercise, or greater than 20 mm Hg 5 minutes postexercise is pathologic. Normal athletes return to resting compartment pressures by 2 minutes after exercise has stopped (8).

The treatment for compartment syndrome is a surgical fascial release. With acute compartment syndrome, a release of all the compartments is warranted. Two longitudinal skin incisions are used. Through a lateral incision, the

fascia overlying the anterior and lateral compartments are incised over the full length of the compartment and through a medial incision the superficial posterior, deep posterior and posterior tibialis fascia are similarly incised. The skin is not closed, because it may act as a constricting compartment. A delayed primary closure of the skin may be performed when the swelling has subsided (84).

For chronic compartment syndrome, only the affected compartments need be released and this may be done through smaller, more cosmetic incisions. To release the anterior and lateral compartments, a small lateral incision is made and a fasciotome is advanced under the skin, splitting the fascia proximally and distally. The deep posterior compartment is released similarly through a medial incision. Postoperatively, a compressive dressing is applied and the patient allowed to ambulate weight-bearing as tolerated with crutches. Early active and passive range of motion is encouraged and light jogging may be started at 2 to 3 weeks as tolerated (84).

Popliteal Artery Entrapment

Popliteal artery entrapment is a very rare condition in which the popliteal artery is compressed at the knee.

There are basically 2 types. In type I, the popliteal artery takes an aberrant course, passing medially and below the medial head of the gastrocnemius. In type II, the popliteal artery runs its normal course but is compressed by an aberrant insertion of the plantaris or the gastrocnemius (64). This condition is most often misdiagnosed as posterior compartment syndrome. Ninety-four percent are males younger than 40 and 25% are bilateral (19).

The occlusion of the artery is intermittent, occurring during active plantar flexion of the ankle. This recurrent arterial compression can lead to intimal damage, aneurysm, stenosis, and thrombosis of the popliteal artery. The athlete presents with intermittent claudication of the lower extremity: cramping, coolness, calf pain, and, at times, paresthesias. It is not unusual for symptoms to be present with walking and relieved with running. This is because with walking the firing of the plantar flexors is prolonged compared to running. The reverse, however, may also be present. On exam, active ankle plantar flexion or passive dorsiflexion with the knee extended obliterates the pedal pulses. Doppler readings with active plantar flexion and passive dorsiflexion are helpful but are also positive in 50% of normal people (19). Compartment pressures are often performed to rule out posterior compartment syndrome. In contrast to compartment syndrome, the compartment pressures decrease during exercise (11). An arteriogram with active ankle plantar flexion and passive dorsiflexion with the knee extended will demonstrate the arterial compression (19,64). The treatment is surgical release of the structures compressing the artery. If significant arterial injury or occlusion has occurred, a reverse saphenous graft is used to replace the damaged vessel (19).

Partial Tear of the Medial Head of the Gastrocnemius

A partial tear of the medial head of the gastrocnemius typically occurs in a middle-aged recreational athlete who makes a sudden move or jump while running. A sudden sharp pain is felt in the posterior medial calf. Significant pain and swelling occurs over the next 24 hours. Development of an acute compartment syndrome has been reported (3). In the past, these symptoms were thought to be secondary to a rupture of the plantaris muscle. The tear occurs at the musculotendinous junction of the medial gastrocnemius. The gastrocnemius is susceptible to tearing because it crosses 3 joints, the knee, ankle, and subtalar joints. The Achilles tendon inserts eccentrically on the calcaneus, so the gastrocnemius is also a supinator of the heel. With isolated heel supination and pronation, the largest change in muscle length occurs in the most medial portion of the medial head of the gastrocnemius. With rapid changes in direction, the knee is actively extending, the ankle is passively dorsiflexing, and the heel passively pronating. Eccentric contraction of the gastrocnemius is

occurring with largest change in muscle length, and therefore highest force, occurring at the medial portion of the medial gastrocnemius. Tension overload causes tearing at musculotendinous junction (96).

Examination of the leg demonstrates tenderness and often a palpable defect in the medial head of the gastrocnemius. Passive dorsiflexion and active plantar flexion exacerbate the symptoms.

This injury is treated with a compressive dressing or neoprene sleeve, elevation, ice, and crutch ambulation weight bearing as tolerated. A one-half-inch heel lift is placed in the shoe. Gentle active assisted and passive range of motion is started the next day. Progressive resistance training is gradually started as the symptoms improve. A gradual return to activity can be expected in 3 to 6 weeks with the mean time to return to sports 6.7 weeks. Achilles taping may be used when initially returning to sports (96).

Achilles Tendinitis

Achilles tendinitis occurs in 6.5% to 18% of runners with men having twice the incidence of women. Athletes involved in sports requiring repetitive jumping are also commonly affected (21). Predisposing factors are overtraining (intensity, duration, and frequency), tibia varum, calcaneal valgus, hyper-pronation of the foot, inadequate shoe heel wedge (heel wedges of 12 to 15 mm are recommended), tight heel cords, and tight hamstrings (92). Common training errors causing Achilles tendinitis are a sudden increase in mileage, a single severe session, increased intensity, hill training and a rapid return after a lay off (22). There are two types of Achilles tendinitis: insertional and noninsertional.

Insertional Achilles Tendinitis

Insertional Achilles tendinitis is secondary to degenerative changes at the Achilles insertion onto the calcaneus and is therefore found in older athletes. It manifests itself as inflammation, thickening, fraying, calcification, and/or reactive ossification within the Achilles tendon (Fig. 16.5A,B). The retrocalcaneal bursitis may also be present. A Haglund's deformity is usually present and the pressure it exerts on the Achilles tendon is thought to be one of the etiologies of the condition. The athlete presents with pain and stiffness with the first steps in the morning and at rest. More acute tendinitis presents with pain on rapid acceleration. A bony protuberance may be present at the Achilles insertion, which is often referred to as a runner's bump. Radiographs may demonstrate a Haglund's deformity, intratendinous ossification, and/or intratendinous calcification. The initial treatment is rest, ice, NSAIDs, heel cord stretching, and a one-half inch heel lift. If a pronation deformity of the foot is present, an orthotic is

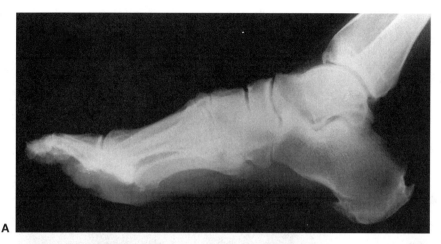

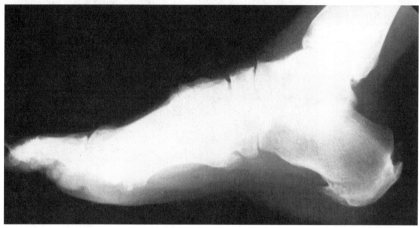

FIG. 16.5. A: Ossification at the insertion of the Achilles tendon and (**B**) within the Achilles tendon.

prescribed (92). Equinus taping decreases the stress on the tendon during activity (Fig. 16.6). A short leg-walking cast or cast boot for 6 weeks may be tried in recalcitrant cases. Steroids should never be injected into the tendon because of the risk of Achilles tendon rupture. If conservative therapy fails, excision of the Haglund's deformity, retrocalcaneal and calcaneal bursa, and intratendinous debridement of any degenerative tendon, calcification, and ossification may be performed. If, after debridement, there is inadequate remaining Achilles tendon, the flexor hallucis longus, flexor digitorum longus, or the peroneus brevis may be used to reinforce the tendon. Postoperatively, a short leg walking cast is worn for 2 to 3 weeks, 6 weeks if tendon reinforcement is done. Heel cord stretching and progressive resistive exercises are started once the cast is removed. Jogging may be started at 8 to 12 weeks and return to competition at 5 to 6 months (21).

Retrocalcaneal Bursitis

Retrocalcaneal bursitis occurs in the area between the Achilles tendon and the posterior calcaneus. It is usually associated with a Haglund's deformity, because the prominence of the posterior calcaneus increases the friction between the calcaneus and the tendon. Insertional Achilles tendinitis is commonly also present. When retrocalcaneal bursitis is present alone, tenderness and swelling are present only anterior to the Achilles tendon. Calcification within the bursa is not uncommon. Conservative treatment is the same previously outlined for insertional Achilles tendinitis. If conservative treatment fails, the next step is to excise the retrocalcaneal bursa and the portion of the posterior calcaneus impinging on the Achilles tendon. A short leg-walking cast is worn for 2 weeks, then stretching and progressive resistive exercises are started, jogging is resumed at 8 to 12 weeks and return to competitive athletics at 5 to 6 months. Seventy percent to 100% are cured or improved (5,90,99).

Noninsertional Achilles Tendinitis

Noninsertional Achilles tendinitis occurs 2 to 6 cm proximal to the insertion of the Achilles tendon on the calcaneus. At this level, the tendon rotates internally. This rotation may cause shear stresses within the tendon leading to tendinitis. Excessive foot pronation increases the internal rotation of the tendon (21,22). At the same level,

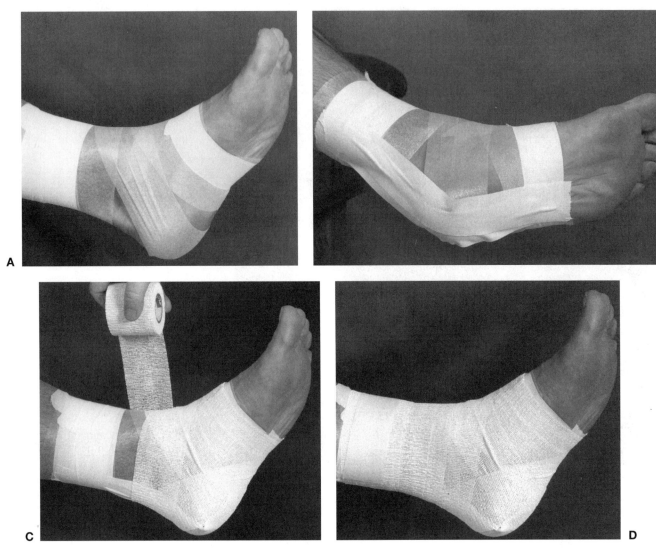

FIG. 16.6 A–D: An equinus taping takes tension off the Achilles tendon.

the blood supply is tenuous, decreasing the ability of the tendon to heal itself once injured (18).

Noninsertional tendinitis can be further subclassified into peritendinitis, peritendinitis with tendinosis, and tendinosis (92).

Peritendinitis involves a thickening of the paratenon with fibrous adhesions to the tendon. It presents as a tender diffuse swelling about the Achilles tendon. Crepitus is often present with ankle motion.

In peritendinitis with tendinosis, the Achilles tendon is thickened, softened, and yellowed with cleavage planes and vascular budding extending into the tendon from the inflamed paratenon (92).

With tendinosis, mucoid degeneration and chronic inflammatory changes are found with the tendon. Calcification within the tendon may be present (see Fig. 16.5), the central portion of the tendon being more involved than peripherally. Clinically, this is seen as a tender focal enlargement of the Achilles tendon. The presence of ten-

dinosis places the Achilles tendon at significantly increased risk of rupture (92).

Initial treatment is the same as for insertional tendinitis: rest, ice, NSAIDs, heel cord stretching, and a heel lift. Equinus taping is used during competition (Fig. 16.6). Pronated feet are prescribed an orthotic. A short period of casting may help recalcitrant cases. Steroid injections should not be used, because of the possible increased risk of tendon rupture.

If the athlete fails to respond to 6 months of conservative care, operative treatment is considered. If there is any question about the presence of tendinosis, magnetic resonance imaging (MRI) or ultrasound of the Achilles tendon is diagnostic. When peritendinitis is present, the thickened adherent paratenon is dissected off the tendon medially, laterally, and posteriorly. The anterior paratenon is left adherent and intact because it is the tendons' source of blood supply. If tendinosis is present, longitudinal incisions are made in the tendon and the degenerative tendon is excised. If the remaining tendon is tenuous, a turn down flap of the proximal Achilles tendon is used to reinforce the area of debridement. Postoperatively, a short leg cast is worn for 2 to 3 weeks with weight bearing allowed after 1 week. After cast removal, Achilles stretching is started. Running is not allowed until 8 to 12 weeks and return to competitive athletics at 5 to 6 months (21). Eighty-six percent of the athletes needing only a paratenon debridement and 73% of those with intratendinous debridement will be cured or improved (21,90).

Achilles Tendon Rupture

Achilles tendon ruptures are most commonly seen in middle-aged athletes. It occurs during forceful contraction of the gastroc-soleus while extending the knee as seen in accelerating for a ball in tennis. Falling from a height is another common etiology. Twenty-five percent are misdiagnosed as an ankle sprain on initial presentation. The athlete feels a pop and pain in the posterior ankle. Ambulation is difficult. The presence of active plantar flexion is not a reliable indicator of a rupture because the posterior tibialis and toe plantar flexors will also plantar flex the foot. A reliable test is to place the athlete in a kneeling position with the knees flexed to 90 degrees and the ankle passively at neutral. The calf is then squeezed just inferior to the area of greatest calf circumference. If the Achilles tendon is intact, the ankle will plantar flex (Fig. 16.7) (39).

Nonoperative treatment consists of placing the athlete in a short leg gravity equinus cast for 8 weeks. After cast removal, Achilles stretching and strengthening are started and a heel lift is worn for 1 to 2 months. With this treatment, the rerupture rate is 8% to 35% and isokinetic

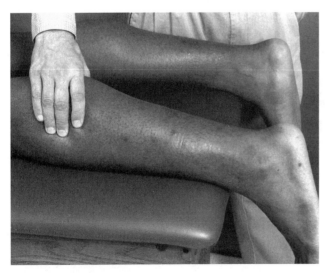

FIG. 16.7. Squeezing the calf just distal to the bulk of the gastrocnemius will cause ankle plantar flexion if the Achilles tendon is intact.

strength is 62% to 73% of the opposite side. If the rupture is treated within 48 hours of injury, the results are significantly better and if treated greater than 1 week postinjury significantly worse. Surgical repair has a 2% to 7% rerupture rate and isokinetic strength 88% to 101% of the opposite side. For this reason, the majority of athletes should have an open repair (39).

An incision is made over the posterior medial aspect of the Achilles tendon and the tendon ends are identified. The proximal tendon end is divided into two bundles and the distal end gathered into a single bundle. The bundles are then sutured together in anatomic position using heavy nonabsorbable sutures (Fig. 16.8). The flexor digitorum longus, flexor hallucis longus, or peroneus brevis are used to reinforce the repair if necessary. A splint is applied with the ankle in neutral. At 1 week, the splint is removed and gentle range of motion started. When 0 degrees of dorsiflexion is obtained a short leg cast or cast boot is worn 3 weeks non–weight-bearing and 3 weeks partial weight-bearing. After cast removal, range of motion, Achilles stretching, and strengthening are begun. An ankle foot orthosis (AFO) is then worn for another 6 weeks. The complications are that 1% will develop an infection and 3% to 5% have some skin necrosis (14,39).

Posterior Tibialis Tenosynovitis

Posterior tibialis tenosynovitis is inflammation and hypertrophy of the synovium surrounding the posterior tibialis tendon from the medial malleolus to the navicular (Fig. 16.9). Athletes participating in sports that require rapid direction changes, for example, basketball, soccer, hockey, and tennis, are most commonly affected. Athletes with pronated feet or a leg-length discrepancy are at increased risk. Activity related medial arch or medial ankle pain is the presenting complaint. Tenderness and swelling are present over the posterior tibial tendon from the posterior medial malleolus to the navicular. Pain is present on performing a single heel raise and on inversion of the foot from a plantar flexed everted position (26).

An MRI is important in recalcitrant cases to rule out tendinosis and tendon rupture. An MRI of posterior tibialis tenosynovitis will show edema and synovial hypertrophy around the tendon. Longitudinal splits in the posterior tibialis tendon may also be present.

This injury may be prevented by proper pre- and postactivity stretching. Runners need to purchase shoes with a flared heel and change shoes when the midfoot cushion and arch support become compressed and ineffective. Worn-out midfoot cushions and arch supports allow increased foot pronation. Runners with pronated feet may benefit from a semirigid orthotic with a medial heel post.

Mild symptoms are treated with decreased activity and a semirigid arch support with a 0.1875-inch medial heel wedge. More severe symptoms are treated for 3 to 4

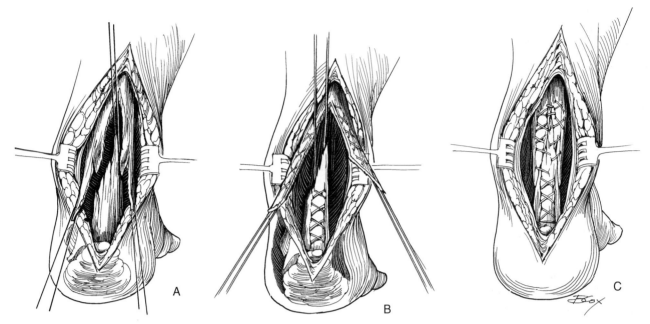

FIG. 16.8. Achilles tendon repair. **A:** The tendon is exposed through a medial incision. **B:** The torn tendon ends are gathered into three bundles with heavy nonabsorbable sutures. **C:** The bundle is secured in anatomic position.

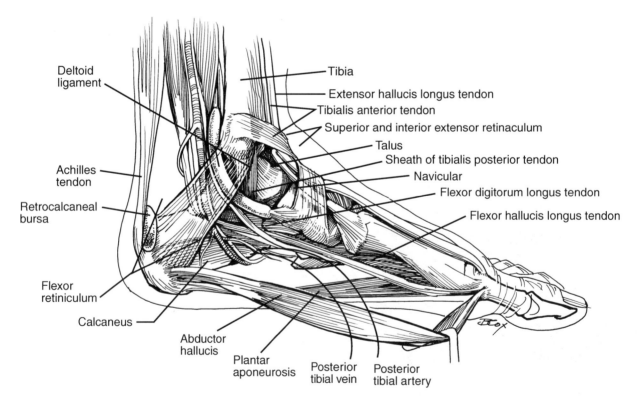

FIG. 16.9. Medial ankle anatomy.

weeks in a short leg walking cast. Initially stretching is started, then specific posterior tibialis strengthening exercises are added as symptoms improve (26).

In recalcitrant cases, a tenosynovectomy from medial malleolus to navicular is performed. If the paratenon is thickened, it is excised. Longitudinal splits in the tendon are often found and they are debrided and repaired. Postoperatively a short leg non–weight-bearing cast with foot in mild plantar flexion and inversion is worn for 3 weeks. The athlete is then changed to a cast boot and encouraged to weight-bear as tolerated. Range of motion is started, and strengthening added at 6 weeks after surgery (26).

Posterior Tibialis Tendon Rupture

Posterior tibialis ruptures are most commonly seen in patients with systemic arthritis, such as rheumatoid arthritis, and are insidious in nature. In athletes, generally older athletes, repetitive microtrauma, for example, running, is the most common mechanism of injury. The rupture can occur acutely from a sudden twisting injury to the foot, and when this occurs it represents the terminal event from ongoing breakdown of the tendon. Symptoms are typically pain and swelling on the medial side of the ankle. On exam, weakness of active foot inversion is found when testing with the foot in a position of plantarflexion and eversion. When the active inversion is tested in maximal inversion, the anterior tibialis may mask the posterior tibialis weakness. On performing a toe raise, the heel normally moves into varus. With a posterior tibialis rupture or deficiency, difficulty performing a toe raise is found and the heel stays in valgus. If a ruptured posterior tibialis tendon is not repaired, flattening of the medial longitudinal arch occurs with weight bearing and the heel may go into valgus. An external oblique radiograph may demonstrate an avulsion of the navicular tuberosity. Ultrasound or an MRI will demonstrate the rupture (25,87,110).

Repair is the treatment of choice for an acute rupture. Pure avulsion fractures are reattached and midsubstance tears are repaired and augmented with the flexor digitorum longus tendon (FDL). In the repair, the FDL is transected at the master knot of Henry. The distal stump is sutured to the flexor hallucis longus and the proximal stump of the FDL passed through a bone tunnel in the navicular (110).

In chronic ruptures secondary to tendinosis with flattening of the medial arch, the athlete must be counseled that surgical treatment at best is a salvage procedure and irrespective may preclude their return to sports. Surgical treatment of chronic ruptures reconstructs the posterior tibialis tendon as previously described and attempts to recreate a normal arch by imbrication of the calcaneonavicular ligament and the talonavicular capsule. A non–weight-bearing short leg cast with the foot plantar flexed and inverted is worn for 4 weeks. A short-leg walking cast is then worn for another 2 to 3 weeks, then range of motion, strengthening, and proprioceptive exercises are started. In chronic tears, this procedure will decrease pain, increase plantar flexion and inversion strength, and stabilize the medial arch. It will not correct a collapsed arch or a significant heel valgus. Success of this operation relates more to relief of symptoms with activities of daily living rather than return to sports (25).

If a moderate or severe degree of medial arch collapse and/or heel valgus are present in a symptomatic individual, a hind-foot arthrodesis is indicated and considered a purely salvage operation (25,110).

Accessory Navicular

An accessory navicular is found in 4% to 14% of the population, but only 0.1% of the population will have pain attributable to it. There are three types of accessory naviculans. In type I, a small ossicle is within the posterior tibial tendon. In type II, a triangular-shaped ossicle is joined to the navicular by a synchondrosis and in type III, the ossicle has a bony union to the navicular. In type II accessory naviculas, symptoms are secondary to injury to the synchondrosis. In type III, accessory navicular, symptoms are secondary to an insertional tendinitis. Type I are usually not symptomatic. The average age of presentation is 12 years with a 3 to 8 male-to-female ratio. The athlete presents with an insidious onset of pain over the medial aspect of the navicular that increases with activity and walking on uneven surfaces. There is usually no history of trauma. Shoe wear may be painful secondary to pressure on the navicular prominence. Tenderness is present with palpation over the navicular prominence, active inversion of the foot, and passive eversion. An external oblique radiograph of the foot best demonstrates the accessory navicular. Mild symptoms are treated with a semirigid arch support with a 0.1875-inch medial heel wedge. Rigid orthotics should not be used because they will apply more pressure to the bony prominence. More severe symptoms are treated with 3 weeks of non–weight-bearing in a short leg cast then another 3 weeks in a short leg walking cast. The results of conservative therapy are poor. In one study, no patient had lasting improvement with an orthotic and only 20% had lasting improvement with casting. Surgical excision of the ossicle or navicular prominence is performed through a longitudinal incision in the posterior tibial tendon. The ossicle is shelled out of the tendon without detaching the tendon from the navicular. Postoperatively, a short leg walking cast is worn for 6 weeks. Ninety-six percent will have resolution of their presenting complaint (26,87,94).

Peroneal Tendon Subluxation and Split

Subluxation and splits in the peroneus brevis occur with forced dorsiflexion against vigorously contracting

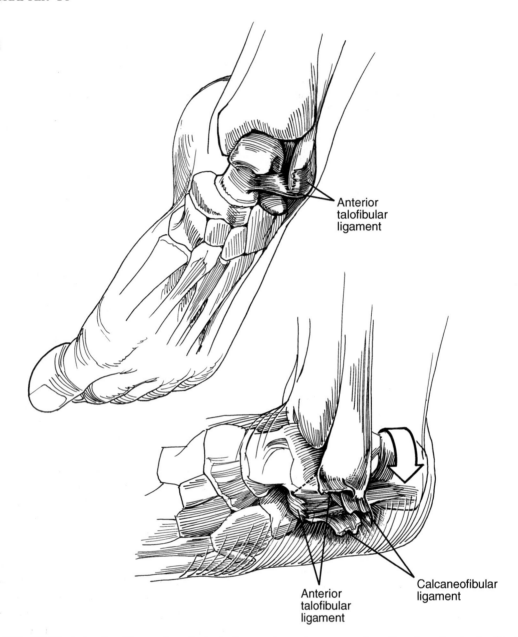

FIG. 16.10. Lateral ankle sprains. A single-ligament sprain occurs when the player's plantar flexed ankle is inverted, tearing the anterior talofibular ligament. If the inversion continues when the whole foot has reached the ground, the calcaneal-fibular ligament rips, producing a double ligament sprain.

peroneals. The peroneus brevis tendon is anterior to the peroneus longus tendon in the peroneal groove. At the level of the lateral malleolus, the superior retinacular pulley holds the peroneal tendons in the groove posterior to the lateral malleolus (Fig. 16.10). Peroneal contraction causes the peroneus longus to compress the peroneus brevis in the fibular groove, flattening it out and pressing it against the superior retinacular pulley. If enough force is present, the flattened tendon partially or completely subluxes out of the fibular groove injuring the superior retinacular pulley. When the peroneus bre-

vis subluxes over the sharp edge of the posterior fibula, a longitudinal split in the tendon may occur. This injury is most commonly found in skiers who fall forward. The ankle will be tender over the posterior aspect of the lateral malleolus. Clicking and popping may be present on ascending stairs. Circumduction of the ankle will reproduce the popping or clicking. Subluxation of the peroneal tendons is palpable at the posterior aspect of the lateral malleolus when the foot is actively moved from plantar flexion inversion to dorsiflexion eversion. If pain and crepitus without subluxation are present with the same maneuver, an isolated peroneal tendon split or peroneal tenosynovitis is present.

Radiographs of the ankle will be normal. An MRI will demonstrate the split in the tendon, if present.

If diagnosed acutely, a short leg cast in 30 degrees of plantar flexion is worn for 6 weeks. If chronic, taping a horseshoe-shaped pad around the lateral malleolus may help to prevent subluxation during activities.

For chronic symptomatic subluxing peroneal tendons and/or peroneal tendon splits, operative intervention is indicated. The superior peroneal retinacular pulley is sharply incised along the posterior border of the fibula. The fibular groove is enlarged with a bur to allow more volume for the tendons captured by the pulley repair. The peroneal tendons are inspected and any splits in the tendon are debrided and repaired. The superior peroneal retinacular pulley is then repaired and reinforced with a flap of the peroneal sheath, a flap of periosteum, or a portion of the Achilles tendon. A short leg cast is worn for 3 weeks, then a cast boot is worn for another 3 weeks. Gentle active dorsiflexion and plantar flexion is started at 3 weeks (98,105).

Anterior Tibiotalar Impingement

The repetitive trauma of forced dorsiflexion of the ankle causes the formation of a reactive osteophyte in the area of contact, the anterior tibia, and the talar neck. The athlete notices initially a vague anterior ankle pain, which with time becomes sharper, occurring when landing from jumping and with dorsiflexion of the ankle. Decreasing ankle dorsiflexion may be noticed. On examination, anterior ankle tenderness, tenderness on forced dorsiflexion of the ankle, and variable degrees of anterior ankle swelling are found. A lateral radiograph of the ankle demonstrates an osteophyte on the anterior surface of the tibia at the joint line and sometimes a corresponding lesion on the talar neck in which the tibial osteophyte impinges (see Fig. 16.5A). Asymptomatic osteophytes are found in 59% of dancers and 45% of football players compared to 4% of the general population (60,93,100). The treatment includes rest until the acute symptoms resolve, NSAIDs, ice, a one-half-inch heel lift and Achilles taping to restrict dorsiflexion (see Fig. 16.6). Arthroscopic removal of the osteophytes has been shown to significantly improve symptoms in all the patients with a return to full activity in an average of 5 weeks. If done as an open procedure, the results are similar, but return to full activity is at an average of 8 weeks.

A second type of anterior ankle impingement is found in long slender dancers with flexible feet. In these athletes, the dorsiflexion force when landing from a jump is not dissipated at the tibiotalar joint but in the midfoot. Once maximal dorsiflexion of the tibiotalar joint occurs, dorsiflexion and foot pronation continues at the midtarsal joint,

stretching the midfoot ligaments and the plantar fascia. The athlete presents with pain over the medial midtarsal joint and plantar fascia after dancing, which resolves after a few hours of rest. Radiographs do not demonstrate any tibiotalar osteophytes. Treatment involves supporting the arch either with taping or an orthotic and technique modification to avoid maximal foot dorsiflexion. The prognosis for return to high level dance is poor. No operative correction is available (60).

Posterior Talotibial Impingement

Posterior talotibial impingement is also known as os trigonum pinch and Stieda's lesion. It is commonly seen in ballet dancers, and also in jumping athletes and kicking athletes (50). An os trigone is found in 10% of the population. In this condition, an os trigone or prominent posterior lateral process of the talus is pinched between the posterior aspect of the tibia and the calcaneus during plantar flexion of the ankle. Typically, the athlete will present with a history of progressive posterior ankle pain made worse by jumping or standing on toes. Forced terminal plantar flexion of the foot and palpation of the posterior ankle is tender. A lateral radiograph of the ankle may show an os trigone, prominent posterior talar process, which may or may not be fractured, and/or soft tissue calcification. The treatment is rest, avoiding full plantar flexion, NSAIDs, and taping to prevent full plantar flexion. If a posterior talar process fracture is present, a short leg walking cast is used for 6 to 8 weeks. A steroid injection of the area may be helpful. If conservative treatment fails, excision of the os trigone, posterior lateral talus and/or calcified tissues through either a medial or lateral incision has had 87% good or excellent results (68,111). Postoperatively, a short leg cast is worn 2 weeks for comfort and activity gradually increased. Return to normal activity can be expected at 12 weeks.

Ankle Sprains

Ankle injuries are the most common sports injury. Of the total injuries in a given sport, ankle injuries are 45% of basketball injuries, 35% of soccer injuries, and 25% of volleyball injuries.

Ninety percent of ankle injuries involve the lateral ligaments, anterior talofibular ligament (ATF) and calcaneal fibular ligament (CFL) (105). Of the lateral ligament injuries, 66% involve only the ATF. The most common mechanism for ATF injury is an forceful inversion of a plantar flexed ankle. This initially injures the anterior talofibular ligament (ATF), which is the primary restraint for inversion with the ankle in plantar flexion. With progression of the injury the calcaneofibular ligament (CFL) is injured (Fig. 16.10). The CFL is the primary restraint to inversion with the ankle at neutral or dorsiflexed.

Although the majority of ankle injuries will involve the only the lateral ankle ligaments, a careful evaluation must always be performed to detect associated or other types of injuries.

The history must include the mechanism of injury, the position of the body during injury, the location of the pain, and the ability to ambulate after the injury. The presence of a rotational component to the injury, whether or not a pop was heard, and if swelling is present whether it occurred immediately or slowly are also important. Often the history alone can be diagnostic. An inversion injury to a plantar flexed ankle with lateral ankle pain indicates a lateral ligament sprain. A pop and immediate pain and swelling in the posterior ankle occurring while pushing off is indicative of an Achilles tendon rupture.

The ankle is inspected next. Areas of swelling, ecchymosis, and deformity are noted.

Sensation is checked especially in the distribution of the superficial peroneal nerve.

The leg, then ankle, are palpated starting from the area least likely injured to the area most likely injured. The fibula is palpated first. The fibula and tibia are then squeezed together. Pain indicates a fibular fracture or syndesmosis injury. The malleoli are palpated for evidence of a fracture. Achilles tendon, peroneal tendons, posterior tibialis, and anterior tibialis tendons are palpated from their insertions to just proximal to the ankle. Tenderness in these areas indicates tendon rupture, subluxation/dislocation, or avulsion fracture at the insertion. The ATF, CFL, syndesmosis, and deltoid ligament are palpated looking for ligamentous injury. The relative tenderness of each ligament is also important.

Isometric muscle testing is performed. Active dorsiflexion tests the anterior tibialis. Weakness of this muscle may be secondary to tendon or a peroneal nerve injury. Eversion from a neutral ankle position tests the peroneal tendons. Palpation of the posterior aspect of the lateral malleolus during testing will detect peroneal subluxation or dislocation. Active inversion with the ankle in comfortable plantar flexion and eversion tests the posterior tibialis tendon. If the posterior tibialis is tested with the ankle inverted, the anterior tibialis may substitute for the posterior tibialis. Active plantar flexion is tested. If any suspicion of a Achilles tendon rupture is present, a Thompson test is performed (see Fig. 16.7).

Ligamentous testing starts with the anterior drawer. The ankle is placed in 20 degrees of plantar flexion. The tibia is held in one hand and the calcaneus in the other. The calcaneus is then pulled anteriorly. Increased anterior translation of the talus in the mortise indicates an ATF rupture.

In the talar tilt test, the calcaneus and the tibia are grasped. The ankle is everted to test the deltoid ligament. Inversion with the ankle plantar flexed tests the ATF and inversion with the ankle in neutral tests the CFL. Things to note while performing these tests are the degree of laxity compared to the opposite side, the quality of the end point, and if it recreates the athlete's chief complaint.

Grasping the tibia and moving the talus side to side without tilting checks the stability of the talus in the ankle mortise, increased play indicates a syndesmotic injury.

If external rotation of the foot with the ankle in neutral and/or squeezing the tibia and fibula together causes pain, a syndesmotic injury must be suspected.

Indications for radiographs: (1) bony tenderness or deformity, (2) suspicion of a fracture or syndesmotic injury, (3) severe pain and swelling that make physical diagnosis unreliable. Initial radiographs should include an anteroposterior (AP), lateral, and mortise view of the ankle. If a syndesmotic injury is suspected, an AP and lateral of the tibia and fibula should also be performed to rule out an associated fibular fracture.

Stress radiographs radiographically document and quantify the laxity of the anterior drawer and talar tilt test. A lateral radiograph of the ankle is taken while performing an anterior drawer. Greater than a 10-mm anterior displacement indicates a complete ATF rupture (Fig. 16.11A,B). An AP of the ankle is taken while inverting the ankle with the ankle at neutral. Greater than 9 degrees of tilt indicates a complete CFL rupture (see Fig. 16.12). Stress radiographs, however, are not necessary with an acute injury.

Ankle sprains are graded by the degree of injury to the ligament. Grade I is a stretch without macroscopic tearing. There is minimal swelling and tenderness, no or slight loss of function, and no mechanical instability. Grade II is a partial tear. There is moderate pain, swelling, and tenderness over the involved ligaments. Ankle range of motion is limited by pain and mild to moderate instability is present. Grade III is a complete tear. There is severe pain, hemorrhage, swelling, and tenderness over the involved ligaments. The athlete is unable to walk on the ankle and significant instability is present. With lateral ankle sprains, the ATF is usually the ligament injured with CFL injury seen with higher grades of ATF injury (15,55).

All grades of isolated lateral ankle sprains are treated with early mobilization and rehabilitation. Studies of complete tears of the lateral ligaments have shown no difference in long-term results between patients treated with early surgical repair versus cast immobilization versus functional rehabilitation. Over the short term, functional rehabilitation returned patients to work and sports two to four times faster (55,61). When comparing early surgical reconstruction to failed conservative therapy with subsequent surgical reconstruction, there is no difference in results. So there is no advantage to early surgical treatment (55,105).

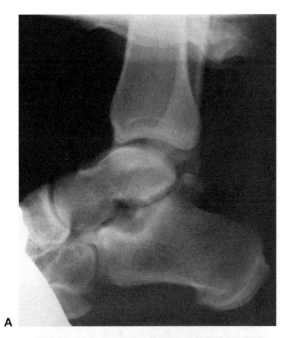

A

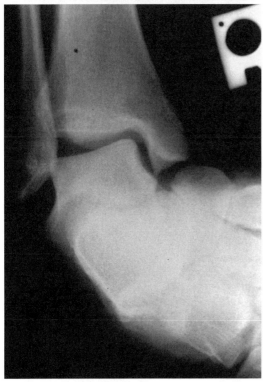

B

FIG. 16.11. A: Anterior drawer is measured by subluxing the talus anteriorly and measuring the distance between the posterior tibia and talar dome. **B:** Talar tilt is the angle formed by a line parallel to the tibial plafond and a line parallel to the talus.

Rehabilitation of an Ankle Sprain

Rehabilitation of the acutely sprained ankle is divided into three phases: the acute phase, the early rehabilitative phase, and the late rehabilitative phase.

The goal of the acute phase is to prevent and control hemorrhage and swelling. The treatment is RICE or rest, ice, compression, and elevation. Cryotherapy is performed for 20 minutes three to four times per day. Ice packs, cold gel packs, ice whirlpool, or cold-compressive pumps may be used. Compression and immobilization are most easily obtained with an ankle brace or gel splint. Open–basket-weave taping with a horseshoe-shaped pad that fits around the malleolus covered with an elastic wrap is another option. An elastic wrap alone is not as effective in controlling the edema around the malleoli. With grade III ligamentous injuries, an ankle brace or other form of immobilization is worn at all times except when bathing for 6 weeks. The leg is kept elevated above the level of the heart as much as possible. Crutch ambulation is used when necessary and the athlete is encouraged to bear weight as soon as possible. While ambulating with the crutches, placing the heel down first and rolling over the foot is emphasized. Gentle active ankle dorsiflexion and plantar flexion is started to regain motion.

When the ankle swelling has stabilized, usually at 48 hours postinjury, the early rehabilitative phase is started. This phase works on decreasing the swelling, increasing range of motion, and increasing weight bearing. Cryotherapy is continued and contrast baths may be added to help decrease the edema. Range-of-motion exercises are performed after cryotherapy. Writing the alphabet with the big toe mobilizes all the joints of the midfoot and ankle. Stationary biking is performed with the seat higher than normal. This requires the ankle to plantar flex at the bottom of the downstroke. The Achilles is stretched with the aid of a towel looped around the foot, progressing to an incline board. Strengthening exercises are started with isometric ankle inversion, eversion, dorsiflexion, and plantar flexion. The athlete progresses to Theraband exercises (Fig. 16.12), then to heel-and-toe raises. Gait training continues to emphasize heel strike and increased weight bearing.

With grade III injuries, an ankle brace is worn during therapy and at all times except while bathing.

When the early rehabilitative phase goals of full weight bearing, minimal swelling, and no pain on palpating ligaments are met, the athlete progresses to the next phase. Grade III injuries must complete 6 weeks of immobilization in an ankle brace prior to progressing to the next phase.

The late rehabilitative phase continues to work on increasing range of motion and strength. Proprioceptive retraining is added. Aggressive range of motion in all planes is started. Gastrocnemius and soleus are stretched using an incline board. Strengthening of the muscles about the

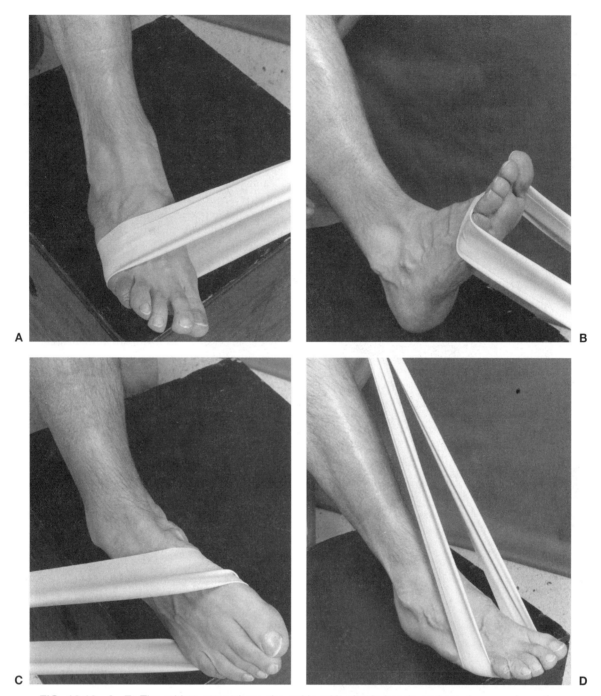

FIG. 16.12. A–F: The athlete strengthens the ankle with elastic bands and regains proprioception by standing on one leg with eyes closed.

ankle using Theraband is continued. Heel raises, seated calf raises, toe raises with foot in inversion, neutral, and eversion, and supinated walking are added as strength improves. When available, isokinetic training is used because it more closely resembles the muscle function during activities (70).

Proprioceptive training starts as soon as full weight bearing is tolerated. It is started with stork stands, standing on one leg. As balance improves, the eyes are closed while doing stork stands. The athlete is then progressed to

a wobble board or other proprioceptive trainer. A wobble board is basically a board with half a crochet ball nailed to its underside. The athlete stands on the board and tries to remain balanced on the ball. Once mastered, the athlete then throws a ball while standing on the board.

The athlete is discharged from therapy when the ankle has 80% to 90% of normal strength, full range of motion and no proprioceptive defect. The use of ankle taping or bracing will decrease the incidence of recurrent ankle sprains (see Chapter 5, Fig. 5.9).

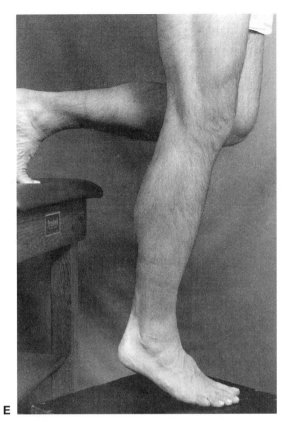

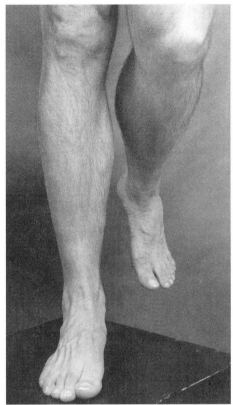

FIG. 12. *Continued.*

Chronic Ankle Instability

Chronic symptoms persist in 10% to 30% of athletes after a lateral ankle sprain. Mechanical instability, peroneal muscle weakness, decreased ankle dorsiflexion, proprioceptive deficits, sural nerve neuropraxia, or peroneal nerve neuropraxia, alone or in any combination, can cause chronic symptoms (105). There are basically two types of chronic ankle instability: mechanical and functional.

Mechanical instability is defined as motion beyond the normal physiologic range and is secondary to ligamentous insufficiency. This insufficiency is demonstrable on exam with a positive ankle anterior drawer indicating an ATF tear and a positive talar tilt indicating a CLF tear. On stress radiographs, greater than 10 mm of anterior displacement on an anterior drawer indicates anterior talofibular insufficiency and greater than 9 degrees of talar tilt indicates calcaneofibular insufficiency. There is, however, no correlation between mechanical instability and symptoms. Many athletes with mechanical instability are asymptomatic (83,105).

The second type of chronic instability is functional. With functional instability, the motion of the ankle remains within a physiologic range, but is poorly controlled within that range. Pain, peroneal muscle weakness and a proprioceptive defect are causes of a functional deficit. Proprioceptive deficits can be secondary to loss of sensory input from the receptors within the injured ligament and/or from neuropraxia of the sensory nerves innervating the ankle. There is no correlation between mechanical and functional instability (83).

Symptoms of chronic ankle instability are pain, swelling, giving way, and recurrent ankle sprains. Difficulty walking on uneven ground and down stairs are also present. Examination of the ankle may or may not demonstrate mechanical instability. The inability to stand on the affected foot with the eyes closed, the modified Romberg test, detects a proprioceptive loss and/or peroneal weakness.

Radiographs, bone scan, and MRI of the ankle may be done to rule out other causes of ankle disability, such as talar OCD lesion, anterior lateral ankle impingement, arthritis, and loose bodies.

Because good functional control of the ankle can stabilize a mechanically unstable ankle, treatment for both types of instability starts with ankle strengthening and proprioceptive retraining. Ten weeks of therapy result in maximum benefit (83). A lateral heel wedge may be helpful. The use of taping or a brace during activities helps in two ways. It provides mechanical stability and proprioceptive feedback of ankle position to the skin. Which of these two mechanisms is more important is still debated. What, however, has been well documented is that taping or bracing a previously injured ankle decreases the incidence of repeat injury. Taping or bracing an ankle that has never been injured has had variable results with some studies showing no change and others a decreased incidence of ankle sprains (97,102).

Surgical reconstruction is considered, if mechanical and functional instability are still present after reaching maximal improvement with functional rehabilitation. There are no differences in the results of later versus early ankle reconstruction so nothing is lost by trying to maximize functional rehabilitation (70). There are two types of ankle reconstruction: anatomic and nonanatomic.

The anatomic repair, modified Brostrom, repairs and retensions the injured anterior talofibular and calcaneofibular ligaments. The repair is reinforced with a portion of the extensor retinaculum. If insufficient tissue is available for repair, the repair is augmented by anatomically placed grafts of the plantaris or a portion of the peroneus brevis (24).

Nonanatomic reconstructions use a portion of or the whole peroneus brevis tendon to stabilize the ankle, the Evans, Watson-Jones, and Chrisman-Snook procedures being the most commonly performed (Fig. 16.13). The success rate is good for all these procedures when used appropriately. The Evans and Watson-Jones procedures do not adequately reconstruct the calcaneofibular ligament, and if performed on an athlete with a significant calcaneofibular ligament tear or subtalar instability, a poor result can be expected. Because of their nonanatomic course and the inclusion of the base of the fifth metatarsal in the tenodesis, all nonanatomic repairs restrict ankle and subtalar motion. This loss of motion may cause some difficulty walking on uneven ground (15,24,83).

The recommended surgical treatment for chronic lateral ligament instability is an anatomic repair with augmentation as necessary. Postoperatively, a short-leg walking cast with the foot in eversion is worn for 6 weeks, then functional rehabilitation is started. Return to sports is allowed at 12 weeks if all rehabilitation goals are met.

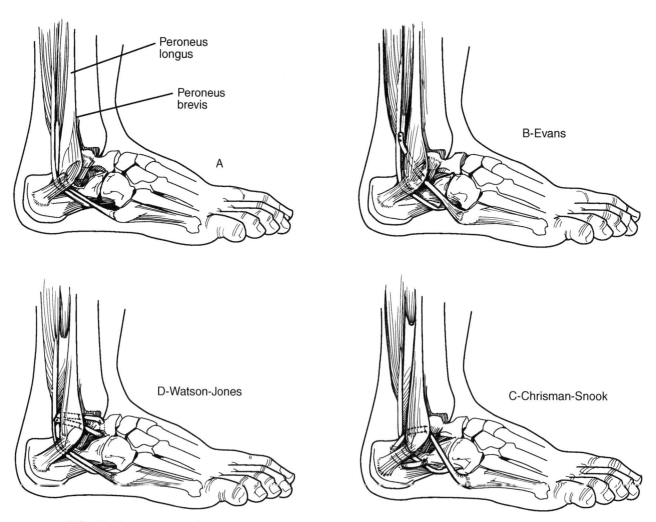

FIG. 16.13. Reconstructive operations to correct ankle instability (**A**), such as the Evans (**B**), the Chrisman–Snook (**C**) and the Watson–Jones (**D**) procedures. Generally, these techniques include a weaving of the tendon of the peroneus brevis through bone. In each of these operations, the tendon of the peroneus brevis is passed through the fibula.

Eighty-seven percent to 95% good or excellent results can be expected with regard to mechanical stability. Fifty percent to 70% will however experience some degree of aches and other complaints after stressful activities (63).

If generalized joint hypermobility or arthritic changes are present, a Chrisman-Snook procedure has been shown to provide better results than an anatomic repair (83).

Syndesmosis Sprain

Approximately 1% of athletes presenting with an ankle sprain have a syndesmosis injury (53). External rotation of the foot with the ankle at neutral is the most common mechanism of injury. This injury is most commonly seen in skiers (1,33). External rotation of the talus within the mortise causes an external rotation force on the fibula and ultimately the tearing of the anterior fibers of the distal syndesmosis. Injury of the deltoid ligament also occurs as the talus rotates away from the medial malleolus. Hyperdorsiflexion also can cause a syndesmosis injury. The talus is wider anteriorly than posteriorly so hyperdorsiflexion drives the talus like a wedge into the mortise, spreading it apart (53).

Maintenance of a normal relationship between the tibia and fibula at the ankle mortise is important because a 1 mm diastasis of the mortise will cause a 42% decrease in tibiotalar contact area (1).

The history is usually one of an external rotation injury. Tenderness is found over the anterior tibiofibular joint and the deltoid ligament. Squeezing the tibia and fibula together at mid-calf causes pain in the anterior lateral ankle. Placing the knee at 90 degrees, the ankle at neutral, and externally rotating the foot causes pain at the syndesmosis. Increased side-to-side motion of the talus in the mortise may be appreciated.

With any injury to the syndesmosis, fracture of the fibula must be ruled out, so an AP and lateral of the fibula must be obtained in addition to the standard AP, lateral, and mortise views of the ankle. The measurement of the tibiofibular clear space on an AP or mortise view is a reliable indicator of a syndesmosis injury. When measured 1 cm above the tibial plafond, any value over 6 mm indicates widening of the syndesmosis (46) (Fig. 16.14). Comparison views of the opposite side are helpful. Axial images of the syndesmosis with CT scan are definitive. A greater than 1 mm increase in the tibiofibular clear space on external rotation stress is abnormal (33). Calcification or ossifications of the syndesmosis or the interosseous ligament commonly occurs after healing of the injury (16,46,53).

Treatment of a stable, no increase in the tibiofibular clear space, syndesmosis sprain is the same as for lateral ankle sprains, although the time to full recovery is usually twice as long when compared to similarly graded lateral ankle sprains (16). If an increase in the tibiofibular clear space is found only on stress radiographs then 6 weeks in a short leg cast with the foot in internal rotation is used (33). If static widening of the clear space is found, the syndesmosis should be reduced and stabilized with a screw through the tibia and fibula approximately 2 cm proximal to the tibial plafond (see Fig. 16.14). The athlete is kept non–weight-bearing in a short leg cast or cast

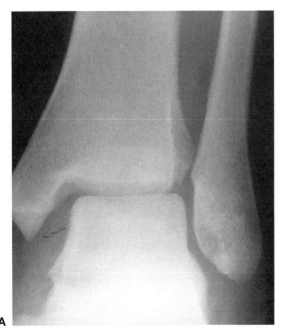
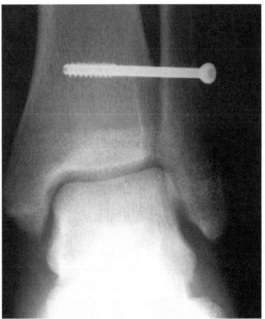

A **B**

FIG. 16.14. Syndesmosis injury is diagnosed by a decreased tibia-fibular overlap in a mortise view (**A**). The syndesmosis is reduced and stabilized with a single screw (**B**).

boot until the screw is removed at 6 to 8 weeks after surgery. Standard ankle rehabilitation is started after screw removal (1,58,79).

Anterior Lateral Ankle Impingement

Anterior lateral impingement, also known as a meniscoid lesion, is a complication of an inversion ankle sprain. It appears as an intraarticular band of white fibrous tissue in the anterior lateral gutter of the ankle. Trapping of the tissue between the talus and fibula with ankle motion is the source of the symptoms. The etiology of the lesion is thought to be residual synovial thickening and exudate from the initial injury, the torn end of the anterior talofibular ligament, or hypertrophy of the anterior inferior bundle of the tibiofibular ligament (36,72,105).

The athlete presents with a history of an inversion ankle sprain and subsequent pain, swelling, giving way, recurrent ankle sprains and weakness. Tenderness is located anterior to the talofibular joint. Snapping may be present on range of motion of the ankle (36,72).

Radiographs and bone scan are negative and an MRI will show synovial thickening in the anterior lateral gutter in 30% to 40% of cases (37,72).

Treatment is an arthroscopic resection of the abnormal tissue within and anterior to the talofibular joint. Weight bearing, range of motion, and strengthening are started immediately and return to activity can be expected in 3 weeks (36,72).

OSTEOCHONDRAL LESIONS OF THE TALUS

Osteochondral lesions of the talar dome are secondary to acute or repetitive trauma. The difference between an osteochondral fracture and osteochondritis dissecans is probably more time-dependent because most lesions are thought to be trauma-related. Osteochondritis dissecans is a more chronic condition. In osteochondritis dissecans, the bony fragment associated with the lesion is necrotic and therefore has lost its blood supply. Medial lesions are more common than lateral. In cadavers, medial lesions are produced by an ankle-inversion injury with the ankle in plantar flexion. The lesion is cup-shaped and located in the posterior one-half of the medial talus (Fig. 16.15A,B). Lateral lesions are produced by an ankle-inversion injury with the ankle at neutral or dorsiflexed. The lesion is wafer-shaped and located on the edge of the anterior one-half of the lateral talar dome (37,38)(see Fig. 16.15B).

The athlete will present with a history of pain, deep aching and swelling aggravated with activity and relieved with rest. Clicking, catching, and crepitus may also be present. Tenderness will be present on palpation of the lesion on the talus. The ankle must also be evaluated for instability. Mortise views with the ankle in dorsiflexion and plantar flexion may detect lesions missed by standard

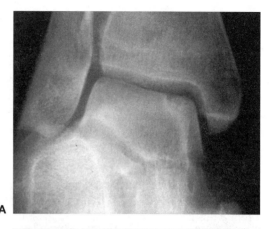

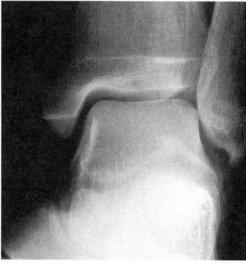

FIG. 16.15. Medial talar osteochondral lesion is seen as a cup-shaped lucency (**A**). Lateral osteochondral lesion is seen as a wafer-shaped radiolucency (**B**).

radiographs of the ankle. The lesion is hot on bone scan. A CT and MRI are useful for evaluating and staging symptomatic lesions.

Berndt and Harty Classification:
Stage I: Small area of compressed subchondral bone.
Stage II: Partially detached subchondral fragment.
Stage III: Completely detached but reduced fragment.
Stage IV: Detached and loose in joint.

If a symptomatic osteochondral fracture is stage I to III, a non–weight-bearing short leg cast is worn for 6 to 8 weeks or until radiographic union occurs. If the fragment is symptomatic and necrotic (osteochondritis dissecans), the results of immobilization are poor for stage II and III (37,38).

Arthroscopic surgery should be considered for stage III and definitely stage IV lesions. If the lesion is stable and the articular surface is intact, 0.0625-inch holes are drilled through the lesion into the underlying cancellous bone to stimulate the healing process. If the fragment is unstable (indicated by a break in the articular surface or motion) or free in the joint, it is removed. The defect is curetted and its base drilled. Large lesions may be placed back into the bed, if the fragment has not overgrown, and secured with small headless screws.

Postoperatively, if the lesion was excised, the athlete is started on early motion and weight bearing as tolerated. If the lesion was drilled or repaired, the athlete is placed in a short leg walking cast with partial weight bearing for 3 weeks and full weight bearing for 3 weeks. One series reported that if a large lesion was reattached, an 84% good to excellent result can be expected (37).

THE FOOT

Biomechanics of Gait

The running cycle is divided into two phases. Stance phase occurs when the foot is in contact with the ground and swing phase when it is not. Stance phase is further divided into heel strike, midstance and toe-off (Fig. 16.16).

Heel strike begins with initial contact of the foot with the ground and ends when the foot is flat on the ground. Initial foot contact may be on the lateral aspect of the heel, midfoot, or in the case of sprinters the forefoot (73).

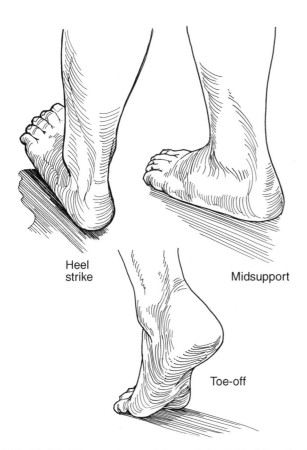

FIG. 16.16. Stance phase of the gait is divided into heel strike, midstance, and toe-off.

The foot is supinated and the tibia externally rotated. As the foot is loaded, the tibia internally rotates and the foot pronates eccentrically, absorbing the impact of heel strike. Weight bearing progresses along the lateral side of the foot and spreads from lateral to medial across the metatarsal heads (7,73). Eccentric knee flexion and eccentric ankle plantar flexion aid in dissipating the impact of heel strike.

Midstance begins with the foot being flat on the ground. Pronation of the foot unlocks the subtalar joint allowing increased flexibility and therefore allowing the foot to accommodate to uneven terrain. As the opposite leg swings past the stance leg, the tibia begins to externally rotate and the foot supinates.

Toe-off starts with the raising of the heel off the ground. Supination of the foot has locked the subtalar joint, making the foot a rigid lever for the gastrocnemius and soleus to work against. Toe-off ends when the foot leaves the ground.

THE TYPES OF FEET

The mechanics of the tarsal joints of the foot allow it to be flexible during midstance to absorb impact and allow accommodation to uneven terrain, and rigid during push-off so it can be an effective lever for propulsion, the flexibility or rigidity is determined by the position of the foot. Pronation unlocks the subtalar joint, increasing the foot's flexibility. Supination locks the subtalar joint, increasing the foot's rigidity.

Cavus feet are relatively supinated and the medial longitudinal arch is elevated (Fig. 16.17). Claw toes and heel varus may be present in more severe cases. Subtalar motion is decreased. The loss of subtalar motion decreases the ability of the foot to pronate and therefore absorb impact. The increased impact on the lower extremity predisposes the athlete to stress fractures, plantar fasciitis, metatarsalgia, and tender plantar calluses. When clawing of the toes is present, the fat pad cushioning the metatarsal heads is pulled distally. The lack of padding of the metatarsal heads increases the tendency for tender calluses under the metatarsal heads. Symptomatic feet will benefit from an orthotic or a shoe with good shock-absorbing qualities. A metatarsal support decreases pressure on the metatarsal heads and a good arch support decreases tension on the plantar fascia (7,73).

Flat feet, also known as pes planus, are pronated and the medial longitudinal arch is depressed (see Fig. 16.17). With greater degrees of foot pronation, the hindfoot goes into valgus. There are two types of pronated feet, flexible and rigid. Flexible pronated feet have a normal range of motion of the midtarsal joints and have a flattened medial longitudinal arch only on weight bearing. When non–weight-bearing or standing on their toes, the longitudinal arch is present. Rigid pronated feet have limited midtarsal

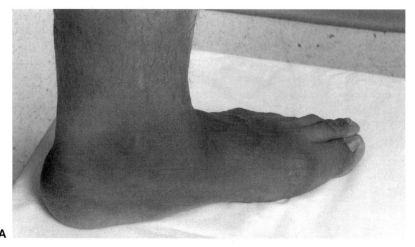

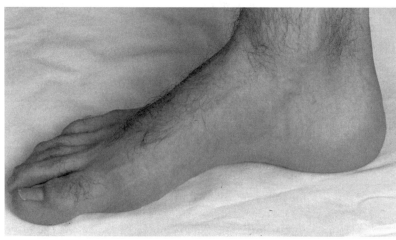

FIG. 16.17. The pronated foot is a flat foot (**A**). Pronation refers to dorsiflexion, abduction and eversion at the subtalar joint. A cavus foot (**B**) is high, arched, and rigid.

motion and continue to have a flattened arch when non–weight-bearing. Only flexible feet will be addressed in this section. Increased pronation increases the excursion of the muscles that control foot pronation and therefore increases the amount of work they do. Work being equal to force times distance. This increased muscular work causes the foot to tire quickly and become uncomfortable when stressed. Orthotics that limit or help to control foot pronation are helpful (7,73).

The Morton's foot has a short hypermobile first metatarsal. The foot goes into pronation during stance phase because the foot must pronate for the first ray to touch the ground. Increased weight is transferred to the second metatarsal, often causing a tender callus under the second metatarsal or a second metatarsal stress fracture. Symptomatic athletes are given an orthotic with an extension under the first metatarsal head, a Morton's extension. This type of orthotic elevates the first metatarsal head transferring more weight to the first metatarsal and decreasing the amount of foot pronation (Fig. 16.18).

Plantar Fasciitis

Plantar fasciitis is an overuse injury in which traction periostitis and micro tears occur in the plantar aponeurosis

where it inserts into the medial tuberosity of the calcaneus and less commonly distally. Among athletes, plantar fasciitis is most commonly seen in runners. The plantar fascia originates from the medial calcaneal tuberosity and flares distally, dividing into five bands, one band for each toe. Each of the five bands further divides into a superficial and a deep band. The superficial band inserts into the intermetatarsal ligament and skin. The deep band inserts into the base of the proximal phalanx. The plantar fascia is the major static stabilizer of the medial longitudinal arch. Because the plantar fascia crosses plantar to the toe MP joints, dorsiflexion of the toes tightens the plantar fascia and increases the height of the medial arch, the windlass effect (Fig. 16.19). Plantar fasciitis is commonly associated with cavus feet, pronated feet, and tight heel cords. Pronated feet cause increased tension on the plantar fascia during midstance when the foot pronates and the arch drops. In cavus feet, the inability of the foot to pronate and absorb some of the impact of heel strike increases the stress on the plantar fascia. Tight heel cords limit ankle dorsiflexion and increase midfoot dorsiflexion (pronation) forces.

The athlete presents with the gradual onset of plantar heel pain, worse with the first few steps in the morning, but quickly improving and gradually worsening as the

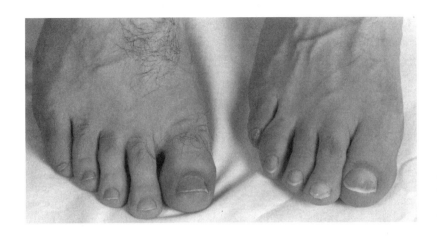

FIG. 16.18. The hyperpronation of Morton's foot (*right*) is secondary to a short first ray, which does not bear weight unless the foot is pronated. A normal foot is shown on the left for comparison.

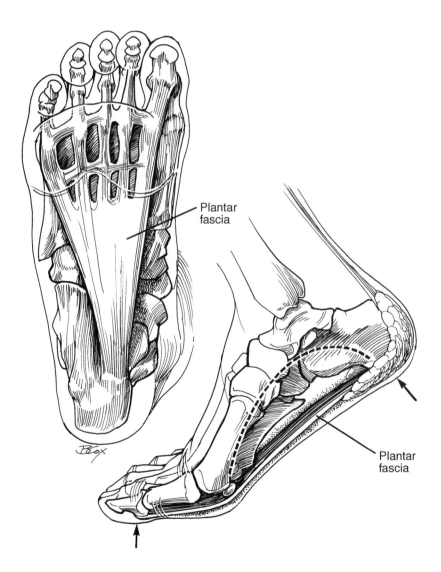

Plantar fascia

Plantar fascia

FIG. 16.19. The examiner palpates the tender plantar fascia with his thumb. *Arrows* show the area that is removed.

day progresses. Standing after prolonged sitting is often very painful. The pain can radiate into the arch or up the leg. Often there is a history of rapid increase in mileage or hill training. On examination, the athlete is tender over the distal medial aspect of the medial calcaneal tuberosity. Occasionally, acute tears of the plantar fascia are seen. These tend to be associated with flexible flat feet and the tenderness extends over the medial plantar fascia in the area of the arch, but this is also rarely seen in plantar fasciitis.

Radiographs may be taken to rule out stress fractures and tumors. Calcaneal spurs seen on radiographs are within the flexor brevis origin, not the plantar fascia. Fifty percent of patients with plantar fasciitis have calcaneal spurs, but 15% of the general population also have spurs and the incidence of spurs increases with age (31). The calcaneal spur is therefore possibly associated with, but not the source of, plantar fascial pain (see Fig. 16.5A).

Rheumatologic workup may be performed on recalcitrant cases to rule out a systemic arthritides as a cause of the plantar fasciitis. Nerve entrapment, heelpad atrophy and gout must also be considered as the etiology of the pain.

Treatment starts with relative rest. Decrease the intensity and duration of training or switch to low-impact exercises, such as biking, swimming, and water running. Icing, NSAIDs, Achilles stretching and viscoelastic heel pads are started. Orthotics are prescribed if pronated feet are found. If there is no improvement in 4 to 6 weeks, a steroid injection or ionophoresis with cortisone cream is considered. Recalcitrant cases are prescribed a night splint, which holds the ankle at 5 degrees of dorsiflexion (108). Four to 6 weeks of cast immobilization may be tried. With conservative therapy, 90% will resolve in less than a year. The recovery is measured in months and the athlete must be informed of the prolonged nature of the recovery period (56).

Surgical treatment may be considered only after 6 to 12 months of adequate conservative therapy. Surgical treatment involves a complete plantar fascial release through a medial incision. Postoperatively, the athlete is placed in a non–weight-bearing cast boot for 2 weeks, then gradually resumes weight bearing and starts a program of strengthening and stretching. Maximum improvement is reached in 3 to 6 months (56).

Lisfranc Joint Sprain

The tarsometatarsal joint is the articulation between the tarsals, the cuneiforms and cuboid, and the metatarsals. The medial three metatarsals articulating with their respective cuneiforms and the lateral two metatarsals with the cuboid. The middle cuneiform is shorter than the other cuneiforms so the base of the second metatarsal is in a recess formed by the three cuneiforms. This is a very

stable configuration. The second to the fifth metatarsal bases are connected by plantar and dorsal intermetatarsal ligaments. There are no intermetatarsal ligaments between the first and second metatarsals. The Lisfranc ligament is a plantar ligament that connects the medial cuneiform to the base of the second metatarsal. The interval between the first and second metatarsal is therefore an area of relative weakness (89).

There are three mechanisms of injury to the tarsometatarsal joint: crushing, abduction/pronation, and axial loading. Abduction/pronation injuries most commonly occur with a quick turn that abducts the foot. Sailboarding is another common mechanism. While sailboarding the forefeet are strapped to the board. Falling backward forces the foot into abduction and equinus rupturing the ligaments of the tarsal metatarsal joint.

With axial loading, the metatarsals plantar flex with respect to the tarsals, and the dorsal, then plantar, ligaments rupture. This occurs either by landing onto an equinus foot or someone falling on the heel of a foot in equinus (6,28,78,89,109).

On examination, there is swelling and tenderness about the midfoot. With the ankle and hindfoot fixed, the forefoot is passively pronated and abducted. Tenderness on performing this maneuver is specific for a tarsometatarsal injury (78).

Radiographic evaluation includes an AP, lateral, and internal oblique. An external oblique is important to evaluate the relationship of the first and second metatarsal bases. Widening of this interval greater than 2 mm indicates an unstable injury. Widening is often associated with the avulsion of a small piece of the medial cuneiform or the second metatarsal. On the AP and oblique views, the medial border of the middle cuneiform should be directly in line with the medial border of the second metatarsal base. On the lateral view, the top of the metatarsal should be in line with the top of the cuneiforms. Weight-bearing or stress views are performed if the routine radiographs are normal (28,78,89).

If no widening or malalignment are present on routine and stress radiographs in suspected grade II or greater sprains, the foot is immobilized in a cast for 6 weeks (28). Our experience has been that it will take 2 to 3 months to return to athletics after this injury. If any widening or malalignment is present, the joint is reduced either closed or through a dorsal longitudinal incision over the first interspace. The joint is held reduced with a 4.0 cancellous or 3.5 cortical screw. The athlete is then placed in a cast boot and allowed toe-touch weight bearing for 6 weeks. The boot is removed daily for gentle active range of motion (ROM) of the foot and ankle. At 6 weeks, partial weight bearing in the cast boot is allowed. At 12 weeks, bracing is discontinued and the screw is removed. Full weight bearing is allowed once the screw is removed (6,28,78,89).

Fractures of the Fifth Metatarsal

There are three common types of fractures that occur in the fifth metatarsal: an avulsion fracture of the tuberosity, a Jones fracture and the previously discussed stress fracture of the diaphysis.

Avulsion Fracture of the Fifth Metatarsal

An avulsion fracture of the fifth metatarsal tuberosity occurs with an inversion injury of the hindfoot. The lateral band of the plantar aponeurosis inserts into the tuberosity of the fifth metatarsal and is responsible for this fracture, not the peroneus brevis as previously thought. This is proven by the fact that the lateral band inserts only into the tip of the tuberosity versus the peroneus brevis, which inserts broadly over the tuberosity. Second, if it was a tendon avulsion, a larger displacement of the fragments would be expected (62). The fracture may be extraarticular or intraarticular. Extraarticular fractures are the most common (Fig. 16.20). An os peroneum is present in 15% of the population and may be mistaken for a fracture (48). The athlete presents with a history of an inversion injury to the ankle and foot, and acute onset of pain in the midlateral foot. Tenderness and swelling are localized to the base of the fifth metatarsal. X-rays will demonstrate an avulsion of the tuberosity. Os peroneum are distinguished from fractures by the following features: Os peroneum have smooth rounded surfaces and do not appear to "fit"

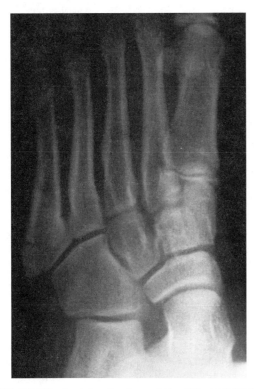

FIG. 16.20. Avulsion fracture of the fifth metatarsal.

back onto the metatarsal. Treatment is symptomatic because even if a nonunion occurs, it is rarely symptomatic. A short-leg walking cast, hard-soled shoe or just a compression wrap may be used. If the fracture is intraarticular and involves greater than 30% of the articular surface, or there is a greater than 2 mm intraarticular step-off, then open reduction and internal fixation is recommended to prevent arthritis of the metatarsal cuboid joint (62). If a symptomatic nonunion occurs, surgical excision of the avulsed fragment is curative.

Rarely, the sural nerve becomes entrapped in the fracture callus causing dysesthesia distal to the area of entrapment and a Tinel's sign is present at the level of entrapment. Surgical release of the nerve from the callus will improve these symptoms (48,62).

Jones Fracture

A Jones fracture is an acute transverse or short oblique fracture at the fifth metatarsal metaphyseal, diaphyseal junction between the insertion of the peroneus brevis and peroneus tertius. Medial comminution is common, but the fracture is usually not displaced (62). There are no prodromal symptoms and the fracture occurs with an inversion injury to a plantar flexed foot. These fractures have a significant risk of nonunion. Treatment is a non–weight-bearing short leg cast for 6 to 8 weeks. Longer periods of immobilization are commonly necessary. Because of the risk of prolonged immobilization and nonunion, primary surgical stabilization is a consideration in an athlete. A single 4.5-cannulated or malleolar screw is placed percutaneously through the tip of the tuberosity, across the fracture site and into the shaft of the metatarsal (Fig. 16.21A,B).

Tarsal Tunnel Syndrome

Tarsal tunnel syndrome is a rare condition caused by the compression of the posterior tibial nerve in the tarsal tunnel. The tarsal tunnel is a fibro-osseus tunnel posterior to the medial malleolus. Because of the lack of compliance of the fibro-osseus tunnel, any condition that increases the volume of the contents within the tunnel will cause a compression of the posterior tibialis nerve. Contained within the tarsal tunnel are the tibialis posterior, the flexor digitorum longus, posterior tibial artery and vein, the posterior tibial nerve, and the flexor hallucis longus (see Fig. 16.9). The etiology of tarsal tunnel includes posttraumatic changes, tenosynovitis, lipoma, ganglion cyst, varicosities, and systemic arthritis (20).

Tarsal tunnel presents with the insidious onset of an intermittent burning sensation and/or anesthesia over the plantar aspect of the foot. Symptoms increase with activity and over the course of the day. Removal of shoes, elevation of the foot, massage, and walking may help to

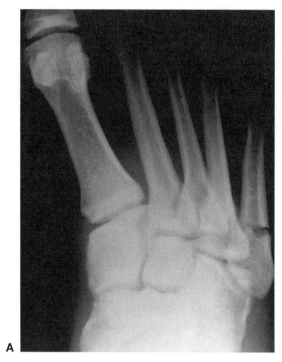
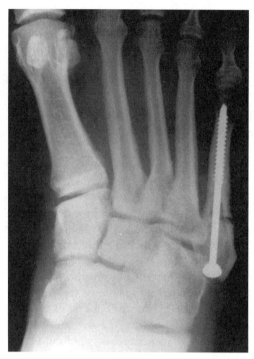

A   B

FIG. 16.21. A: Fracture of the fifth metatarsal at the metaphyseal-diaphyseal junction. **B:** Fixation of the fifth metatarsal fracture with a malleolar screw.

relieve the symptoms. Night pain may be present and the pain may radiate proximally. Motor weakness is uncommon and difficult to demonstrate. Percussion of the tibial nerve within the tarsal tunnel may reproduce the symptoms, Tinnel's sign. Compression to the tarsal tunnel for 60 seconds is another provocative maneuver. Inversion or eversion of the foot occasionally recreates the symptoms.

Electrodiagnostic studies are specific for tarsal tunnel, but not very sensitive. At best, using sensory nerve conduction, the sensitivity is only 90.5%. Meaning 9.5% of the time the diagnosis will be missed. Motor conduction is worse, being only 54.4% sensitive. So although a positive study confirms the diagnosis, a negative study does not rule it out (20).

Conservative therapy involves rest, NSAIDs, immobilization, steroid injections, and orthotics to correct any heel varus or valgus deformity (20).

Approximately 65% will fail conservative therapy and require surgical intervention. Surgery involves incising the flexor retinaculum, which makes up the posterior aspect of the tarsal tunnel, thereby decompressing the tarsal tunnel. Any mass lesions present are also excised. Although some studies have shown 90% will have a good or excellent result, we have found the results of a decompression to be unpredictable (20).

Morton's Neuroma

A Morton's neuroma is a neuroma incontinuity caused by irritation of the common digital nerve as it courses plantar to the deep transverse intermetatarsal ligament. It most commonly affects the third interspace where the medial and lateral plantar nerves coalesce. This is also the most mobile interspace. The second interspace is the next most common (41).

A Morton's neuroma presents with the gradual onset of pain and paresthesia in the affected web space with weight bearing. It is relieved by removing the shoe and massaging the foot. Pain radiates between the toes and decreased sensation in the web space may be noted. When severe, the pain may radiate up the foot or leg.

On exam, the foot is maximally tender between metatarsal heads. Palpation of the affected interspace will cause radiation of the pain to one or both toes. Hypesthesia may be present at the affected interspace (66). The finding of a Mulder's click is diagnostic. This exam is performed by alternately squeezing and releasing the metatarsals together while pressing on the plantar aspect of the tender interspace. If a neuroma is present, the plantar pressure will press the neuroma into the interspace and squeezing the metatarsals will squeeze the neuroma out of the interspace causing pain and a clicking sensation. A click without pain is a negative exam.

Initial treatment consists of shoewear modification. Flat-heeled shoes with a wide toe box and metatarsal pads placed just proximal to the metatarsal heads are used. Steroid injections may be helpful with 30% getting complete relief and 50% temporary (42). The number of steroid injections should however be limited because of the risk of fat-pad atrophy.

For refractory cases, excision of the neuroma carries an 80% chance of success, but only 25% can wear any type of shoe at any time. Most will be limited in their ability to wear narrow high-heeled shoes. The approach to the nerve can be either plantar or dorsal. A dorsal incision removes the possibility of a tender plantar scar. With the dorsal incision the metatarsals are spread apart and the intermetatarsal ligament is incised. The neuroma will be just plantar of the intermetatarsal ligament. The nerve is then transected 1 to 2 cm proximal to the neuroma and the neuroma excised. A compressive dressing and wooden shoe are used until 3 weeks postoperatively (66).

Sesamoid Injuries

Sesamoid injuries are most commonly found in long-distance runners with medial sesamoid being most commonly involved. Sesamoiditis, osteochondritis, stress fractures of partite and nonpartite sesamoid and metatarsal-sesamoid arthritis all present similarly. The athlete complains of pain over the affected sesamoid. Tenderness is reproduced by direct pressure on the sesamoid and forced passive metatarsal phalangeal (MP) extension. Radiographs and a bone scan are useful in diagnosis of sesamoid problems.

Sesamoiditis is an inflammation of the sesamoid. Radiographs are normal, but the bone scan is hot.

Osteochondritis is avascular necrosis of the sesamoid. Radiographs show mottling, fragmentation, and collapse of the sesamoid, but in early cases may be negative. The bone scan is hot. When diagnosed, it is important to bone-scan the opposite foot to determine if it is also involved or ''at risk.''

Sesamoiditis and osteochondritis are treated with a custom orthotic with a firm arch support, a J pad and a Morton's extension. The orthotic controls pronation, decreasing the pressure on the medial sesamoid. The J pad provides a relief for the tender sesamoid, and the Morton's extension prevents MP dorsiflexion. The orthotic should be worn for a minimum of 6 months even if the symptoms quickly resolve. If the symptoms are not relieved by a minimum of 6 months of full-time orthotic wear, excision of the sesamoid is considered. After excision, the athlete is kept non–weight-bearing in a splint for 1 week. Gentle range of motion is started at 1 week postoperatively and toe stands, toe curls, and aggressive range of motion started at 2 weeks. Return to full activity is gradually started after 6 weeks (85).

Nondisplaced fractures and stress fractures are treated with the same orthotic or a short leg cast with dorsal and plantar toe plates depending on the degree of symptoms. A fracture is distinguished from a partite sesamoid radiographically. Bipartite sesamoids have sclerotic, smooth margins. Ten percent of the population have a bipartite tibial sesamoid. If one side is bipartite, there is a 25% chance of the other side also being bipartite. The fibular sesamoid is rarely partite (1%). Stress fractures may or may not radiographically demonstrate callus formation, but the bone scan will be hot (85,86). If the fracture does not heal with 3 to 4 months of casting or orthotics, a complete or partial excision is considered.

Metatarsal-sesamoid arthritis is demonstrated best on a sesamoid axial. The bone scan is also hot. Sesamoid arthritis is treated symptomatically with the orthotic and NSAID.

Sesamoid bursitis is distinguished from sesamoid injury by the tender area being tender to lateral pinch. Erythema and swelling are also commonly present. It is treated with rest, ice, NSAID and occasionally a steroid injection or steroid ionophoresis. Recurrent protracted bursitis over the tibial sesamoid may benefit from a excision of the sesamoid.

Sesamoid osteomyelitis must be considered in all cases of sesamoid pain. The athlete should be asked if any puncture wounds to the foot have occurred. The athlete's erythrocyte sedimentation rate will be elevated and a bone scan hot. This is treated by excising the infected sesamoid.

Turf Toe

Turf toe is a dislocation or subluxation of the first metatarsal phalangeal joint secondary to hyperextension. The incidence of this injury significantly increased with the increased use of artificial turf. It is most commonly seen in offensive linemen, tight ends and wide receivers. With forced hyperextension of the first metatarsal phalangeal joint, the dorsal proximal portion of the proximal phalanx impacts against the dorsal metatarsal head, occasionally causing a compression fracture of the metatarsal head, which may progress to hallux rigidus. With further hyperextension, the plantar plate and metatarsosesamoid ligaments tear, progressing to tearing of the collateral ligaments. Sesamoid fractures rarely also occur. Initial treatment is ice, elevation, NSAIDs, gentle motion, and a hard-sole shoe. Taping the toe to prevent extension, placing a spring steel plate in the forepart of the shoe or fabricating an orthotic with a Morton's extension will protect the injury on returning to competition (88,89).

Hallux Rigidus

Hallux rigidus is an arthritic condition of the first metatarsal phalangeal joint in which osteophytes are present on the metatarsal head dorsally and laterally (Fig. 16.22). This causes pain with dorsiflexion, swelling, and loss of dorsiflexion. Irritation of the dorsal medial sensory nerve is also common. For athletes, hallux rigidus may be secondary to repeated metatarsal phalangeal joint injuries, such as turf toe. The majority will have an insidious onset of symptoms without any history of a specific injury.

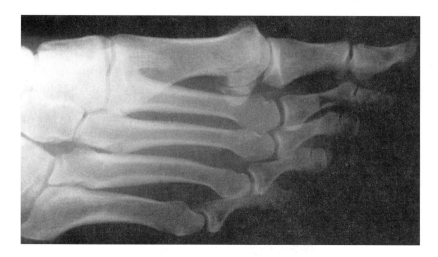

FIG. 16.22. The early radiographic manifestation of hallux rigidus is a dorsal osteophyte.

Conservative treatment involves preventing dorsiflexion of the toe and increasing the size of the toe box to accommodate the increased size of the joint. Rocker bottom shoes, orthotics with a Morton's extension, and a spring steel insert into the sole of the shoe are treatment options. The goal of operative treatment is to relieve the dorsal impingement. A chilectomy works well in the majority of athletes with mild to moderate loss of dorsiflexion. With a chilectomy, the lateral osteophyte is debrided and the dorsal 20% to 30% of the metatarsal head is excised. The dorsal metatarsal head being excised until 60 to 70 degrees of dorsiflexion is possible. Postoperatively the athlete wears a stiff-soled shoe for 7 to 10 days and immediately works on active and passive range of motion of the MP joint. Maximum improvement is seen by 3 to 4 months. If after the chilectomy, dorsiflexion is still not adequate, pain continues on MP dorsiflexion and good MP plantar flexion is present, a Moberg procedure is indicated. A Moberg procedure is a dorsal closing wedge osteotomy of the proximal phalanx. Up to 25 degrees of dorsiflexion may be obtained with this procedure. This should not be performed at the same time as the chilectomy because a chilectomy requires early motion and a Moberg procedure requires immobilization. If severe arthritic changes are present or other operative procedures have failed, an MP fusion is indicated. After a fusion, the athlete will be able to return to athletics but probably not at a highly competitive level. A Keller resection arthroplasty may also be considered, but does not do as well compared to fusions and should be considered only in relatively inactive individuals (67).

Hallux Valgus

Hallux valgus, also known as a bunion, is defined as lateral deviation of the great toe at the MP joint with prominence of the first metatarsal head medially. Complaints are initially attributable to the inflamed tender bursa that forms over the medial prominence secondary to pressure from the shoe. With progression of the great toes' lateral deviation, the joint becomes incongruous, resulting in arthritic changes in the joint, and the toe flexors become ineffective. Shoes with a small toe box, pointed toe box and/or high heels increase symptoms and probably cause progression of the deformity. Pronated feet and feet with a short first metatarsal also contribute to symptoms and progression of the deformity.

The treatment is proper fitting shoes with an adequate toe box and a good arch support. A shoe-maker's swan may be used to selectively stretch the shoe in the area of the bunion. If excessive foot pronation is present, an orthotic is prescribed. If a short first metatarsal is present, an orthotic with an extension under the first metatarsal head or Morton's extension is prescribed. Web space pads placed between the first and second toe may be helpful. If the symptoms are not controlled by conservative means surgical correction may be considered. Severe or progressive deformities need to be addressed early because arthritic changes or functional rigidus may ensue. In the majority of cases, a chevron ostotomy is our procedure of choice (Fig. 16.23). Postoperatively, the athlete wears a wood-sole shoe for 4 weeks, then a wide, deep running shoe for 6 to 8 weeks. Return to athletics can be expected at 4 to 6 months. Even after surgical correction, proper shoe fit and orthotics are necessary to prevent recurrence of the deformity.

Lesser Toe Deformities

The mallet toe deformity is flexion of the distal interphalangeal joint. The second toe is the most commonly affected because it is usually the longest. Direct pressure of the shoe box against the tip of the toe causes the toe to flex. Pressure is placed on the tip of the toe rather than the toe pad causing a callus on the tip of the toe and/or a nail deformity.

The hammer toe deformity is a flexion of the proximal interphalangeal joint as it is flexed with or without hyper-

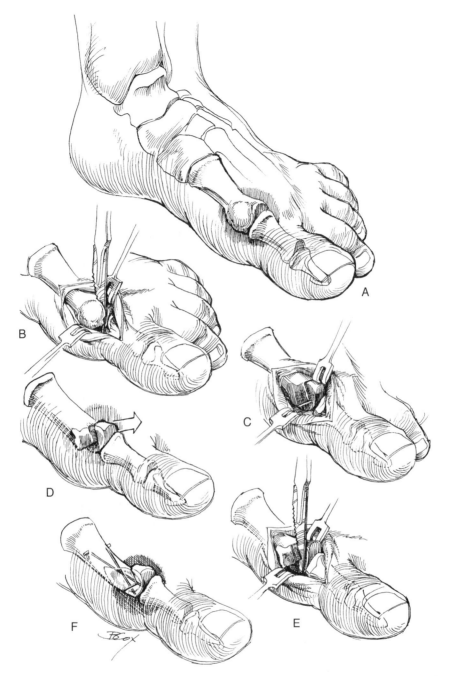

FIG. 16.23. Chevron osteotomy. **A:** Medial skin and capsular incision. **B:** Removal of the medial eminence. **C:** Chevron osteotomy. **D:** Lateral displacement of the distal fragment. **E:** Removal of the prominent portion of the proximal metatarsal. **F:** Stabilization with K-wires.

extension of the metatarsal phalangeal joint. Again the second toe is most commonly involved and the most common etiology is buckling of the toes secondary to poor shoe fit. A bunion deformity may cause the second toe to hammer. Tender calluses form over the dorsal proximal interphalangeal (PIP) joint and the plantar metatarsal head.

The claw toe deformity is a flexion of both the proximal and distal interphalangeal joint and hyperextension of the metatarsal phalangeal joints. Generally, all four toes are

involved and is secondary to a muscle imbalance between the intrinsic and extrinsic muscles of the foot. Simultaneous contraction of the long toe flexors and extensors without contraction of the intrinsics will produce clawing of the toes. Claw toes may be associated with neuromuscular disorders (e.g., Charcot-Marie-Tooth, Friedreich ataxia, and multiple sclerosis), arthritis (e.g., rheumatoid and psoriatic), insensitive feet (e.g., diabetes), or be a residual of a posterior compartment syndrome. The majority of athletes are idiopathic. Clinically, athletes present with painful calluses over the dorsum of the PIP joints and the plantar aspect of the metatarsal heads.

Treatment of lesser toe deformities begins with improving shoe fit. The toe box must be wide and high enough to accommodate the toes. With claw toes, a custom shoe may be necessary. Metatarsal pads or a metatarsal bar are placed just proximal to the symptomatic metatarsal head or a custom-molded shoe insert made. This relieves some of the pressure on the metatarsal heads. Adhesive pads may be placed over tender dorsal calluses and the tip of the toe. Tubular cushions are also helpful. Daily manipulation of the toes is performed to prevent a fixed deformity.

If shoe modifications fail and a fixed deformity is present, a resection arthroplasty is performed on the contracted PIP or distal interphalangeal (DIP) joint. An extensor tenotomy is performed at the MP joint if necessary to correct the MP hyperextension deformity. The resected joint is reduced and a K-wire is used to immobilize the joint. At 6 weeks. the K-wire is removed and normal activity resumed. The resected joint will usually have a 15-degree arc of motion. Full activity can be expected at 3 months.

Rarely, claw toe deformities are dynamic and no fixed contractures are present. In these cases, we perform a Girdlestone procedure. The long toe flexors are detached from their insertion and reattached dorsal to the proximal phalanx. This reverses the deforming forces. The transferred tendon flexes the MP and extends the PIP joint.

SKIN PROBLEMS

Blisters

Blisters are caused by friction on the skin. The resultant shear stress separates the skin into two layers with fluid exuding into the space between the layers. In areas where the skin is thin, such as over the Achilles tendon, the separation occurs between the epidermis and dermis. Where the skin is thick, such as the sole of the foot, the separation occurs within the epidermis (Fig. 16.24). Blisters are prevented by proper fitting shoes, gradual breaking in of new shoes, placing moleskin/adhesive tape over areas at risk and lubricating friction areas with petroleum jelly. Acrylic socks are better at preventing blisters than cotton.

Once a blister has occurred, treatment is tailored to its size and location. Small blisters, which are not causing much discomfort, may be protected with a felt or foam donut. Larger blisters, greater than 5 mm, especially those on weight-bearing surfaces, are drained with a sterile needle. The overlying skin is left in place as a biological dressing. Antibiotic ointment is applied and a dressing taped over the blister. Second skin or similar synthetic porous membranes when applied over the blister will help to decrease friction. If the blister is ruptured, the blister roof is excised to the edge of the normal tissue. The presence of the torn loose skin could cause extension of the tear into normal skin if not removed. Antibiotic ointment and second skin are then taped over the open wound. This dressing should be changed twice a day (12).

Callus

A callus is an area of thickened skin, more specifically stratum corneum, formed in response to abnormal pressure over a bony prominence or in response to shear stress. The treatment is relief of the abnormal pressure or shear stress and paring down of the callus. The callus may be removed either mechanically, shaving with a razor or sanding with a file or pumice stone, or chemically with salicylic acid impregnated pads or plasters. The pressure is relieved from a plantar callus by placing a metatarsal pad just proximal to the metatarsal head or by fabricating a shoe insert with a relief in the area of the callus. Calluses over the dorsal PIP joint of the toes, found in athletes with hammer or claw toes, are treated with high toe box shoes and stick-on or tubular pads. Pinch calluses are relieved filling the corner formed by the sole and the upper with liquid rubber.

Soft calluses are usually found in the fourth web space and are secondary to pressure between the lateral portion of the fourth proximal phalanx and the medial portion of the head of the fifth proximal phalanx. Treatment is to keep the lesion clean and dry, and place lamb's wool or a pad in the affected web space.

Plantar Warts

Human papilloma virus causes warts. It is spread through direct contact and fomites, such as shower floors. Auto-inoculation causes the spread of warts in a given person. Pressure stimulates their growth and 87% are found over bony prominences. This is probably because the virus gains access through tiny breaks in the skin and these breaks in the skin are more prevalent over weight-bearing or prominent areas. Athletes present with complaints similar to those of calluses. The distinguishing features between a plantar wart and a callus are that warts are tender to lateral pinch and on paring down a wart, tiny capillaries are found within its substance. The natural history is for spontaneous resolution of 60% at 2 years. Paring down the wart may give temporary relief. Over-the-counter salicylic acid preparations may be used with a 45% to 84% chance of permanent cure. If this fails a multitude of other prescription preparations are available. Laser ablation and cryotherapy with liquid nitrogen are

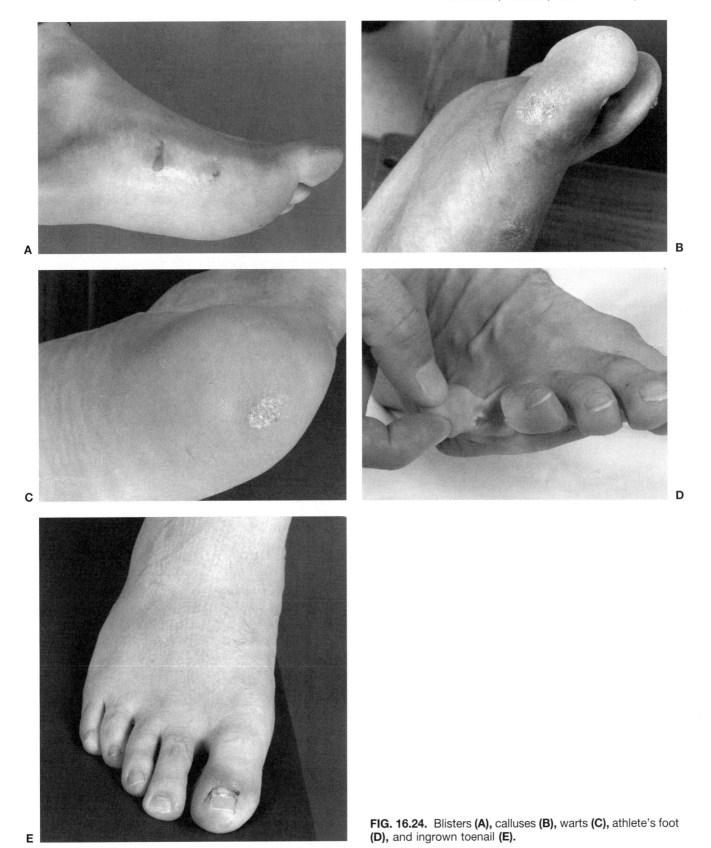

FIG. 16.24. Blisters **(A)**, calluses **(B)**, warts **(C)**, athlete's foot **(D)**, and ingrown toenail **(E)**.

acceptable surgical options. Excision and cauterization have led to the formation of painful scars and are therefore not recommended. No treatment has been found to be 100% effective (40,43).

Athlete's Foot

Athlete's foot is caused by fungi: *Tricophyton rubrum*, *Tricophyton mentagrophytes*, or *Epidermophyton floccosum*. Fungi thrive in the dark, warm, moist areas—showers, locker rooms, towels, and sweaty socks. Transmission is through exposure in common showers and locker rooms. The athlete presents with pruritic vesicular lesions, maceration, blistering, cracking, and/or peeling of the skin of the feet, especially in the warm damp areas between the toes. Contact dermatitis, eczema, and psoriasis may present with similar complaints. If there is any question of the diagnosis, skin scrapings placed on a potassium hydroxide prep will show fungi. Treatment entails gentle removal of the loose skin by gentle rubbing with a towel and the use of an antifungal agent: Lotrimin (clotrimazole), Tinactin (tolnaftate), Miconazole. If no improvement is noted after 4 days of treatment, change the antifungal agent. The antifungal agent should be used for 2 weeks after the symptoms have resolved, otherwise they may recur. In severe cases, oral griseofulvin or ketoconazole may be used. Prevention entails routine cleaning of the showers and locker rooms with a disinfectant, the use of footwear while in showers and locker rooms, thorough drying of the feet after showers, and regular sock changes (43,52).

NAIL PROBLEMS

Subungual Hematoma

A subungual hematoma is a collection of blood or serous fluid under the toenail. It can be produced by direct trauma such as dropping a weight plate onto a toe, which causes a laceration of the underlying nailbed and bleeding under the nail. Indirect trauma as seen in runners with a shoe toe box that is too short is another etiology. The toes move forward in the shoe while running and jam against the front of the toe box, causing a shear stress between the nail and nail bed that can lead to the separation of the nail from its bed and the filling of that potential space with serosanguineous fluid. Having a shoe with adequate space in the toe box will prevent this problem. With either mechanism, a subungual hematoma is painful. Drainage of the hematoma by drilling a hole or burning a hole in the nail with a heated paper clip will relieve the pain. Care must be taken not to remove the nail from its bed or if it is detached to reattach it with a couple of sutures. If the nail is detached and a large nail bed laceration is present, the nail bed laceration should be repaired

with 6-0 chromic sutures prior to reattaching the nail. Reattachment of the nail is important because it acts as a splint for the injured nail bed. Without this splinting a deformity of the nail may occur.

Ingrown Toenail

With an ingrown toenail, the edge of the nail cuts into the nail fold, causing an inflammatory reaction, which often leads to an infection. Poor-fitting shoes and improper nail-trimming are the primary etiologies. When the shoes are too tight the nail is squeezed into the medial and lateral nail folds. Trimming the nail too far back produces a sharp corner, which cuts into the nail fold. Prevention entails proper-fitting shoes and allowing the nail to grow beyond the nail fold. If an ingrown nail becomes infected, the edge of the nail should be elevated out of the nail fold and cotton or gauze placed between the edge of the nail and the nail fold. If the nail cannot be elevated out of the nail fold secondary to swelling or overgrowth of the nail fold, the portion of the nail within the nail fold is longitudinally split off the rest of the nail and removed. Warm soaks and antibiotics are then started. If the problem is recurrent, the offending portion of the nail is removed along with its associated nail matrix.

PEDIATRIC ANKLE AND FOOT EXTREMITY

Ankle Sprain

With ankle injuries in children with open physis, a physeal fracture must always be considered. Tenderness over an open physis, even with a normal radiographic examination, should be treated as a fracture. Normal-appearing initial radiographs may be found with minimal or nondisplaced physeal fractures. Treatment of an ankle with a tender physis and negative radiographs is a short leg walking cast with reexamination in 2 weeks. If the physis is nontender on repeat evaluation, the cast is discontinued. If it continues to be tender, casting is continued for another 2 to 4 weeks. Nondisplaced fractures of the distal fibular or distal tibial physis are treated in a short leg walking cast for 6 weeks.

Kohler's Disease

Kohler's disease is avascular necrosis of the tarsal navicular. Fifty percent will report a single trauma or repetitive trauma as the inciting event. It is most commonly found in children ages 3 to 8 years with a 6-to-1 male-to-female ratio. Females are affected at a younger age than males. Level of activity and body habitus have not been correlated to the occurrence of the disease. Twenty percent to 30% are bilateral (103,106).

The athlete presents with pain in the medial aspect of the longitudinal arch and an antalgic gait. The athlete walks bearing weight only on the lateral side of the foot. Initially the symptoms are intermittent but with progression become continuous. Tenderness is present over the navicular and the talonavicular joint. Soft tissue swelling, synovitis, and joint effusion may be present. If the navicular has not ossified, radiographs of the foot may show nothing except soft-tissue swelling. In ossified navicula, the earliest signs are condensation and increased density of the ossific nuclei. This progresses to flattening and fragmentation and ultimately to restoration of nearly normal contour (Fig. 16.25). The athlete's symptoms correlate with the amount of synovitis and effusion present, not the radiographic stage or level of involvement. The synovitis is secondary to the mechanical distortion and the inflammation secondary to the healing process. Decreasing the synovitis usually decreases the symptoms regardless of the radiologic picture.

Treatment is conservative with varying degrees of immobilization used to decrease the synovitis and an arch support to decrease the forces on the navicular. If significant pain and synovitis are present, treatment is started with 4 to 6 weeks in a short leg walking cast with a well-molded arch. UCBL orthotics are used after casting or in less severe cases. In athletes with mild symptoms and little or no synovitis, medial longitudinal arch supports of felt or rubber can be used. Non–weight-bearing has no effect on the duration of symptoms or the final outcome. Repeat radiographic evaluation should be performed every 3 months with the healing process generally taking 9 to 12 months. The prognosis is very good with the majority having no residual deformity or disability (103,106).

Freiberg's Disease

Freiberg's disease is avascular necrosis of the metatarsal head. The second metatarsal head is involved 62% to 82% of the time. The third metatarsal is the next most commonly affected. It is most commonly found in the 11- to 17-year age range and has a 5-to-1 female-to-male ratio. This is the only osteochondrosis more common in women than men. It is bilateral in 6.6% of cases (51,57).

Dorsal trabecular stress, the impingement of the proximal phalanx on the metatarsal head during MP dorsiflexion, is thought to be the etiology of the avascular necrosis. The second MP joint dorsiflexes the most during the toe-off phase of gait because the second ray is usually the longest. This accounts for the predilection for second-ray involvement.

This condition may be completely asymptomatic and found only incidentally. When symptomatic, the athlete complains of activity-related forefoot pain. On examination, there is synovitis about the affected joint. Tenderness is found with palpation of the involved metatarsal head and at the extremes of the metatarsal phalangeal joint range of motion. An antalgic gait with avoidance of weight bearing on the involved metatarsal may be present. Symptoms may wax and wane. Increased symptoms may be noted with trauma or increased activity. If the condition progresses, the joint becomes enlarged, the range of motion decreases and the pain becomes more constant.

In its early stage, radiographs may be normal. A bone scan with pinhole collimation will, however, show an area of hypoactivity surrounded by a hyperactive collar. With progression of the disease, collapse and flattening of the head, then loose body formation and arthritic changes occur (Fig. 16.26).

Treatment is initially conservative. A short leg cast and/or non–weight-bearing may be used for severe symptoms. Metatarsal pads, metatarsal bars, and orthotics are used to decrease the pressure on the involved metatarsal head. Surgical treatment is a dorsiflexion osteotomy that elevates the metatarsal head, thereby reducing the pressure on the head and debridement of the joint, removing the loose bodies, and trimming the osteophytes (51,57).

Sever's Disease

In the past, Sever's disease was thought to be avascular necrosis of the calcaneal apophysis. Subsequent studies have shown that the increased density and irregular ossification of the calcaneal apophysis are normal findings (Fig. 16.27). Sever's disease is therefore not an osteochondritis or osteochondrosis, but instead Achillis tendi-

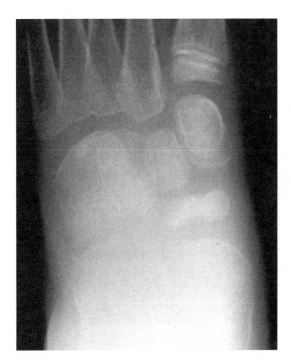

FIG. 16.25. Kohler's disease is seen radiographically as collapse and sclerosis of the navicular. (Photograph courtesy of Perry L. Schoenecker, M.D.)

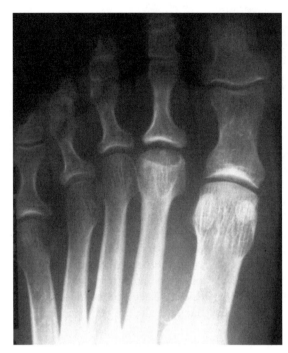

FIG. 16.26. Freiberg's disease is avascular necrosis of the metatarsal head that leads to collapse and flattening of the metatarsal head.

nitis, subcutaneous bursitis, or retrocalcaneal bursitis. It is seen in children 7 to 10 years of age. It is more commonly seen in males and associated with very active obese or stocky children. The condition is usually unilateral.

The athlete presents with activity-related posterior heel pain with associated limping. Tenderness is most often found at the insertion of the Achilles into the calcaneus. Tight heel cords are commonly present.

The treatment is symptomatic. Activity is decreased. A $^1/_4$-inch heel lift is used and the heel counter is modified to reduce pressure on the tender area. Heelcord stretching is started and continued until the athlete has an easy 15 to 20 degrees of dorsiflexion (104,107).

Tarsal Coalition

A tarsal coalition is a failure of segmentation between two bones of the foot. The union between the two bones may be fibrous, cartilaginous, or bony. It is present in 1% to 2% of the population and bilateral in approximately 50%. Calcaneonavicular and talocalcaneal coalitions are equal in incidence and together make up 90% of all coalitions in the foot. Only 33% to 53% of coalitions are symptomatic. Talocalcaneal coalitions usually become symptomatic between the age of 12 to 16 years and calcaneal navicular between the age of 8 to 12 years. The occurrence of symptoms is correlated with ossification of the coalition. The coalition restricts the motion of the

subtalar joints causing abnormal motion and forces across the other joints of the foot (13,82).

The athlete presents with the insidious onset of pain about the subtalar and tarsal area. An ankle sprain or other injury may be the precipitating factor. Symptoms are often related to weight gain, increased activity or athletic participation and alleviated with rest. On examination, the majority present with a rigid planovalgus foot, but rarely it presents with a rigid cavo-varus foot (82,101). The athlete will have decreased to absent motion of the subtalar joint. Peroneal spasticity may be present.

Radiographic evaluation begins with AP, lateral, and internal oblique views. The internal oblique radiograph will demonstrate a calcaneonavicular coalition (Fig. 16.28A,B). A talonavicular coalition or other coalition should be suspected if talonavicular beaking, flattening of the lateral talar process, increased trabeculation under the sustentaculum tali (halo sign), poor visualization of the middle or posterior subtalar joint, or beaking of the calcaneus at the calcaneal cuboid joint is found. A Harris-Beath view visualizes the posterior and middle subtalar joint and should demonstrate a talocalcaneal coalition. A CT scan or MRI will best demonstrate the anatomy of a coalition (82) (see Fig. 16.28B).

Conservative therapy consists of NSAIDs and shoe modifications. Modifications include a Thomas heel with medial wedge and arch support or a soft Plastizote insert. If this fails, the foot is placed in a short leg walking cast for 3 to 6 weeks followed by shoe modifications (13,82). Return to competitive athletics is usually not possible with only conservative management (75).

If the athlete has failed 2 courses of casting, surgical

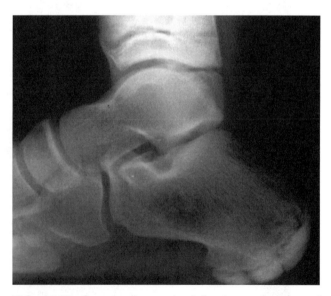

FIG. 16.27. Sever's disease is defined as sclerosis and fragmentation of the calcaneal apophysis. This was originally thought to be secondary to avascular necrosis, but is now known to be a normal variant. (Photograph courtesy of Perry L. Schoenecker, M.D.)

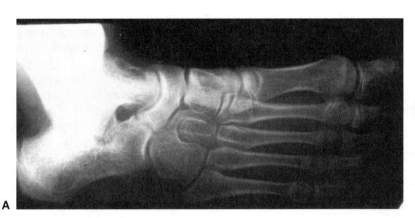
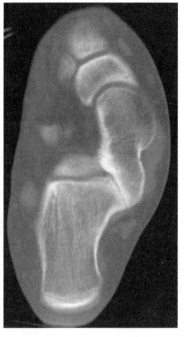

FIG. 16.28. A: Calcaneo-navicular coalition is well demonstrated on an internal rotation oblique radiograph. **B:** Talocalcaneal coalitions are best seen on computed tomography (CT) scan. (Photographs courtesy of Perry L. Schoenecker, M.D.)

intervention is considered. Surgical treatment depends on the condition of the adjacent tarsal joints, if they are arthritic, a triple arthrodesis is performed and a return to athletics should not be expected. The presence of a talar beak without associated arthritis is not a contraindication to a resection (74). If there are no significant arthritic changes, calcaneonavicular bars may be resected and the muscle belly of the extensor brevis interposed. Calcaneo-navicular bar excision in a foot without arthritic changes can expect an 85% chance of a good or excellent result and an 80% to 100% chance of returning to competitive sports (34,74,75).

If no arthritic changes are present and less than 50% of the joint is involved, talocalcaneal bars are treated with resection and fat interposition. A return to competitive athletics can be expected (34). A subtalar arthrodesis or a Grice extraarticular arthrodesis is performed if there is greater than 50% involvement of the joint (82). Return to athletics is usually not possible after a fusion.

RUNNING SHOES

The choice of an appropriate running shoe is important in both treating and preventing injury. A running shoe must be comfortable, cushion the impact of heel strike, provide stability and help control motion (27). Because of the variability in types of feet, running style, and terrain, no one shoe is ideal for every person. By knowing the anatomy of the running shoe, the different characteris-

tics of each shoe may be appreciated and a shoe selected to best fit the runner's needs (Fig. 16.29).

The sole of the shoe is divided longitudinally into the heel, shank, and forepart.

Heel flare width is the width of the heel at its base. Increasing the heel flare width spreads the impact of heel strike over a larger area and increases heel stability. A wider heel flare is of benefit to hard heel runners and athletes with recurrent ankle sprains (54,65). Athletes with pronated feet are adversely affected by a wide heel flare because it increases the rate of foot pronation, which can lead to anterior knee pain and Achilles tendinitis (80).

Heel height: The heel height should be at least 12 to 15 mm. Training shoes have a higher heel than racing shoes. A higher heel increases the shock absorption on heel strike and decreases the tension on the Achilles tendon, but increases overall shoe weight. Athletes who wear high heels daily, have tight heel cords, or have Achilles tendinitis should select shoes with higher heel height (65).

Forepart of the sole: The forepart of the sole should be easily bent and this is an important characteristic. If the forepart is stiff, increased forces are transmitted to the Achilles tendon, tibia, and calf muscles (65).

The sole is also divided into the outsole, midsole, and insole. The outer sole is made of a durable flexible material and comes in many designs. The aggressive tread designs, that is, waffled or studded, are good for both pavement and grass running, whereas the less aggressive designs are not as good for running on grass.

The midsole and wedge: The midsole and wedge are

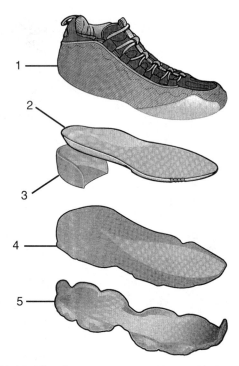

FIG. 16.29. The five components of an athletic shoe. **1. Upper:** the part that covers the foot. It provides comfort, protection, support, and style. **2. Insole (sockliner):** the inside of the shoe on which the foot rests. It provides comfort, cushioning, and arch support. **3. Heel counter:** located in the heel area of the upper, it circles the heel and helps to keep the foot centered and stable. **4. Midsole*:** located underneath the sockliner, it is designed to absorb shock, control motion, and cushion the foot. **5. Outsole*:** the bottom part of the shoe. It provides traction and durability. (*The combination of the midsole and outsole together are crucial in determining the shoe's overall flexibility, stability, and weight.) (Courtesy of Reebok Shoe Company)

the shock absorbers of the shoe. The midsole should run the entire length of the shoe. This shock absorption is particularly important in athletes with cavus feet or metatarsal problems. In pronated feet, a thinner, firmer midsole allows for better control of motion. In the heel, either the midsole thickens or a heel wedge is present. This area absorbs the impact of heel strike. The heel cushion has been shown to lose 30% of its impact-absorbing qualities after 500 miles of running (27). The presence of an air bladder in the heel and midsole may prevent this loss. For any given athlete, the optimal midsole for running on pavement is thicker and more shock-absorbing than one for running on grass or softer surfaces.

The insole: The insole rests between the foot and the midsole. It absorbs perspiration, cushions impact, and supports the foot. The arch support is part of the insole. Having a removable insole is important because it allows the athlete to tailor the shoe to his or her needs through the use of inserts and orthotics.

The arch support: Foot type determines the appropriate arch support. Pronated feet require a low, firm arch sup-

port and cavus feet require a relatively higher, softer arch support (65).

The last: The last is the mold over which the shoe is assembled. A curve-lasted shoe is one in which there is an angle between the heel and forepart. The average runner's feet are moderately curved and most companies' shoes have a 7-degree curve. Higher curves are needed for runners with cavus feet. A straight-lasted shoe is one in which there is little or no angle between the rearfoot and forefoot. Straight-lasted shoes are adequate for most runners and preferred for runners with pronated feet (35) (see Fig. 16.29).

The upper: The upper is the part of the shoe that covers the foot. The upper should be made of lightweight material that allows cooling of the feet.

The heel counter: The heel counter cradles the heel, stabilizing the subtalar joint and preventing excessive heel valgus. A firm heel counter is particularly important in athletes with pronated feet. Extension of the heel counter medially increases the support of the medial longitudinal arch. When selecting a running shoe, it is essential that good heel control is present. The heel should not excessively pronate, slip up and down, or slide back and forth (65,73).

The rear wall depth: The rear wall depth is the height of the heel counter. The rear wall depth must be great enough to control the heel, but not so great that the shoe rubs the medial or lateral malleolus.

The Achilles pad: The Achilles pad is the portion of the heel counter that contacts the Achilles tendon. It should not bite into the Achilles tendon nor irritate the skin.

The tongue: The tongue extends under the laces and should be adequately padded to protect the dorsum of the foot from irritation from the laces.

The saddle: The saddle is the area between the laces and the sole. It tightens the shoe over the instep and helps to support the arch.

The vamp: The vamp is the area between the laces and the toe box. It provides support to the midfoot. This area must be flexible to allow free motion of the metatarsal phalangeal joints.

The toe box: The toe box gives shape to the shoe distally. Increased depth of the toe box is necessary in runners with lesser toe deformities, such as claw toes.

A running shoe should be selected on the basis of comfort, fit, and qualities complementing the runner's foot type. Runners with pronated feet should select a straight-last shoe with a firm midsole and low-firm arch support. Runners with cavus feet should select a curved-last shoe with a soft midsole and a high arch support.

It is best to shop for a shoe in the afternoon, preferably after running because feet can swell with activity from a half to a full size (65). Fitting is started by checking the heel counter. It should be snug and firm, and not dig into the Achilles tendon or malleoli. The calcaneous should not slip or rub excessively. The toe box needs to be roomy enough to allow the toes to wiggle comfortably. There should be at least one-quarter of an inch between the front of the toe box and the longest toe (35). The shoe should be wide enough at the forefoot to allow for the swelling that occurs while running. Once a well-fitting shoe is found, walking and jogging in the shoe determines if it is comfortable and has the desired combination of motion control and cushioning.

REFERENCES

1. Amendola A. Controversies in diagnosis and management of syndesmosis injuries of the ankle. *Foot Ankle* 1992;13(1):44–50.
2. Andrish JT, Bergfeld JA, Walheim J. A prospective study on the management of shin splints. *J Bone Joint Surg* 1974;56-A(8):1697–1700.
3. Andrish JT. The leg. In: DeLee JC, Drez D, eds. *Orthopedics and sports medicine*. Philadelphia: WB Saunders, 1994:1621–1622.
4. Andrish JT. The leg. In: DeLee JC, Drez D, eds. *Orthopedics and sports medicine*. Philadelphia: WB Saunders, 1994:1612.
5. Angermann P. Chronic retrocalcaneal bursitis treated by resection of the calcaneus. *Foot and Ankle* 1990;10(5):285–258.
6. Arntz CT, Veith RG, Hansen ST. Fractures and fracture dislocations of the tarsometatarsal joint. *J Bone Joint Surg* 1988;70-A(2):173.
7. Athletic training and sports medicine. *Am Acad Orthop Surg* 1984:321.
8. Awbrey BJ, Sienkiewicz PS, Mankin HJ. Chronic exercise-induced compartment pressure elevation measured by a miniaturized fluid pressure monitor. *Am J Sports Med* 1988;16(6):610–615.
9. Barrow GW, Saha S. Menstrual irregularities and stress fractures in collegiate female distance runners. *Am J Sports Med* 1988;16(3):209–216.
10. Beals RK, Cook RD. Stress fractures of the anterior tibial diaphysis. *Orthopedics* 1991;14:869–875.
11. Bell S. Intracompartmental pressures on exertion in a patient with popliteal artery entrapment syndrome. *Am J Sports Med* 1985;13(5):365–366.
12. Bergeron BP. A guide to blister management. *Phys Sportsmed* 1995;23(2):37–46.
13. Berman AT, Finn CA, Van Horne J, Fye MA. Tarsal coalition. *Orthopedics* 1990;13:910.
14. Beskin JL, Sanders RA, Hunter SC, Hughston JC. Surgical repair of Achilles tendon ruptures. *Am J Sports Med* 1987;15(1):1–8.
15. Boruta PM, Bishop JO, Braly WG, Tullos HS. Acute lateral ankle ligament injuries: a literature review. *Foot Ankle* 1990;11(2):107–113.
16. Boytim MJ, Fischer DA, Neumann L. Syndesmotic ankle sprains. *Am J Sports Med* 1991;19:294–298.
17. Brill DR. Bone imaging for lower extremity pain in athletes. *Clin Nucl Med* 1983;8:101–106.
18. Carr AJ, Norris SH. The blood supply to the calcaneal tendon. *J Bone Joint Surg* 1989;69B(1):100–101.
19. Casscells SW. Another young athlete with intermittent claudication. *Am J Sports Med* 1983;11(3):180–183.
20. Cimino WR. Tarsal tunnel syndrome: review of the literature. *Foot Ankle* 1990;11(1):47.
21. Clain MR, Baxter DE. Achilles tendinitis. *Foot Ankle* 1992;13(8):482–487.
22. Clement DB, Taunton JE, Smart GW. Achilles tendinitis and peritendinitis: etiology and treatment. *Am J Sports Med* 1984;12(3):179–184.
23. Clemmente CD. *Anatomy: a regional atlas of the human body*, 3rd ed. Baltimore: Urban & Schwarzenberg, 1987.
24. Colville MR, Grondel RJ. Anatomic reconstruction of the lateral ankle ligaments using a split peroneus brevis tendon graft. *Am J Sports Med* 1995;23(2):210.
25. Conti S, Michelson J, Jahass M. Clinical significance of MRI in preoperative planning for reconstruction of posterior tibial tendon ruptures. *Foot Ankle* 1992;13:208–214.
26. Conti SF. Posterior tibial tendon problems in athletes. *Orthop Clin North Am* 1994;25(1):109–121.
27. Cook SD, Kester MA, Brunet ME. Shock absorption characteristics of running shoes. *Am J Sports Med* 1985;13(4):248.
28. Curtis MJ, Myerson M, Szura B. Tarsometatarsal joint injuries in the athlete. *Am J Sports Med* 1993;21(4):497.
29. Dameron TB. Fractures of the proximal fifth metatarsal: selecting the best treatment option. *J Am Acad Orthop Surg* 1995;3(2):110.
30. Davey JR, Rorabeck CH, Fowler PJ. The tibialis posterior compartment. *Am J Sports Med* 1984;12(5):391–397.
31. Davis PF, Severud E, Baxter DE. Painful heel syndrome: results of nonoperative treatment. *Foot Ankle* 1994;15(10):531–535.
32. Detmer DE. Chronic shin splints. *Sports Medicine* 1986;3:436–446.
33. Edwards GS, DeLee JC. Ankle diastasis without fracture. *Foot Ankle* 1984;4(6):306–311.
34. Elkus RA. Tarsal coalition in the young athlete. *Am J Sports Med* 1986;14(6):477.
35. Ellis J. The match game. *Runner's World* 1985;Oct:66.
36. Ferkel RD, Karzel RP, Del Pizzo W, Friedman MJ, Fischer SP. Arthroscopic treatment of anterior/lateral impingement of the ankle. *Am J Sports Med* 1991;19:440–446.
37. Ferkel RD, Fasulo GJ. Arthroscopic treatment of ankle injuries. *Orthop Clin North Am* 1994;25(1):17–32.
38. Flick AB, Gould N. Osteochondritis dissecans of the talus: review of the literature and new surgical approach for medial dome lesions. *Foot Ankle* 1985;2(11):165.
39. Frymoyer JW. Orthopedic knowledge update 4. *Am Acad Orthop Surg* 1993.
40. Glover MG. Plantar warts. *Foot Ankle* 1990;11(3):172–179.
41. Graham CE, Graham DM. Morton's neuroma: a microscopic evaluation. *Foot Ankle* 1984;5(2):150–153.
42. Greenfield J, Rea J Jr., Ilfeld FW. Morton's interdigital neuroma. Indications for treatment by local injections versus surgery. *Clin Orth* 1984;185:142–144.
43. Griffin LY. Common sports injuries of the foot and ankle seen in children and adolescents. *Orthop Clin North Am* 1994;25(1):83–93.
44. Griffin LY. The female athlete. In: DeLee JC, Drez D, eds. *Orthopedics and sports medicine*. Philadelphia: WB Saunders, 1994:362.
45. Grogan DP, Gasser SI, Ogden JA. The painful accessory navicular. *Foot Ankle* 1989;10(3):164–169.
46. Harper MC, Keller TS. A radiographic evaluation of the tibiofibular syndesmosis. *Foot Ankle* 1989;10(03):156–160.
47. Heckman JD. Fractures and dislocations of the foot. In: Rockwood CA, Green DP, Bucholz RW, eds. *Rockwood and Green's fractures in adults*, 3rd ed. New York: JB Lippincott 1991–2060.
48. Heckman JD. Fractures and dislocations of the foot. In: Rockwood CA, Green DP, Bucholz RW, eds. *Rockwood and Green's fractures in adults*, 3rd ed. New York: JB Lippincott, 1991:2156–2159.
49. Heckman MM, Whitesidee TE, Grewe SR, Rooks MD. Compartment pressure in association with closed tibial fractures. *J Bone Joint Surg* 1994;76-A(9):1285.
50. Hedrick MR, McBryde AM. Posterior ankle impingement. *Foot Ankle* 1994;15(1):2–8.
51. Helal B, Gibb P. Freiberg's disease. *Foot Ankle* 1987;8(2):94–102.
52. Hoffman TJ, Schelkun PH. How I manage athlete's foot. *Phys Sportsmed* 1995;23(4):29–32.
53. Hopkison WJ, St. Pierre P, Ryan JB, Wheeler JH. Syndesmosis sprain of the ankle. *Foot Ankle* 1990;10(6):325–331.
54. James SL, Bates BT, Osternig LR. Injuries to runners. *Am J Sports Med* 1978;6(2):40–49.
55. Kannu P, Renstrom P. Treatment for acute tears of the lateral ligaments of the ankle. *J Bone Joint Surg* 1991;73A:305.
56. Karr SD. Subcalcaneal heel pain. *Orth Clin North Am* 1994;25(1):161–173.
57. Katcherian DA. Treatment of Freiberg's disease. *Orthop Clin North Am* 1994;25(1):69.

58. Kaye RA. Stabilization of ankle syndesmosis with a syndesmosis screw. *Foot Ankle* 1989;9(6):290–293.

59. Khan KM, Fuller PJ, Brukner PD, Kearney C, Burry HC. Outcome of conservative and surgical management of navicular stress fractures in athletes. *Am J Sports Med* 1992;20:657–666.

60. Kleiger B. Anterior tibiotalar impingement syndrome in dancers. *Foot Ankle* 1982;3(2):69–73.

61. Konradsen L, Holmer P, Sondergaard L. Early mobilizing treatment of grade III ankle ligament injuries. *Foot Ankle* 1991;12(2):69–73.

62. Lawrence SJ, Botte MJ. Jones fracture and related fractures of the fifth metatarsal. *Foot Ankle* 1993;14(6):358–365.

63. Li GP, Zhang SD, Chen G, Ghen H, Wang AM. Radiographic and histologic analysis of stress fractures in rabbit tibias. *Am J Sports Med* 1985;13:285–294.

64. Lysens RJ. Intermittent claudication in young athletes: popliteal artery entrapment syndrome. *Am J Sports Med* 1983;11(3):177–179.

65. Mann RA, Baxter DE, Lutter LD. Running symposium. *Foot Ankle* 1981;1(4):190–224.

66. Mann RA, Reynolds JC. Interdigital neuroma—a critical analysis. *Foot Ankle* 1983;3(4):238–243.

67. Mann RA. Disorders of the first metatarsal phalangeal joint. *J Am Acad Orthop Surg* 1995;3(1):34–43.

68. Marotta JJ, Micheli LJ. Os trigonum impingement in dancers. *Am J Sports Med* 1992;20:533–536.

69. Martens MA, Backaert M, Vermaut G, Mulier JC. Chronic leg pain due to recurrent compartment syndrome. *Am J Sports Med* 1984;12(2):148–151.

70. Mascaro TB, Swanson LE, Rehabilitation of the foot and ankle. *Orthop Clin North Am* 1994;25(1):147.

71. Matheson GO, Clement DO, McKenzie DC, et al. Stress fractures in athletes. *Am J Sports Med* 1987;15(1):46–58.

72. McCarrroll JR, Schrader JW, Shelbourne KD, Rettig AC, Bisesi MA. Meniscoid lesions of the ankle in soccer players. *Am J Sports Med* 1987;15(3):255–257.

73. McKenzie DC, Clement DB, Tauton JE. Running shoes, orthotics, and injuries. *Sports Medicine* 1985;2:334–347.

74. Micheli LJ, O'Neill DB. Tarsal coalition: a follow-up of adolescent athletes. *Am J Sports Med* 1989;17(4):544.

75. Morgan RC, Crawford AH. Surgical management of tarsal coalition in adolescent athletes. *Foot Ankle* 1986;7(3):183.

76. Micheal RH, Holder LE. The soleus syndrome, a cause of medial tibial stress. *Am J Sports Med* 1985;13(6):87–94.

77. Mubarak SJ, Gould RN, Lee YF, Schmidt DA, Hargens AR. The medial tibial stress syndrome. *Am J Sports Med* 1982;10(4):201–205.

78. Myerson M. The diagnosis and treatment of injuries to the Lisfranc joint complex. *Orthop Clin North Am* 1989;20(4):655.

79. Needleman RL, Skrade DA, Stiehl JB. Effect of syndesmotic screw on ankle motion. *Foot Ankle* 1989;10(1):17–25.

80. Nigg BM, Morlock M. The influence of the lateral heel flare of running shoes on pronation and impact forces. *Med Sci Sports Exerc* 1987;19(3):294.

81. Orava S, Karkpakka J, Taimela S, et al. Stress fracture of the medial malleolus. *J Bone Joint Surg* 1995;77-A(3):362.

82. Pachuda NM, Lasday SD, Jay RM. Tarsal coalition: etiology, diagnosis, and treatment. *J Foot Surg* 1990;39(5):474.

83. Peters JW, Trevino SG, Renstrom PA. Chronic lateral ankle instability. *Foot Ankle* 1991;12(3):182.

84. Philips BB. Traumatic disorders. In: *Campbell's Operative Orthopedics* 8th ed. St. Louis: Mosby Year Book, 1992:1985.

85. Richardson EG. Injuries to the hallucal sesamoid in the athlete. *Foot Ankle* 1987;7(4)230–245.

86. Rodeo SA, Warren RF, O'Brien SJ, Pavlov H, Barnes R. Diastasis of bipartite sesamoid of the first metatarsal phalangeal joint. *Foot Ankle* 1993;14(8):425–434.

87. Rosenberg ZS, Cheung Y, Jahss MH, Noto AM, Norman A. Rupture of posterior tibial tendon. *Radiology* 1988;169:229.

88. Sammarco GJ. Turf toe. *Instr Course Lect* 1993;42:207–212.

89. Schenck Jr RC, Heckman JD. Fractures and dislocations of the forefoot. *J Am Acad Orthop Surg* 1995;3(2):70–78.

90. Schepsis AA, Leach RE. Surgical management of Achilles tendinitis. *Am J Sports Med* 1987;15(4):308–315.

91. Schils JP. Medial malleolar stress fractures in 7 patients. *Radiology* 1992;185:219–221.

92. Scioli MW. Achilles tendinitis. *Orthop Clin North Am* 1994;25(1):177–182.

93. Scranton PE, MC Dermott. Anterior tibiotalar spurs. *Foot Ankle* 1992;125–129.

94. Sella EJ, Lawson JP. Biomechanics of the accessory navicular synchondrosis. *Foot Ankle* 1987;8(3):156–163.

95. Shelbourne K, Fischer D, Rettig A, McCarroll J. Stress fracture of the medial malleolus. *Am J Sports Med* 1988;16(1):60–63

96. Shields CL, Redix L, Brewster CE. Acute tears of the medial head of the gastrocnemius. *Foot Ankle* 1985;5(4):186–190.

97. Sitler M, Ryan J, Wheeler B, et al. The efficacy of a semirigid ankle stabilizer to reduce acute ankle injuries in basketball. A randomized clinical study at West Point. *Am J Sports Med* 1994;22(4):454.

98. Sobel M, Geppert MJ, Olson EJ, Bohne Walker HO. The dynamics of peroneus brevis tendon splits. *Foot Ankle* 1992;13(7):413–422.

99. Stephens MM. Haglund's deformity and retrocalcaneal bursitis. *Foot Ankle* 1994;25(1):41–45.

100. Stoller SM, Hekmat F, Kleiger B. A comparison of the frequency of anterior impingement exostoses of the ankle in dancers and nondancers. *Foot Ankle* 1984;4(4):201–203.

101. Stuecker RD, Bennett JT. Tarsal coalition presenting as a pes cavo-varus deformity: report of three cases and review of the literature. *Foot Ankle* 1993;14(9):540.

102. Surve I, Schwellnus MP, Noakes T, Lombard C. A five fold reduction in the incidence of recurrent ankle sprains in soccer players using the sports-stirrup orthosis. *Am J Sports Med* 1994;22(5):601.

103. Tachdjian MO. *Pediatric orthopedics*, 2nd ed. Philadelphia: WB Sanders, 1990:1003.

104. Tachdjian MO. *Pediatric orthopedics*, 2nd ed. Philadelphia: WB Sanders, 1990:1016.

105. Trevino SG, Davis P, Hecht PJ. Management of acute and chronic lateral ligament injuries of the ankle. *Orth Clin North Am* 25(1):1–16.

106. Trott AW. Developmental disorders. In: Jahass MP, ed. *Jahass disorders of the foot and ankle. Medical and surgical management*. Philadelphia: WB Saunders, 1991:607.

107. Trott AW. Developmental disorders. In: Jahass MP, ed. *Jahass disorders of the foot and ankle. Medical and surgical management*. Philadelphia: WB Saunders, 1991:609.

108. Wapner KL, Sharkey PF. The use of night splints for treatment of recalcitrant plantar fasciitis. *Foot Ankle* 1991;12(3):135–137.

109. Wiley JJ. The mechanism of tarso-metatarsal joint injuries. *J Bone Joint Surg* 1971;53-B(3):474.

110. Woods L. Posterior tibial tendon rupture in athletic people. *Am J Sports Med* 1991;19:495–498.

111. Wredmark T, Carlstedt CA, Bauer H, Saartok T. Os trigone syndrome: a clinical entity in ballet dancers. *Foot Ankle* 1991;11:404–406.

The Injured Athlete, Third Edition,
edited by D. H. Perrin.
Lippincott–Raven Publishers, Philadelphia © 1999.

Appendix A

Sports Medicine Organizations

American Academy of Family Physicians
8880 Ward Parkway
Kansas City, Missouri 64114
816-333-9700

American Academy of Podiatric Sports Medicine
1729 Glastonberry Road
Potomac, Maryland 20854
800-438-3355

American Chiropractic Association Council on Sports Injuries
   and Physical Fitness
2240 NE 202 Street
North Miami Beach, Florida 33180
800-593-3222

American College of Sports Medicine
401 West Michigan Street
Indianapolis, Indiana 46202
317-637-9200

American Medical Society for Sports Medicine
7611 Elmwood Avenue, Suite 203
Middleton, Wisconsin 53562
608-831-4484

American Optometric Association/Sports Vision Section
6430 South Pulaski Road
Chicago, Illinois 60629
708-598-1322

American Orthopaedic Society for Sports Medicine
6300 North River Road, Suite 200
Rosemont, Illinois 60018
847-292-4900

American Osteopathic Academy of Sports Medicine
7611 Elmwood Avenue, Suite 203
Middleton, Wisconsin 53562
608-831-4484

American Physical Therapy Association/Sports Medicine Section
505 King Street, Suite 345
LaCrosse, Wisconsin 54601
800-285-7787

Canadian Academy of Sports Medicine
1600 James Naismith Drive, Suite 502
Gloucester, Ontario K1B 5N4 Canada
613-748-5851

National Athletic Trainers' Association
2952 Stemmons Freeway, Suite 200
Dallas, Texas 75247
800-879-6282

United States Olympic Committee/Sports Medicine Society
One Olympic Plaza
Colorado Springs, Colorado 80909
719-578-4546

The Injured Athlete, Third Edition,
edited by D. H. Perrin.
Lippincott–Raven Publishers, Philadelphia © 1999.

Appendix B

Accredited Athletic Training Programs

These programs are accredited by the National Athletic Trainers Association or by the Commission on Accreditation of Allied Health Education Programs (CAAHEP). For detailed information, contact the program director at the college or university.

Four basic plans of education for athletic training are listed in the following key:

(1) Undergraduate Athletic Training Educational Programs (NATA)
(2) Graduate Athletic Training Educational Programs (NATA)
(3) Entry-level (undergraduate) Athletic Training Educational Programs (CAAHEP)
(4) Entry-level (graduate) Athletic Training Educational Programs (CAAHEP)

ALABAMA

Samford University (1)
Exercise Science and Sports Medicine
Box 292448
Birmingham, Alabama 35229
205-870-2574

University of Alabama (1)
Professional Studies
Tuscaloosa, Alabama 35487-0312
205-348-8683

ARIZONA

University of Arizona (2)
Exercise and Sports Sciences
Tucson, Arizona 85721
602-621-6988

CALIFORNIA

California State University, Fresno (1)
Department of PE and Human Performance
Fresno, California 93740-0027
209-278-2400

California State University, Long Beach (1)
Department of Physical Education
Long Beach, California 91330
818-885-4738

California State University, Northridge (3)
Department of Kinesiology
Northridge, California 91330
818-885-4738

California State University, Sacramento (1)
Department of HRP
Sacramento, California 95819-2694
916-278-6401

San Jose State University (2)
Department of Human Performance
One Washington Square
San Jose, California 95192-0054
408-924-3019

COLORADO

University of Northern Colorado (1)
Department of Kinesiology and Physical Education
Greenley, Colorado 80639
970-351-2282

CONNECTICUT

Southern Connecticut State University (3)
Physical Education Department
501 Crescent Street
New Haven, Connecticut 06515
203-392-6091

DELAWARE

University of Delaware (1)
Physical Education Department
Newark, Delaware 19716
302-831-2287

FLORIDA

Barry University (3)
Sport and Recreational Services
11300 N.E. Second Avenue
Miami Shores, Florida 33161
305-899-3497

University of Florida (2)
Department of Exercise Science and Sport Science
Gainesville, Florida 32611
904-392-0584

GEORGIA

Valdosta State University (3)
Department of Physical Education and Athletics
Valdosta, Georgia 31698
912-333-7161

IDAHO

Boise State University (1)
Department of Physical Education, Health and Recreation
Boise, Idaho 83725
208-385-3709

ILLINOIS

Eastern Illinois University (3)
Department of Physical Education and Athletics
Charleston, Illinois 61920
217-581-3811

Southern Illinois University
Department of Physical Education
Carbondale, Illinois 62901
618-453-5482

University of Illinois (2,3)
Department of Kinesiology
Urbana, Illinois 61801-3895
217-333-7699

Western Illinois University (1)
Physical Education and Athletics
Macomb, Illinois 61455
309-298-2050

INDIANA

Ball State University (3)
Department of Physical Education
Muncie, Indiana 47306
317-285-5128

Indiana University (1,2)
Department of Kinesiology
Bloomington, Indiana 47405
812-855-4509

Indiana State University (1,2)
Athletic Training Department
Terre Haute, Indiana 47809
812-237-3961

Purdue University (3)
Health, Kinesiology, and Leisure Studies
West Lafayette, Indiana 47907
317-494-3167

Anderson University (3)
Athletic Training
Anderson, Indiana 46012-1362
317-641-4491

IOWA

University of Iowa (3)
Department of Exercise Science and Physical Education
Iowa City, Iowa 52242
319-355-9393

KANSAS

Kansas State University (3)
Secondary Education
353 Bluemont Hall
1100 Mid-Campus Drive
Manhattan, Kansas 66506-0302
913-532-6757

KENTUCKY

Eastern Kentucky University (3)
Department of Physical Education
Richmond, Kentucky 40475-3103
606-622-2134

MARYLAND

Towson State University (1)
Athletic Training Education
Towson, Maryland 21204-7097
410-830-3174

MASSACHUSETTS

Boston University (1)
Sargent College of Allied Health Professions—PT
635 Commonwealth Avenue
Boston, Massachusetts 02215
617-353-7507

Bridgewater State College (1)
Movement Arts, Health Promotion, and Leisure Studies
Bridgewater, Massachusetts 02325
508-697-1200 x2072

Northeastern University (1)
Athletic Training
Boston, Massachusetts 02115
617-373-4475

Springfield College (1)
Physical Education and Health Fitness
Springfield, Massachusetts 01109
413-748-3231

MICHIGAN

Central Michigan University (3)
Department of Physical Education
Mount Pleasant, Michigan 48859
517-774-6687

Grand Valley State University (3)
Department of Physical Education and Athletics
Allendale, Michigan 49401
616-895-3140

Western Michigan University (2)
Department of Health, Physical Education, and Recreation
Kalamazoo, Michigan 49008
616-387-2678

MINNESOTA

Gustavus Adolphus College (3)
Department of Physical Education
St. Peter, Minnesota 56082
507-933-7612

Mankato State University (1)
Human Performance
Mankato, Minnesota 56002-8400

MISSISSIPPI

University of Southern Mississippi (1)
Department of Human Performance and Recreation
Hattiesburg, Mississippi 39406-5142
601-266-5577

MISSOURI

Southwest Missouri State University (3)
Sports Medicine and Athletic Training
Springfield, Missouri 65804-0094
417-836-8553

MONTANA

University of Montana
Department of Health and Human Performance
McGill 126
Missoula, Montana 59812
406-243-5246

NEVADA

University of Nevada, Las Vegas (1)
4505 Maryland Parkway
Health Education and Sports Injury Management
Las Vegas, Nevada 89154-3032
702-895-3209

NEW HAMPSHIRE

University of New Hampshire (1)
Department of Kinesiology
Durham, New Hampshire 03824
603-862-1831

NEW JERSEY

Kean College of New Jersey (1)
Department of Physical Education
Union, New Jersey 07083
908-527-2103

William Paterson College of New Jersey (1)
Department of Movement Science
Wayne, New Jersey 07470
201-595-2267

NEW MEXICO

New Mexico State University (1)
Department of Physical Education, Recreation, and Dance
Las Cruces, New Mexico 88001
505-646-5038

University of New Mexico
Physical Education
Albuquerque, New Mexico 87131
505-277-5114

NEW YORK

Canisius College (1)
Athletic Training/Physical Education
Buffalo, New York 14208-1098
716-888-2952

State University of New York, Cortland (1)
Department of Physical Education and Recreation
Cortland, New York 13045
607-753-4962

Ithaca College (1)
Department of Exercise and Sports Science
Ithaca, New York 14850
607-274-3178

Hofstra University (1)
Health, Physical Education, and Recreation
Hempstead, New York 11550
516-463-6952

NORTH CAROLINA

Appalachian State University (3)
Department of Health Education, Physical Education,
    and Leisure Studies
Boone, North Carolina 28608
704-262-6303

East Carolina University (1)
Health Education
Greenville, North Carolina 27858-4353
919-328-4560

High Point University (3)
Sports Medicine Program
University Station
Montlieu Avenue
High Point, North Carolina 27262
910-841-9267

University of North Carolina (2)
Department of Physical Education
Chapel Hill, North Carolina 27599-8700
919-962-5174

NORTH DAKOTA

North Dakota State University (1)
Department of Health, Physical Education, and Recreation
Fargo, North Dakota 58105-5600
701-231-8093

University of North Dakota (1)
Department of Sports Medicine
Grand Forks, North Dakota 58202
701-777-3102

University of Mary (3)
Physical Education
7500 University Drive
Bismarck, North Dakota 58504
701-255-7500 x456

OHIO

Marietta College (3)
Department of Sports Medicine
Marietta, Ohio 45750-3058
614-376-4772

Miami University of Ohio (1)
Physical Education, Health, and Sport Studies
Oxford, Ohio 45056
513-529-3813

Ohio University (1)
Recreation and Sports Sciences
Athens, Ohio 45701
614-593-1169

University of Toledo (1)
Department of Health Promotion and Human Performance
Toledo, Ohio 43606
419-530-2752

Capital University (1)
Health and Sports Sciences
Columbus, Ohio 43209
614-236-6569

Mount Union College (1)
Department of Health, Physical Education,
   and Sports Management
Alliance, Ohio 44601
216-823-4882

OKLAHOMA

University of Tulsa (1)
School of Nursing
Tulsa, Oklahoma 74104-3189
918-631-2316

OREGON

Oregon State University (3)
Exercise and Sports Sciences
Corvallis, Oregon 97331-3302
503-737-6801

University of Oregon (2)
Department of Exercise and Movement Science
Eugene, Oregon 97403
503-346-3394

PENNSYLVANIA

California University of Pennsylvania (1,2)
Department of Sports Medicine
250 University Avenue
California, Pennsylvania 15419
412-938-4562

Duquesne University (3)
Athletic Training
111 Health Sciences Building
Pittsburgh, Pennsylvania 15282
412-396-5695

East Stroudsburg University (1)
Movement Studies and Exercise Science
East Stroudsburg, Pennsylvania 18301
717-424-3065

Lock Haven University (3)
Department of Health Science
Lock Haven, Pennsylvania 17745
717-893-2383

Mercyhurst College (1)
Sports Medicine
Erie, Pennsylvania 16546
814-824-2444

Messiah College (1)
Sports Medicine
Grantham, Pennsylvania 17027
717-766-2511 x6037

Pennsylvania State University (1)
Exercise and Sports Science
University Park, Pennsylvania 16802
814-865-2725

University of Pittsburgh (1)
HPER
Pittsburgh, Pennsylvania 15261
412-648-8261

Slippery Rock University (3)
Allied Health
Slippery Rock, Pennsylvania 16057
412-738-2261

West Chester University (1)
215 South Campus
Department of Sports Medicine
West Chester, Pennsylvania 19383
610-436-2969

Waynesburg College (1)
Department of Sports Medicine
Waynesburg, Pennsylvania 15370
412-852-3295

Temple University (1)
College of Health, Physical Education, Recreation, and Dance
Philadelphia, Pennsylvania 19122
215-204-1950

Temple University (2)
Department of Physical Education
Philadelphia, Pennsylvania 19122
215-204-8836

SOUTH CAROLINA

University of South Carolina (1)
Department of Physical Education
Platt Physical Education Center
Columbia, South Carolina 29208
803-777-7301

SOUTH DAKOTA

South Dakota State University (1)
Department of Health, Physical Education, and Recreation
Brookings, South Dakota 57007
605-688-5824

TENNESSEE

East Tennessee State University (1)
Department of Physical Education, Exercise, and Sports Science
Johnson City, Tennessee 37614-0634
615-929-4208

TEXAS

SW Texas State University (1)
Department of Health, Physical Education, and Recreation
San Marcos, Texas 78666-4616
512-245-2561

Texas Christian University (3)
Health, Physical Education, and Recreation
Box 32924-TCU
Forth Worth, Texas 76129-3292
817-921-7984

UTAH

Brigham Young University (1)
College of Physical Education and Sports
Provo, Utah 84602
801-378-4670

VERMONT

University of Vermont (3)
College of Education
Burlington, Vermont 05405
802-656-7750

VIRGINIA

James Madison University (1)
Department of Health Sciences
Harrisonburg, Virginia 22807
540-568-6510

Old Dominion University (2)
Health, Physical Education, and Recreation
Norfolk, Virginia 23529-0197
804-683-3383

University of Virginia (2)
Department of Human Services
Curry School of Education
Charlottesville, Virginia 22903
804-924-6187

WASHINGTON

Washington State University (3)
Kinesiology and Leisure Studies
Pullman, Washington 99164-1610
509-335-0307

WEST VIRGINIA

University of Charleston (1)
Department of Sports Medicine
2300 MacCorkle Avenue, S.E.
Charleston, West Virginia 25304
304-357-4902

Marshall University (1)
Department of Health, Physical Education, and Recreation
Huntington, West Virginia 25755
304-696-2412

West Virginia University (3)
Department of Health Promotion
Morgantown, West Virginia 26506-6116
304-293-3295 x148

WISCONSIN

University of Wisconsin, LaCrosse (1)
Exercise and Sports Science
LaCrosse, Wisconsin 54601
608-785-8190

The Injured Athlete, Third Edition,
edited by D. H. Perrin.
Lippincott–Raven Publishers, Philadelphia © 1999.

Appendix C

University of Virginia Intercollegiate Athletics Substance Abuse Policy

The Department of Athletics at the University of Virginia, its coaching personnel, physicians, athletic trainers, and administrators, strongly believe that the abuse of alcohol and illicit use of drugs (excluding those drugs prescribed by a physician to treat a specific medical condition) can be detrimental to the physical and mental well-being of its student-athletes, no matter when such use should occur during the year. Additionally, use or abuse of alcohol and use of drugs can seriously interfere with the performance of individuals as students and as athletes and can be extremely injurious to student-athletes and their teammates, particularly when participating in athletic competition or practice.

Various forms of alcohol and drugs have worked their way into practically every segment of modern society, and athletics apparently are not immune to this phenomenon. Furthermore, because athletes are so often in the public eye, alcohol/drug-related activity on their part is cause for extremely adverse attention. Numerous studies have indicated that the problem is not limited to any particular group but rather touches all segments of our society.

In light of health, safety and social concerns, the Athletic Department at the University has implemented a mandatory program of alcohol and drug education, drug testing, and counseling/rehabilitation efforts to assist and benefit the men and women athletes at the University of Virginia. In addition, a mandatory counseling/rehabilitation program will be required of any athlete involved in alcohol abuse with resultant social misbehavior (e.g., DWI, destruction of property, assault, disorderly conduct). The athlete's parents will be informed of these actions if the athlete is a minor. (''Minor'', for purposes of this policy, shall mean any student who is declared as a dependent on his or her parent(s)' federal income tax return.)

Purpose of the Program

The purpose of the University of Virginia Intercollegiate Athletics Alcohol and Drug Education Program is to inform and help the student-athlete at the University. This program is based on the Athletic Department's policy that alcohol abuse and drug use are detrimental to the student and a violation of team rules. Specific goals of this program are:

1. To educate University of Virginia athletes concerning the associated problems of alcohol abuse and drug use and abuse.
2. To discourage any drug use or alcohol abuse by University of Virginia athletes.
3. To identify any athlete who may be abusing alcohol or using drugs, to identify the drugs and to provide any substance abuse education as may be needed by the student athlete.
4. To educate any athlete so identified how such usage may affect the athlete and his or her team and teammates.
5. To see that any chronic dependency is treated and addressed properly.
6. To provide reasonable safeguards that every athlete is medically competent to participate in athletic competition.
7. To encourage discussion about any questions the athlete may have, either specifically or generally, about use of alcohol or drugs.

Implementation of the Alcohol and Drug Education Program

At the beginning of the academic year a presentation will be made to all intercollegiate athletes at the University of Virginia to outline and to review the Intercollegiate Athletics Alcohol and Drug Education Program, its purposes, and its implementation. Copies of this program will be mailed to each student-athlete and to the parent(s) or legal guardian(s) of the first-year athlete. Each athlete will be asked to sign a form acknowledging receipt and understanding of the program, providing consent to the administration of the urinalysis testing required by the program, and permitting release of drug-testing information to a limited, defined group of individuals. Each athletic team shall participate in one substance abuse education program each semester.

It is hoped that no University of Virginia athlete has a problem with drug or alcohol abuse; however, alcohol and drugs have touched practically all occupations and age groups, with some exceptionally respected persons found to be abusers. Drug testing, if for no other reason,

467

should enhance the feeling of trust among athletes and their teammates.

The Substance Abuse Testing Program

The head athletic trainer is charged with implementing the substance abuse testing program.

As part of the annual health assessment, at the beginning of the academic year, athletes will be subject to substance abuse testing. Athletes will be randomly and regularly tested, announced and unannounced, during the academic year for substances which may include, but are not necessarily limited to, the following:

- Alcohol
- Amphetamines
- Barbiturates
- Cocaine
- Methaqualude
- Opiates
- Morphine
- Codeine
- Steroids
- Clenbuterol
- PCP (Angel Dust) and analogues
- Tetrahydrocannabinol (THC or marijuana)
- Masking agents
- Diuretics

With reasonable suspicion of drug usage, the head athletic trainer may require a student-athlete to be tested independent of the random sample. Suspicion of use may come from a number of sources: teammates, coaches, the dean of students' office, judiciary committee, resident staff, and the community. We have specifically requested that the office of the dean of students and the judiciary committee inform the athletic department of incidents of substance abuse by student athletes.

Furthermore, all members of teams participating in NCAA-sanctioned post-season competition or individual team members participating in such competition will be tested prior to that competition. The NCAA will also conduct year-round testing of football and track and field. Those who at any time experience a positive test can expect further screening to be done on a more regular basis. For the athlete's and teammates' safety every athlete who tests positive must be retested to obtain medical clearance before participation in a practice session or competition.

The drug-testing shall consist of a collection of a urine specimen from the athlete under supervision. Specimens will be stored in a locked refrigerator prior to transport to the University of Virginia Clinical Chemistry lab by their courier. Each urine sample shall be analyzed for the presence of drugs by an agency employed by the University to provide this service. Each athlete's sample will be

identified by code rather than by name, and the code and all records relating to testing will be kept in a safe confidential place.

The University of Virginia Clinical Chemistry Lab analyzing the samples by gas spectrometry/mass chromatography will report all test result screens. This will be reported in the initial screening, but the athlete's test will not be considered positive until the results of a confirmation is obtained. At this time the Athletic Director and student health physician will also be notified in writing. For purposes of this program, a positive result is one which indicates, in the opinion of the outside agency performing the testing, the presence of one or more of the above-listed drugs in the athlete's urine. Steps will be taken to maintain the accuracy and confidentiality of the test results, including maintaining a documented chain of specimen custody to establish the identity of the sample throughout the collection and testing process.

The provisions of this program are subject to change, but only through formal action by the Athletic Director. Such changes will not be applied retroactively.

Self-disclosure

The Athletic Department encourages any of its student athletes to voluntarily seek help if the athlete feels that he or she has a problem with substance abuse. Self-disclosure at any time will be seen as a request for help. The head athletic trainer will assist in referring the athlete for counseling. If self-disclosure occurs prior to any upcoming drug testing, the athlete may continue as a member of the team if he or she is deemed medically able to continue. The athlete must remain substance free while receiving assistance to avoid the imposed sanctions. The athlete will be tested at regular intervals to ensure that he or she remains substance free.

Effect of Positive Test Results

Each athlete will be immediately notified if the test result is positive. Every athlete with a positive result must be retested prior to participation in practice or an event, and evaluated by a student health provider to ensure that he or she is medically fit to participate. The athlete has the right to challenge the test result and may request a conference to present his or her side of the story. If the student continues to dispute the result, the student may submit a statement setting forth the reasons for disagreement. Thereafter, any time the results are disclosed to the parties specified herein, the athlete's statement must be disclosed as well. See alcohol section for sanctions for alcohol.

Drug use will be deemed a violation of team rules. A positive test result will have the following consequences:

First Positive during the Athlete's National Collegiate Athletic Association (NCAA) Eligibility

On the first positive test, the head athletic trainer will be contacted by the University of Virginia Clinical Chemistry Lab. The student-athlete and their head coach will be notified by the head athletic trainer. If the athlete is a minor, he or she will participate in a conference telephone call between the athlete, the athlete's parent(s) or legal guardian(s), and the team coach and/or the Athletic Director wherein the parent(s) or legal guardian(s) will be advised of the first positive test result. The athlete will be required to attend a mandatory psychological assessment at the Student Health Center. The Student Health substance abuse counselor will determine the length and manner of counseling best suited to the athlete. Every athlete with a positive result will be suspended from practice and competition and must be retested and be negative on retesting prior to participation in practice or a game.

Second Positive during the Athlete's Four-Year National Collegiate Athletic Association (NCAA) Eligibility

On the second positive test, the head athletic trainer will again be contacted by the University of Virginia Clinical Chemistry Lab. The student-athlete and his or her head coach will be notified by the head athletic trainer. Any athlete who is a minor will participate in a conference telephone call between the athlete, the athlete's parent(s) or legal guardian(s), and the team coach and/or the Athletic Director wherein the parent(s) or legal guardian(s) will be advised of the second positive test result. The restrictions placed on the student at this time are dependent upon the drug identified as well as the assessment of the individual by a Student Health substance abuse counselor and retesting will be required, with a negative result, prior to participation in practice or a game. A meeting between the athlete, coach, and head athletic trainer will be conducted to determine the appropriateness of continued athletic participation.

Third Positive during the Athlete's Four-Year National Collegiate Athletic Association (NCAA) Eligibility

If a student's third test is positive, it must be assumed that the athlete has a very significant problem or has made some conscious value judgments as to his or her behavior, and this must be treated extremely seriously. This information will be shared with the head athletic trainer, the Student Health substance abuse counselor and physician, the student's coach, and the Director of Athletics, as well as the student's parents where the athlete is a minor. The third offense will dictate an indefinite suspension of the student from practice and athletic competition, and the individual will be asked to return for frequent testing. Whether he or she will be allowed to reenter the athletic program will depend on recommendations of the Student Health substance abuse counselor and physician. Prior to suspension the athlete will have the opportunity to discuss the matter with the Athletic Director and to present evidence of any mitigating circumstances.

Sanctions

The student-athlete may be suspended indefinitely after the second or third positive test at the discretion of the team coach following consultation with the athlete, head athletic trainer, Director of Athletics, and Student Health substance abuse counselor.

The athlete who tests positive for alcohol will be required to meet with the Student Health substance abuse counselor to determine if an alcohol problem is present. Recommendations by the counselor will be followed prior to and after returning to practice and competition.

All suspensions will be explained as a "violation of team rules" unless made public by the student athlete.

The Alcohol Program

The University of Virginia does not condone the illegal or otherwise irresponsible use of alcohol. Alcohol abuse is a progressive disorder in which physical dependency can develop. The negative physical and mental effects of the abuse of alcohol are well-documented. Even low doses of alcohol impair brain function, judgment, alertness, coordination, and reflexes. Very high doses cause suppression of respiration and death. Chronic alcohol abuse can produce dementia, sexual impotence, cirrhosis of the liver, and heart disease, and sudden withdrawal can produce severe anxiety, tremors, hallucinations, and life-threatening convulsions.

Therefore, it is the responsibility of every member of the University community to know the risks associated with alcohol use and abuse. This responsibility obligates students and employees to know relevant University policies and federal, state, and local laws and to conduct themselves in accordance with these laws and policies.

Violation of state alcohol laws is a criminal misdemeanor which is punishable by suspension of driver's license, imprisonment for up to twelve months, and/or fines up to $2,500. Any member of the University community who violates state alcohol control laws is subject to prosecution. Whether or not criminal charges are brought, all students are subject to University discipline for any violation of state alcohol laws that occurs (i) on University-owned or leased property, (ii) at University-sponsored or supervised functions, or (iii) under other circumstances involving a direct and substantial connection to the University. Any student found to have engaged in such conduct is subject to the entire range of University sanctions described in the University Standards of Conduct, including suspension and expulsion.

The consumption of alcohol by student-athletes is prohibited in connection with any official intercollegiate team function. An official team function for purposes of this policy is defined as any activity which is held at the direction of or under the supervision of the team's coaching staff.

A student-athlete who consumes alcohol will be accountable for any alcohol-related incident in which he or she is involved. In such cases, the student-athlete is subject to University Athletic Department or team disciplinary action dependent upon the incident having or not having legal implications.

If a student-athlete is involved in an alcohol-related incident in which there are no legal implications, the head coach of that team and the athletic administrator supervising that program will determine if the circumstances warrant suspension of the student-athlete from practice and/or game competition.

If a student-athlete is involved in an alcohol-related incident which has legal implications (violations of University regulations, violations of local, state, and/or federal laws), the student-athlete's case will be handled in a manner consistent with a student-athlete's positive drug test. Therefore, the first time a student-athlete is found guilty of an incident involving excessive use of alcohol, the individual will be suspended from practice and competition until he or she has completed mandatory alcohol-abuse counseling and the student-athlete has received a written release to rejoin the team by the counselor.

All matters related to subsequent proven guilty alcohol-related offenses during the student-athlete's four-year NCAA eligibility will be handled in a manner consistent with the second and/or third positive drug tests.

As noted above, student-athletes are subject to University Judiciary Committee sanctions for conduct associated with the illegal and/or irresponsible possession and use of alcohol. In the event the Judiciary Committee imposes disciplinary sanctions against a student-athlete, the head coach and the administrator supervising that sport will review the findings and recommend whether the alcohol offense warrants suspension or dismissal from the team.

Finally, the Athletic Department prohibits the purchase of alcoholic beverages to be used by any department-affiliated person who is under the legal drinking age. This applies to prospective student-athletes while visiting the University and their student hosts. Regardless of whether a student-athlete or student host has reached the legal drinking age, purchasing alcohol for consumption by a person under the legal drinking age (a teammate or, in most cases, a prospective student-athlete) is a violation of state law.

Tobacco Policy

The University of Virginia does not condone the use of tobacco. Tobacco use often results in a physical dependency in the form of nicotine addiction. The negative effects of tobacco abuse are well-documented in the high incidents of oral, lung, and other forms of cancer. Even casual users may become addicted. Smokeless tobacco is included in this policy.

The use of tobacco is prohibited in connection with any intercollegiate team function. A team function is defined as any activity which is held as a team whether it be meetings, practices, games, or informal workouts on and off the grounds of the University of Virginia.

The University of Virginia also strongly encourages its athletes to abstain from tobacco use in their private lives.

NCAA Legislation Prohibits Use of Tobacco Products: Effective August 1994, NCAA legislation prohibits use of tobacco products, a ban that has applied to NCAA championship events since 1991. "One of the responsibilities of membership is to comply with the rules," says Stephen A. Mallonee, NCAA Director of Legislative Services. If you know a student-athlete is using tobacco (during a practice or game, the institution is obligated to apply the rule (just like any other bylaw in the NCAA Manual).

"If one school allows (its student-athletes or coaches to use) tobacco and another school reports that to the enforcement department, and it can be proven that tobacco was used, the (potential) penalty will likely be more severe, just as with other violations (where rules are knowingly violated and not self-reported)."

Substance Abuse Policy Committee

The athletic director shall appoint a committee chaired by the head athletic trainer to annually review these policies and procedures. The committee shall consist of representatives of the athletic department, student affairs, athletes, student health and others as deemed necessary.

Conclusion

It is believed and hoped that implementation of this University of Virginia Intercollegiate Alcohol and Drug Education Program will serve to benefit all connected with intercollegiate athletics at the University. Further, we believe that participation in this program will make the men and women who participate in athletics at the University and who represent the University in various areas of athletic competition better students, better athletes, and better able to make individual, informed, and intelligent decisions with reference to alcohol, drug, and tobacco usage, both now and in the future.

Subject Index